Contents

Couples in Care and Custody

Editors

Pamela J. Taylor and Tom Swan

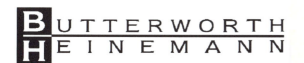

BUTTERWORTH
HEINEMANN

OXFORD   AUCKLAND   BOSTON   JOHANNESBURG   MELBOURNE   NEW DELHI

Butterworth-Heinemann
Linacre House, Jordan Hill, Oxford OX2 8DP
225 Wildwood Avenue, Woburn, MA 01801-2041
A division of Reed Educational and Professional Publishing Ltd

Ⓡ A member of the Reed Elsevier plc group

First published 1999

British Library Cataloguing in Publication Data
A catalogue record for this book is available from the British Library

ISBN 0 7506 3618 1

Typeset by Keytec Typesetting Ltd, Bridport, Dorset, UK
Printed and bound in Great Britain by Biddles Ltd, Guildford and King's Lynn

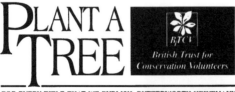

Contributors

Maggie Cole RNMS SRN RMN (Forensic)
(Formerly of Broadmoor Hospital, Berkshire, UK)

Andrew Coyle BA PhD
Director, International Centre for Prison Studies, School of Law, King's College, London, UK

Colin Dale MA RN DipN (Lond) Cert Ed RNT DMS
Senior Research Fellow, University of Central Lancashire, Ormskirk, UK

Sophie Davison MA MB BChir MRCPsych MPhil DFP
SHSA Clinical Research Fellow and Honorary Lecturer in Forensic Psychiatry, Institute of Psychiatry, London, UK
(Also Broadmoor, Bethlem Royal and Maudsley Hospitals)

Conor Duggan PhD MD MRCPsych
Professor, Section of Forensic Mental Health, University of Leicester, UK

Edward Fitzgerald QC
Barrister, Doughty Street Chambers, London, UK

Harvey Gordon BSc MBChB FRCPsych
Consultant Forensic Psychiatrist, Broadmoor Hospital, Crowthorne, UK

Anthony Harbour Solicitor
Scott-Moncrieff, Harbour & Sinclair, London, UK

Tracey C. Heads MBChB MD MRCPsych DFP
Clinical Lecturer in Forensic Psychiatry, Institute of Psychiatry, London, UK
(Also Broadmoor Hospital)

John E. Hodge BSc MPhil
Head of Professional Practice, Rampton Hospital, Retford, UK

Ilona Kruppa BSc MSc
Consultant Clinical Psychologist, Royal Edinburgh Hospital, Edinburgh, UK

Fiona L. Mason MBBS MRCPsych DFP
Consultant Forensic Psychiatrist, Broadmoor Hospital, Crowthorne, UK

Tom Swan MSc, RNMH, RMN, RNT, CertAd Ed
Course Director for the Centre of Aggression Management, Ashworth Hospital
Authority, Merseyside, UK

Pamela J. Taylor MB BS MRCP FRCPsych
Professor of Special Hospital Psychiatry, Department of Forensic Psychiatry,
Institute of Psychiatry, London, UK
(Also Broadmoor Hospital and Bethlem Royal and Maudsley Hospital)

Louise Tobin BA MA CQSW
Guardian *ad litem* and Independent Social Worker, c/o Institute of Psychiatry,
London, UK

Eithne V. Wallis BA (Econ) MA (Social Studies) CQSW
Chief Probation Officer for the Oxfordshire and Buckinghamshire Probation
Service, Aylesbury, UK, and member of National High Security Psychiatric
Services Commissioning Board

Anne Walt Cert Ed
Senior Lecturer, Patients' Education Department, Broadmoor Hospital,
Crowthorne, UK

Trevor Walt RMN RNT Cert Ed Cert Biblical and Religious Studies
Hospital Chaplain and formerly Psychiatric Nurse and Nurse Tutor, Broadmoor
Hospital, Crowthorne, UK

Preface

Pamela J Taylor and Tom Swan

'The parents of each forbade their child
To marry the other. That was that.
But prohibition feeds love,

Though theirs needed no feeding. Through signs
Their addiction to each other
Was absolute, helpless, terminal.

And the worse for being hidden.'

(Hughes, 1997)

Once society takes it upon itself to require people to live in purpose designed communities, in some cases against their expressed wishes, it has to assume responsibility for many aspects of their lives. People who run secure hospitals and prisons, and to a lesser extent those who run open hospitals, hostels and other managed accommodation, have a responsibility to their residents for their safety and overall well-being while resident. As such they seek to regulate against overtly harmful acts, such as violence, and to have clear policies and procedures for dealing with breaches of such regulations. Managers adopt almost a parental role, and as part of that have tended also to forbid their 'children' sexual, erotic or even emotional partnerships. As they are forbidden, most such organizations have seen little reason to develop policies or procedures for managing such relationships. Those charged with looking after the residents have therefore tended to collude with the notion that they do not exist. Our first main point is that denial and ignorance of relationships in such circumstances is unhealthy and even dangerous. We do not pretend to any simple solutions to the complexities of their management, but seek to encourage recognition and debate and research in the field. Occasionally we and many of our colleagues in this exercise have been deliberately provocative, but mostly we have sought simply to present established information, such as it is, and to share practical experiences. Although we have not commissioned a chapter from a patient or offender with relevant experience, we have listened to many and hope that their voice comes through too.

'Les and Sue Stocker, who run the hospital out of their garden in Aylesbury, Buckinghamshire, have launched a $1.8 million expansion drive. Part of the money will be used for rooms to keep the patients separate. In a triumph of instinct over infirmity, recuperating male hedgehogs tend to treat the wards like honeymoon suites.'

(TIME, Nov 16, 1987)

As lay people in the matter we may smile at the plucky little hedgehogs here, many recently half squashed on the road, reasserting their capacity for a full life. Nevertheless, those charged with their care evidently saw good reason to ensure better separation during hospitalization. The same tensions undoubtedly arise when the patients are humans. Just three years after Broadmoor (high security psychiatric) hospital was opened, on the 2nd of March 1866, the 'female staff defaulters' book' records:

'Passing through the wash-house at about 10 am today, I found two men cleaning the washing machine and two female patients (W and M) without a laundry maid. On enquiring from Mrs Bevan, she had left Ellen Francis with instructions not to leave the wash-house so long as the men were employed there. Francis had gone into the drying closet with a patient (L.T.) and had shut the door. Mrs Bevan further stated that she had had a good deal of trouble with Francis who requires to be told repeatedly every small matter connected with her duty. She is no laundry maid. E. Francis's appearance much against her – manner flighty. Notice to leave in 14 days from this date.'

It is not recorded whether W or M subsequently had any need of the cradle that is now also in the Broadmoor hospital archives, but we do not believe so. Nor is it clear whether, whoever L.T. may have been, it was E. Francis's own sexual proclivities or that of her charges that so outraged Mrs Bevan and the disciplinarians. It is clear, however, that in the mid-nineteenth century, patients were not wholly segregated by sex, and that there was recognition that they might engage in sexual activity and need protection, and that the hospital staff were liable to disciplinary action if they fell short in providing it.

Our second main point, then, is that relationships will happen, and that a presumption that a statement of prohibition prevents, or that illness may be its own safeguard in the matter is false and naive. There is, though, remarkably little information about wishes, needs and therefore informed safe practice in the matter. Avoidance of the issue is by no means simply a feature of secure institutions. As we set up an investigative working group for the special hospitals, we found that enquiry about practice or procedure in other regulated communities, particularly other psychiatric hospitals, was not very productive. Further, community based staff were generally hostile to the recognition even of well established relationships. It was a particularly salutary experience to find, in 1994, that when a husband and wife pair became ready to leave one of the special hospitals, no hostel or group home anywhere in England could be found to accept them as a couple. Attempts to negotiate that position were far from successful; the situation is however, now slightly changed.

Dickens (1852) had perhaps been shown a more sanitized version of relationships in a psychiatric hospital, maybe a picture in which many would still prefer to believe. Writing of the state hospital for the insane in Boston, Massachusetts, he notes similarities with English facilities of the period, such as the Hanwell asylum.

'Once a week they have a ball, in which the Doctor and his family, with all the nurses and attendants, take an active part. Dances and marches are performed alternately ... and now and then some gentleman or lady (whose proficiency has been previously ascertained) obliges the company with a song ...

Immense politeness and good breeding are observed throughout. They all take their tone from the Doctor; and he moves a very Chesterfield among the company. Like other assemblies, these entertainments afford a fruitful topic of conversation among the ladies for some days; and the gentlemen are so anxious to shine on these occasions, that they have sometimes been found "practising their steps" in private, to cut a more distinguished figure in the dance.'

Perhaps the doctors and nurses and attendants of the twentieth century are falling short as role models, but we no longer recognize or choose to recognize this kind of institutionalization of social skills. Finding appropriate alternatives, however, is not easy for residents of institutions, most of whom almost by definition have recognized problems in relationship formation and activities. Wider society, with a superficially more casual structure, does not care to extend that to hospitals, prisons or other institutions. Professional attempts to recognize and work with relationships is made more difficult by the often very public climate in which new approaches must be developed. In the summer of 1994, despite the whole national and international potential for newsworthy items, the front page of one of the tabloid newspapers of the time was almost entirely taken with a story trumpeted in headlines about 2 inches high – BROADMOOR LOVE CHILD. There followed a remarkable piece alleging that one of the patients was 3 months' pregnant and that the hospital's management had spent £3 million to 'make sure that behaviour leading to this sort of situation does not occur.' (*Today*, Aug 1, 1994) She wasn't, they hadn't and, as an interesting footnote and potential warning to tabloid survivors, that newspaper shortly met its demise. Untrue, sensational reporting may not command the kind of public support that some news editors have imagined. In fact the hospital had already begun the much more sensitive business of considering how to assess and manage close personal and romantic relationships, the risk of pregnancy being just one issue. The work had been, in essence, forced by the trickle of marriages between special hospital patients following the adoption in the UK of the European Convention of Human Rights (especially article 12; see Fitzgerald and Harbour, this volume). Trevor and Anne Walt (this volume) were pioneers in helping secure hospital patients in this situation. While they naturally began from a Church of England perspective, their sensitivity extended policy and practice far beyond any specific creed.

So, our third point is that there is nothing about trying to formulate policy in this area that is easy. There are a few absolute rights and wrongs – the right to form a marriage is now clarified in law, at least in Europe; in these circumstances people have spiritual and cultural needs which must be taken into account; staff–patient or staff–offender relationships are clearly wrong, and coercive and abusive relationships, or those in which one person cannot give real consent are undisputed targets for prevention and control. The evidence base for other actions in facilitating or limiting social mixes with patients in hospital or offenders in the criminal justice system, or for assessing or managing relationships that form in whatever climate, is small, and some of it poor. At first sight an experience in this matter founded mainly, although by no means exclusively, in secure hospitals may seem too specialist to be of interest more generally in mental health and criminal justice services, but we would argue that few of the problems in security hospitals are qualitatively different from other settings. They are simply the more intense and urgent because of the immediacy and seriousness of some of the risks if there is no recognition, assessment and management strategy in place, and because the length of confinement and nature of observations even in medium security units rarely gives residents the opportunity to develop relationships without the institutional gaze. In any event, we have also drawn as widely as possible on published literature and included relevant material from a range of other settings and countries and cultures too.

'She hadn't reformed him, but she was waiting for him to come out so she could try again.'

(Chandler, 1950)

Although so much of the concern on the part of people running institutions or communities is about relationships that become sexual, our fourth point in this brief introduction to what we have tried to do is that people make and maintain special, affectionate, romantic, or erotic relationships for all sorts of reasons, and not sexual consummation alone. It is vital not only to be sensitive to the wide range of potential in important relationships, but also of a wide range of relationship types – heterosexual and homosexual, relationships formed before admission and new ones forged during residency, legal marriages and other long standing relationships, those made through ordinary social contact and those through the special nature of the contacts that the individual's circumstances have brought about. Casual or short term relationships may need just as much help or attention as more long standing associations, albeit potentially of a rather different kind.

By no means everyone in a long term institutional placement who forms an affectionate relationship wants to remain celibate, but many do, at least for the remainder of their time 'inside'. It is important that in considering management or treatment of relationships, that the prospect of sexual activity does not overwhelm other considerations. People who have a mental disorder, or who have committed a criminal offence, or both, are certainly seeking many of the same sorts of things from such relationships as any healthy or law abiding citizen – a sense of being valued, companionship, fun, a wish to give or do something positive for someone else, and so on. Nevertheless, expectations of a relationship, often too great in ordinary society, can be so out of proportion to what it can deliver when at least one party is chronically ill, antisocial or both, that the relationship may require special attention on these grounds alone. Nor is it always the patients or offenders or their partners that become, at times, over-optimistic. Recognizing that for such people *as a group* a marriage or similar relationship may apparently interrupt a tendency to recidivism, individuals may be very disappointed, and professionals unconsciously entering this variable into a risk assessment process may encourage inappropriate or unhappy relation-ships. There is some evidence from long-term birth cohort study that all working in this field should heed: As men apparently break off from violent careers in the context of a marriage or stable partnership, many may simply be transferring the object of their violence from someone outside the family circle, when an act is more likely to lead to prosecution, to someone within, where the violence becomes less visible and prosecution is much less usual (Moffitt, 1997). Conversely, unremitting pessimism is similarly uncalled for. Some individuals really do change in the context of a satisfying relationship, and one study confirmed the extent of benefit in marriage for a group of chronically ill and rather disabled people with schizophrenia who had been advised against it (Shanks and Atkins, 1985).

Our final point must be, then, that in this work little can yet be assumed except that, for each person who has or who forms an intimate relationship of any kind within a 'made' community, whether that is closed and secure or open and as integrated in the wider community as it is possible to be, that relationship must be recognized. In conjunction with those people in that relationship, its potential for good or harm must be assessed as objectively as possible and any management strategy based on that assessment. Assessment and management are likely to be more complex according to the importance given to the relationship. 'Importance' is a judgement that will certainly take account of the views of the participants, but includes staff judgements about its longevity, depth, and likely interpersonal risks. We seek to offer in more detail what we and our colleagues have learned about that. Few of us are prepared to engage in tasks without the necessary framework and skills. To that extent policy and or practice guidelines are likely to be helpful for patients in psychiatric services and offenders in the criminal justice system as well as the staff charged with their care and supervision. We present some examples. In this area lack of evidence for much of the practice together with the strong ethical and moral connotations of much of the work conspire to make consensus difficult. This, however, is not a reason for not formulating guidelines or implementing policies, but rather one for exposing them to further debate, regular review and adjustment as better knowledge emerges. We hope readers will join in these processes.

Acknowledgements

After a few marriages among special hospital patients, the then managing authority – the Special Hospitals' Service Authority (SHSA) – recognized a need to consider the formation and development of close personal relationships within the hospitals. A working party was set up with the following terms of reference:

> 'To reconsider Department of Health advice on permitting legal marriages between patients detained in Special Hospitals at the time of the proposed marriage and the nature of pre-marital counselling and investigation of competence to contract marriage.
>
> To advise the SHSA on facilities that should be made available to married couples and what for these purposes should be taken to constitute a marital relationship.'

We are particularly keen to acknowledge all who contributed to that work, including the then Chief Executive of the SHSA, Charles Kaye. Without that experience, important as much for the gaps in knowledge that it revealed as for the things we found out, this book would not have been written. We were both members of that working group, which reported to the Authority in 1992. Our co-workers in that exercise were not only essential to the task itself, but also sufficiently stimulating and challenging to drive us further. They were the late Richard Derby, former Bishop of Southwell and Chairman of the Hospital Advisory Committee at Rampton Hospital; Alan Franey, then Unit General Manager at Broadmoor Hospital; Harvey Gordon, then Director of Medical Services for Broadmoor Hospital; Jo Green, then personal assistant to the Chief Executive of the SHSA, and secretary to the group; Anthony Harbour, solicitor; and Renee Short, former Member of Parliament and Chair of the Parliamentary Select Committee for Social Services (1979–87).

Thanks are then further due to all those who gave so freely of their time in informing this group, and therefore in part this book.

Foremost among these are patients and offenders in many settings from whom we learned a lot; some allowed lengthy interviews about their experiences and from some we have also drawn illustrative material. None of these people can be publicly acknowledged. As most of the situations that we have chosen to illustrate are not uncommon, we have been thus able to draw collectively from a number of very similar cases. In the interests of protecting privacy, therefore, none of the names refers to an individual we have known in such circumstances and no vignette includes a real person, but each is rather a composite.

We can acknowledge professional colleagues more openly and will list them all, although it will be apparent that some were recruited to join the task of producing the book as well, and in that case we will not specify their affiliations here. Shane Thompson, then Director of Personnel in Broadmoor Hospital, and John Hodge were principal among those who facilitated site visits, in their roles chairing local hospital based groups (T.S. chaired a comparable group at Ashworth Hospital). Both patients and staff approached gave unstintingly of their time and experiences. Of people outside the service who gave advice at the time we were particularly grateful to Edward Fitzgerald QC, for additional legal advice. Julie Feldbrugge from the van der Hoeven Kliniek, Utrecht, Holland, introduced us in some detail to policies and procedures in that setting, very much more accepting of patient relationships and indeed their full consummation than anywhere in Britain then or now. Gwen Adshead, then with the Institute of Psychiatry Traumatic Stress Project and Prue Stevenson of Women in Special Hospital (WISH), provided a standing sounding board as the work developed.

In working on subsequent policy development we were advised and supported by many others including: Dawn Batcup from the Maudsley Hospital; Jane Branston from the Effra Trust, Brixton; Colin Dale; Sophie Davison; Conor Duggan; Stephen Firn, Royal College of Nursing; Anthony Harbour; John Hodge; Dilys Jones, in transition between Broadmoor Hospital and becoming Head of Medical Services for the SHSA; Ilona Kruppa; Ian Keitch, Rampton Hospital; Tom Mason, Ashworth Hospital; Gill McGauley, Broadmoor Hospital and St George's Hospital Medical School, London; Margaret Orr, Broadmoor Hospital; and Louise Tobin. We are further and particularly grateful to Eric Byers and to Sheila Foley, Chief Executives respectively of the Bethlem and Maudsley NHS Trust and of Rampton Hospital Authority, for permission to publish their hospital policies on relationships.

As we have struggled with the process of writing and editing, Maggie Cole asked us particularly to acknowledge the assistance of Murial Dunnigan, Graham Durkin, Margaret Harrison, Mollie Jackson, Helen Murphy and M. Tonkinson in her work. Bernard Huckstep, pharmacist at Rampton Hospital was, as ever, generous in his advice about medication matters. George Stein gave us additional advice and a preview of one of his overviews in the field for the pregnancy chapter. Michael Loughlin, of HM Prison Service gave us information about some overseas prison developments.

In a phase when books seem to count so little for employers in the bureaucracy of research assessment exercises and systems for funding health service provision, they have become more truly 'spare time' initiatives. This book has therefore taken far longer than we meant. For that we apologize to our contributors and thank them again for their patience. Above all we want to express our gratitude to Susan Devlin of Butterworth-Heinemann who has shown the patience of a saint, but nevertheless kept us at it. Without her discreet but ever present deadlines and support, we would perhaps never have finished.

As ever, though, the people who have suffered and given most are our wonderful secretaries Gerrie Gane, Sandra Pendleton and the ever ready go-between, keeper of the files and disks, and manuscript maker – Christine Tonks.

Pamela J. Taylor and Tom Swan

The couples in care or custody

Pamela J. Taylor

Couples and their societies

Human societies generally have some sort of law setting limits on the making and breaking of eroticized partnerships, and often highly visible rituals or ceremonies that go with making them. Some such relationships are explicitly prohibited, others just tolerated, and others widely accepted. Some attract a formal contract, the breach of which will require legal or formal resolution. Some societies attempt more regulation of such bonding than others. In any one society fluctuating patterns of liberality and rigidity in attitudes and approach can commonly be seen over time; at any one time it is generally possible to see a wide range across cultures and countries worldwide.

Rules for humans are in many ways not so very different from those for other social animals. More often than not they are about the safeguard of property and territory, of the interests of any male required to contribute to the support of progeny, and to limit the burden of the latter on the wider society if the 'approved' systems fail. Fertility and the capacity to control it are probably important factors in influencing bonding patterns, as may be the life expectancy of adults and young, and the nature and extent of property or territory. There is a certain face validity in the notion that belief systems, perhaps religion particularly, profoundly affect laws and customs for humans, but so many bonding patterns seem originally based on pragmatism with respect to survival that perhaps the influence of abstract ideas should not be overemphasized.

In most western societies, while the observational and management skills described in Edith Warton's 1920 novel *The Age of Innocence* now seem to be applied both less impressively and less oppressively, the family remains an institution. It may take different shapes from those in previous generations, but family members often do still seek to influence if not control the pair bonding of their members. Families are not, however, alone in this. They have competitors in such regulated societies as schools, hostels, religious communities, the armed forces, and other occupationally bonded groups, particularly where these may from time to time separate the individual from his or her family, for example international airlines. Membership of these, however, is generally chosen in the first instance, and beyond the scope of this book. Hospitals, nursing homes, hostels and prisons in varying degrees imply less freedom of choice even at the point of entry.

People with physical illnesses are rarely under legal obligation to be in hospital, but persons with quadriplegia or debilitated by terminal cancer are bound to their carers even more definitively. There is insufficient space here to take up their problems in any detail, but some of the general principles discussed apply. Then, some people apparently living independently in the wider community are subject to the kind of supervision that allows or even requires an official interest, and thus possibly intrusion on any eroticized partnership formed. People serving a life sentence, returned to the community under licence, prisoners on parole or patients under restriction orders (the latter under British mental health legislation) may be required to disclose to any partner the nature of previous offending. This is especially likely if that might be held to indicate potential for harm to that partner and/or others likely to be intimates as a result of such a liaison, such as previous children or children conceived in the relationship. These people together with those in psychiatric hospitals, specialist hostels or prisons form the principal focus for this book. It is useful to recognize separately the implications of detention for such relationships, and of such relationships on the closed community. The former may lie in the reasons for detention, or in the detention itself, but will need acknowledgement and management. In similar settings but without compulsion, the differences in this are mainly of degree, the choice to be resident may have been only nominally free and the managers, supervisors or carers have duties of care.

Becoming or remaining a couple when mental disorder intrudes

Difficulties in reliable, valid and useful measurement of what occurs

Very little is known about how mental disorder affects the making and maintenance of a marital type relationship. What little has been recorded tends to refer to one extreme or the other – whether people make a marriage *per se*, or whether they engage in sexual activity in hospital. This in itself hints at the difficulties in establishing any data base in this area. Marriage, a legal contract, provides an easy measurement regardless of what it excludes or what it actually means in terms of quality of relationship. For the first time the 1991 census of household and family composition in Great Britain (Office of Population Censuses and Surveys (OPCS), 1994) included 'living together as a couple' as a consistent category, conceding simultaneously, however, that family relationship information is 'more difficult to code' and could only be processed for a 10 per cent sample. It appears, too, that the cohabitation measure was applied only to the 'household of 2+ unrelated adults' category. The survey of 'communal establishments', by contrast, appeared to rate marriage in only the strict legal sense (OPCS, 1993).

Davison (this volume) deals with the more explicitly sexual acts and attitudes of people in 'communal establishments'. Sexuality more generally is scantily researched. British Government funding was withheld during the Thatcher years from a proposal to research sexual attitudes and behaviours in the general population. Anxieties about such work, and attitudes to sexual activity including anyone who does not conform to a rather bland, fit, youthful standard were well illustrated by some of the response to the 1990s US survey. This was the first such study to employ a random community sample (Laumann *et al.*, 1994;

Michael *et al.*, 1994). A remarkable 79 per cent of those approached ultimately cooperated, and 4369 people were interviewed by rigorously trained researchers. The survey, in common with almost all much vaunted 'community samples' excluded anyone who did not live in a 'household', thus excluding those likely to be of particular interest here – the 3 per cent or so adult Americans in institutions or who are homeless. The most powerful objections, however, were emotional (Lewontin, 1995):

> 'If I can believe even half of what I read in *The Social Organization of Sexuality*, my own sex life is conventional to the point of being old-fashioned and I wouldn't have cooperated for any price the NORC [National Opinion Research Center] was likely to find in its budget.'

> '... why should anyone lie? ... After all, complete confidentiality was observed. It is frightening to think that social science is in the hands of professionals who are so deaf to human nuance ... Only such deafness can account for their acceptance, without the academic equivalent of a snicker, of the result of a NORC survey reporting that 45 per cent of men between the ages of eighty and eighty-four still have sex with a partner.'

Lewontin is a scientist. A geriatrician (Cassel, 1995) highlighted his mistakes at least about the elderly. Other, independent studies of non-institutionalized men over the age of 65 had suggested similar findings (Mulligan and Moss, 1991; Pfeiffer *et al.*, 1969; Rowland *et al.*, 1993), with more than twice the prevalence of sexual activity (nearly 74 per cent) among those married than those not (Kaiser, 1991). Further, even in a residential community for healthy 'upper-middle-class' men between the ages of 80 and 102 years and with a mean age of 86, more than half had a sexual partner (Bretschneider and McCoy, 1988). On the positive side, here at least is one community which appears to avoid suppressing the sexuality of its residents without apparent adverse effect. The main point of this discussion though is that, if such prejudice about healthy sexual relations can exist even among thoughtful scientists, how much more difficult it is to develop knowledge and promote understanding of the sexuality of couples with mental disorders, serious offending careers or both. It is right to be cautious when considering research based exclusively on self report, but not right to dismiss it. Further, when studying intimate relationships, potential bias introduced by attempting direct observation of certain aspects might be more misleading.

Mental disorder limiting opportunity for relationships

Birtchnell and Kennard (1983) compared 240 depressed or neurotic women attending psychiatric services in north east Scotland with 44 similar women and 230 control women in the South of England. Seventeen per cent of the Scottish women were unmarried and 14 per cent of their Chichester peers, but less than 2 per cent of the community controls had remained single – a very significant difference. Census figures (OPCS, 1995) suggest a much lower rate of marriage nationally than this control figure, although the comparison may still be valid because of the geographically matched sampling in Birtchnell and Kennard's series. Further, social patterns are changing, and marriage is generally less prevalent in the 1990s than the 1970s. In 1993 the proportion of interviewed census women aged between 18 and 49 years who were married was only 59 per cent, and the proportion cohabiting was 22 per cent, but in 1979 the figures were 74 per cent and 11 per cent respectively. The National Census figures for people in 'communal establishments' are not presented in a form so that national psychiatric figures can easily be extracted. There were about 35 000 people resident in psychiatric hospitals of a communal total of 1.5 million, but psychiatric cases would also have appeared in prisons, hostels and homeless groups. Census communal establishments also included children's homes, schools, defence establishments and civilian shipping, but ignoring minors and employees allows an estimate of the wider group of interest here. Excluding those of 15 years and under (the youngest age for marriage in Britain is 16), 31 per cent of the non-staff resident men and 18 per cent of the non-staff women were married. This fell to 20 per cent of men and 18 per cent of women in the 18–44 year age bands (most likely to be affected by imprisonment or non-dementing psychiatric disorder). Any communal living seems to be associated with a lesser likelihood of marriage per se, but perhaps this affects men less in those groups with least contribution from imprisonment and psychiatric hospitalization.

By implication, almost all the marriages in the Birtchnell and Kennard series had been contracted well before the onset of psychiatric disorder, so the interaction between disorders and marriage was probably less to do with the capacity to make a marriage than to maintain it. Poor marriage tended to be associated with earlier breakdown and a more neurotic rather than endogenous type of depression. A comparison of the poor marriages just among the Chichester women showed that they had a lot in common, regardless of health status, but the patients demonstrated significantly more disturbance of sexual relationships and had relatives who were more disapproving of the marriage than the controls.

The depressive women just described had illnesses that had almost invariably been delayed in their onset at the very least into their 20s, generally later, and that were intermittent and often self limiting. Their disorder seemed to have only a small effect on ability to contract a marriage. It might be expected that people who develop a serious psychiatric disorder at a very much younger age, when pair-bonding is generally at its peak, would be much less likely to make satisfactory relationships of this kind, and the evidence bears this out.

One fairly early indicator of this came from Steven's (1969) study, again focusing on women. Women with an affective psychosis were less disadvantaged in finding a long term partner than women with schizophrenia. If the illness were an affective psychosis, the marital patterns of men and women proved very similar, but women with schizophrenia were much more likely to make a marriage than men with schizophrenia. The peak age of onset of schizophrenia is during the late teens and early twenties for men, but mid to late twenties for women. Affective psychosis and/or major depressive illnesses tend to have a later onset still for either sex.

In Finland, Salokangas (1983) studied samples of men and women for up to 8 years after their first episode of schizophrenia. As expected, the men were more likely than the women to have fallen into the earliest age of onset group (38 per cent men between 15 and 24 years), and never to have had a social relationship with anyone of the opposite sex (40 per cent male : 16 per cent female). They were also rather less likely to have been married at the time of first admission to hospital (30 per cent : 40 per cent), the difference slightly exaggerated for cohabitation. The men were significantly more likely, in fact, still to be living with their parents at the time of first admission. In spite of little apparent difference in symptom presentation or illness subtype recognized during the 8 years of study, this balance in social relationships persisted. Although there was a slight decline in the number of men living with parents, the alternative appeared to be living in institutional settings. Overall the men were coping less well socially, less likely to hold a job and more likely to be dependent on social security.

In a sample selected at a similarly early age (18–45 years) attending a New York teaching hospital, Goldstein (1988) found similar differences between men and women in prognosis of illness and in general social adjustment, but little difference in marital status per se. This was, however, a group of people expected by definition to return to live with family or spouse. In Wisconsin, USA, the more familiar picture of disproportionate male disablement in this regard was clear (Test et al., 1990). The group studied was of men and women between 18 and 30 years who had been ill for at least 1 year with a relatively pure form of schizophrenia and had spent some time in hospital or penal institutions prior to entry into the study. They were followed for up to 5 years. Only about 40 per cent of either sex were readmitted over 2 years, with a median of 15 days in hospital per episode but few attained success as a couple. Seventy per cent of the women but 95 per cent of the men had never married. This order of difference was reflected in every aspect of such relationship measures. At the time of study entry, a minority of women were living with a partner, or had dated in the month prior to interview or had had sexual intercourse in that time. A bare majority (54 per cent) had managed to qualify for any one of these ratings. Men were less likely to have done or be doing any of these things, although the only statistically significant difference at this stage was for marriage. At 6, 12, 18 and 24 months after entry, a significantly greater proportion of women than men were engaging in partnership activities, although the numbers cohabiting changed very little. The men, as a group, were stuck on a plateau of isolation. Only heterosexual partnerships were studied, although there was an observation that about 20 per cent each of men and women reported no close friends at all.

Test and colleagues emphasized their difficulty in collecting information about intimate relationships; the women were initially less likely to answer questions about this than the men, but this changed during the follow-up. The other point worth stressing was that the women as a group were perhaps atypically young for a diagnosis of schizophrenia. They may have been a more seriously ill group than most women with the illness, and the social and partnership potential of women, thus underestimated and male : female differences minimized. By the end of the 2-year follow-up 38 per cent of the women had had children, and most were parenting them while struggling with persistent illness, poverty and attempts to work. The implications for effective hospital and community services are considerable. The authors were also sensitive to the possibility that indications of more 'dating' behaviours and sexual activity than supposed, perhaps with greater opportunities for living outside hospitals, might not necessarily be positive indicators; the disease might have rendered the women more disinhibited or vulnerable to victimization. Asked 'how satisfied are you with the kind and amount of contact you have had with the opposite sex?' at each stage of the inquiry, initially there was little difference between the sexually active and non-active women, but this changed towards the 2-year mark, with the sexually active recording significantly more satisfaction. There was a similar trend for the smaller proportion of sexually active men. 'Not having a girl friend' was a prominent source of distress for many of the men. The authors commend their experience of men's groups directed at discussion of these and other relationship issues as being particularly helpful in this regard. Sirkin *et al.* (1988) reported an evaluation of such work, demonstrating its advantages.

In a Chicago based sample, Miller and Finnerty (1996) found disproportionate evidence of risk of harm in the relationships of women with schizophrenia. Comparing forty-six 18–45-year-old women with schizophrenia with 50 demographically matched women without major mental illness, they found that the women with schizophrenia, as a group, had more transitory relationships and chaotic sex lives. They were significantly less likely to have a current partner, to have been physically or emotionally satisfied with sexual relations, and significantly more likely to have been raped or engaged in prostitution. They had had significantly more sexual partners over their lifetime up to the study, and were significantly more likely to have had a same sex partner. Concerns about resulting children were also drawn out; the women with schizophrenia were significantly more likely to have had unplanned pregnancies, problems during pregnancy and to be unsupported and in difficulty with child-rearing later.

The introduction of routine questions about relationships, and of a specific needs assessment and linked management strategy for individuals who report relationships or relationship needs should perhaps follow from these findings alone.

The major group of mental disorders for which it is even more difficult to disentangle disorder-relationship association or effects is that of the personality disorders. Concepts of personality disorder include disorder or disability in relationships, and particularly intimate relationships as definitional criteria. Paranoid personality disorder, for example requires 'recurrent suspicions, without justification, regarding sexual fidelity of spouse or sexual partner' (presuming there is one) (ICD-10: WHO, 1992). Schizoid personality disorder criteria include 'little interest in having sexual experiences with another person (taking into account age); ... lack of close friends or confiding relationships and or desire for such relationships'. Dissocial personality disorder includes the 'incapacity to maintain enduring relationships, though having no difficulty in establishing them;'. The US version of disorder classification (DSM-IV: American Psychiatric Association, 1994) is rather more entertaining if not necessarily any more effective for this diagnosis in its catalogue of anti-relationship possibilities than the more modest ICD-10. Borderline personality disorder carries the criterion of 'A liability to become involved in intense and unstable relationships ...'; and so the list goes on.

If disordered relationships are so much at the heart of the disorders themselves it seems to make little sense to dwell on numbers of relationships made or maintained as an indication of how far the disorders impair opportunity for such relationships. For what it is worth, in a sample of men with personality disorder entering Grendon, a psychiatric prison in England, half (58) had experienced marriage at the time of entry, of whom only about half were planning even at that stage to return to their wives on release (Gunn *et al.*, 1978). The finding that, on release, those men who resumed antisocial behaviour were more likely to have no partner, or a broken or unhappy partnership, is similarly difficult to interpret in this context. Was the absent or unhappy partnership indicative of continuing disorder, and a reasonably satisfactory partnership indicative of 'cure', or was the partnership in either case in the 'permissive role' – poor relationships compounding other aspects of antisocial behaviour, but good relationships allowing the potential for improvement and stability to emerge as prominent. Suffice it to say that assessment, and probably management and/or treatment of relationships are more than usually important among people with a personality disorder; here, estimation of overall frequency with which a marriage or cohabitation occurs is rather sterile, and assumptions about the value of such a partnership are likely to need testing.

Disorder limiting the choice of partners

Choice of an intimate partner is inevitably limited by availability, the question is whether people with a mental disorder may suffer disproportionate problems because of the disorder. It may be that their social circle is entirely restricted to others with a mental disorder, and this is dealt with more fully below. There is a view, however, that, among people with a mental disorder, certain kinds of choices are more likely to be made regardless of any institutional dimension.

Miller (1997) describes the complexities both in choosing a partner and in researching the process of people 'finding the best mate who will accept them.' The latter simple statement immediately introduces the concept of mutuality into the process. The 'Pleistocene tropical fantasy' of a single virgin picking favourites from a line-up of passive strangers on a desert island is not what happens in real life. The importance of wider social context is acknowledged, in the point that attempts to study relationship formation under laboratory conditions are unlikely to have much ecological validity. Moving then to the protagonists as the centre of interest, Miller presents models for considering the interactional psychology of the process. Physical characteristics, so often studied as measures of 'attractiveness', may indeed have some sort of screening role in the preliminary ascertainment of a prospective mate, but choice and attainment are essentially emotional and cognitive – for example recognizing feelings, making judgements, decision making and reasoning. Such processes hold different implications for long and short term relationships. People may start relationships with others who they find physically attractive, or who fulfil some fairly superficial need, but continue relationships only with those who they find psychologically compatible. Further, the 'settlement' no longer rests with the proposer alone, but with the receiver of the proposal, and, within any group of proposers and receivers, members of each side begin to allow in the scheme for the implications of mutual choice. In thinking about relationship development in this sort of way, the scope for limitation in the process, or by error, by someone who has a mental disorder becomes apparent. Inability to give, receive or process psychological cues in even one party will hold the potential for failure to achieve a relationship, or maladaptive partnerships; in both people it could render the process almost impossible.

Miller's approach, though of interest, is almost entirely theoretical, and certainly untested in any institutionalized population. For some understanding of the impact of unusual or abnormal psychological characteristics or of abnormal environments on the making and maintaining of relationships, it is necessary to look elsewhere.

Assortive mating means that there is a tendency for mated pairs to be more similar for a particular trait or presentation than if the choice of a partner occurred at random. Sometimes this may be secondary to some environmental factor, such as sharing in an artificial community, sometimes the partners may share a common stressor, sometimes become more like each other over time. Also, though, there may be some sort of primary phenomenon of attraction to intrinsic psychological traits, or perhaps characteristics of disorder. Merinkangas (1982) extensively reviewed the literature, concluding that assortive mating does occur for personality traits, intelligence, attitudes and values. She emphasized, however, that there are methodological differences between studies, not least in definition of traits or, in the case of disorder, of diagnosis. She cautions too that having consistent evidence for concordance between spouses for psychiatric illness still leaves the task of determining for which aspects assortive mating may occur and for which marital interaction has led to observed concordance.

Kreitman (1969) studied couples in which both partners had been patients in psychiatric hospitals. It is hard to tell from the sampling technique, which relied on colleagues in south-east England to respond to his requests for referral, and case exclusion if the medical records were poor, produced a sample that is representative of anything. Nevertheless, being able to distinguish between a group of 23 couples who had had at least their first admission to hospital before marrying each other and 43 pairs who had first become ill after marriage meant that he was able to offer some informed observations on the assortive mating: developing similarity debate in such a special group. Those marrying after illness and hospitalization showed a considerable scatter of diagnoses, with concordance for diagnosis within just six pairs. By contrast, in 19 (44 per cent) of the pairs who were first admitted to hospital after marriage, each had the same diagnosis. Manic depressive psychosis was most likely to be 'shared' (12), with reactive depression following (4 cases). Kreitman then compared the presentations of all those who were concordant for diagnosis. In the majority of these cases (74 per cent) the clinical symptomatology was very similar between spouses, regardless of diagnosis. He advanced an assortive mating hypothesis to account for the psychotic pairings, but an interactive model to account for similarity between spouses for neurotic symptoms or personality traits.

Hagnell and Kreitman (1974) studied mental illness in husbands and wives from two total population surveys from semi-rural southern Sweden, derived in 1947 and 1957. In the population of 3300 people interviewed by 1957 there were 328 married couples with each partner under 60 years. Fifty were pairs in which both partners had some sort of mental disorder during the marriage, about 40 per cent more than would be expected by chance. Inevitably in a sample of this kind most had a neurotic disorder (33), a few a personality disorder (11) and only three had psychosis among the wives; there was a similar distribution with the additional intrusion of alcoholism for the husbands. Overall, the majority of sick husbands had a sick wife but most sick wives had a healthy husband. There were 269 couples seen in both surveys. Their concordance for disorder appeared to have emerged over time, with no excess of husband and wife pairs in the 1947 sample, but a very significant excess in 1957. The wives of sick husbands tended to show an increase in morbidity with increase in length of marriage. The study thus yields some evidence that neurotic and personality traits may lead to partnerships in disorder; the sample of people with psychosis was too small to comment further on direction of illness–partnership morbidity.

Fowler and Tsuang (1975) focused on the 293 married people in a sample of 525 with a functional psychosis who had been discharged from one Iowa hospital in 1940. Each spouse was evaluated blind to the presentation of the patient. Sixty of them were given a diagnosis – 19 (39 per cent) of the spouses of those with schizophrenia, 10 (17 per cent) of those with mania and 31 (17 per cent) of those with unipolar depression, a very significant difference. Most of the disorder in the spouses was accounted for by personality disorder or alcoholism (42 cases; 70 per cent), suggesting that their disorder was well established at the time of pairing. Rosenthal (1974) had found an even higher rate of mental disorder (58 per cent) among spouses of a population of people with schizophrenia, employing blind ratings of the spouses.

Parnas (1985) studied the partners of mothers with schizophrenia who had been identified for the Danish–American high-risk study of their offspring (Mednick and Schusinger, 1965). Sufficient information was available on 97 of the 134 men to be able to make a lifetime diagnosis and compare that with the diagnoses of 63 demographically matched male partners of women without schizophrenia. The mates of the schizophrenic mothers were more likely to have acquired any diagnosis than the controls, but the differences were again most striking with respect to personality disorder. Schizophrenia itself occurred in only one man, but the combined frequency of psychotic illnesses and the 'sub-psychotic character disorders' (schizoid, paranoid, narcissistic and borderline personality disorders) was very significantly higher among the partners of the women with schizophrenia. The frequency of so-called anti-social personality disorders was also significantly increased. The age of the woman at onset of illness was important; the younger the woman at onset of illness, the more likely that a mental disorder would be identified in the man. As an important footnote, there were already serious concerns about the implications of such relationships for any children. Parnas demonstrated an increased risk of major mental disorder (schizophrenia, any other psychosis or schizophrenic spectrum disorder) among the children when the father had one of these disorders. Brennan *et al.* (1996) noted that a higher risk of violence among the adopted away sons had been reported in an unpublished PhD thesis by Moffitt in 1984. This echoed Heston's (1996) report of increased risk of violent crime in an independent, American sample of adopted away children of mothers with schizophrenia. Brennan and colleagues observed that the opposite association also holds true – that a violent male partner of a woman with schizophrenia increases the chance of schizo-phrenia in the adopted away offspring (Brennan *et al.*, 1996).

Partnerships in pathology

This is an understudied area, perhaps for the rarity of cases, but even that is not clear. This is where the special problems of people with personality disorder perhaps cry out particularly for further study. The Committee on the Family Group for the Advancement of Psychiatry (GAP) (1995) has proposed a system of classification, modelled on DSM-IV, that would allow recognition of rela-tional disorders independently of individual pathology. According to the propo-sal, disorders of marriage and cohabitation would be classified as:

I. Relational disorders within one generation
   A. Severe relational disorders in couples

      1. Conflictual disorder with and without physical aggression
      2. Sexual dysfunction
      3. Sexual abuse
      4. Divorce dysfunction
      5. Induced psychotic disorder (folie à deux)
    B. Severe relational disorders in siblings
II. Intergenerational relational disorders

'Conflictual disorders with aggression' and other abuse will be discussed further below; sexual dysfunction and indeed divorce dysfunction may well be relational disorders within a psychiatric or offending population, but psychiatric patients who are taking psychotropic medication may have individual problems with sexual dysfunction as a result. Conventional neuroleptics are particularly likely to be a problem in this regard, affecting libido in men and women but also with potential for causing erectile failure and impairment of ejaculation in men. Fertility may also be affected by drugs, such as neuroleptics which tend to raise prolactin levels. Antidepressants, particularly the serotonin specific re-uptake inhibitors (SSRIs), are more likely to create problems for men than women, as libido is not generally impaired, indeed likely to be improved if the drug is effective (for reviews see Gitlin, 1994; Parkinson and Bateman, 1994).

    The syndrome of folie à deux, in which the psychosis of one is taken on, reinforced and entered into a cycle of exacerbation by the other, is rare, and perhaps particularly so among married or cohabiting couples. In one series of 118 cases, about one fifth were accounted for by married couples (Gralnick, 1942). The vast majority of the rest were blood relatives, with just seven people other than spouses who were unrelated.

    The GAP Committee on the Family did not consider another rare condition, which has many of the qualities of a folie à deux, but which is not generally considered in that category – those who appear to engage in partnerships of sadism and in serial killings – the Hindley/Bradey partnership and the Wests have been presented as among the best known such couples of late twentieth century in Britain. Capp (1996) points to such couples as a rare but consistent feature of history. They may be the subjects of serious study by journalists, but academic researchers seem to avoid them, and clinicians tend to avoid involvement. Perhaps it is easy to see why the most extreme cases, if studied, are not reported, since the maintenance of confidentiality, a guiding principle for clinical researchers, could hardly be protected given their presumed rarity. The importance of making such studies seems real, however. There was a time before the killings and abuse started when these people may have been giving indications of their need for help. If those needs had been met then, much tragedy might have been prevented.

    For the few who work regularly with people who have a serious personality disorder, clinical impression further reinforces this area as one ripe for research. For those who maintain a capacity to make relationships, probably the majority, the patterns with which some select their putative mates come to seem very stereotyped. Often finding direct personal contact initially difficult, whether environmentally compromised, for example by being in an institution, or not, the first step in assuring a deviant or disabled partner is that they seek them from a group which is more likely than not to have similar kinds of problems. Their 'ascertainment' process tends to be in environments likely to yield damaged people, say among heavy drinkers, or perhaps through specialist penfriend columns. Almost unerringly men and women alike tend to pick a potential partner who has experienced a deprived if not frankly abusive childhood, and while the man tends to pick someone who has graduated to a position of recidivist victim, the woman tends to find a man for whom an important defence is repeating victimizing behaviours. This is clinical impression within a selected field of work; systematic enquiry is needed. Enough is known, however, to suggest that while individual assessments remain important, they may be dangerously incomplete.

White and Mullen (1989) provide a model for understanding jealousy which would bring it within a relational disorder classification and which might be extended to assist description and understanding of some of the other relationship pathology just touched on. In the case of jealousy, the jealous, the beloved and the rival are each seen as having interrelated thoughts, feelings and actions, and thus each with the potential for influencing the complex in the others. Although the rival may be imagined rather than real, the feelings arising in the jealous from sense of loss or threat to the relationship are more often than not projected on to a real person, and so even the 'innocent' rival may effectively fill the role allocated. White and Mullen go on to explore the demographic social and personality characteristics that are most likely to predispose to jealousy, particularly disruptive and pathological jealousy. They attempt to make distinctions between 'normal variants of jealousy' allowing that even these can be 'furious passions', and 'pathological', 'morbid' jealousy or 'Othello syndrome', and delusions of infidelity, but the states seem to be along a continuum.

Jealousy is undoubtedly a major force in domestic violence, even though far from the only one. At one extreme, jealousy has been shown to be an important motivation for homicide; Gibbens (1958) studying 195 cases of homicide found jealousy alone to be the motive in 22 per cent. In Wolfgang's (1958) larger series of 588, jealousy was the third most common motive.

Perhaps violence is one of the factors that leads the couple to begin defining for themselves their jealousy as pathological. Mullen and Maack (1985) studied a cohort of 138 psychiatric patients with jealousy as a principal problem. Only 27 (20 per cent) had not acted aggressively towards their partners. Thirty-three had issued threats to kill, 18 of these going so far as to brandish weapons, but not inflicting physical injury. Seventy-eight (57 per cent) had committed an act of violence. Just two people in the sample had ever been charged with a crime of violence in relation to this behaviour.

Disorder as a stressor

It seems intuitively inevitable that a mental disorder of any seriousness or longevity will pose stresses on intimate relationships, but such a hypothesis has not been well studied, and is probably also rather ill dealt with clinically. Quinton et al. (1976) offered evidence that marriages were more likely to be rated as poor among a patient sample than in a comparable community sample. There have been attempts to introduce marital therapies as part of the essential treatment of depressive illnesses. They follow from the presumption that marital problems are contributing significantly at least to the maintenance of depression, but have not yet been demonstrated as useful in this regard (Bloch et al., 1994). Uptake by partners was a principal limit here; perhaps it might be improved by greater acknowledgement of the stresses of living with a depressive. The popularity of 1960s accounts of relationship pathology, perhaps particularly family pathology, leading to disorder in a scapegoated individual (Laing and Esterson, 1964) or at least exacerbating established disorder (Brown *et al.*, 1962, 1972; Vaughn and Leff, 1976) have perhaps tended to mask this other side to the problem.

Impact of partnerships on disorder

Special benefits of partnerships for progress of disorder

Marriage is generally regarded as holding out the prospect of benefit for the participants, and has been shown to have certain measurable advantages in areas which might be taken as indicators of mental health. Whether cohabitation has precisely the same effects is not clear. Men, for example, although not women, who are married are less likely to kill themselves (Registrar General, 1971). By contrast death of a spouse ranks as the most adversely stressful life event, followed closely by divorce.

Among people with most serious disorders not only is there evidence that social networks generally have a powerful influence on well-being (see also Hodge and Kruppa, this volume) but also that marriage can confer advantages. Blumethal *et al.* (1982) studied patients discharged from a psychiatric hospital in New York State in 1975. There were 50 000 discharges in total, but counting each patient only once, and excluding the compulsorily detained, those with a primary diagnosis of alcohol or drug addiction, mental retardation or organic psychosis, the sample size was reduced to just over 20 000 and results reported for half of these. Involuntary patients were excluded, they said, because so many of them had had constraints on living arrangements imposed on discharge. Patients were followed for 7 months or until readmission to hospital, whichever came first. People with schizophrenia accounted for the largest group in the sample (61 per cent), affective psychosis for 11 per cent and neurosis or personality disorder for the rest. While the number of previous hospital admissions was the most robust predictor of rehospitalization, there was no evident disadvantage for placement on discharge with family. Specifically there appeared to be considerable advantage for those returning to a marital setting.

Shanks and Atkins (1985) acknowledged that marriage between psychiatric patients with chronic disability is unusual; they found just one example of a two-patient marriage among 250 individuals randomly selected from all those who had first made contact with the Maudsley Hospital in South London 5 years previously. From various sources they identified 22 couples who were willing to be interviewed who were current hospital service attenders, having had at least 5 years' continuous hospital contact, and a marital relationship of at least 2 years' duration. Nearly two-thirds of the couples had been advised against the marriage by at least one of the workers in their case. Evaluation of the marriages revealed 18 of the husbands and 20 of the wives as 'happier now than before'. Objective measures were simply time spent in hospital – which was significantly less in the 2 years following marriage than before, and the number of outpatient appointments – which was unchanged. In these respects there were no differences between those who had been counselled against marriage and those who had not. The couples tended, however, to maintain an emotional distance from each other.

Marriage between people with a mental retardation has similarly been shown to be much less risky and much more beneficial for many such couples than previously suspected (Berry and Shapiro, 1975; Craft and Craft, 1979; Mattinson, 1970). As more and more people with such disabilities are encouraged to live life outside large institutions and as far as possible within the general population, so expectancies for romantic attachments rise, and sexual activity as part of that. Craft (1994) focuses on recognizing vulnerabilities to abuse when cognition is grossly impaired, but provides models for achieving a balanced approach.

Partnerships and disorder if pregnancy follows

The interests of any child of a partnership are, as a matter of principle, paramount and in practice, both through pregnancy and after birth, every effort is made to honour this. Most of the issues are dealt with in Tobin and Taylor (this volume). Suffice here to emphasize that the effects on the parents also need assessment and, where necessary, management. A mother may discontinue medication for the duration of the pregnancy and this itself is likely to affect her mental state, but she, like any other mother, is also subject to hormonal changes and the stresses imposed by a demanding, dependent but separate human being. Relationships which are tenuous may break under the additional burdens, and violence or abusive capacity, well contained during a mutually supportive relationship, may erupt with the distraction and intrusion of a 'rival', however small. The risks to the child and the parental relationship are higher when the parents have a mental disorder than when not, but still some relationships may be sustained and rewarding, perhaps even more so for the presence of the child. Each case has to be taken on its own merits, and monitored over time as dynamics change and evolve. Automatic pessimism is not justified, and much can be achieved within the biological family with appropriate, sustained professional attention.

Other long term interactions between chronic mental disorder and marital partnerships

It is difficult to know the extent to which any marriage or cohabitation meets the ideal of equality in partnership. Perhaps there are many in which each at least brings a sufficient balance of strengths and weaknesses that, overall, neither partner can be considered to be particularly dominant or particularly dependent. In still others patterns may change according to circumstance, so that acute injury, short term illness or even pregnancy may result in a period in which the usual balance of the relationship is changed, but the shifts even out over time as each partner variously assumes the role of the more needy or of the stronger, so that overall, equality is maintained. Chronic illness or disability creates the potential for a very different kind of dynamic.

All too often, if there is a spouse or cohabitee it is simply assumed by caring agencies that one will assume the care of the other partner at every possible opportunity – in western tradition at least the philosophy of sticking together 'in sickness and in health' remains powerful at least in public policy. It is in the interests of those who hold the purse strings of health care – whether public or private – that it should, since anything else would add to costs. Many 'carers', spouses or not, will testify to how difficult it is even to gain respite care for the sick or disabled person. The problem is not, however, much studied, despite the fact that the sick person's very survival may depend on the qualities of the carer, for example after major spinal injury; realization of his or her full potential commonly does.

The use of the word dependency here is important. Not only is it likely to indicate a major aspect of the relationship in these circumstances, but it has the potential for creating its own pathology on both sides. If one member of a previously healthy partnership becomes sick or disabled, a marriage of equals may then be transformed into a sort of parent/child relationship, or a patient/ therapist relationship; elements of authoritarianism may creep in if some measure of coercion is required – or used anyway – to ensure maintenance of treatment or function. Worse, the couple may be trapped in the double bind of healthy partner simultaneously being real saviour but effective tormentor for the unpleasant tasks that may have to be performed.

This can be a particularly important issue for people with mental disorder where one partner, sick or no, may have to exert their legal rights and responsibilities in respect of the placement of the other or the management of their property (see also Fitzgerald and Harbour, this volume). In the dependent role it is often difficult to deal with or even express such emotions – perhaps because of feeling gratitude for care and attention received, or at least sensitive to an expectation of it, perhaps through fear that antagonizing the carer could result in worse experiences or, literally, failure to survive. Conversely the carer will have a range of feelings – some not so very different. Fear of failing the sick partner may be prominent, surrogate suffering may be depressing, and time taken from other activities and self-fulfilment resented. It is known, although not known how often, that carers and recipients alike, even in the absence of psychiatric disorder, may feel murderous toward the other partner from time to time. This can be purely from an altruistic position, with the goal of limiting the suffering of the other, but may be from darker motives too. Occasionally there may be pressure from the sick partner to assist death. In most cases the presumption seems fairly sound that angry or murderous feelings are rarely enacted in these circumstances, and yet such a belief in itself may be dangerous. Child abuse has been a problem for a very long time – probably throughout human existence – but was barely formally recognized until 1962, when Kempe *et al.* published the first description of 'the battered child syndrome' in a professional journal. Problems of 'elder abuse' were first professionally documented even more recently.

Not all harm is inflicted willfully or maliciously, but the dangers may be none the less great for that. People with a learning disability may be particularly prone to accidents, especially if their disability is complicated by frank manifestations of organic brain damage, such as epilepsy or physical disability. While the most usual problem is almost certainly harm to self, others may become vulnerable by association, and it seems plausible to suppose that the chances of this becoming true are highest if the partner is similarly disabled. Such conditions, though, tend to be very stable, which increases the probability of developing an accurate assessment of risk, a management strategy that will minimize it, and discussion with the couple, generally in such cases over a long period of time, about the level of acceptable risk. Perske (1972) wrote both movingly and wisely about according certain groups (and here he was principally referring to those with a learning disability) 'the dignity of risk'. It is not possible for anyone to be safe at all times, and as far as possible it is important for those with illnesses and disabilities, as anyone else, to choose the risks that they will take.

The risks become proportionately more alarming for any professional people that may be involved, and variably so for the spouses, when disorder or disability is so great that the sick person's capacity for making judgements about his or her behaviour and/or the relationship is specifically and gravely impaired or distorted. Psychotic depression, particularly if nihilistic delusions are strong in the absence of depressive retardation, may be particularly dangerous between couples and within families. Although rare, whole families have died in 'extended suicide'; the concern is that even this may be rather commoner than is sometimes supposed – since, if the depressed person dies too, then official statistics could be misleading. Such cases would not come to criminal trial, and, unless there is a clear suicide note, a coroner's verdict of misadventure, or an open verdict, may be recorded, masking the extent of the problem. When homicide is established, severe depression creates the one group in which women outnumber men (Häfner and Böker, 1973); the elderly may be another unusually vulnerable group (Taylor and Parrott, 1988). In one particularly tragic case a loving husband, father and grandfather and a highly respected member of the local community had a recurrent depressive illness. Previously successfully treated, during this relapse he wished only to die, but deferred suicide because his wife was becoming increasingly physically disabled. He had classical diurnal swings of mood. Early one morning, the solution came to him. He would take her with him. She died, he did not. His grief was profound and prolonged. A special worry in such cases is that, even when such a possibility is articulated, given their generally loving and responsible state when well, the partner finds it impossible to conceive of any dangers, or to be objective about safety.

Several studies have shown that marriage or cohabitation may hold its dangers when one partner has schizophrenia. Häfner and Böker's comparison between a 10-year collection of people with schizophrenia who had killed or nearly killed and a non-violent hospitalized group showed that 39 per cent of the homicidal schizophrenics had been married, compared with 28 per cent of the others, a significant difference. Planansky and Johnstone (1977) found that in a hospitalized sample of men with schizophrenia, 41 per cent of a group that had made homicidal attacks or threats were married at the time compared with just 28 per cent of a non-aggressive group. In a sample of 121 pre-trial prisoners with schizophrenia or other functional psychosis (Taylor, 1993), one of the social factors that best distinguished the men who had been most seriously violent to others and delusionally driven in their violence was close proximity in relationships – be that living with a marital or marital type partner or another family member. In that study, however, which included extensive interview data, it was clear that the interactional effect of such relationships was quite complex. First, simply the greater physical availability of a victim was a factor for those living in a family situation compared with those living an anomic existence. Secondly, those living in close social proximity with another or others appeared to have generally higher drive and to have retained more skills than the itinerant or more institutionally based men, including the skill of 'effective' use of violence; there was a relative incapacity for 'effective' violence in the more generally disabled group, which seemed just a part of their general impairment. Then, in addition, there was the force of the more specific relationship factors – for example the incorporation of a partner into a delusional system which necessarily in the psychotic man's mind meant that attack or death had to be an option. Passivity and paranormal delusions seemed particularly dangerous, with the perpetrator's sense of the partner perhaps unduly influencing or 'making' the psychotic man's behaviour, or being a potential object of sacrifice to spare him, or additionally incorporated in a persecutory delusional system. Häfner and Böker (1973) observed a high prevalence of delusional qualities in the relationships between couples in their more exclusively homicidal sample of people with psychosis.

Abusing partnerships

Marital violence

From time to time general medical services (including general practice and hospital casualty departments), psychiatric and criminal justice services are confronted by the problem of violence between partners. Any apparent increase is most probably related to a greater acknowledgement of the existence of such problems, and, perhaps more importantly, the case for intervention. While professional involvement in cases of suspected violence or sexual abuse against children has risen since the 1960s, attention to violence or sexual abuse between spouses or other sexual partners was less ready. Such behaviour tended to be construed as 'justifiably' private, or cases too hard to prosecute because of the reluctance once a particular episode was over of the more victimized or injured partner to pursue complaints or charges. Further, some relationships are by their nature covert, and in some cases illegal, for example involving a woman under 16, or a man of under 18 in a homosexual partnership, increasing the reluctance of the injured partner to go to law or even disclose. Such cases raise worries about breach of confidentiality for professionals if they force further disclosure, or of collusion in illegal behaviour if they do not. This sort of dilemma is also apparent in the ambivalent approaches to safe sexual practices in closed institutions (see Cole and Taylor, this volume).

Unofficial police policy for many years was to minimize or ignore domestic disputes but this changed, at least in England, in the 1980s. A factor in this was a comprehensive parliamentary review of violence in marriage in Britain in the mid-1970s (House of Commons, 1975). Even then estimates were of up to 6500 reported wife assaults and 20 or more husband/wife killings each year in the London area alone. In the 1992 British Crime Survey (Mirrlees-Black, 1995), which included confidential interviews with women in a randomly selected, nationwide household sample, 11 per cent of women who were living with a partner reported physical violence against them in that partnership. In Britain through the 1990s the police started to take a more vigorous role in relation to domestic violence, to offer specialist training to some officers, and to set up domestic violence units in some areas. Another example of how awareness of the issues and readiness to help has grown lies in the Probation Service. The Service has a long tradition of family welfare work, but more explicitly in the context of the divorce court and custody hearings. It followed that if the police were likely to follow up more cases, other elements in the criminal justice system would have to respond too. In 1996, for example, the Inner London Probation Service produced guidance on the recognition, assessment and management of marital and other family violence.

It is important to be clear that neither the perpetrators nor the victims of marital violence necessarily have a psychiatric disorder. Smith (1989) was particularly keen to emphasize this, writing from a feminist and criminological perspective. Without dissenting from that principle, it is also vital to acknowledge that clinicians, particularly general practitioners and accident and emergency staff, are in a particularly strong position to recognize that violence has occurred and make a preliminary assessment of need in the participants. Indeed, the American Medical Association (1992) has recommended that doctors should routinely ask all women questions about abuse. Then, there is more than one way to become a clinical or psychiatric 'case'. There are some degrees of reliably diagnosable disorder that bring people within such a category, almost regardless of their wishes, but it is also possible for people to define themselves as 'cases' where their problems do not readily fit a diagnostic model such as ICD-10, but they have sought help. In these circumstances a person has a legitimate expectation that the clinician will assist, if only as a triage agent.

All that said, much violence between spouses or cohabitees that is of a sufficient order to come to the attention of health, social or criminal justice services has its origins in such maladaptive experiences and entrenched beliefs and patterns of behaviour, that it is hard to identify many cases in which mental health service intervention would not be of potential benefit. People who become caught up in persistently violent marriages, whether as perpetrator or victim of violence, or as mutually escalating contributors, tend to have had considerable experience of violence or other major trauma as children. Some may have modelled on violent parents, some inherited traits of, say, impulsiveness that predispose them to exercising certain kinds of destructive solutions to perceived threat or challenge, some may have unexpired rage resulting from direct victim experiences, or combinations of all these, or still other factors again. They should be able to expect a systematic assessment of the evolution of their victim or violent career and the offer of a consequently informed strategy for help.

The presumption in marital violence, or violence between heterosexual couples, is that the woman is almost invariably the victim. It is true that, on the whole, men are stronger than women and may be able to inflict more serious harm by physical contact. They may also be more likely to assume frankly violent rather than merely aggressive methods of resolving disputes. It is dangerous, though, to assume that all violent transactions are in this direction. In a 1970s study of over 1500 reported cases of family violence, although the vast majority of victims were women, as many as 25 per cent of them were men battered by their wives or fathers thrashed by their sons (Martin, 1978). Violence at its most serious emphasizes where the main violence risks lie. In Britain, for women, they are in the home, with about 45 per cent dying by homicide being victims of their partners; risks for men are elsewhere, with just 6 per cent killed by spouses (Home Office, 1995). In a series of monographs Stacey and colleagues seek to provide as complete a picture as possible, this time from an American (Austin, Texas) base. Starting with a focus on women (and children) as victims (Stacey and Shupe, 1983), then offering an exploration of the origins of the abusive behaviour and role of the men (Shupe *et al.*, 1987) they go on to explore the wider dynamics of violence within the couple, and the particularly destructive potential of mutually violent mates (Stacey *et al.*, 1994). It may not surprise many practitioners in the field that struggles around power and its inequalities accounted for much of the driving force behind psychological and physical abuse alike, and evidence for this clearly presented. Some strategies for intervention are offered and results evaluated, leading to strong recommendations for treatment and rehabilitative models to be offered, albeit in many cases within a criminal justice system framework. Effective monitoring in conjunction with reliably imposed sanctions in the event of breakdown are seen as important components of the model.

Multiplication of destructive behaviours

Violence may, then, occur within couples when neither partner has a recognizable mental disorder, when one or both have such a history of deprivation or abuse and/or such entrenched patterns of using violent solutions that a disorder model in approaching them is helpful, or when one or both has a reliably diagnosed mental disorder, but there is evidence that alcohol or other drug misuse may be an important problem within any of these groups, and in all of them increase the risk of violence. Swanson *et al.* (1990, 1994) highlighted this point for violence more generally, but there remains the problem of unpicking the precise role of alcohol or other drugs. At one extreme one or both partners may be dependent, or maintain such a habit that it dominates much of their interactions of any kind. At the other, occasional overindulgence may release violence in a partnership where it is otherwise contained, and then there are all the shades in between, and the risk for some that chronic misuse may be complicated with additional binges or extra substance use. Further, some substances have such a powerful mind altering effect that secondary psychiatric syndromes become apparent, some with particular implications for couples. Pathological jealousy is one such state, by no means invariably rooted in or compounded by alcohol abuse, but not uncommonly so.

Displaced abuse

It is beyond the scope of this book to do any more than touch on other forms of relationship abuse, but it is important to recognize that the abuse of children and other weaker family members, such as the elderly, may not uncommonly be symptomatic of a marital disorder. Violent abuse is perhaps particularly likely to be associated with frustrations or imbalances in the marital dynamics. A particularly dependent partner, for example – usually the man – may find too much competition from an infant who inevitably usurps the dependent role. Traditional role reversal between the couple – so that the woman is in outside paid employment and the man housekeeping and childminding – can increase the risk. The violent or abusive step-parent is not invariably confined to nursery tale myth. In some non-human species a male routinely kills the offspring of his predecessor before consummating the relationship with his new partner, who is generally very receptive despite the treatment of her previous brood. Such behaviour is not unknown among humans. Step-children are at much higher risk than natural children both for violence in general (Daly and Wilson, 1996) and fatal violence (Clarke, 1989). Further, most professionals who have worked with families in difficulty know of cases in which, when violence against the 'resident parent's' biological children starts, that parent will allow the children to be taken out of the home and into care rather than ask the abuser to leave. While it is arguable that this sort of dynamic may simply emphasize that man's social structures may sometimes be no more sophisticated than those of supposedly 'lower' animals, more deviant patterns are also well recognized. It is known, for example, that some men target and subsequently marry or cohabit with single mothers in order to gain access to their children. Further, such women, often themselves deprived and previously victimized in this way, may fail to recognize the hidden agenda in such approaches or suppress their knowledge.

When illness, disability or absenteeism becomes too much for one parent, the other may coerce a child into taking on domestic duties which come to include sexually satisfying that parent. While it is believed that this form of abuse is more often perpetrated by men, it is increasingly recognized that women may be direct sexual abusers (e.g. O'Connor, 1987). It has long been acknowledged also that women in such partnerships not uncommonly collude to some extent with the man; this may result from their own self-preoccupation and inaccessibility to the child, their failing to acknowledge warning signs or refusing to believe a child's complaint, conscious denial or, occasionally, open procuring of the child's cooperation. In a few extreme cases the couple may take mutual pleasure from sexual abuse of the child. Incestuous families, in Western countries at least, tend to be very isolated from any society beyond the walls of the home, and to be generally chaotic, with loose inter-generational boundaries (Herman and Hirschman, 1981).

Enforced separations

One of the reasons why people are admitted to a secure hospital or to a prison is that they have killed their spouse or partner, or their children, or, more rarely, some other family intimate. Despite the circumstances of the death there is almost always bereavement work needed with the survivor (Curle, 1990), and because of the circumstances this is an exceptionally difficult task. Where the perpetrator had a serious depressive or psychotic illness, the first stages of effective treatment may bring him or her into an exceptionally vulnerable state, in which suicide becomes an even higher risk as insight is restored.

States of morbid jealousy or some sorts of personality disorder may pose problems of a different order as the individual perhaps gains some understanding of past events, but insight into the capacity for repetition remains elusive. Consolation is rapidly sought at the first possible opportunity in a new relationship, often of a very similar kind. For many, most serious or pathological violence may be confined to such relationships, or triggered by them, so that the only way of preventing future tragedy is at some stage to work within some form of relationship. To some extent some types of psychotherapy – the dynamic psychotherapies – offer this possibility in the therapy with the individual, as transference occurs. This may not be without its own risks.

Substance abuse may also have been marked around the time of a killing, which tends to increase difficulties in attaining an understanding of events, recall often being genuinely patchy, or 'state dependent' (only subject to recall if the subject is again in the same mental state, in this case intoxicated). In brief, the details of the work may be directed by the nature of the disorder or disorders that prevailed around the time of the killing, but the 'couple-work' cannot be ignored in these circumstances because one is dead.

Where there was non-fatal violence against the partner, some of the matters for attention may be very similar. Both in these circumstances, though, and others where, notwithstanding criminal convictions, mental disorder or both, the problems within an established couple were unremarkable, the couple have to cope with separation enforced by the resulting institutionalization. In these circumstances absence rarely makes the heart grow fonder, but rather the partner who remains free is often worn down by having to take on lone responsibility for survival, or single parent duties while attempting to maintain contact with the incarcerated partner. Not uncommonly it is the man and the breadwinner that is imprisoned or hospitalized, and so the circumstances are much strained financially. The 'free' partner feels as trapped as the institutionalized partner and not uncommonly develops a sense of resentment, as an 'innocent party' nevertheless punished. The incarcerated partner, however, can often only see the riches of freedom, and is at best unsympathetic. At worst he (usually) may become profoundly jealous, perhaps to begin with in rather general terms, but often focusing specifically on imagined or real substitute partners. These issues are dealt with more fulsomely in the chapters by Tracey Heads and Andrew Coyle.

With the exception of the dementias, most of the mental disorders that result in long term hospitalization or separation into specialist community facilities affect younger people and this is also true for the vast majority of the kind of serious crime likely to result in imprisonment. Whether or not there is an established relationship at the time of the incarceration, it is thus people who are particularly likely to be at their peak for interest in forming romantic and sexual partnerships who are most affected. Frustration of need and substituted activities are among the resultant management issues for the individuals concerned, their existing partners if they have them, and the institutions. Some of the later chapters in the book – particularly including those on the family, prisons, practical management of sexual activity and general management of relationships, take these matters further.

Regulated communities, mandated professional relationships and the couple

Restricted choices

People tend to meet through having their immediately local community or workplace in common. For those, even in western society, who find such opportunity too limited, there is the option of 'arranged matches', through dating agencies or marriage bureaux, or simply the chance of the personal ads columns in a variety of newspapers or magazines.

The more regulated and closed a community the proportionately greater its influence on choice. In a psychiatric hospital, for example, people who are already restricted by disabilities, which may include severe social phobias or florid psychosis find that almost all of their time is spent in the company of people with similar problems and that they are relatively cut off from the healthy. In a prison, no matter what the offence or alleged offence, the offender/ accused will find him or herself mainly in the midst of others who may variously have been violent, sexually offensive, dishonest or dependent on alcohol or drugs, even all of these things. In special hospital, mental disorder and antisocial tendencies are combined. There are other restrictions too. Prisons are almost invariably single sex institutions; in the special hospitals, men outnumber women by a ratio of 4 : 1 – women thus having a rather better peer group than in other forensic psychiatry inpatient units, but being in a small minority compared with other NHS hospital units. Between them, the three special hospitals have just two mixed-sex wards, but planned educational, occupational and recrea- tional activities may occur regularly for most patients on a mixed sex basis (see also Swan and Taylor, this volume).

Little is known for sure about 'arranged partnerships' with people in secure hospitals or prisons. It is an important area for research. There is no doubt that some of the men and women who seek befrienders, volunteers or penfriends choose routes in doing so which are reflective of their fundamental pathology and that they may be profoundly dangerous to the people they contact. There is no doubt that some of the men and women who respond have their own serious problems, and that while some may be inadvertently destructive to the prisoner or patient, at least a few are knowingly damaging. Cheque-book journalism is one motive for a tiny minority; the excitement, perhaps even specifically sexual excitement, of having a relationship with a notorious person may be the attraction for others. Thus, even when seeking relationships from outside the institution, people may be terribly limited to finding others with disorders and disabilities. Nevertheless, there is no question that some people who come forward to befriend are stable and appropriately motivated. Sometimes from within this group a lasting and successful relationship may develop. MccGuire (1994) presents first person accounts from mothers, daughters, sisters and wives already married to men who killed. She also interviewed four women who met and married such men. These women were not 'murder groupies' as MccGuire calls the many women who write or propose to notorious criminals, but women attempting a serious relationship. One marriage failed in acrimony, but the others survived despite all the restrictions on the inside and the mix of expected and unforeseen problems as two of the men were released. There was little or no professional support for these relationships; one woman found Aftermath – a charity set up for the relatives of offenders – helpful in the circumstances. This is further illustrative of the range of possibilities in this sort of situation, but still takes us little further than the point that sometimes it works, and sometimes it can be devastating. Information-based guidelines on assessment and appropriate support in such circumstances are needed more and more urgently as attempts progress to introduce more truly appropriate rehabilitation into closed institu- tions.

Restricted opportunities

The more secure or specialist a unit, whether health, social services or criminal justice, the more likely it is that the individuals resident there will be dislocated from their home communities. This is not invariably a bad thing, for example if they have been involved in abusive relationships as victim or perpetrator.

However, where there are marital type relationships that are even partly successful prior to one partner being subject to admission, the geographical separation can mean the death of that relationship.

The more regulated the community also the more regulated are the activities possible, even within chosen and acknowledged relationships. Privacy for the individual or couple is invariably compromised by any kind of communal living, but in secure institutions it is more often than not explicitly denied. In many instances this is with good reason, but is a blanket denial of privacy appropriate – or even safe? There is no doubt that some of the more able will find ways of restricting observation. Simple privacy is all that many, if not most, ask – to talk without being overheard, for example – but some may be more openly sexual, perhaps in the haste and covertness of the acts compounding pre-existing difficulties, perhaps extending risks which under other circumstances might be rather ordinary – of pregnancy or of infection – into extraordinary and serious risks. A 'blind eye' on the part of staff may have short term convenience, but in the longer term safeguard none of the individuals and jeopardize the institution itself which has a responsibility to provide a safe environment.

Conclusions

This book is influenced by my personal experiences and those of my co-authors. Most of us have worked in a wide variety of settings and services. For many of us this has most recently been or currently is within the special hospitals. They are the best of places and the worst of places from which to attempt such a piece of work. The patients have problems to extremes, and the environment is artificial, but the differences from other settings in the nature and quality of relationships and their problems do seem to be more of degree than quality. The concentration of the problems, the clinical professional expertise of most of the staff, and the length of time for which the patients remain in hospital, provide both an observational and experiential base that are more likely than not to be generalizable in many aspects. Where there are data from other settings, we have drawn on it. If reading and practice together have so far raised more questions than they have answered, then we hope that what follows may stimulate other clinicians and practitioners to join the quest for a more information-based approach to work with couples in regulated and secure communities.

2

Marriages and partnerships for psychiatric patients or prisoners: European rights and law in the UK

Edward Fitzgerald QC and Anthony Harbour

The right to marry

Most psychiatric texts are curiously silent on the issue of a contract of marriage between people with a mental disorder, or detained in hospital. Even texts specifically on the family avoid the subject. When it receives mention, at most a couple of paragraphs refer darkly to the possibility that a contract of marriage may not be valid if, at the time of the marriage, either party was so mentally disordered as not to understand the nature of the contract. Many lay people might consider a contract of marriage as difficult as any other legally binding agreement; there are legal responsibilities within such a contract – not least to do with the care and control of a partner in the event of a mental disorder requiring compulsory detention – while the legal withdrawal from such a contract, if desired, may take years of expensive negotiation.

Article 12 of the European Convention of Human Rights says:

> 'Men and women of marriageable age have the right to marry and found a family according to the national laws governing the exercise of this right.'

Two leading cases involved British prisoners Hamer and Draper: the European Commission held that a convicted prisoner 'deprived of his liberty under Article 5 remains in principle entitled to the right to marry and any restriction of this exercise of that right must be such as to injure its substance' (paragraph 63 of *Hamer*). The result was that English law had to change so that detained persons were not *de facto* deprived of their right to marry merely because they were detained in a prison or secure hospital and therefore denied access to 'prescribed places' for a marriage ceremony. The Marriage Act 1983 allowed for variance in where a marriage could take place, so that those who were bedridden or housebound, in prison or detained in hospital were not prevented from marrying merely by virtue of their confinement. The principles established by *Hamer* and *Draper* go further, however. No restriction of the right to marry will be permitted simply because the person has been convicted of a crime and is indefinitely detained in prison or hospital. Nor will any domestic law be tolerated which is inconsistent with the universality of the right recognized by Article 12.

Requirements for consent under European law

Although nowhere clarified, it seems overwhelmingly likely that the European Commission and Court would interpret Article 12 as applying only to those of marriageable age who are capable of giving a valid consent to marriage. In all European states, marriage is envisaged as a contract and a contract requires contractual capacity. According to *Hamer*:

> 'The essence of the right to marry, in the Commission's opinion, is the formation of a legally binding association between a man and a woman.'

So that part of English/UK national law which requires a basic consensual capacity would undoubtedly be upheld by the European Commission and Court.

The Matrimonial Causes Act 1973 lists the following grounds for a marriage being void:

1. the marriage has not been consummated owing to the incapacity of either party to consummate it;
2. the marriage has not been consummated owing to the wilful refusal of either party;
3. either party did not readily consent to it, whether in consequence of duress, mistake, soundness of mind or otherwise;
4. at the time of the marriage either party though giving valid consent was suffering (whether continuously or intermittently) from mental disorder within the meaning of the Mental Health Act 1983 of such a kind or to such an extent as to be unfitted for marriage.

Psychiatric disorder may contribute to impotence, wilful refusal or incapacity to make the contract, but evidence of such disorder is very rarely called in these circumstances. It is the incapacity or the refusal in itself which is legally important. The level of understanding required by English law to establish capacity to render a marriage valid is, however, indeed basic. The test was put by Lord Justice Singleton in the case of *Park*:

> 'The question, I think, is this: was the deceased on the morning of May 30, 1949, capable of understanding the nature of the contract into which he was entering, or was the mental condition such that he was incapable of understanding it? To ascertain the nature of the contract a man must be mentally capable of appreciating that it involves the responsibilities normally attaching to marriage.'

Additional limit permissible under European law

In the case of *Draper*, the European Commission left it open whether national law could limit a person's right to marry on some other consideration of public interest than those embraced in the general 'rules concerning capacity, consent, prohibited degrees of consanguinity or the prevention of bigamy'. It may be permissible to prohibit the marriage of a person with a mental disorder in the most exceptional circumstances on the basis of the special dangerousness of an established crime combined with a prediction of future high risk that they would pose to any partner (or, conceivably, their children). It is possible that in this context it might be considered appropriate to contest a marriage, for example on the basis that a man had an already established pattern of selecting partners who had been abused by other men, with children who had been similarly abused, and had himself killed at least one of these partners or children. Such people, retaining their own optimism for a new marriage, certainly exist, but there has been no test case.

Void and voidable marriages

Part of English law which requires an ability to make a valid contract to marriage is, then, consistent with the Articles of the European Convention. So it is a ground for the refusal of permission to marry that a patient lacks basic consensual capacity. The mechanism for preventing a marriage from proceeding is to enter a caveat with the Superintendent Registrar under Section 29 of the Marriage Act 1949. In addition, as already noted, Section 12 of the Matrimonial Causes Act 1973 (the MCA) indicates when a marriage may be voidable on mental health grounds.

It seems clear that Section 12(a) of the Act as now amended (4. above) introduces a concept of 'unfitness for marriage' which is broader than the unfitness of the person incapable of giving a valid consent. It must be wide enough to include those manifestly incapable of sustaining a marriage by reason of their mental disorder and may also include those so dangerous and ostensibly antisocial as to be 'unfit for marriage'. The compatibility of this provision with the European Convention has not been tested, but is likely to be critically scrutinized by the Commission and Court if it is not given a very narrow construction. Under English law all hospital patients and prisoners must be permitted to have the right to marry other such patients, prisoners or outsiders unless it can be shown that they lack the basic capacity to give a valid consent to marriage.

In hospitals, if thought that either partner lacks capacity for the contract or is 'unfit for marriage' it will be for the responsible medical officer (rmo) to raise an objection on this ground with the Superintendent Registrar (Section 29(1) of the Marriage Act 1949). It will then be for the Superintendent Registrar to decide whether to issue a certificate or licence. The purpose of the caveat procedure, though, is to stop a marriage taking place which would be *void* from the outset. The unfitness concept is broader and, if established, would allow either party to what was, at its inception, a lawful marriage, to argue that the marriage was *voidable*. 'The general reason for making a marriage voidable rather than void is to allow the parties themselves to decide whether they wish to continue it or not' (Hoggett, 1990). The caveat procedure should not, therefore, be used to try and prevent a marriage taking place that an rmo simply does not consider to be in the best interests of the patient or spouse.

Appropriate pre-marital counselling

There is no legal requirement to counsel. This is not to say that it is not good clinical practice to counsel any patient during their contemplation of marriage or, indeed, of any long term relationship.

Investigation of competence to contract marriage

The responsible medical officer could reasonably request an interview with every patient proposing to marry in order to form an opinion on this issue. Even if a patient refuses, the rmo would be entitled to express an opinion to the Superintendent Registrar on the basis of his or her knowledge of the patient. Patients should be informed of the rmo's intended action and invited to make representations and, if appropriate, be legally represented. The hospital managers could, in addition, intervene in an appropriate case.

Facilities to which married couples are entitled

Formal rights deriving from legal status

A patient spouse will attain all the formal rights that derive from the legal status of marriage. In particular, when two patients marry they will become each other's nearest relative for the purposes of Section 26 of the Mental Health Act 1983, and will acquire all the rights to information and notification (particularly in relation to Mental Health Review Tribunals) that derive from the primacy accorded to married relationships by Section 26(1)(a) read in conjunction with Section 26(3). The only way to prevent a patient from exercising his or her rights would be to apply to a County Court to have them removed as nearest relative on one of the grounds specified in Section 29(3). Section 29(3)(b) is particularly relevant:

> 'that the nearest relative is incapable of acting as such by reason of mental disorder or illness'.

There are comparable rights under the related legislation for Scotland and Northern Ireland.

Such issues do not arise for prisoners unless or until they become liable to mental health legislation, when their rights under this and with respect only to this apply.

Rights to association and correspondence

Special hospital patients, other detained patients and prisoners married to one another – or indeed to a person still free in the community – are entitled to a reasonable degree of association, phone calls and to private correspondence. However, this right is not absolute or unlimited even under European Convention Law. Article 8(2) of the European Convention permits a limited interference with the citizens' 'right to respect for his private and family life' by a public authority where that interference is:

> 'such as is in accordance with the law and is necessary in a democratic society in the interests of national security, public safety or the economic well-being of the country, for the prevention of disorder or crime, for the protection of health or morals or for the protection of the rights and freedoms of others.'

It would not be incompatible with Article 8(2) to impose the kind of restrictions on association and correspondence between two married inpatients in hospital or two prisoners as are imposed in relation to the association and correspondence of a married patient or prisoner with a spouse who is free in the community. Any restrictions would have to be justified in the individual case with reference to the prevention of disorder or crime, which includes the security of the institutions, 'the protection of health or morals', which would include the protection of the mental health of one or both of the parties or 'the protection of the rights and freedoms of others'.

The Mental Health Act 1983 also contains provisions for controlling correspondence with or from any compulsorily detained patients. Section 134 provides that a postal package addressed to a patient detained in a special hospital may be withheld from the patient if, in the opinion of the managers of the hospital, it is necessary to do so in the interests of the safety of the patient or for the protection of other persons. The same section also contains restrictions in relation to the mail of other detained patients who are not in special hospitals.

Right to sexual relations and to found a family

This is undoubtedly a matter of some controversy and concern. The position is entirely unclear under domestic law which recognizes no such general right. The issue would have to be tested by reference to administrative law principles and to the principle that applies to those convicted of crimes and/or detained in a special hospital (the substantial majority of patients in special hospitals have been convicted of a serious crime) – that they retain all civil rights not taken away by necessary implication.

People who are inpatients in open psychiatric hospitals are also likely to be so restricted while in the hospital premises. When allowed leave away from the premises, whether prisoner or patient and subject to continuing restrictions on liberty or not, then people are likely to be able to find the requisite privacy. It is partly for this reason that prisons prefer to grant occasional home leave if safe to do so, than to make available facilities in a prison for the exercise of conjugal 'rights'. For psychiatric patients, not only questions of safety but also the level of activity of mental disorder may complicate decisions in favour of such leave, but in principle more natural arrangements through leave may be preferable to any within institution arrangements for patients, as for prisoners. Such leave arrangements would also have to be properly sanctioned. For patients this would mean leave authorized by the doctor in charge of the case (technically the responsible medical officer under Section 17 of the Mental Health Act 1983). For prisoners, permission from the Home Office would be necessary. European Convention law is itself not clear on the issue of such activities within institutions. The decided cases for the most part concern convicted prisoners and do not accord to them any general right to conjugal relations. A case of relevance is X and Y. The Commission found that the denial of conjugal rights to a husband and wife detained in the same penal institution constituted no violation of their rights under Article 12 (which guarantees the right to marry and found a family) or Article 8 (which guarantees a general right to private and family life) subject to the exceptions listed in Article 3 8(2). In this case the Commission placed particular emphasis on the exception contained in Article 8(2) to the general right to privacy and family life when it is necessary to restrict those rights for 'the prevention of disorder or crime.'

The requirements of the European Convention and Commission are a helpful starting-point; the law specific to the European country concerned remains the primary consideration. There is certainly nothing in the law of England and Wales that specifically authorizes any general restriction on sexual relations between hospital patients in general or even special hospital or other compulsorily detained patients. Such a general restriction would be upheld only if the detaining authority was prepared to justify it as reasonable and necessary for the prevention of disorder, the security of the institution, or the protection of patients from serious harm. Similar principles apply in Scotland and Northern Ireland, so patients from all parts of Britain requiring treatment in security would be in a similar position.

It would therefore follow that a policy to permit sexual relations between patients might, subject to certain exceptions, be lawful. Indeed it is suggested that any limitation on sexual relations between detained patients would, strictly, have to be justified. The basis for any such justification would be that to permit sexual relations would give rise in a particular class or category of cases to a serious threat to security or to the physical and mental well-being of patients. The risks in a high security hospital are exceptionally high given established patterns of predatory behaviour in many of the men and substantial histories of traumatic abuse and continuing vulnerability among many of the women and some of the men, over and above a serious but sometimes coincidental mental disorder. Nevertheless it may be possible, under both English and European law, to frame a policy that permits sexual relations in secure hospitals in well-defined circumstances.

Under existing statute law, however, there remains a major problem in the way of such a development. That is contained in the provisions of the Sexual Offences Act 1956, which makes it a criminal offence for a man to have sexual intercourse with a 'mental defective' [Section 7(1) of the Sexual Offences Act 1956]. A defective is defined to mean 'a person suffering from a state of arrested or incomplete development of mind which includes severe impairment of intelligence and social functioning' – so that the prohibition against all men in this regard would seem to be limited to sexual intercourse with a person with severe mental impairment (see also Section 25 of the Sexual Offences Act 1956, as amended). It would seem to follow from these provisions that health service providers must establish clear policies and procedures to deal with these prohibitions. It should also be noted that Section 27 of the same Act makes it an offence for the person who owns, occupies, manages or controls any premises to 'knowingly suffer' a woman 'to be on those premises for the purposes of having sexual intercourse with men or with a particular man'. Though the words were probably not intended to deal with a responsible authority that comes to a reasonable decision not to prohibit sexual intercourse between, say, patients in a hospital or residents in a group home who have established a relationship, the words of the Act would appear to ensure that the managers do take consideration of the protection of the vulnerable.

Partnerships other than marital relationships

Article 12 of the European Convention which guarantees the right to 'marry and found a family' confines its protection to heterosexual relationships of a formal legal nature. Indeed, the essence of Article 12 is to confer the right to acquire the legal status of being married on all citizens subject to the limited exceptions generally recognized by national laws in relation to the contractually incompetent and prohibited degrees of consanguinity. The protection of Article 8, however, which guarantees the right to privacy and family life, extends beyond the legally married heterosexual couple to the common-law marriage of two long-term cohabitees in a heterosexual relationship, and also to homosexual couples in some situations. It would therefore be necessary in order to comply with Article 8 to give some recognition to the right to correspond and associate (if not to have sexual relations) of those who are involved in a common-law heterosexual or homosexual partnership before detention, and also to those who develop long-standing and responsible relationships of this kind after being detained.

Conclusions

English law follows the European Convention of Human Rights to which all countries in the European Community have subscribed. Interpretation or clarification of the law, as in case precedents, or increasingly through judicial review of provider authorities, generally aims to assist in the facilitation and establishment of sensible and humane policies. New issues regularly emerge; the hypothetical and the real merge. Some patients who have married within a hospital have had to consider legal separation or divorce, and found that usual grounds may not apply because of their unusual circumstances. In the matter of 'right to found a family', particularly difficult questions may arise where there is a healthy, law abiding partner who wants to stay in the partnership but who does not want to give up the prospect of having children. If such a woman, for example, asks whether, if her husband were to remain incarcerated and she were to continue to be denied sexual intercourse with him, she may be artificially inseminated using his semen, what rights cover her position and to what law can she or a conscientious hospital or prison turn? The law, like other aspects of care and service for prisoners and people with a mental disorder, is an evolving process and, as new issues arise, the legal aspects of the problems will need constant re-evaluation and updating.

Cases cited

Draper versus United Kingdom [1981] 24 D & R 72.
Hamer versus United Kingdom [1981] 4 E.H.R.R. 139.
D & R 23 [1981] page 72.
Park, In the Estate of [1953] 2 All ER 1411.
X and *Y versus Switzerland* [1979] 13 D & R 241.

Glossary

D & R Decisions and Reports (Council of Europe)
E.H.R.R. European Human Rights Reports
All ER All England Law Reports

3

In sickness and in health: Making and sustaining marriage against all odds
Experience in one high security psychiatric hospital

Trevor and Anne Walt

Concepts of marriage

Whether one begins from the Christian viewpoint that marriage is a sacrament of the Church and 'a gift of God in creation and a means of his grace' (*The Alternative Service Book*, 1980) or from the secular position that it is a legal contract, marriage is understood, throughout Western society, as the union of one man and one woman, freely entered into with the primary intention of the union being lifelong. Most other societies, whether or not principally mono-gamous, also recognize, formalize and celebrate certain unions. In the 1980s and 1990s the institution of marriage in many Western countries has been under threat of decline, with a corresponding increase in the numbers of people opting for alternatives to conventional marriage, such as co-habitation or forms of communal living. There has been what most commentators would describe as an alarming rise in the rate of divorce and legal changes designed to facilitate and normalize the ending of unhappy marriages, and yet the rate of re-marriage has also risen substantially. Although our experience has been requested for and principally with couples seeking a legal contract of marriage, much of what we discuss may equally apply to any long term partnership.

Whether or not following a period of experimental co-habitation, the decision to marry involves some uncertainties and the possibility of failure, even when a couple's situation is ideal. Couples who enjoy full employment, financial stability, good standards of physical and emotional health and the support of their respective families, can still be susceptible to marital instability. It is, therefore, not surprising that the prospect of a marriage involving those with certain kinds of special problems invokes reaction, particularly among those who are in professional caring roles and who have responsibility for the detention, care and treatment of such people. People who raise such a response include those detained in custody, and who may have committed serious offences against other people, indeed perhaps a former spouse or partner; those who may have health problems such as severe forms of mental disorder; those whose social histories may show an alarming catalogue of exposure to depriva-tion, violence and instability in domestic relationships; and/or those with little or no family support. We too have felt such caution and concern, but we also see the importance of maintaining a balanced approach after experience over the last 7 years listening to detained special hospital patients asking permission to marry, and supporting them from the first request through a process of marriage preparation, and facing up to the reality of being a married couple whilst remaining in hospital.

What follows is a description of the development of the marriage process at Broadmoor Hospital and a reflection on the experience of helping those who 'in sickness and in health' aim to make and sustain marriage against all odds.

> 'Marriage is given, that husband and wife may comfort and help each other, living faithfully together in need and in plenty, in sorrow and in joy.'
>
> *(The Alternative Service Book, 1980)*

As described in the previous chapter, the Marriage Act 1983 made changes to the law so that detained persons were not deprived of their right to marry merely because they were detained in an institution and therefore denied access to 'prescribed places' of marriage. Broadmoor Hospital staff became concerned that there would be a torrent of requests from patients with unsuitable motives for marriage. There was also an uneasy feeling that such change could bring further legal, clinical and social complexity to an already difficult and potentially volatile environment. In fact, in each of the years 1986 and 1987, one male patient requested permission to marry a female visitor. Both of these marriages were civil ceremonies, the first taking place at the local registry office and the second within the hospital secure perimeter and attended by the local Registrar. It is worth noting that the level of intrusive media attention in the former case led to the decision to allow the hospital premises to be used in the second case, thus setting the precedent that civil marriages should take place within the hospital on grounds of security and to minimize the risk of compromising patient confidentiality.

Between January 1988 and the end of 1995 there were three further marriages between a patient and a partner from outside and ten patient–patient marriages, from an available population of 215 women and 754 men. All but one of these marriages have been civil ceremonies carried out by the Registrar of Marriages from the nearby town. Often couples have asked for a church blessing after civil marriage, and this has occurred immediately after the ceremony. On one occasion a full Church of England marriage ceremony took place in the Hospital Chapel. This was the marriage between a male patient who was near to discharge and a woman who was an ex-patient who had already been discharged into the community with the support of her parents. On this occasion they had requested such a marriage and this seemed appropriate as there was an imminent opportunity for this couple to be able to set up home together and fulfil the vows of marriage. In most other cases, at least one of the people intending to marry has been subject to indefinite restriction on discharge under the provisions of the Mental Health Act 1993. It is our view, endorsed by the local Anglican bishop, that in these circumstances with the likelihood of several further years in a high secure placement after the marriage, the fulfilment of marriage vows is not forseeably attainable and this creates an impediment to marriage in Church.

Developing a hospital policy

The many valid reasons for concern about such marriages are aired elsewhere in this volume (e.g. Chapter 1), but as also noted it is extremely unlikely that either serious mental disorder or a history of serious violence would in themselves be sufficient to mount a successful legal challenge to the marriage taking place. It would be fair to acknowledge, too, that some of the articulated concerns even of professional staff were, in fact, based on feeling states that had little to do with a recognized body of factual information about either the circumstance generally or the pair proposing to marry. Nevertheless, even for those couples where the prospects of the marriage contributing positively to rehabilitation seemed better than average, the pressures on attempting marriage within a competing institutional system seemed to constitute a distinct dimension which would be likely to call for development of special, additional work in any preparatory counselling.

After the first two marriages, and only after them, the first hospital policy for the guidance of staff handling a request from patients to marry was produced. Although subject to minor revisions, it still forms the basis of current practice.

Pre-marital counselling: support and preparation

Since 1988, all Broadmoor Hospital patients intending to marry have been offered a programme of pre-marital support and counselling as a couple. They may refer themselves or be referred by their clinical team. In general, outside hospitals or prison, any couple seeking a marriage ceremony within a Christian church would be expected to engage in one or more preparation sessions with the clergyman or woman who would in due course conduct their marriage service. In some respects, therefore, the Broadmoor approach of initiating this area of work within the chaplaincy was quite 'normal'. Not all people, however, either want or are suited to a religious ceremony and it is important to make some assessment of the broad spiritual, cultural and social needs of each couple. Marriage is an important and emotional life experience, a rite of passage which calls for particular sensitivity on the part of those involved. Hospital chaplains are well suited to undertaking this work or facilitating others from other faiths or cultural backgrounds to do so. Coincidentally, the current Broadmoor Hospital chaplain, one of us (T.W.), is also a registered psychiatric nurse and nurse tutor of long experience at the hospital and has been well placed to facilitate the development of a programme of support and counselling. Several other staff of other disciplines are now able to offer couple counselling and the choice of counsellor is made dependent upon the needs of the couples concerned.

The counselling completed with the first pair of patients presenting for marriage set a precedent for others, and provided a basis for policy development. Finding a suitable place which provided privacy and establishing the principles of confidentiality, without compromising the hospital's basic principles of security, were troublesome first tasks. Ward staff advised against meeting on the ward of one of the patients and the wisdom of finding a neutral place was easily agreed. Accommodation was booked, as needed, in the Patients' Education Centre. In Broadmoor, patient movement through the hospital depends upon staff escorts being provided. At first, sessions were therefore timed to coincide with other activities in the Centre to minimize staffing requirements and maximize cooperation. As the importance of working with patients in this situation became more widely accepted, gradually it became possible to tailor the accommodation and timing for the counselling to fit more precisely with the needs of each couple.

Following preliminary meetings between the counsellor and each patient individually, a series of joint sessions timed to provide counselling and support during the months leading up to the proposed date of marriage is offered. The aims of such counselling are several:

First, to help patients talk about the origin and quality of their relationship and how it has developed

Second, to examine the decision to marry, the motivation behind it and to check out that each partner understands the nature and purpose of marriage

Third, to help the couple gain insight into the problems and difficulties associated with being married whilst remaining in a special hospital

Fourth, depending on individual ability to engage in therapeutic work, to facilitate an exploration of the expression of sexuality within their relationship

Fifth, to assist patients to grow in personal knowledge of each other in relation to life history, criminal history, previous relationships, if any, and the events which led to special hospital admission. A major anxiety of staff is that one partner may enter into marriage without full knowledge of the destructive capacity of the other, or indeed recognition of their own.

People in special hospital have almost invariably expressed their distress or mental disorder or sought solutions to their perceived problems in extremely dangerous acts. The counsellor always observes total confidentiality with each partner in the relationship, and would not disclose information about one to the other. A prime purpose of counselling, however, is to ascertain the extent of mutual knowledge and to encourage further disclosure where necessary. The basic ethical principle followed is that marriage cannot, and should not, be built on anything other than full knowledge and trust of one another.

It has not always been easy to convince professional staff in the clinical team of each patient that joint relationship counselling is of benefit to their patient. It is feared that in some cases the counselling itself may be perceived as tacit encouragement of a pathological or even dangerous relationship. However, all agree that, in other cases, not only is counselling advisable while considering marriage, but that this counselling may be of general and mutual holistic benefit. From time to time, there have been conflicts between the two clinical teams involved: one may believe that the relationship is helpful to their patient's progress, the other that progress is being hindered; one team may acknowledge not only that marriage is taking place but also that they must take account of it when designing or updating care and treatment plans, the other team insisting that the marriage must have minimal impact on the planning of care for their patient. This may be both a form of counter transference and a partially realistic response, since it seems particularly likely to happen when an individual patient announces his or her refusal to be treated as an individual any longer and demands that she/he and partner are considered only together.

One further area of concern has been the involvement and views of close family members when decisions to marry are being taken. In our experience, the declared intention to marry has resulted in a wide range of reactions by family members, from total approval and a high level of support to active discouragement and even the threat of severing contact. In general, however, although close relatives have often been surprised and shocked at the news, many have agreed to attend weddings and offered ongoing support.

The wedding day

> 'In marriage, husband and wife belong to one another and they begin a new life together in the community.'
>
> *(The Alternative Service Book, 1980)*

In the final weeks leading up to a wedding day, the couple concerned are offered further counselling and support, and finally help with practical matters to do with festivities such as organizing a wedding reception, inviting family members where appropriate, and photographs. For the couple this tends to be an important and sometimes anxious time as they will not be subject to the range of family attention and support that couples in the community would expect, and yet those reaching this stage need to be able to mark the importance of the step they are taking. Some patients have reported it was difficult to feel entirely happy through the wedding day, particularly if they felt some degree of disagreement or displeasure from staff. On the whole, though, wedding days themselves have gone well, without incident, and most couples have felt content with the way that the hospital has facilitated the event. On more than one occasion, patients who have had no close family have asked members of nursing staff to stand as witness for the ceremony and contract. The range of staff responses in this long-stay hospital is perhaps, after all, not so different from the range in families.

Each wedding day must end with painful and inescapable separation. Relatives and other outside guests are escorted back to the hospital entrance. More poignant – particularly in view of the sentiments read out for those who choose an Anglican religious ceremony, but which in any case reflects a universal expectation – the new couple must go their separate ways too. However well prepared to face up to the challenge of being married whilst in hospital, the resumption of separate status is suddenly and sharply a harsh reality.

One further issue remains important on wedding days. As with most other major events concerning special hospital patients, it is possible that information about the event may 'leak' from the hospital and create media interest. This may happen in a number of ways.

The contract of marriage, whether religious or secular, is made only after steps have been taken to ensure that there is no legal impediment to marriage such as the existence of a surviving spouse from a previous marriage. In England, for civil marriages, this involves the local Registrar taking notice of the intention to marry 21 clear days in advance of the proposed marriage and publically posting the relevant information at the registry office. For marriages in the Church of England, similarly, this involves the publication of banns on three consecutive Sundays prior to a wedding date. Both systems are designed to alert the general public to the proposed marriage so that any objection regarding a local impediment can be made. For detained persons, especially those considered to be of high public profile, this can lead to unwanted media attention. For this reason it may be important to consider with the couple whether this should influence them towards a choice of marriage by licence, avoiding the need to display information publically and which would thus limit the knowledge of the event to those with a direct and relevant interest. Even so, on wedding days it may be necessary to have prepared a press release with the assistance of the hospital's public relations manager. It is worth noting that the chaplain, on more than one occasion, has had to walk through a bank of reporters and television crews to enter the hospital whilst trying to hide his clerical collar! Few general psychiatric hospitals might expect such problems, but the advice may be pertinent for prisoner marriages in prison.

It has been suggested on occasions that hospital staff may have passed information to the press. Each special hospital is a large organization, employing well over one thousand people, not all of whom have a professional qualification or code. It is hardly surprising if one or two, often out of misguided altruism seeking to prevent something they fear can only be disastrous, break a hospital rule. For any member of staff, professional or no, such a breach of confidentiality if established would be a disciplinary matter likely to result in dismissal.

Post-marital support

As indicated, the end of a wedding day may be somewhat of an anticlimax and care must be taken over the next days and weeks to continue the support of the patients concerned, both as individuals and as a couple. It is good practice to arrange further counselling during these weeks to continue the process of relationship awareness, to avoid any unnecessary communication difficulties and to assist patients to affirm their 'married couple status' within the bounds established by the hospital community.

As more couples have been married, the hospital has gradually developed policies to increase the opportunities for couples to meet and communicate with one another. In so doing it appeared very important to staff to try and avoid giving other patients cause to consider that the hospital was giving special privileges to those who married. It was feared that this might encourage others to marry simply to obtain greater opportunity for recreational social activities. It is now normal practice for patients, whether married or not, whether in a long lasting relationship or not, whether male or female, to be allowed to visit one another in the visiting area as well as meeting, as appropriate, at work, at occupational therapy, in the education centre or at other organized activities.

In 1992, as the presence of patient couples became more accepted within the hospital, we gained hospital management support to establish a 'couples support group'. While the number of marriages remained small, slightly larger numbers of people came forward wanting a way of expressing their serious intent in a long term partnership, or support for it. The Couples Group was for couples, whether married or not, to discuss with one another the problems and difficulties of maintaining a relationship in a special hospital. It was not restricted to heterosexual couples. It principally attracted couples both of whom are patients in the hospital but this was not a criterion for membership.

Clinical teams were asked to identify all patients whom they thought might have a significant partner, using assessment criteria based on the stated importance, apparent stability and durability of the relationship. The couples identified were invited to attend fortnightly evening sessions in the Patients' Education Centre. Up to six couples attended and time was given during each session to discuss practical issues and hospital policy relating to the domestic and social lives of patients. The forum was used by couples to gain mutual support from others experiencing the same problems and frustrations in their daily lives. Common concerns relating to 'couple identity' were debated, including patient–patient communication within the hospital, clinical team acceptance of the interest of one partner about the other, joint visiting arrangements and staff perception of demonstratively affectionate behaviour at hospital social functions. Another recurring topic was an appreciation of staff attitudes about patient relationships; patients were aware that many staff of all disciplines were openly against this development on grounds of the risk of encouraging sexual behaviour. However, it became clear that, although couples regarded physical sexual expression as very important, most patients gave a higher priority to being able to enjoy periods of relative privacy within the hospital for quality private conversation and simply to relax and 'be together'. What they wanted most was to be allowed to visit each other's wards, cook a meal together and then curl up on a settee and watch television! After several months, it became clear that once the process of change had begun to allow couples better access to one another and to encourage better cooperation between clinical teams, the support group itself became less important and did not continue. It did, however, create a forum for debate at the right time during the process of development.

Rehabilitation of couples

Facing temporary separation

It is highly likely that one partner in a two-patient marriage in hospital (or two-prisoner in prison) will be ready for transfer or discharge before the other. One criticism of marriage in special hospital expressed by clinical teams involves the situation created by a married partner who is ready for transfer but who is reluctant to leave because of the resulting enforced marital separation. In most cases it would be counterproductive to delay transfer for this reason, but there are times when the benefits of moving on need to be weighed against the risk of instability caused by separation.

When such a separation is planned, it is good practice to support the couple by planning with them, well in advance, a programme of communication and contact to minimize the risk of isolation and misperception. If possible, a visit to the new accommodation of the departing partner by the one who will stay may also help. It is imperative that detailed reports about the relationship, agreed with the couple, are given to the receiving clinical team.

Considering all factors, it would be fair to suggest that any marriage which begins within the confines of a special hospital will be at its most vulnerable when such separation occurs. However, one male patient when facing such separation and asked to comment stated, 'we would prefer that staff held the view, as we do, that our relationship is "trying to survive" after transfer rather than "doomed to fail!"'

Difficulties with receiving agencies

Most special hospital patients who are considered ready for transfer or discharge are frustrated by the time taken to obtain a bed in a regional secure unit, or to arrange accommodation and supervision in the community. Couples who have married whilst in hospital and who hope, eventually, to be rehabilitated together face what sometimes seems like the impossible. The Special Hospitals' Service

Authority–Inner London Probation Service liaison probation officer completed a national survey of local authorities, by phone, and found that none was aware of any such community accommodation (Cameron, personal communication). Other hospitals proved no better at setting up facilities for married couples and there is some reluctance in accepting responsibility even for longer term supervision in these circumstances.

Despite this, three couples who previously were patients in Broadmoor Hospital are now living together in the community or are being accommodated within the same regional secure hospital facility. One couple, the only couple to have had a church wedding, are living together in independent accommodation and are supported by the woman's family. This couple did not leave the hospital together but the male patient was able to join his wife several months after their marriage. Their marriage is now in its sixth year. A second couple were transferred together to independent accommodation within a privately run hostel. They have continued to live in the same place and are now in their third year since discharge. They remain the only couple to have been discharged simultaneously. A third couple is now in the same regional secure unit, but in separate wards. They spend much time together and it is hoped that their further rehabilitation can be simultaneous.

Conclusions

> 'It is a way of life that all should honour; and it must not be undertaken carelessly, lightly or selfishly, but reverently, responsibly, and after serious thought.'
>
> *(The Alternative Service Book, 1980)*

Marriage remains a popular institution and is probably seen by most people to be the ideal foundation for domestic life. A good marriage can bring long-lasting mutual support and stability to the life of each partner and their families, whereas a bad marriage can lead to unhappiness and harm. Elsewhere the evidence is predominantly that this is as true for psychiatric patients and/or offender marriages as for the more healthy and generally socially adjusted (see Taylor, this volume). Any long term human relationship should only be entered into with care and after serious thought, and yet all too often in the wider community marriages fail. Within special hospitals, relationship formation usually follows a distinctly different pattern than in the wider community. The environment of the secure hospital imposes on couples what can be best described as a 'traditional courtship'. Contact with one another is limited to certain public areas and begins and ends at set times controlled by others. However unobtrusive the observation, there is a constant 'chaperoning effect'. Physical contact is controlled by policy and sexual behaviour is not allowed. Under such circumstances relationships not destined to survive usually remain superficial or fail quickly.

For some couples, the environmental controls may lead to comparatively slow progress in relationship formation, with a higher level of verbal interaction than is usual. Such patients tend to sit together for 2-hourly visiting sessions holding hands and talking to one another. For some, this can lead to a gradual development of cognitive and emotional insight of one another without a rapid progression to physical experimentation. For patients with previous experience of loneliness, rejection and of abusive relationships, this pattern of development may have great therapeutic benefit. An opposite view is that within the choice of partners available, patients with experience of bad relationships only and with poor role models will seek out new relationships which may simply repeat abusive patterns of the past. Marriages could occur, which not only would have difficulty surviving the transition to the community, but may become physically dangerous for one partner or the other. The full range is seen in practice and it is essential that staff become better attuned to recognition, and the kind of acceptance which can lead to professional guidance or treatment appropriate to each situation. With the establishment of a good working alliance, counselling may assist separation in the latter type of case before harm is done, as well as support and growth in the future for the former.

Of the fifteen marriages which have taken place at Broadmoor Hospital, five have been between a patient and an outside visitor and ten have been patient–patient marriages. Of the five, three marriages have ended in divorce and the other two are continuing with relative stability. Of the ten patient–patient married couples, four remain in hospital and their marriages have continued. One couple have been rehabilitated together and remain stable. One couple are being rehabilitated together but from separate wards in a regional secure unit. One couple are divorced after being separately rehabilitated. Three couples are now separated, with one partner remaining in Broadmoor Hospital and one partner transferred or discharged. Of those three, one couple have divorced and the other two are surviving with regular visits. Overall, of the fifteen marriages, five have ended in divorce. It is difficult to draw any meaningful conclusions from such a small sample but the picture is one not dissimilar to that of the population at large.

The legal changes brought about by the Marriage Act 1983 triggered a challenge to special hospitals which has not only resulted in the development of services to meet the needs of the small but important group of patients who decide to marry, but also in a much greater awareness of patient relationships in general, from the need for basic friendship to the need to express mutually exclusive intimacy. The presence of an increasing if still small number of married couples and others in long lasting relationships has provided the opportunity for much debate and changes in policy. Joint case conferences for couples and regular contact between key members of clinical teams have now become widely accepted. The incorporation of assessment, management and in some cases treatment of relationships into the care and treatment plans and into pre-discharge planning is now seen to be important to the process of overall improvement or recovery and rehabilitation. When problems occur within a relationship or when a marriage appears to be failing, there is now general support for the notion of 'relationship therapy'.

There remains one major dilemma. Special hospitals are able to fulfil the requirement of law and allow patients to marry but, as yet, are unable to allow married patients to live together in the sense understood in marriage, or to have full conjugal visits. However stable and near to discharge or transfer patients may be, there is no provision for married accommodation within the high-security environment. Some secure psychiatric facilities in other European countries have advanced further, allowing conjugal visiting and the provision of married accommodation reflecting their own cultural position (see Gordon, this volume), but this does not occur in the United Kingdom in the 1990s. Consequently, the legal, clinical and ethical debate continues.

Despite all the institutional complexity of special hospitals, some patients detained within them have made and sustained marriage against all odds.

4

Social context of relationships: Working with the family

Tracey C. Heads

Partnerships do not occur in isolation. The social environment may include family, friends and other social contacts involving, for people who are ill or in jail, professional contacts. A new relationship emerges out of and continues within this social context. In earlier societies and currently in a number of non-western societies, there is an important and well-defined role for the family when an individual member enters into a partnership; indeed in some it may be the family that determines entirely the relationship. In contemporary Western culture the emphasis on individual autonomy and exclusivity of romantic love has resulted in a rather ambiguous role for the family in such a situation.

The interactions between a couple and their combined social networks are complex and involve not only the impact of family and friends on a partnership but also the effect the couple has on the social network. This complexity is given a further dimension by the contribution of early experiences of family life to personality development and adult behaviour. Of particular relevance is the suggestion that relationship styles established in childhood are of an enduring nature. Evidence also suggests a degree of intergenerational continuity in relationship styles (Hartup and Rubin, 1986; Hinde and Stevenson-Hinde, 1988; Parkes *et al.*, 1991).

The social aspects of a relationship are even more complex in the context of an individual with a psychiatric disorder and a history of offending. In such a situation a detailed family history and description of the early social environment is essential for an understanding of the development of both illness and offending, and is particularly relevant in an assessment of the possible difficulties which may be encountered in a new partnership. The current nature of relationships within the family is also of importance, particularly in the light of influence of social environment on the prognosis of some psychiatric illnesses (Lam, 1991; Leff *et al.*, 1982; Leff *et al.*, 1990a) and the importance of the social context in violent behaviour (Estroff *et al.*, 1994; Monahan and Klassen, 1982).

A new relationship involves a redefining and renegotiation of relationships with family and friends and developing new relationships with the social network of the partner (McGoldrick, 1989). This is likely to be stressful for both the individuals involved, and their friends and families. Difficulties with 'in-laws' are particularly renowned (Apter, 1986). For families with relatives who are mentally ill, such a redefining of relationships may be particularly difficult, but potentially even more so in the case of a prospective partner who is mentally ill and has a history of offending. Successful negotiation of this difficult process is important for both the patient and his or her family and friends. Much of what is said in this chapter is likely to be helpful background in relation to prisoners and offenders as well as patients in hospital, but it does draw particularly from the latter, while such qualities more specific to relationships in a prison setting are dealt with further in Coyle, and in relationship to pregnancy in Tobin and Taylor, this volume.

Importance of family and social network to development of a romantic or sexual partnership

A confusing variety of theoretical approaches contributes to an understanding of the importance of family and friends in relation to adult romantic relationships. There is a considerable social psychology literature reporting on the nature of contemporary interactions between the couple and their combined social networks. The work of family therapists, emphasizing the location of an individual within the family system, is also of relevance. An understanding of such contemporary influences can be enhanced by a consideration of the effects of past experiences in shaping personality development and, in particular, relationship style. Such issues have been considered of fundamental importance by many of those of a psychodynamic orientation and by developmental psychologists. Certain schools of family and marital therapy have also emphasized family of origin issues in understanding contemporary difficulties experienced by couples and families. Although much of the literature about the social context of relationships relates to populations different from the ones of interest here, a number of issues highlighted are of relevance.

Direct influence on a new relationship

Interaction between the couple and their combined social networks is complex and depends on characteristics of both the individuals and their networks (Ridley and Avery, 1979). This is of relevance for special hospital and prison populations, where network characteristics are likely to be distinctive. Social influences may be direct and practical, such as arranging introductions, facilitating meetings and couple privacy (important in a custodial setting), or more subtle (Bates, 1942). The reaction of family and friends to a new partnership may also vary depending on the stage of the relationship. Early tolerance may change to increasing opposition when there is a realization of the seriousness of the relationship. Conversely, early opposition by family and friends may give way to realization of the need to come to terms with the situation in order to preserve their own relationship with the individual. Individuals, sensing antagonism to the relationship, may well try and influence opinions of family and friends (Leslie et al., 1986).

A number of studies have examined the influence of social networks on relationships (Bates, 1942; Driscoll et al., 1972; Leslie et al., 1986; Lewis, 1973; McGoldrick, 1989; Parks et al., 1983; Ryder et al., 1971; Sprecher and Felmlee, 1992; Sussman, 1953). Although interpretation is difficult due to methodological limitations, the results suggest that social networks may influence not only partner choice but also the quality and stability of relationships. Support from the network has been shown to affect positively the relationship, with opposition having the converse effect (Felmlee, 1990; Johnson and Milardo, 1984; Lewis, 1973; Sprecher and Felmlee, 1992). A variety of theoretical models have been proposed to explain such influences (Sprecher and Felmlee, 1992). One possible mechanism is the labelling by others of the partnership as successful or unsuccessful being internalized and acted on by the individuals involved (Lewis, 1973; Ryder et al., 1971). A further factor may be the value that the partner's social network acquires for an individual (Ridley and Avery, 1979). This network may also provide information about the partner, and in doing so reduce uncertainty about the partner (Sprecher and Felmlee, 1992). In addition, the development of an overlapping network may act as a barrier to relationship dissolution (Milardo, 1982; Parks et al., 1983).

Driscoll et al. (1972), in contrast to the studies referred to above, found parental interference enhanced relationship development (an effect they termed the 'Romeo and Juliet effect'). The authors explained this finding in terms of the motivating affect of frustration and increased emotional dependence on the partner resulting from social opposition. Such opposition can lead to an idealization of the forbidden partner (McGoldrick, 1989). This situation may result in anger and aggression, which may be directed towards critical family or friends or redirected toward the partner (Driscoll et al., 1972; McGoldrick, 1989). This is an issue of possible special importance among people with a mental disorder, who have offended, or both, where social and professional resistance to relationships is not unusual and anger control and violent behaviour may be identified problems.

Effects of new relationship on existing family and social networks

Evidence suggests that the formation of a new partnership significantly affects the networks of both individuals involved (Johnson and Leslie, 1982; Johnson and Milardo, 1984; Leslie et al., 1986; Milardo et al., 1983; Slater, 1963). In general, results point to reduced involvement with the social network as the partnership progresses (Johnson and Leslie, 1982; Milardo et al., 1983). This withdrawal by a couple from the social group as they become 'wrapped up in each other' has been analysed from a psychodynamic perspective by Slater (1963). In this model, as the partnership develops, libido is withdrawn from the social group and invested instead in the partner. Slater (1963) described such libidinal withdrawal as causing social anxiety related to the threat to group solidarity. He described a variety of ways in which such anxiety could be expressed, including anger, moral indignation, ridicule or scorn. Johnson and Milardo (1984), recasting Slater's theory in the language of social psychology, reported that social anxiety produced by network withdrawal was expressed in attempts to interfere with the relationship. Slater (1963) described such social anxiety as especially prominent in groups and societies formed on the basis of common interests and proposed that the strongest opposition to partnerships would be within totalitarian collectives. Such ideas are of interest in considering some of the professional resistance to relationships in prisons and hospitals.

The views of family and friends about a partnership may be coloured by their own experiences of romantic relationships. In addition, aspects of their own relationships with the individual concerned and relationships within the family are likely to influence attitudes to the partnership. Particular problems may be likely in families characterized by a lack of clear boundaries between individuals, with over-involved, intrusive relationships, a situation referred to as enmeshment (Minuchen, 1974). Individuals in such families may not be allowed space for their own individual development and a partnership, as a symbol of independence, serves to highlight such difficulties. A situation where parents have failed to accept that their child has become an adult and are reluctant to relinquish the parenting role may be particularly problematic. These issues are likely to be especially relevant in the context of a family member suffering from a serious mental illness, particularly where overinvolvement and criticism are thought to be particularly damaging (see below). Some of these issues have been highlighted in the 1993 film Benny and Joon, in which a brother who has cared for his mentally ill young sister for many years has difficulty coming to terms with her relationship with a somewhat eccentric young man.

Effect of family and social networks in influencing patterns in new relationships

Both partners bring to the relationship their own past experiences. A variety of paradigms, including psychological, psychodynamic and social, have described the important contribution of early childhood experiences, particularly relationship experiences, to personality development and adult behaviour. The relationship with the primary caregiver has received particular emphasis; however other relationships, such as those between siblings and the observation of the parental relationship, are also likely to be important. It has been proposed that individuals show a degree of continuity in the style and quality of their relationships (Hinde and Stevenson-Hinde, 1988; Parkes et al., 1991). Repeating patterns of relationships, for example in quality of parenting, child abuse, marital violence and marital instability, have also been described across family generations (Hinde and Hinde-Stevenson, 1988; Rutter, 1988). The connection between early experiences and later relationship behaviour is complex and other factors relating both to the individual and subsequent social experiences are also likely to be of importance. Endless repetition is certainly not inevitable and an examination of the degree of continuity and change in relationship style is essential in assessment.

One route to explaining continuity or repetition in relationship styles is attachment theory (Ainsworth et al., 1978; Belsky and Pensky, 1988; Bowlby, 1969; Bowlby, 1973; Bowlby, 1980; Holmes, 1993; Parkes et al., 1991). Attachment theory proposes that early patterns of attachment behaviour result in 'internal working models' of the relationship between the self and caregiver, which become integrated into the personality structure. These working models are carried forward, and, in colouring expectations and interpretations, guide social interactions. Where there is a degree of ambiguity in a relationship, these effects are likely to be particularly pronounced (Ainsworth, 1991). Concepts of attachment have been applied to adult romantic relationships (Bartholomew, 1993; Weiss, 1986). A number of studies have described the significant influence of perceived early attachment patterns on partner selection, marital adjustment, relationship satisfaction, couple communication and conflict resolution (Bartholomew, 1993; Collins and Read, 1990; Feeney and Noller, 1990; Hazen and Shaver, 1987; Kobac and Hazan, 1991; Pistole, 1989; Senchak and Leonard,

1992; Weiss, 1991). Of special relevance is the concept of repetition of early dysfunctional attachment styles in adult relationships. In addition, attachment theory has been applied to concepts of vulnerability to development of adult mental illness (Holmes, 1993; Patrick et al., 1994).

A number of family and marital therapists have emphasized the contribution of conflicts within the family of origin to current difficulties experienced by couples and families (Boszormenyi-Nagy and Spark, 1973; Bowen, 1978; Framo, 1981). Such conflicts may be acted out within the context of the current relationship (Framo, 1981; McGoldrick, 1989). Bowen (1978), working initially with families of patients with schizophrenia and later extending his findings to other families, described a situation where there was inadequate differentiation between family members, with a lack of individual autonomy. He referred to the 'undifferentiated ego mass' of these families (a concept which overlaps to an extent with the notion of enmeshment) and described the difficulties which arise within families and couples when individuals are still part of the 'undifferentiated ego mass' of their family of origin.

Framo (1981), incorporating ideas from object-relations theory (Fairbairn, 1952) has emphasized psychodynamic issues in relation to marital difficulties. Framo emphasizes the individual's perception of their partner in terms of unconscious expectations relating to their own primary object relationship. There are unconscious hopes that the partner will contain aspects of the self which have been denied or split off (Dicks, 1967). Such expectations, not based on who the partner actually is in reality, may well create problems. An individual may also fight against disowned parts of themselves which they have projected on to their partner (Framo, 1981).

Importance of family and social network to mental disorder and offending

Early social environment is important in understanding development of mental disorder and offending, and thus is of indirect relevance to the special relationships considered here. For a recent review of family influences on the development of psychiatric disorder, the reader is referred to Bloch et al. (1994). A number of family and social risk factors have also been identified in relation to later development of delinquency and offending behaviour (Farrington, 1993; Loeber and Stouthamer-Loeber, 1986; Robins et al., 1978; Rutter and Smith, 1995; West and Farrington, 1977). It is perhaps hardly surprising that there is overlap in the nature of problem backgrounds, and that indeed a small minority of people have both mental disorder and the capacity to offend seriously.

Although there is little research examining the early social environment of mentally disordered offenders, clinical experience suggests that a seriously disturbed childhood is common in this population. A history of childhood sexual abuse may be particularly important, although the deprived and chaotic environment in which such abuse commonly occurs is also likely to be relevant (Mullen, 1993). A history of serious physical abuse, often associated with use of alcohol, is also common. Some will also have had parents suffer from mental illness, possibly requiring repeated hospitalization. There is some evidence that those with schizophrenia and a history of offending are likely to have experienced poor parental relationships and a lack of affectionate relationships with parents (Addad et al., 1981). In a series of special hospital patients with schizophrenia (who had either offended or been seriously violent) adverse experiences in childhood were recorded for just over one quarter, but some aspects of poor parenting were much more common. About half of the women and over 40% of the men, for example, experienced parental conflict (Heads *et al.*, 1997).

The current social network indirectly affects the relationship by having an important influence on the course of the mental illness. Social support is widely viewed as beneficial, especially in enhancing an individual's ability to cope with adversity, the work of Brown and Harris (1978) demonstrating the importance of a confiding relationship. Deficits in social networks have been suggested as of causal and prognostic importance in a variety of psychiatric illnesses (Henderson *et al.*, 1978; Henderson, 1980; Brown and Harris, 1978; Brugha, 1989; Brugha, 1990). This aspect of illness has relevance for treatment in terms of social reintegration and support (Beels, 1979; Brugha *et al.*, 1993; Eber and Riger, 1990; Goldstein and Caton, 1983; Hammer *et al.*, 1978; Holmes-Thornicroft and Breakey, 1991; Pattison and Pattison, 1981).

While an individual is in a special hospital, especially for those with lengthy admissions, there is a risk of isolation and alienation from the outside world (Vaughan, 1980; Vaughan, 1981). The practical difficulties involved in visiting by family and friends are often considerable and in addition such contact may be associated with emotional distress. Although it may be thought that chronically ill long stay hospital patients inevitably become socially isolated, investigation has demonstrated a considerable amount of social interaction in such groups (Dunn *et al.*, 1990; Leff *et al.*, 1990b). Many special hospital patients receive social support not only from their family, but also from other social contacts, both within and outside the institution. McCann (1993) has described an initiative in one of the special hospitals aimed at enhancing the social aspects of patient care. The project has emphasized maintaining and increasing patient social networks, improving communication between social network members and staff, and decreasing the stress that many relatives and friends experience when dealing with the hospital. Such measures are likely to enhance the ability of family and friends to provide support for the patient. Such ideas are of relevance when considering social attitudes to patient partnerships.

Although emphasis has been given to the positive influence of social support, negative and upsetting effects of social interactions are inevitable (Fiore *et al.*, 1983; Pagel *et al.*, 1987; Rook, 1984; Thompson and Sobolow-Shubin, 1993). Social support may appear to a patient to be overprotective, dependency inducing and frustrating. More extreme examples include emotionally charged arguments and actual physical violence. Negative interactions with members of the social network may aggravate mental disorder and may in fact outweigh the protective effects of positive social support (Fiore, 1983; Rook, 1984). The negative effects of a certain style of family interaction, termed 'high expressed emotion', have been recognized particularly in relation to schizophrenia (Brown *et al.*, 1972; Vaughn and Leff, 1976). High expressed emotion environments are characterized by emotional over-involvement and expression of criticism and hostility by key relatives. A link has been proposed between concurrent high levels of expressed emotion and early dysfunctional attachment styles (Holmes, 1993). Levels of expressed emotion have been found to influence the course and relapse rate of schizophrenia, especially if there is close contact between the patient and family members (Vaughn and Leff, 1976). A variety of family interventions aimed at changing family behaviour and attitudes have proved successful in reducing relapse rates (Falloon *et al.*, 1985; Lam, 1991; Leff *et al.*,

1982; Leff *et al.*, 1985; Leff *et al.*, 1990a). Although levels of contact with family members are much lower for patients in hospital, this is still likely to be an important issue, especially where potentially highly emotionally charged issues such as romantic relationships are being discussed (see also Hodge and Kruppa, this volume).

There has been little investigation of social networks and social support in mentally disordered offender populations. Family and friends may well influence not only illness prognosis, as discussed above, but also offending and violent behaviour. Appropriate support and intervention may serve to reduce the risk of such behaviour, with the converse applying to negative social interactions such as those characterized by high levels of expressed emotion. Estroff *et al.* (1994) have demonstrated that some aspects of the social network of seriously mentally ill patients (larger network size, networks composed predominantly of relatives and living with unrelated persons) are associated with violent behaviour. Evidence also suggests close relationships pose a risk for violence for those suffering from a psychotic illness (Mullen *et al.*, 1993b) and family members and partners may well be at risk.

Working with families

General issues

Illness and/or offending on the part of one family member are likely to have had an enormous impact on others in the family and, not unusually, family members have been victims. Admission of a relative to a psychiatric hospital, frequently a painful and traumatic experience for the family, is likely to be particularly so in the case of a compulsory admission, and worst still admission to a secure facility. Families are likely to have strong feelings, particularly anger and guilt, about the patient, the admission and the institution, and may mistrust and resent both staff and the institution. Families of those in special hospitals and prisons are likely to have particular needs (Matthews, 1983; McCann, 1991; McCann, 1993; NACRO's National Policy Committee on Resettlement, 1995).

There are a number of difficulties with family work carried out in secure facilities (Bruce, 1982; Pilgrim, 1988; Robinson *et al.*, 1991). Many institutions have found the involvement of the family in assessment and treatment to be threatening, and the lack of such family involvement has been publicly criticized in one English high security hospital (Committee of Inquiry into Complaints about Ashworth Hospital, 1992). Difficulties also include issues of conflicting roles for therapists, and concern about families and individuals feeling coerced into participation. Compliance may be only superficial with a view to being seen to be cooperative in order to improve chances of discharge. Traditional family work is often difficult in an inpatient setting as there is little chance for formal homework, or developments within the family outside sessional work. There are additional problems in the case of special institutions providing a national service – in England special hospitals and prisons – with the family often residing at a site far distant from the hospital, restricting visiting and therapy possibilities. In many cases multiple family members, often geographically distant, need to be contacted. For special hospital patients, for example, resident during 1993, in Broadmoor Hospital in Berkshire the median distance between the hospital and their home community was 54 miles, with a range of 4 to 608; in Rampton in Nottinghamshire it was 129 miles with a range of 12 to 486; and in Ashworth near Liverpool 119 miles with a range 9 to 373 (Ferraro *et al.*, submitted). Meetings may be highly emotionally charged and the family may be left after meetings feeling angry and resentful with no ongoing support available for themselves.

Meetings may be held with individual informants or with several family members present. There are advantages to the latter in that observation and assessment of family interactions are possible. Such meetings may take place at the hospital or at the family home. If meetings occur at the hospital site, either for assessment or for work relating to specific issues, there needs to be a decision regarding whether or not the patient should be present. Although the presence of the patient does allow for a fuller assessment of family interactions, their absence in the first instance may allow for a more frank discussion. In addition, the mental state and dangerousness of the patient need reassessment, keeping in mind the potentially highly agitating nature of family meetings.

An initial difficulty may be refusal by the family to be involved in assessment or management issues. Equally, the patient may refuse permission for the family to be involved, or may set specific limits on the work – for example they may not wish to inform their family of a new relationship. There may be a variety of reasons for such refusals and time needs to be taken for these to be fully explored. The reasons why such involvement is likely to be helpful need to be explained, and the family informed of how their involvement will allow for a more comprehensive understanding of the patient's problems and have an impact on management. There are always ethical issues to consider regarding confidentiality and sharing of information (Bloch *et al.*, 1994). After such discussion and with considerable persistence, cooperation is frequently obtained.

The initial contact is very important in establishing a good relationship with the family. Obtaining knowledge of background issues prior to the interview is useful. Attempts should be made to build rapport, and a non-blaming, sympathetic, interested and objective manner is helpful. There should be an emphasis on developing a collaborative relationship between the family and staff (McCann, 1993). Although in initial sessions staff may be seeking specific information, the family may need time to express their particular concerns. It is important to bear in mind the extreme emotions which family members may experience in such meetings and which may underlie resistance to addressing certain issues. Challenge to family views, particularly in early sessions, is likely to alienate families further – families who may already be suspicious and resentful.

Family work on specific issues should be carried out within the general context of the potential beneficial and detrimental effects of the social network described above. Specific issues, such as a new relationship, provide opportunities to address negative styles of family functioning. Education is often an important part of family work. Helping family members to understand their relative's illness and/or behaviour and the provision of advice about particular issues can enable the family to be maximally supportive. For those with a relative suffering from schizophrenia, for example, education about the benefit of a calm, supportive, non-critical atmosphere and the damaging effects of an argumentative, hostile atmosphere is likely to be helpful (Kuipers *et al.*, 1992). Of particular note in reports of family work in secure facilities is the description of an association between increased trust between relatives and staff, improved understanding of mental illness by the family, and an improvement in family communication on the one hand, and reduction in levels of anger and hostility and an increased ability to articulate feelings on the other (McCann, 1991; Robinson *et al.*, 1991).

Working with families: past history and current functioning

Family work during the initial assessment period involves extensive gathering of detailed information regarding the patient's past. The family, with their life-long knowledge of the patient, are a unique source of information about the patient's relationships, illness and offending. Such gathering of information overlaps to an extent with the assessment of current relationships within the family and serves as an introduction to therapeutic work. A detailed history of the family of origin is important and the construction of a genogram (family tree), including extended family, is a common starting point (Barker, 1992). This allows for a description of who is in the family and some factual information about them. If several family members are present, conflicting views about family members may become apparent and be able to be explored. It is useful to discover the ways in which the family worked as a whole to deal with issues and the ways different family members responded to change, problems and crises.

An assessment of relationship patterns and the social atmosphere within the family, both currently and in the past, has particular importance when considering new relationships. It is important to understand how early relationships are remembered in real terms and in fantasy. Informants may consciously or unconsciously conceal or distort information and it is helpful to be able to verify information or to observe for oneself family interactions. Differences in perception between informants may become evident and tactful exploration, while adequately controlling any conflict, may contribute to an understanding of how such differences have arisen. It may also become evident that there are taboo topics within the family, which may well relate to relationship issues, and full and open communication should be encouraged (Robinson *et al.*, 1991). It is important to be aware of major conflicts between family members and how others in the family respond to such conflict. Information on whether relationships have changed and, if so, how such change has occurred, is useful. Related to such work with the family are instruments used with individuals to assess retrospectively early relationships. The Parental Bonding Instrument (Parker, 1979) examines two dimensions: 'care', ranging from warmth and empathy to coldness and indifference, and 'overprotection', ranging from intrusive overprotection to promotion of autonomy. The Adult Attachment Interview (George *et al.*, 1985) examines current representations of early attachment.

A variety of theoretical approaches have been described for assessing current family functioning (Barker, 1992; Bloch, 1994). A number of areas are usually assessed including problem solving techniques, communication styles, family roles, methods of influence and control of behaviour in addition to patterns of interactions and family relationships. Relationships may be described in terms of closeness or distance and by qualities such as warmth or hostility (Bloch, 1994). Types of affective involvement between family members include: uninvolved, interested but devoid of feelings, narcissistic involvement (involved with another for own reasons rather than concern for interest in another), empathic involvement, and enmeshment (Barker, 1993). A particular style of interviewing known as circular questioning, developed by the Milan group, focuses on relationships and interactions between family members. Circular questioning involves asking a member of the family about the interaction between two other members of the family or about aspects of their own relationships within the family. Questions focus particularly on differences between individual responses. Further questions are then asked in response to the new information discovered. Such assessments of family interactions will also allow an estimation to be made of levels of expressed emotion, perhaps particularly important for patients with a schizophrenic illness.

A knowledge of family interactions is also of relevance for staff–patient relationships. Britten (1981), utilizing Freudian concepts of transference and repetition compulsion, described how professionals may unconsciously re-enact family dynamics. Moore *et al.* (1992) have compared staff–patient interactions with family–patient interactions in regard to expressed emotion. As with family interactions, staff over-involvement and criticism is likely to be damaging.

Working with families: new partnerships

Work with families in relation to new intimate partnerships may well need to cover a range of more general issues first; some of these have been described. This is complex work and considerable time is likely to be required for it. Family members may have their own views on the relationship, ranging from the extremely hostile to the unrealistically positive. Their responses may well be emotional and they may be uncertain as to their own role in the situation. Working with the family involves recognizing and exploring family views and emotions and aims to help the family come to terms with the relationship, while still maintaining or even improving their own relationship with their relative.

Family opinions may well mirror social attitudes to relationships and sexuality within institutions and a number of concerns are likely to be present. First, they may fear their relative is unable to cope with any such relationship, and believe a deterioration in mental state is likely to follow. Their views may be based on knowledge of previous relationships which have been distressing or destructive for one or both of the partners. They may have concerns primarily about the new partner in terms of mental illness, dangerousness and/or reputation and coping abilities. Particular concern may be present about partners who have a history of violence, sexual offending or offending against children. Family members may have held long cherished hopes of their relative having a long term relationship with a very different type of individual. Other fears may include possible pregnancy, the birth of a child, child care, passing a tendency to inheritance of mental illness to another, and/or the risk of acquiring sexually transmitted disease.

Issues relating to current family relationships, such as over-involvement and lack of acceptance of the relative as an adult, may well be relevant. In one case the overt signs of this were a maternal figure who, over a number of years, brought a monthly supply of comics suitable for young teenagers to a man nearing 30. Unable to say anything directly to his relative, he invariably threw them away in a mini rage attack. An important step in his maturation and rehabilitation took place when, after discussion and rehearsals with nursing staff, he was able to tell her that the magazines had long since ceased to be of interest to him and why. It is nevertheless important to acknowledge that, in other senses, one reason for the continuing presence of a patient in a long stay hospital is that in some respects they have not yet been able to take on successfully the full responsibilities of healthy adult life. The family may feel their relative still requires 'parental' guidance and may consider they have handed such responsibility, including the sanctioning of relationships, to the institution. They may be angry or unclear that the institution is able, as they themselves have been, to control some aspects of patients' lives but not others.

Past difficulties in relationships within the family are also important to explore in the context of individual and intergenerational continuity of relationships styles. Robinson *et al.* (1991) report a case where offending against a partner appeared to be linked to childhood experiences, particularly of abandonment. Boszormenyi-Nagy and Spark (1973) have also described how such early experiences of abandonment may leave the individual with feelings of worthlessness, inadequacy and underlying yearnings for love which may be minimalized or hidden by anger and resentment. These aggressive emotions may then be projected on to a current relationship. A shared understanding of the importance of such past experiences by the families, as well as the couple, may well prove beneficial to the new relationship (Framo, 1981; McGoldrick, 1989). The family are also likely to have views, in the context of past relationship difficulties, of the possibility of change. Family members may be able to make useful suggestions for avoiding past difficulties, thus improving the chances of the relationship being a success. On a final word of caution, however, the more dysfunctional the early family experiences, the less clear it is that anyone in the family network should be accepted as having an accurate perception of the current situation or a wise suggestion with respect to the patient, and the greater the importance of work with the family as a unit where possible. Occasionally, a break with family of origin may be essential.

Conclusions

The social context is an important consideration in the assessment and management of a relationship formed while in prison or a secure psychiatric facility. Information obtained regarding past and current relationships and interactions within the family can add a further dimension to an assessment of potential difficulties and risks. Family work directed at helping the family come to terms with a new relationship can enable relatives to continue to develop a healthier relationship with their sick or troubled relative, and improve their supportive role for the new partnership where appropriate.

5

Achieving the impossible
Maintaining relationships in prison

Andrew Coyle

There's my Daddy

In April 1995 the Royal National Theatre collaborated with Brixton Prison, a large local prison in South London, in a 6-week workshop which culminated in a number of productions of Hamlet. With the exception of the two female leads, all parts were played by prisoners. Prisoners also shadowed the backstage staff and were responsible for music and artwork. It was an exciting venture which showed the prisoners that they had considerable talent. Properly harnessed by self-discipline and hard work, it could be put to extremely positive use in a manner which was both entertaining and instructive.

There were many amusing and instructive cameos during the 6 weeks. One in particular is relevant here. Prisoners were allowed to invite members of their families to one of the performances. They were determined to show their wives, partners, parents and children what they had achieved. In one of the final scenes of the play the ghost of Hamlet's father walked on to the stage accompanied by the ghost of Ophelia. It was a forceful scene and the audience, including a large number of prisoners, was giving its full attention. The silence was broken by a small voice exclaiming, 'There's my daddy; and he's with another woman'. There were a few embarrassed titters but there was no widespread open reaction. The comment was too near the bone.

Reality of imprisonment

Prison is a place of exile from society. One of its original purposes was to separate the prisoner from all contact with the outside world, with his or her community, with his or her family. Such a separation was a key element in the punishment which was at the centre of imprisonment. Considerable attempts are made nowadays to minimize this part of the deprivation of liberty and to help the prisoner to maintain and to develop contact with his or her family. This is an admirable objective, but it is one which is made more difficult precisely because it goes against one of the tenets on which the original concept of imprisonment was based.

There is a great deal of symbolism in prison life. This is never more obvious than at the point when the prisoner is first received into prison. He is brought directly from court under escort. Having passed through the gates of the prison he is taken to the reception area where he is subjected to a process which is highly symbolic. His clothes and personal possessions are taken from him. He is required to shower or bathe and is given a set of prison uniform clothing. And he is given a number. Henceforth this number becomes almost more important than his own name. It is unique to him and will be an infallible identifying mark. In all of this process the prisoner is a passive object. He is required to do nothing other than conform. This reception is very little different for women as they become prisoners.

When the reception process has been completed the prisoner is taken to a small room, known as a cell. Here he will spend the major part of his sentence. In the local prison to which he has first come he will probably be required to share this small room with a total stranger with whom he has nothing in common other than the fact that they are both in prison. Until the mid 1990s in the UK they would each have been required to perform their bodily functions into a plastic bucket while the other turned discreetly away. Nowadays there is likely to be a toilet in the cell, but not much greater privacy.

The fact that the man in prison is a father, a husband, a son goes virtually unrecorded at this stage. Indeed, as part of the process of initiation into prison the prisoner's responsibility for supporting his family is taken away from him. For the duration of the sentence it is likely that the state, through social security benefits and other provisions, will take over financial responsibility for his family. Nevertheless, through all this process we tell the prisoner that we will teach him to be a responsible citizen, who will come out of prison more able to support his wife and family. The logic is not immediately obvious.

Coercive nature of prison

Prison is an abnormal institution in many respects. One of these is that it is predominantly a single sex community. In many prisons for men there is now a small number of female staff, but generally speaking the human dynamics of a prison consist of one group of men who deprive another group of men of their liberty. Virtually every moment of the day is pre-ordained. When a person rises in the morning, when he goes to wash, when he collects his meal, how he passes his time, perhaps even when he may perform his bodily functions. In such an environment the insensitivities of an all-male organization are never far below the surface.

Personal survival is the first priority. One requirement for ensuring personal survival is to suppress any sign of emotion. Any demonstration of personal feeling or sensitivity is likely to be interpreted as a sign of weakness. Any concession to another may well be seen as an indication of softness, to be exploited as far as possible. Any display of emotion is to be confined to a private moment, of which there are very few in a prison. In public a sense of bravado is the order of the day. This will often be expressed through selfishness in petty matters. Prison is a place where detail looms large, where issues which would pass unnoticed in normal life take on an importance far beyond what can be justified.

One of the most interesting recent commentaries on what it is like to be in prison has been given to us by Vaclav Havel, President of the Czech Republic. Between 1979 and 1983 Havel was imprisoned in his own country because of his human rights activities. The letters which he wrote to his wife during that period have been published (Havel, 1990). They give a fascinating insight into the reality of imprisonment:

> 'I used to think prison life must be endless boredom and monotony with nothing much to worry about except the basic problem of making the time pass quickly. But now I've discovered it's not like that. You have plenty of worries here all the time, and though they may seem "trivial" to the normal world, they are not at all trivial in the prison context. In fact you're always having to chase after something, arrange something, hunt for something, keep an eye on something, fear for something, hold your ground against something, etc. It's a constant strain on the nerves (someone is always twanging on them), exacerbated by the fact that in many important instances you cannot behave authentically and must keep your real thoughts to yourself.'

As in every aspect of life, there are exceptions to the norm. From time to time one comes across an example of the unselfishness of the human spirit. It may be the older man who takes a volatile young prisoner under his wing to help him avoid the mistakes which he made years before. It may be the prison officer who befriends the inadequate man who cannot read or write. It may be the way a group rallies round to protect a mentally disordered offender and helps him to survive.

Women in prison

Most of the previous references to prisoners have been made in the masculine. That is because about 95 per cent of people in prison in England and Wales are men. This figure is amazingly consistent across the world, with women making up between 2 and 6 per cent of the prison population in most countries.

There can be little argument that the trauma of imprisonment is more extreme for a woman than for a man. This is partly because of the kind of women offenders who end up in prison. They are very likely to be vulnerable, to have been subject to personal and institutional abuse, to have been exploited by men. They are more likely to have difficulty in coping with daily living and to be mentally disordered in some way.

The fact that there is a relatively small number of women in prison means that there are fewer women's prisons. This brings an additional form of punishment in that women are likely to be held in prisons which are some considerable distance removed from their home and family. Broadly speaking, any women who is sentenced to prison in the northern half of England will initially be sent to Styal prison near Manchester. Any woman sentenced in the south will go initially to Holloway prison in London. That makes contact with family, and particularly with children, exceedingly difficult, adding to the punishment of imprisonment for the woman herself and also for her family.

The nature of family relationships in our society means that the imprisonment of a mother usually has more direct consequences for other members of a family than does imprisonment of a father. The reality in our society is that the mother, rather than the father, is at the centre of the daily dynamics of most families. She is the one who organizes the daily necessities and who makes the family operate. If the father is removed, there will be immediate problems, particularly if he is the breadwinner. But, after a period of reorganization, the mother takes on board the part which he previously played and ensures that the family continues to operate as a unit.

It is a different matter when the mother is imprisoned. The family will only be able to continue to operate with great difficulty unless a substitute mother figure is found. That may well be an older daughter, an aunt or a grandmother. In extreme cases it may be that the family unit cannot continue without the presence of the mother. The father either cannot cope on his own or is thought by those in authority to be unable to do so. The family will then be broken up and the children taken into care (see also Tobin and Taylor, this volume).

The mother who is in prison is aware of these realities and has to cope, not only with the fact that she has been deprived of her liberty, but also with the consequences of this for her family. One woman has described the pain of being visited in prison by her children as follows:

> 'After the visits I'd think it was so painful, seeing the children and then coming away from them again, telling yourself that it would be six or nine months before you'd see them again. It was so painful that I used to have to try and cut them out of my life for that time. I wrote to them every week, but it was as if I was writing to – I don't know how to explain it – I had to push them away from me, because I couldn't survive any other way.'
>
> (Padel and Stevenson, 1988)

The dilemma of how to arrange matters so that women prisoners might be kept in prisons closer to their homes is a difficult one to resolve. Given the numbers involved, it would not be economically viable to build small prisons in each large centre of population exclusively for women. One suggested alternative is that in each large local prison there should be an autonomous unit for women: in effect, a prison within a prison. A similar argument is sometimes put in respect of young offenders. Arguments for such an arrangement include the fact that women would have access to a better range of facilities for work, education, exercise and other activities. The contrary argument is that women would take second place to the greater number of men in using such facilities. A more powerful argument is that many women who are in prison have had damaging relationships with men, which might well have resulted directly in the offence which led to imprisonment. The one thing which they need while in prison is to feel secure and safe from male pressure.

Some commentators argue that the experience of so called co-ed prisons in the USA (see Gordon, this volume) indicates that with rigorous planning, supervision and management there can be some positive consequences from mixed gender prisons. One would have to be very cautious about reaching this conclusion, since such a mix goes against all international norms.

Partner's perspective

Prisoners are less likely to have an intimate partner than others in the general population, even allowing for the fact that prisoners as a group are younger. Nevertheless, about half of all men and only a slightly lower proportion of women will have been living with a spouse or partner immediately prior to imprisonment (Walmsley *et al.*, 1992).

It is a truism to say that the family of the prisoner suffers deprivation every bit as much as and sometimes more than the prisoner himself. One of the key elements of the family unit is taken away. This is likely to have a major effect on its financial situation. The family's disposable income will be significantly reduced. More significantly, there will undoubtedly be major emotional consequences. Morris (1965) reported that among a national sample of prisoners' wives nearly 30 per cent reported receiving medical treatment for a 'nervous condition' and 50 per cent in total had some sort of mental or physical illness. Many more complained of 'nerves' for which they were not attending a doctor.

The balance of the relationship between the prisoner and his partner will inevitably change. The person who is not in prison will become more dominant in the relationship than she may previously have been. The prisoner will be the passive partner, dependant on the other for most aspects of the continuing relationship, having no option but to trust his partner in respect of many features of their relationship.

If there are children in the family, their relationship with their father will be altered. They will see him irregularly, if at all, in the extremely artificial setting of the prison visiting room. His significance in their lives will become very distorted. There will also be important changes in the social standing of the family. In some cases the family may attempt to conceal the fact that the husband/father has been sentenced to imprisonment. They may present a facade that he is working away from home. The maintenance of this pretence will place additional strain on the family. It is probable in most cases that those with whom the family comes into contact will know of the imprisonment. Some people will break off contact. Others may be openly critical. This will be particularly difficult for the children, who may be subject to taunts and abuse from other young people. They, the most vulnerable of those affected, will be open to the greatest abuse. They are also likely to be the most exposed and to have the least support.

All of this can be summed up in what one might describe as guilt by association. The family are tainted as a result of the husband/father's imprisonment. They are seen as guilty at one step removed. They are directly affected by his conviction and sentence. The partner of a man who was in prison summed it up in this way:

'People give you a body swerve. No support at all. Treat you as though you were also guilty. Like a funeral without the body. People don't know how to respond to you, therefore avoid you.'

(Save the Children, 1992)

Maintaining the relationship

All of these factors put great strain on the relationship between the prisoner and his partner. Even if the marriage was strong at the start of the period of imprisonment it will now be subject to exceptional pressures, while at the same time attracting minimal support. The reality, however, is that many of these relationships will already have been subject to great pressure and uncertainty before the imprisonment of one of the partners. Morris (1965) reported that between 70 and 80 per cent of married prisoners, whether or not they were recidivists, reported serious marital conflict prior to imprisonment.

In many partnerships the husband had the dominant role in name and by tradition. This dominance, however superficial, was important to him. The wife is now able to take on publicly the role for which she was previously responsible in private. The reality was that she was always the one who ensured that there was a meal on the table, that bills were paid, that the children were ready to go to school, but she had the added complication that she had to pretend that she was acting on behalf of her husband. This charade has now been eliminated and the reality can be recognized. That makes life much more honest for her and perhaps for the children. It is likely to create major difficulties in her relationship with her husband.

The husband is now totally dependent on the wife for anything which is outwith the ambit of the prison. The implications of this are quite complex. On the one hand, he may well attempt to retain his sense of dominance. He will do so by demanding that his every little need is met. The pettinesses and coercions of life in prison are passed on. It may be that prisoners are allowed to wear their own training shoes, for example. This would be one of the few expressions of individuality which are allowed. In that case, it is important that each person should have the best pair available. It does not matter that their cost represents the equivalent of one week's income for the family. The wife is expected to provide them, and usually she will.

Another example arose in Brixton Prison a few years ago. According to prison rules, untried prisoners are entitled to a visit of 15 minutes each day. A new arrangement was introduced which allowed prisoners to convert these visits into two sessions of 45 minutes or one of 90 minutes each week. This allowed a visit of reasonable length and also reduced the pressure on the partner to trek to the prison each day. Most men welcomed this change but one or two insisted on their statutory entitlement. They took no account of the fact that their partner faced a 1 or 2 hour journey each way across London, often with a couple of small children in tow. They were entitled to a visit each day and they were determined to have it, whatever the implications for other people. In passing, it is worth noting that such times and distances involved in visiting are common in England and Wales. The 1991 National Prison Survey found that of those visited (60 per cent), nearly one third said that their most important visitor had to travel more than the average of about 60 miles; for nearly one quarter the travelling time was two and a half hours and for a further quarter in excess of one and a half hours (Walmsley et al., 1992).

Even when both partners cooperate fully in arrangements for visiting, there are likely to be stressful periods. For most convicted prisoners they will be limited to two or at best three visits each month. They will generally take place in a very impersonal visiting room, around one of 40 or 50 tables. Prison officers are stationed at various corners watching in case anyone attempts to pass drugs or any other item which is forbidden. The whole area reeks of stress and unhappiness.

In some prisons genuine attempts are made to help people relax. This may be through longer visits and a more relaxed setting in which the prisoner can be more at ease with his or her children. But whatever the setting, there is no disguising the fact that the visits take place in a prison and that they represent only a short break in the period of separation. Despite this stress, visits bring a moment of the real world into the prison. Their presence or absence is extremely important to the prisoner, as underlined by Vaclav Havel (1990) in a letter to his wife:

'Dear Olga
First of all, I'm grateful to you and Ivan for the visit. It was very successful, I'm still under its beneficial influence and I realise once more what an enormous significance even such a brief encounter has for someone here: suddenly, you realise that your "other", normal world is not just a dream or a memory, but that it physically exists.'

Richards *et al.* (1994) provide a range of similar views from English prisoners and an account of their contact and visiting conditions.

To a significant extent the relationship between a prisoner and his or her partner can best be described as one-dimensional. One hears talk nowadays about 'normalizing' the experience of imprisonment. Such talk is at best unwise, at worst dishonest. It is important to recognize that the world of the prison is abnormal. The best that can be done is to minimize the abnormality. There are several ways in which this can be done in respect of family relationships. One of the most important changes in recent years in the prisons of the United Kingdom has been the introduction of pay telephones for prisoners. Most prisoners now have the opportunity for a short daily conversation with their families. But even in this case things are more complex than they may appear at first sight.

I remember having a conversation in the mid 1980s with a man in a Scottish prison when pay telephones were first introduced. Most of the men in that prison came from within a fifty mile radius. They got into the habit of making a ten pence telephone call home each evening. This man pointed out how the change had significantly altered his conversations with his wife. Previously they had met twice a month for one hour in the prison visiting room. By unspoken agreement they had discussed only 'safe' subjects: Britain's place in the Common Market, which football team was likely to win the league, favourite television programmes. But when they got into the habit of speaking each day, even for a short period, the subjects of their conversation expanded. Matters which had previously been taboo were raised. His wife mentioned that their teenage daughter did not come home until the small hours of the morning; that their son was truanting from school. Suddenly, said the man, he felt that he was close to the core issues of his family again. But at the same time the reality of his separation was magnified. He could go only so far into the family life before being faced with the fact of his impotence to influence anything. He was not suggesting that the pay telephones should be taken away. He was simply pointing out that innovations brought a new set of problems.

If we are serious about encouraging men and women who are in prison to maintain and to develop family relationships we have to recognize that this will best be done in the home environment. This means that prisoners who are not a threat to the security of others should be allowed home from time to time to adopt the role of wife/husband, mother/father, daughter/son. Such an arrange-ment can be part of a strategy to reduce future offending but it sits uneasily with a philosophy which sees prison merely as exile from the community, in which separation from family is one of the direct purposes of imprisonment. For many other prisoners there is not an option of going home to be with their families. The families have to come to them in prison.

In many countries authorities go to great lengths to encourage prisoners to maintain contact with their families (see also Gordon, this volume). In some jurisdictions, such as Poland, prisoners are given leave to visit their families after having completed a relatively short period even of a long sentence. Almost all of them return to prison; absconding is very rare. Apart from anything else, peer group pressure will ensure this. The privilege is too important to be put at risk. The statistical evidence from across the world seems to be that between 97 and 94 per cent of prisoners return on time from home leave, regardless of the total numbers involved. The important thing is to make a proper assessment of the risk which a man or woman may pose if he or she does not return. Length of sentence or even length of time already served is not the only indicator of such risk. This sort of leave may be exceptionally important. The 1991 National Prison Survey covering England and Wales found that the longer a sentence, the less likely it was that a marriage or partnership would survive. Of those serving under 6 months only 12 per cent changed their marital or cohabiting status but after 5 years it was over 50 per cent (Walmsley *et al.*, 1992). Practical, and monitored if not yet fully tested, approaches to risk assessment and management are in increasing use (e.g. HM Inspectorate of Probation, 1995; Inner London Probation Service, 1995; Tidmarsh, 1997).

In many countries arrangements are made for families to spend extended periods visiting the imprisoned person. This is a sensitive matter and public reaction to it says a great deal about cultural attitudes. In northern Europe such visits are often seen solely in terms of conjugal visits. In prisons in several Scandinavian countries, for example, a suite of small rooms is set apart where prisoners and their partners can meet in private for an hour or two (see also Gordon, this volume). The whole atmosphere is almost clinical and must be particularly demeaning for the partner who is obliged to come to the prison in such circumstances.

In other countries the arrangement is for family visits, which will last typically for 48 or 72 hours. In most of the countries of the former Soviet Union, prisons or camps have a number of small flats. In Canada and some of the United States trailers or mobile homes sit in a corner of the prison surrounded by a ranch style fence. Three or four times a year the families of prisoners come to visit them. Very often it will be a spouse or partner accompanied by children. Sometimes it will be parents or a sibling. For that short period the family live together again. The prisoner will have to report to a guard several times a day but otherwise he lives with his family. Such an arrangement is a powerful incentive to good behaviour on the part of the prisoner. More importantly, it gives the family a better chance of maintaining some greater semblance of cohesion than would otherwise have been possible.

After release

The vast majority of men and women who are in prison will one day be released. For most of them the period of imprisonment is relatively short. The damage done to family relationships is likely to be much longer lasting. In certain respects relational problems will increase rather than be resolved once the prisoner is released, particularly if the released member of the family is male.

In his absence the family will have found a new style of living. It will have become more self-sufficient. In some instances, the wife for the first time will have been able to take control of the family finances. She will know how much income the family has. She will be able to control the budget without having to concern herself first with her husband's spending power. When the husband returns he is unlikely to be willing to allow this arrangement to continue. He will wish to resume his position as head of the family. There will be a new sense of disharmony which will place the relationship under new strain.

Just as comparatively little is done to help a family to come to terms with the pangs of separation when one of its members is taken into prison, so the family receives very little preparation for that member's return.

The financial dimension may be the most obvious example of the need for re-adjustment but there are likely to be others which reach into every aspect of the family. The children may be unwilling to accept support or guidance from a father who has caused them so much distress, who has been shown to have feet of clay. At the very least, relationships will not be as they were before.

Conclusions

This chapter began with an anecdote about Hamlet and the National Theatre in Brixton. Let me end with another story about a 2-week workshop led by the English National Opera in Brixton Prison in 1993, which culminated in produc-tions of the opera 'Street Scene'. The reader should not be left with the impression that imprisonment is all about collaborations with major artistic companies. The reality of prison life is quite different, but from time to time there is an opportunity to unleash creative talent in these highly challenging ways.

As with Hamlet, prisoners involved with this project were given the opportu-nity to invite members of their families to see one of the actual performances. I remember having a conversation with one of the actors. His 13-year-old son was coming to the performance. 'You know,' said the man, 'this is the first time my son will have seen me doing anything positive.' I watched the two of them during and after the performance. In each of them one could sense a pride and satisfaction and a certainty that their relationship meant a great deal. I never discovered what happened to the man when he left Brixton. It might have been too much to hope that the experience of appearing in 'Street Scene' ensured that he was never involved in crime again. There is no doubt that it would have changed his relationship with his son. On this occasion one trusts that it was for the better. If so, that was surely the exception.

Prisons have no inbuilt right of existence. They are there because we, as members of society, want them to be there. As a society we are very ambivalent about how we want them to operate. On the one hand, we see them as places of punishment where criminals are sent to pay the penalty imposed by the court for the crimes they have committed. In this context they should be places of exile from the community where austerity is the order of the day and where strict discipline is imposed. On the other hand, we expect them to be places of rehabilitation where, having learned the error of their ways, prisoners will prepare themselves for a return to the community as law-abiding citizens, able and willing to support their families and to contribute to the well-being of society. In this context it is important that prisoners should be able to maintain and, if possible, develop relationships with their families. This can only happen if there is regular and worthwhile contact between prisoners and their families. This fact is not in dispute:

> 'The Prison Service recognises the importance of helping prisoners to maintain their family ties. Good contact with the outside world helps them to cope better inside prison and prepares them for their return to freedom.'
>
> (HM Prison Service, 1995)

This is easily stated. As with so many aspects of prison life its implementation is extremely complex.

6

Assessment and management of relationships in adolescent facilities

Fiona L. Mason

'I would there were no age between ten and three and twenty, or that youth would sleep out the rest, for there is nothing in between but getting wenches with child, wronging the ancientry, stealing, fighting . . .'

(*The Winter's Tale*, Act III, Scene iii)

Introduction

The development phase that begins with puberty, and ends at a less easily defined point called adulthood, is referred to as adolescence. It is a time of great change, in terms of biological and cognitive functioning, and in emotional, social, sexual, and moral development. The age boundaries are influenced by legal, cultural, biological and societal factors; however, most authors would agree that adolescence includes the ages of 11 to 18 years in girls, and 13 to 19 years in boys.

The development of sexual awareness and the formation of intimate relationships are an integral part of adolescence. These are areas that often lead to conflict, both internally for the individual, and externally in the surrounding peer group and among the adults who care for them. Adolescents living in residential settings will inevitably form relationships with each other and although, on occasions, these may be entirely appropriate, they may also be abusive, damaging and highly inappropriate. Such relationships are often a source of enormous difficulty for all involved. Rutter *et al.* (1976), in their extensive study of 14–15 year olds in the Isle of Wight, concluded that adolescent turmoil, as represented by feelings of misery, self-depreciation and ideas of reference, was a fact, not a fiction.

Winnicott (1990) argued that during adolescence the individual does not at first know if s/he is homosexual, heterosexual, or narcissistic. He said that the only 'cure' for this lack of established identity was the passage of time. Whilst this may be true, institutions are often poor at coping with situations involving uncertainty, inner turmoil and confusion, and may react with unreasonable and, at times, harmful responses.

Those caring for such adolescents need to be able to distinguish the normal from the abnormal and have the skills, knowledge and resources necessary to assess, understand, and manage the issues that may arise. Any attempt to generate pertinent policies and procedures needs to give consideration to a wide range of factors, including patterns of relationship formation in the 'normal' adolescent, the nature and purpose of the residential facilities involved, and of all people involved – staff and residents and families, and outside contacts too.

This chapter attempts to inform, rather than dictate in such a complex area. Consideration is given to related literature and suggestions generated. It would be naive, however, to believe that there are any easy answers.

Development of sexuality and relationship formation in adolescence

In pre-adolescence and early adolescence, peer relationships, especially close friendships, tend to be restricted to others of the same sex. As maturation occurs, self-preoccupation and the importance of family relationships diminish, and sexuality develops. Generally, interest in the opposite sex increases (unless the individual is of homosexual orientation), and relationship formation becomes a possibility.

Most authors, whatever their background, would argue that such relationship formation is intricately linked with the emotional and sexual development of the adolescent. The influences on such development are yet to be fully understood, but they appear to be multifactorial, and are subject to the interaction of inborn characteristics and environment.

Steinberg (1987) reviewed the psychodynamic theories relating to emotional development in adolescence. He concluded that a common strand could be drawn from this wide body of literature, namely that the adolescent is someone who could contemplate achieving a number of goals that in earlier life were only fantasy. He illustrated this point by considering sexual drive, as discussed by Sigmund Freud. In childhood, it is argued, sexual drive is expressed through talk and play but, with the onset of adolescence, it becomes possible for this drive to be expressed more directly in the form of sexual activity. This drive, Steinberg argued, is not only directed towards genital sexuality, but also towards the establishment of relationships with peers of the opposite sex.

Theoretical models of adolescent development patterns are not, however, limited to this one body of literature. Bancroft's Eclectic Interactional Model (1989), for example, provides a useful, non-psychodynamic framework for considering sexual development. The model has two dimensions – strands and stages. The strands are described as:

1. Differentiation into male or female, and development of gender identity
2. Development of sexual responsiveness
3. Capacity for close dyadic relationships

and the stages as:

1. Prenatal
2. Childhood
3. Adolescence and early adulthood
4. Marriage or the establishment of a stable sexual relationship
5. Early and late parenthood
6. Mid-life.

The strands of sexuality coalesce as the individual proceeds through the life stages, under the influence of two further factors, namely sexual preference and the functions or consequences of sexual behaviour.

These latter two factors are those that often generate the most difficulty for the carers of adolescents, whether they are the individual's own parents, or the staff of a residential facility. Whether a particular behaviour is considered to be acceptable may be influenced by the gender of the individual under considera- tion, social norms, the law, institutional policies, and the attitudes of individual carers. Attitudes towards sexual behaviour and preference vary enormously and issues such as homosexual behaviour, overt sexual activity and promiscuity often lead to heated debate and discussion.

Residential facilities for adolescents

Facilities for the accommodation of the adolescent outside the family home are provided by a number of different organizations including the National Health Service, local authorities and the independent sector. The welfare of these adolescents is the responsibility of the local authority and to a lesser extent other organizations. The Children Act 1989 contains a formulation of the welfare duty which governs decisions of local authorities in England and Wales in relation to an adolescent in their care. The over-riding purpose of the Act is to promote and safeguard the welfare of those under 18 years, although the responsibility of local authorities for those leaving care extends to the age of 21. In Britain, and many other countries, adolescents may also be sent to prison, but in England and Wales they also fall under the Children Act, and should be able to expect standards of care accordingly. Although these facilities vary enormously, it is important to emphasize that there is one important and relevant factor that links them all. For many of the residents these facilities become their home, and as such should be aiming to provide stability, permanence and care.

The organizations that run such facilities have to consider issues such as staffing, policies, rules, and statutory obligations. Situations may arise, there- fore, where the aims of the facility appear to conflict with those of the organization running that facility. Such conflicts can potentially mirror those the adolescent left behind, and it is vital that such conflicts are recognized and discussed so that potential divisions are avoided, and the individual continues to receive consistent, nurturing care.

Adolescents who require residential care, particularly those within secure settings, present many challenges to the organization responsible for them. Most individuals placed within such settings will experience loss as well as gain when they move into the facility, and these factors will undoubtedly influence their behaviour. In addition, the adolescent living within a residential facility con- tinues to develop and, in common with all adolescents, will experience a growth in sexuality and a desire for relationship formation. Despite the importance of such issues to the adolescent, it is notable how little this topic is considered and discussed in many residential care facilities (Parkin, 1989), and how much anxiety is generated in staff when the issues are discussed (Rose, 1990). It is also notable that the Children Act 1989, although specifically considering issues of race, culture and linguistic background, gives little attention to sexuality apart from reference to consent to marriage in those aged 16 or 17.

Although often ignored within individual facilities, debate about sexuality in institutions has occurred, particularly in the wider context of discussions about the advantages and disadvantages of single sex versus mixed sex units. Gabbidon (in Bailey and Higginbotham, 1994), summarized the discussions held on this topic at a conference in 1992. Participants included young women held in secure units across the country. Most expressed concerns in relation to privacy and subsequent vulnerability in mixed units, and strong views were also expressed in relation to placing the abused (women) with abusers (men).

At the same conference, Morton, from the Social Services Inspectorate, also considered issues relating to single *versus* mixed sex units. He concluded that although mixed sex units were 'normal', in that they recreated society and allowed for interaction between different sex residents, single sex units were more likely to create an atmosphere of trust and safety, particularly for female residents. He noted that many adolescent females within residential care settings have suffered physical, emotional, and/or sexual abuse before entry, and mixed sex units (particularly if the unit admits male abusers) risk replicating the environment from which the young women have been removed and from which they require sanctuary.

Adolescents in residential facilities

Packman (1986) divided children in care into the 'victims', the 'villains' and the 'volunteered'. Add to these groups the 'ill', and this constitutes a broad description of the residents of adolescent facilities. Whilst it is difficult to generalize across groups, all have, for one reason or another, been removed from their families, with the subsequent inevitable disruption in relationships. For many, family relationships will have already been severely disturbed prior to leaving home, and this may well be the reason for the adolescent's placement in a residential facility. Bowlby (1979) considered the value of relationships for the individual, writing of the importance of a secure base 'from which he can explore both himself and his relations with all those with whom he has made, or might make an affectional bond'. Given the previous absence of a 'secure base' for most of those placed within residential facilities, it is hardly surprising that their ability to engage in future successful relationships may be disrupted, whatever the immediate precipitant of their placement. Other factors that influence relationship formation there include: psychiatric illness; limited, and often single sex, peer group; poor social skills; physical, emotional and/or sexual abuse and its common accompaniment – low self esteem – however brash the superficial presentation.

These factors were investigated in a study by Bullock *et al.* (1994), who examined the characteristics of those in English Youth Treatment Centres (YTCs), and other specialized services for difficult and disturbed young people. YTCs were secure, special units incorporating education, but run under the auspices of an executive unit of the Department of Health. They took girls as well as boys, but boys were in the majority by about 4 : 1. In their reports, the authors highlighted that the family relationships of YTC entrants were, on the whole, severely disrupted. Although almost all (92 per cent) of the population they studied had a notional parental home on reception to the YTC, less than two-thirds (60 per cent) had been able to live there. Strained and abnormal patterns in parent/child relationships were a feature in two-thirds of the cases examined.

In addition, these authors found that the young people in YTCs had many educational and social deficits which handicapped their wider social relationships. Sixty-two per cent had been assessed as emotionally immature and 50 per cent had a poor self-image. Many had difficulty relating to peers and adults. On leaving the YTC, 48 per cent of leavers were considered by their after-care agencies still to have a poor capacity to make personal relationships. In addition, these authors reported that 49 per cent of males and 80 per cent of females studied had reported the recent stress factor of abuse or neglect at home immediately prior to entry to the YTC. Since the publication of this study one YTC has closed, and the remaining facility, Glenthorne, is now known as The Youth Treatment Centre Service.

It is extremely difficult to get an accurate estimate of the population rates of child abuse in any country. Much is concealed. In the UK there is a system of child protection registers. Where abuse has been suspected, established or is thought to be a high risk, a child protection conference may be called to consider formulation of an inter-agency plan to protect that child and placement of the child's name on the register. Figures from this system cannot provide an accurate estimate of the prevalence of various kinds of child abuse, but they provide a useful indicator and one that is certainly better than using criminal statistics. Annual figures fluctuate, but within a fairly narrow range for England, after a high of 45 300 in 1991, and a low of 32 500 in 1993, figures have been increasing again (Department of Health, 1995). With some overlap between certain categories, because some children experience multiple forms of abuse, in the 12 months up to 31st March 1995, for every 10 000 members of the population under the age of 18, ten were recognized as sufficiently neglected to be on a protection register, and 12 subject to physical abuse, 8 to sexual abuse and 4 to emotional abuse with similar needs.

If estimates of prevalence of abuse are difficult, then a full understanding of the impact of it is even more so. Most such studies suggest that a link between early abuse and later problems depends on retrospective recognition of the abuse, but potentially more difficult to unravel are the multiplicity and complexity of adverse experiences for many if not most children who come to the attention of social services, child protection registers or into secure accommodation. In their prospective study of 672 children who had suffered verified abuse and 518 controls matched for factors including parental problems and poverty, Widom and White (1997) found that the impact of abuse per se appears to differ between male and female children growing up. Violent crime, for example, was more likely to be associated with childhood abuse among the women.

Mrazek and Mrazek (1981) reviewed the short- and long-term effects of such abuse on the victims and found problems and preoccupations with sexual matters frequently reported as an outcome for young people. Writing about the therapeutic community of Peper Harow, Rose (1990) noted that many of the youngsters within that community had been abused in ways that were thought to have affected their ability to develop a clear sense of sexual identity, and that the resultant behaviour frequently disrupted the community. These issues are given further consideration by Itzen (in Bailey and Higgenbotham, 1994) who noted the heightened sensitivity of abused adolescents to sexual stimuli, and their inappropriate sexual signalling.

Assessment

As with other areas in the assessment of adolescents, the assessment of relationships cannot simply be a matter of labelling, given the complex interaction of factors involved. Assessment therefore requires a far wider appraisal of who is involved, who is concerned about what, and why. It is also vital that the purpose of assessment is clearly understood. The gathering of information to see if a crime has been committed should not be confused with accurate assessment of sexuality and relationship formation. Information should be gathered from all those involved with the individual, as well as the individual. Observation of behaviour must be detailed, and self-assessment tools may also be of use.

In most Western cultures adolescent relationships will, almost inevitably, involve some level of sexual contact. Such sexual behaviour can arouse very powerful emotions, and will quite possibly require institutions to examine complex issues such as moral beliefs, taboos, religious, cultural and legal factors. It is important, both for the adolescent and the institution, that any assessment carried out is not influenced by individual or institutional bias and that, given the extremes of personal reaction, legal response and variations of perception that occur in relation to this topic, such assessment is accurate, careful and considered (Steinberg, 1987).

All institutions, therefore, must first recognize that the vast majority of adolescents will be sexually active (Zelnik and Katner, 1980) and that such activity does not, in itself, constitute abnormal behaviour. Institutions must, however, guard against complacency, and recognize problems when they arise. Whilst most observers would agree that substantial and significant changes have occurred in the sexual practices of the young during the last 20 years, and that some problems in relationship formation are common in normal adolescents, promiscuity, chaotic relationship formation and abnormal sexual practices are not a part of normal adolescent development and therefore should not be ignored. McConaghy (1993) provided a useful and comprehensive review of adolescent sexuality, considering both normal and deviant behaviour. For those presenting aggressive sexual behaviour, there may well be an underlying history of sexual victimization (Shaw et al., 1993).

Difficulties in assessment arise, however, as behaviour which is acceptable to one is considered unacceptable to another. Social norms and attitudes also change with time, as illustrated for England and Wales by the recent lowering of the age of consent for male homosexual activity (Criminal Justice and Public Order Act 1994), and the new legal acceptance that boys under the age of 14 are capable of sexual intercourse (Sexual Offences Act 1993). The issues relating to the 'new sexual morality' in Western culture is well reviewed in Coleman and Hendry (1990), who examined how changing attitudes have influenced sexual behaviour, and what implications these changes have for adolescents and those caring for them. If illegal activity is suspected, legal issues can further complicate assessment, given that the phase of adolescence does not conveniently coincide with the age bands applicable in law.

Barlow (1977) outlined three components of sexual behaviour, namely arousal, social skills and gender role. This model provides a useful framework for inclusion in any assessment of sexual functioning and relationship formation, and incorporates many of the factors delineated in Bancroft's model outlined earlier.

Altschul (1978), in considering child and adolescent disturbance in the context of social relationships, developed a systems approach to the assessment of the pattern of relationships within which the individual operates. Included in the systems of which the individual is a part were the family, peer group, biological and psychological personal system, and work group. Such an approach has the advantage of broadening focus, and thus guarding against narrow assessment of isolated elements of any problem. The special difficulty for facilities created for adolescents, secure or otherwise, and for those who use them is that these environmental issues become confrontative and compressed within the institution. It is further likely that an assessment in these circumstances must allow for this and incorporate other factors specific to the institution, and the other residents within it. Any assessment developed also needs to be within the capability of the staff working within the organization.

Management

It would be both impractical and naive to attempt to produce a rule book on this topic; however, absence of guidance has also been experienced as problematic. Given the many factors influencing sexual development and behaviour, as already emphasized, good management is complex, must be flexible, and involves supporting and promoting normal, healthy expression as well as reduction and limitation of problems (Steinberg, 1987). Rose (1990) argued that management of burgeoning sexuality is important both from the point of view of behaviour control and treatment.

The age at which sexual intercourse is considered proper is decided by society and laid down in legislation. At present in England the age of consent for heterosexual intercourse is 16 and that for male homosexual intercourse 18. The law does not, however, determine at what age other sexual activity is permissible when both parties consent. Avoidance of these difficult issues does not mean that they go away. The importance of defining clear boundaries between what is acceptable and what is unacceptable behaviour (limit setting) is emphasized in a wide range of texts concerning children and adolescents. The boundaries must be explicit, and it should be the responsibility of any institution or agency caring for adolescents to ensure this, and to provide sufficient resources to ensure that the limits are respected.

The aim of limit setting is as much to teach the individual acceptable modes of behaviour, and thus assist their development, as to ensure safety. For many of those in residential facilities, their previous experience of such limit setting will have been minimal. Certain characteristics of limit setting have been shown to be more effective than others in subsequent alteration of behaviour achieved. Thus staff in any organization that aims to achieve changes in the resident adolescents must give careful consideration to achieving these factors, which are consistency, frequency of response, praise for positive behaviour, modelling, reasonableness and reasoning (Wilkinson, 1983).

Difficulties relating to management and staff responses to issues of sexuality in residential care were highlighted in the research undertaken by Parkin and Green (1994). Steinberg (1987) also recognized that certain cases, particularly within residential settings, could arouse strong and conflicting feelings, and suggested that in such cases it could be helpful for staff to have support and supervision meetings chaired by a person otherwise independent of the organization.

For a behaviour to be managed, it must first be observed, and yet those who will be managing, or indeed those with experience of residence, are rarely consulted on building design. Morton (in Bailey and Higgenbotham, 1994) reported that The Social Services Inspectorate had commissioned a *design guide*, which not only gave technical specifications but also made reference to issues of good practice. Consideration was given, for example, to the need for en-suite bathrooms, quiet areas, and an appropriate range of educational and leisure areas. Morton suggested that it is essential that the design elements to units should be flexible in order that the units can respond accordingly to the needs of the individual, if necessary dividing the unit up into separate wings where smaller groups could live. Whilst this may be advantageous to the residents, it is important to remember that issues relating to safety and observation should also be incorporated into designs, so that, for example, sight lines can always be maintained. Initiatives such as these are to be encouraged in that they allow local authorities to learn from the experiences of others when considering new designs for adolescent resident facilities.

In recognition that adolescents will have sexual feelings and drive, all staff in any facility caring for them should receive appropriate training and education. For some it may be sufficient to develop observational and environmental management skills. Certain staff, it could be argued, should receive a level of training that enables them to initiate group discussion with residents and provide education, information and counselling as required. This would ensure that sexuality was no longer a hidden issue, which would, in turn, promote open, appropriate management. Were staff to undertake such a role, special consideration may be needed in their selection (see also Dale *et al.*, this volume) and appropriate supervision should be provided.

Morton, (in Bailey and Higgenbotham, 1994) also expressed the view that it is important to consider the gender mix of staff within units, and stressed the importance of providing residents with 'safe male appropriate role models'.

Conclusions

Numerous theoretical models relating to child and adolescent development exist. Different institutions may adopt different individual models, or incorporate a number of models into their philosophy of care. Full knowledge and understanding of normal sexual development is an important element. Consistent application of the model or models chosen is vital if they are to be of benefit to the individuals who live in the institution. Any approach must be applied to the individual, not the individual to the approach.

Institutions must balance the rights of individuals to engage in relationships and certain forms of sexual behaviour with the rights of others, and the need to protect the vulnerable from physical and/or psychological damage. They cannot ignore the emerging sexuality of the young people in their care, but equally have an absolute duty to protect them from further harm. Rights *versus* protection and duty of care issues, as discussed by Commons *et al.* (1992), provide one of the most complex ethical debates, and need to be considered in detail with each case that arises. It may be, in the most complex of cases, that legal authority for decisions will need to be sought, and/or that residents will 'test' their legality.

Sexuality

Sophie Davison

A discussion of couples in care and custody is incomplete without consideration of the issues surrounding sexuality, as the relationships under examination in this book involve sexual attraction, whether or not the relationship is actually consummated. There are both similarities and differences between psychiatric hospitals and prisons in this regard, which will be explored separately, but for both it is often, in practice, the sexual aspects of a relationship which give rise to the most anxiety amongst staff dealing with people who pair off in institutions.

Sexuality and psychiatric patients

Attitudes to sexual behaviour by patients

In the nineteenth century sex was considered both a cause and a symptom of mental disorder and was therefore banned in institutions (Andrau, 1969; Bourgeois, 1975). Some authors at that time suggested that psychiatric patients should not be allowed to reproduce so they could not pass on their defective genes (Andrau, 1969). Total separation of the sexes within institutions meant that many of the issues surrounding heterosexuality could easily be ignored.

A number of factors have led to a gradual change in attitude towards the sexuality of psychiatric patients and a need for a reappraisal of the topic. The attitude of society to sexuality in general has become more liberal. There has been a growing awareness of the importance of sexuality as a part of an individual's overall psychosocial adjustment. Much of the thinking underpinning social psychiatry has been the concept of normalization. Emphasis is placed on rehabilitating patients in hospital for their full reintegration into all their social roles in the community, including their roles in sexual relationships (Eiguer *et al.*, 1974; Kretz, 1969).

As psychiatric hospitals generally unlocked their facilities through the 1950s, followed by the creation of mixed sex general psychiatric wards in the 1960s and 1970s, leading to men and women living in close proximity, the issue of heterosexuality ought to have been a factor in planning the changes in service, but often it was not. Perhaps partly as a result, there has been something of a backlash against men and women sharing residential accommodation.

In recent years there has also been an increasing emphasis on psychiatric patients' rights, including the right to privacy, the right to make choices about their own lives and the right to have the fewest restrictions placed on their freedom as is clinically necessary to protect themselves or others. Patients are no longer considered to have relinquished all their rights when detained in hospital against their will. Nor are they automatically considered incompetent to make all choices related to running their lives.

Nevertheless, those who are competent need information in order to be able to make informed choices and those who may not be able to look after themselves, for whatever reason, need protection from unwanted sexual advances, unwanted pregnancy, sexually transmitted disease and from deterioration in mental state as a result of inappropriate sexual activity (Binder, 1985; Greenberg, 1993).

Notwithstanding generally more liberal attitudes to sexuality, society as a whole still has difficulty in accepting the sexuality of the mentally ill (Akhtar *et al.*, 1977; Eiguer *et al.*, 1974). The staff of hospitals and other institutions form a microcosm of society generally.

In secure psychiatric hospitals there are particular concerns about safety, as most patients have been admitted because they are considered a danger to others, and a number have committed sexual offences. In addition, many patients have themselves been the victims of sexual abuse in the past. Patients are deprived of their liberty for much longer than most general psychiatric patients, separated from any pre-existing sexual partner, with few, if any, opportunities for intimacy. They are forced to live in close proximity with others they have not chosen for long periods of time. In addition, society takes an even harsher view of such patients' sexuality as prejudices and fears about both mental illness and crime come to the fore. Most medium secure units in England and Wales currently have mixed sex residential accommodation, but with women very much outnumbered. Though two of the three special hospitals in England each have a mixed sex ward, the majority of living accommodation is single sex, with patients having the opportunity to mix only at occupational therapy, education and social activities.

Patients' attitudes and interest in sexuality

Though it is no longer believed that mental illness is caused by sexual activity *per se*, it is not uncommon for psychiatric patients to have a history of early abusive sex and relationships. Even when there is no such history, there is no doubt that many psychiatric patients do have psychosexual difficulties which may need assessment and treatment, or help as part of rehabilitation. These may be highlighted, or even present for the first time, if a patient becomes involved in a new relationship during treatment.

Some psychiatric illnesses may present with symptoms interfering with sexual functioning. A decrease in sexual interest and enjoyment is a common symptom of major depression (Howell, 1987). Mania may lead to indiscriminate or increased sexual activity. People with schizophrenia may present with a range of delusions, hallucinations and abnormal experiences on a sexual theme (reviewed in Akhtar *et al.*, 1980).

Many mental disorders can have a more general effect on sexual functioning. Observations on those hospitalized with chronic schizophrenia indicate an apparent lack of interest in sexual matters in many patients with negative symptoms, with the lack of interest increasing as the illness becomes more chronic. A study by Luckianowicz (1963) showed, however, that in the early stages of a schizophrenic illness, male patients tended to show an increase in their sexual desire and frequency of gratification, particularly by masturbation. He further found that among women with schizophrenia, the psychosis was more likely to break down moral and social inhibitions leading to unrestrained sexual behaviour.

Rozensky and Berman (1984) surveyed chronic psychiatric day-patients and found that over half the subjects did not think that sexuality was a positive part of human life. The group as a whole was not very sexually active and had little knowledge of birth control. Nearly 12 per cent reported having been raped at some time in the past and a further 9.8 per cent had received money for sex. Bourgeois (1974) quotes a French study which found that only half of psychiatric patients surveyed by questionnaire had any sexual life and that this was generally unsatisfactory.

Few studies have specifically examined the sexual orientation of psychiatric patients. Zubenko et al. (1987) found that patients with borderline personality disorder had a much higher rate of homosexuality and of paraphilias than a depressed control group or than the general population. This was particularly marked in male patients.

Some chronically mentally ill patients may have deficits in problem-solving, planning and judgement that might increase their vulnerability to casual, coercive, risky or exploitative sexual relationships (Kelly et al., 1992). An early study found a high rate of coitus unprotected by contraception and unwanted pregnancy among women being admitted to an inpatient unit (Abernethy, 1974). More recently, a number of American studies have shown high rates of high risk sexual behaviours among psychiatric patients (e.g. Kelly et al., 1992), in particular of multiple sexual contacts and infrequent use of condoms. These researchers also found that many chronically ill schizophrenic patients from the inner city reported trading sex for money, for a place to stay or for drugs, coercion to engage in unwanted sex, as well as a history of casual sexual encounters. One fifth had met their sexual partners on the streets, in parks or in other public places. One third had been treated for sexually transmitted disease and many showed substantial deficits in their understanding of HIV risk or risk reduction measures.

In addition to psychosexual difficulties related to mental disorders, most of the medications used in psychiatry have adverse sexual side effects. Few affect fertility per se, apart from some conventional neuroleptics. The principal effects include decrease in sexual desire, failures of erection, lubrication, ejaculation or orgasm (for general reviews see Gitlin (1994) and Parkinson and Bateman (1994); for a more specific review of the effects of neuroleptics see Collins and Kellner (1986)). Such problems may have serious implications for compliance with treatment, especially if the patient concerned becomes involved in a relationship. In some cases, insofar as medication reduces libido, patients may welcome a relief from intrusive, distressing sexual thoughts, but this is relatively unusual.

Studies of sexual activities of psychiatric inpatients

Psychiatric patients may have partners outside hospital and for acute services this may not be much of a problem as the services are generally quite close to home, and any admission short. Particular care may have to be taken if the partner is caught up in any delusional system, or a focus of morbid jealousy, but in general it is perhaps not surprising that there has been little research in this area. For some patients, however, the admission may not be brief and yet they may have partners from whom, therefore, they may be separated for long periods with no facilities for private visits. On surveying the literature, the absence of research or commentary on this is notable. The subject of the day-to-day sexual activity of psychiatric inpatients has received very little more attention, even though it is a very real aspect of ward life and is an area about which many professionals feel uncertain and uncomfortable. Although some authors have claimed that sexual activity does not occur within psychiatric hospitals (Kretz, 1969; Ortega, 1972), there is clear evidence that sexual activity does occur, even where hospital policies specifically ban it.

Several studies have depended on staff report. Akhtar et al. (1977) identified 34 patients out of 1086 on a general psychiatric unit over a 2-year period who had displayed overt sexual activity of some kind. Young, single, personality disordered patients were most likely to have engaged in sexual activity, the majority of which was heterosexual and non-genital. Two thirds of the activity was 'discovered' by nurses in the evenings in patients' rooms. Modestin (1981) found that 16 of a total of 1060 patients on four mixed wards were involved in sexual activity of some kind.

Keitner et al. (1986) studied an acute psychiatric hospital. Over a 2-year period staff reported 64 relationships involving 102 patients, amounting to 10.7 per cent of patients. Once again it was found that patients involved in relationships were more likely to be young, single and have a diagnosis of personality disorder, eating disorder, or bipolar disorder. Most relationships noted were heterosexual but same-sex relationships did occur and were more common between women than between men. Thirty-three per cent of relationships were judged to be emotional only, 9 per cent physical only and 58 per cent both. Physical involvement in this study included anything from flirting to sexual intercourse. Twenty-six patients had multiple relationships. These were mainly women with eating disorders.

An English study by Morgan and Rogers in 1971 involved a retrospective survey of a psychiatric facility where male and female patients were accommodated separately but mixed for social and work activities. Staff reported that 18 per cent of patients had associated with the opposite sex, ranging from casual flirtation to marriage. Of the 51 couples formed, 30 had broken up by the time of discharge. Four couples married after discharge, one as a result of pregnancy. One association ended with the man being admitted to Broadmoor special hospital after killing the woman with whom he had associated. No specific comment was made in this study about sexual activity.

Schneider et al. (1964) interviewed psychotic inpatients in a French hospital (42 women and 42 men, with an average length of stay of 5–6 years) and found that 8 men and 7 women had been involved in heterosexual activity, ranging from kissing and cuddling to sexual intercourse, during their admission. Two women and four men had been involved in homosexual activity during admission. Four more men had been approached for homosexual intercourse during admission but had refused.

It is unclear to what extent one can generalize from the actual numbers, as units vary and staff may underestimate the level of sexual activity if patients conceal it from them. Most of the units studied have been short stay general psychiatric units. The situation may differ on long stay units (Keitner *et al.*, 1986) as is the case in prisons (see below). On the one hand patients spend longer together with fewer opportunities to visit partners outside, but on the other hand they are generally much more closely supervised, with fewer opportunities to engage in sexual activities.

Most studies have concentrated on heterosexual activity in mixed settings. There is a notable lack of information about homosexual activity on single sex wards. So called 'situational homosexuality' has been written about in relation to prisons (see below) but has been largely ignored in the psychiatric literature. Nevertheless, on talking informally to staff on single sex wards one becomes aware that, whatever the hospital's policy, homosexual activity does occur. Hickling (1993) wrote that male homosexual activity is 'fairly frequent' on single sex wards in a long stay Jamaican psychiatric hospital, though it occurs in a much more clandestine manner than heterosexual activity because of the cultural taboos.

Risk of pregnancy

One of the concerns about sexual activity in psychiatric hospitals is that of unwanted pregnancy. Hickling (1993) states that pregnancy among long stay patients in a Jamaican mental hospital is 'frequent'. Despite an official policy forbidding sex, patients create opportunities to meet in the extensive grounds and sometimes the local community intrudes. This report reminded one of the editors (P.J.T.) of a practice which had been very common in the 1970s in at least one large South of England mental hospital too, often with goods (in lieu of money) exchanged for sexual favours. Bourgeois' paper (1975) confirms this is not purely an English problem. Baillard-Lapresle (1975) reported on eight illegitimate pregnancies in a mental hospital in Western France. In no case had contraception been used. Despite concerns about the high rate of unprotected sex reported in community samples, Wignall and Meredith (1968) found, in a survey of state institutions in the USA, that the rate of illegitimate pregnancies was only one fifth that of the general population. They comment that despite this low rate, a single pregnancy in a hospital can threaten a whole programme because of adverse publicity. The experience of one of the English special hospitals is that a story of pregnancy does not even have to be true to warrant nearly full occupancy of the front page in a tabloid newspaper.

Despite fears about the transmission of sexually transmitted disease there are no exact figures as to the prevalence of these disorders in psychiatric hospitals. Anecdotally they do occur, but even where they are easy to treat, they can compromise the therapeutic atmosphere by reinforcing the rigidity of staff defences (Bourgeois, 1975). With the advent of HIV, the possibility of sexually transmitted disease has again become particularly anxiety provoking.

Sexual relationships: detrimental or beneficial?

There is a notable lack of objective evidence as to the effect of sexual activity and relationships on psychiatric patients (Pinderhughes, 1972). In addition, it is almost impossible, if a relationship has been established, to separate out the sexual element and its effect, though it is often the sexual activity which causes the most concern among staff. Some authors have written about the psychological and dynamic factors involved in sexual relationships between inpatients, and it is interesting to speculate on the extent to which they are merely reporting counter transference. There are claims that such relationships represent acting out staff expectations, proving masculine identity, meeting dependency needs, expressing anger through sexual activity, anger at staff, compensating for feelings of loneliness or boredom, response to delusions or hallucinations and acting out transference feelings about therapists (Binder, 1985; Easson and Kan, 1967; Harticollis, 1964).

Easson and Kan (1967) and Harticollis (1964) argue that the consequences of patient sexual relationships are nearly always destructive and interfere with treatment, though Harticollis does acknowledge that it is possible that a relationship might be turned into a therapeutic asset. Modestin (1981) observed three types of sexual relationships in his study: one approaching normality, one where the relationship developed at the insistence of one partner and was terminated as soon as that partner recovered, and a third purely physical, non-emotional relationship. Are we to believe that this is so very different from healthy people?

There is an argument that a good sexual relationship can have very beneficial effects such as enhancing well-being and self-esteem (Payne, 1993). Keitner and Grof (1981) point out that hospital romances may in fact have a reconstitutive effect on patients who often feel better as a result, and that such relationships often involve positive personality aspects. It has also been suggested that, in some circumstances, relationships being played out in the safe therapeutic environment of the ward, under the supervision of skilled therapists, could be used as an opportunity to understand a patient's difficulties and work on them in a constructive way (Modestin, 1981).

If staff are to rehabilitate patients with psychosexual difficulties, it is a potentially paradoxical situation whereby they may be encouraging the patient to work towards a fulfilling sexual life whilst banning all activity until after discharge. It is not clear what effect this may have on rehabilitation. Mentally disordered sex offenders are a particularly complicated group. It is imperative to try and rehabilitate them, whilst not allowing them to harm others in hospital any more than in the wider community. What should be done if a paedophile starts a sexual relationship with an adult male for example? Is this a desirable change in behaviour to be encouraged or undesirable ward behaviour to be discouraged? There are no easy answers to these questions but they must be considered.

Non-consensual sexual activity

There has been a growing concern about sexual assaults on psychiatric wards (Averbruch, 1992; Tonks, 1992). Once again research has concentrated almost exclusively on heterosexual harassment and assault on mixed wards, though it is known that homosexual assaults do occur on single sex wards. Nibert *et al.* (1989), in a survey of 28 men and 39 women on four psychiatric wards, found that 38 per cent of them reported having been sexually assaulted in a psychiatric institution. The sampling was, however, not random, with subjects self-selecting. In an anonymous letter to the BMJ (Anonymous, 1988) a psychiatrist reported that out of 12 female psychiatric patients she interviewed in outpatients, five reported unsolicited sexual advances whilst in hospital. Keitner *et al.* (1986), in the study mentioned previously, found that 25 per cent of relationships observed by staff were not reciprocal. In these non-reciprocal cases women were more likely to be the recipients, especially sad, withdrawn patients with personality disorder or schizophrenia. Batcup (1994) reported that, in a mixed psychiatric hospital in South London, there were 1290 untoward incidents of all kinds reported in   six months. Sixteen of these incidents were classified as sexual assaults and 146 were assaults on women by men, the nature of which is not specified.

It is essential to differentiate consensual sexual activity from coercive sexual activity in order to protect patients, although this can be very difficult in practice. It may be fairly clear if an acutely psychotic patient is temporarily not competent to consent to sexual intercourse and is behaving irrationally or out of character. In the absence of acute disturbance, or during recovery assessment, it can be more difficult (Cournos *et al.*, 1980) and so also the balance between autonomy and protection. Patients with long histories of sexual abuse and abusive relationships may enter into further abusive and apparently destructive relationships; further, they may claim that this is their choice and they are consenting.

Staff–patient sexual relationships

Just as patients do not abandon all sexual feelings at the front door of a hospital, nor do staff. Although all codes of medical practice explicitly forbid a doctor to have sex with a patient, it is well documented that doctors do enter sexual relationships with patients on occasions (Fahy and Fisher, 1992). In a survey of 1442 North American psychiatrists, 7 per cent of male and 3 per cent of female respondents acknowledged having had sexual contact with their own patients (Gartrell *et al.*, 1986). Doctors are not alone in this; any professional may have difficulties. Nursing staff in particular spend a great deal of time in very close contact with inpatients, like social workers visiting patients at home, making boundaries particularly difficult to maintain.

Fahy and Fisher (1992) suggest that professionals may enter into sexual relationships with patients deliberately to exploit their position of relative power, as an early symptom of mental illness, or because of their own unacknowledged psychological or psychosexual vulnerabilities. They also suggest that patients with profound personality disturbances who have diffi- culty defining or accepting psychological and social boundaries may be at most risk of entering into sexual contact with a professional caregiver. Victims of sexual abuse may attempt to repeat, often unconsciously, the sexualization of relationships with therapists and caregivers, who must be prepared to manage this without inappropriate responses or overtures (Fahy and Fisher, 1992). It is arguable that secure psychiatric settings have a particularly large number of patients with difficulty maintaining boundaries and who have been abused.

The overwhelming evidence is that sexual contact between patient and professional is harmful to the patient (Fahy and Fisher, 1992). They suggest that the cornerstone to prevention of such sexual contact is education and training. Mental health staff should be able to talk to their peers and supervisors about these issues without fear of ridicule (see also Dale *et al.*, this volume).

Staff attitudes to patient sexual relationships

Given the paucity of information about sexual activity on the part of psychiatric patients, it is hardly surprising that staff attitudes to, and decisions about it are varied and greatly affected by their own prejudices about sexuality (Binder, 1985; Commons *et al.*, 1992). This, in turn, may inhibit the research needed. Staff experience a range of emotions including anger, disbelief, embarrassment, restrictiveness, indifference, denial and pessimism (Akhtar *et al.*, 1977; Eiguer *et al.*, 1974; Keitner and Grof, 1981). A French study of the attitudes of staff from various disciplines towards the formation of couples in a mixed psychiatric institution found that opinions were divided (Eiguer *et al.*, 1974). Staff who were tolerant to it felt that it was normalizing and reduced social isolation. Those who were opposed to the formation of couples were concerned that relationships between patients would worsen their mental state, might pass on their mental illness by heredity and might lead to unwanted pregnancies. Many who were tolerant of heterosexual couple formation were opposed to homosexual couple formation. The majority of staff surveyed (89 per cent) felt that couple formation had an effect on treatment: 34 per cent considered the effect positive and 33 per cent negative. Pinderhughes (1972), in a survey, found that 66 per cent of responding psychiatrists felt that sexual activity might retard recovery in most categories of mental illness. In the study of Keitner *et al.* (1986), staff felt that about half the relationships they observed were destructive, in particular those where a patient became involved in multiple relationships. Studies in Finland (Vartiainen, 1993) and Egypt (Loza and Zaki, 1993) have found a range of staff attitudes to sexual relationships. Most were tolerant, even where the law or hospital policies banned it. Keitner and Grof (1981) found that staff on long stay units in Canada were less likely to separate patients involved in sexual relationships and more likely to use the situation therapeutically than those on short stay units.

Commons *et al.* (1992) found that staff decisions about institutionalized patients' sexual activity were not influenced by professional norms of competence of a patient or engagement in sexual activity or degree of consent. They were instead influenced by conventional norms of the nature of the sexual activity, location of the sexual activity, sex of initiating patient, and sex of the other patient. The main implication is that mental health professionals should re-examine their own prejudices (e.g. homophobia) to clarify their decisions about institutional policies.

It is notable that few psychiatric hospitals in Britain have formalized policies regarding sexuality, though many have unwritten rules banning all sexual activity. Where policies are available, they tend to concentrate on the negative side of sexual relationships and play down the positive aspects (Payne, 1993). With specific regard to sexual activity, Holbrook (1989) and Keitner and Grof (1981) both give very good accounts of the difficulties facing institutions and staff in formulating policies. Holbrook (1989) draws particular attention to the lack of clear guidelines for assessing competency to consent to sexual intercourse, the legal and clinical difficulties of distinguishing consensual from non-consensual, the confusion surrounding issues of patients' rights to confidentiality, privacy and safety and the affect-laden nature of the whole issue. Keitner and Grof (1981) demonstrate the complexity of taking account of both patient variables (e.g. mental state) and milieu variables, such as the feelings of other patients, the current conflicts on the unit and the ability of professional staff to deal therapeutically with patients and their relationships. For a fuller discussion of the formation of policies regarding patient relationships see Swan and Taylor, this volume, and, for a sample of policies, the appendices.

Staff training

Staff receive little or no training in sexual matters (Payne, 1993) and often feel very uncomfortable and unsupported in dealing with these issues (Thomas, 1990a; Withersty, 1976). Without guidance and training they are often having to deal as best they can using common sense with very complex issues. Withersty (1976) found that a continuing staff education programme on the sexual needs of patients improved the quality of patient care and Thomas (1990a) describes a model for setting up a workshop to help staff explore their attitudes and prejudices towards sexuality. See Dale *et al.* (this volume) for a fuller discussion of the selection and training needs of staff.

Prisons and sexuality

Many of the practical issues in prisons are very similar to those in secure psychiatric hospitals. A large number of young, physically healthy, sexually experienced people, many of whom are considered dangerous to others in some way, are detained for what can be lengthy periods, living in close proximity to one another, with no opportunity for intimacy or privacy with partners outside. Nevertheless there has been a different emphasis in the way sexuality has been considered in relation to prisons. This is for a number of reasons. First, all prisons in the UK are single sex and, unlike the psychiatric literature, nearly all that has been written has therefore concentrated on homosexual activity. Second, there has not been the same emphasis on rehabilitation, normalization and rights. This is probably because of the different role of prison and the different attitude of society to prisoners. Deprivation of sexual activity is considered by many as part of the deprivation of freedom associated with prison (Aldridge, 1983). Most of what has been written has been about sexual aggression and, more recently, about the potential transmission of HIV.

Sexual activity in prisons

Because sexual activity in prison is officially forbidden, some professionals deny that any sexual activity occurs (Farmer *et al.*, 1989) and the Home Office has maintained that it is very rare (*Lancet*, 1991; Thomas, 1990b). However, it is clear from the literature that, as in psychiatric hospitals, sexual activity can and does occur (Thomas, 1990b). There remains, nevertheless, a paucity of accurate information as to the exact nature and extent of sexual relationships in prisons.

Until recently, more was written about sexual activity in American prisons, where a series of different studies estimated that between 30 and 50 per cent of prisoners had some form of homosexual relationship whilst in prison (reviewed in Thomas 1990b). One study found that as many as 80 to 90 per cent of long stay prisoners were involved in homosexual relationships.

Since the late 1980s there have been a number of British studies confirming that sexual activity is not uncommon. Some have surveyed the sexual activities of all prisoners, whereas some have concentrated only on drug users because they are most at risk of contracting or spreading HIV.

The National Association of Probation Officers (NAPO) interviewed probation officers from 40 prison establishments in England and Wales (NAPO, 1989). The majority of the probation officers reported that sexual relationships were not unusual within prison establishments, although the extent was difficult to assess. In their opinion the degree of sexual activity depended on the degree of surveillance and privacy within the institution. Sexual activity was reported as being low in open prisons with dormitory provision and in young offender establishments with a high degree of staff surveillance. This was not the case in local, remand or long term prisons. The Prison Reform Trust (1988) reports that estimates from prisoners and from some prison staff suggest that up to 20 to 30 per cent of prisoners may be involved in sexual activity in long term prisons.

Curran and Morrissey (1989) conducted a survey of 30 prisoners and 16 staff members at HMP Wormwood Scrubs and found that prisoners estimated that between 20 and 30 per cent of induction life sentence prisoners have some kind of homosexual experience during their time on the long term wing. Staff estimates varied from 10 to 50 per cent. As in the NAPO (1989) study, sexual activity was reported as being much rarer in the remand wing than in the long term wing. The sexual contacts or relationships on the long term wing were described as generally covert, as inmates were hostile to overt homosexuality. The culture, however, did not appear to outlaw homosexuality altogether. For example the most an inmate could expect at discovery was verbal ridicule and signals evolved to indicate when visitors to a cell would not be welcome.

Turnbull et al. (1991) surveyed 450 ex-prisoners in a widely quoted study. They found that 10 per cent had had sex with an average of three partners in prison. Women were twice as likely as men to report having had sexual contact whilst in prison. These figures cannot be used as a basis for generalization, as the sample was not representative of the prison population as a whole. They recruited a substantial part of their sample deliberately because of their homosexual or bisexual orientation and another because they were injecting drug users. Severely dependent drug injectors have high rates of high risk sexual behaviour, including anal sex (Strang, 1993). About three quarters of those who did report sexual activity were from the homosexual/bisexual group, though a small number were of stated heterosexual orientation. What is interesting is that, despite having been incarcerated in single sex institutions, four people reported heterosexual intercourse, sometimes involving staff members. Just over a fifth of those reporting sexual activity, all male, reported having been pressurized into having sex, some having been threatened with violence. None had felt able to report it as they were known as homosexual within the prison and feared either not being taken seriously or reprisals.

Dolan et al. (1990) interviewed a group of injecting drug users and found that 6 per cent of those who had been in custody reported having engaged in sexual activity whilst in custody, with a number of partners ranging from one to thirty. Subsequent interviews revealed that about half of those reporting male to male contact had engaged in anal sex. Carvell and Hart (1990) also asked a group of injecting drug users retrospectively about any sexual activity whilst in custody. One woman out of a total of eight and four men out of 42 had had sex in custody. The number of partners ranged from two to 16 for the men.

These English studies are in stark contrast with the findings of Power *et al.* (1991). They surveyed 559 remand, short-term and long term prisoners in eight penal establishments in Scotland and found that only one male inmate reported being sexually active during a period of incarceration. He had engaged in anal intercourse. Four women reported homosexual activity. They attributed these low rates to the high rates of single cell occupancy in Scottish prisons and the lack of acceptance of homosexuality by the prison population in Scotland. The latter may, however, only make it less likely for people to admit to it.

Types of sexual relationships in prison

Studies have found that, generally, factors that have an influence on the level of sexual activity are length of stay, type of accommodation, level of overcrowding and prison regime. Sexual activity may be less frequent in large dormitories or single cells and is less likely to occur where there is a high level of staff supervision (Curran and Morrissey, 1989; NAPO, 1989). Factors that have been identified as making short-term prisoners less likely to engage in sexual activity are the relatively short period of heterosexual deprivation, the sight of a release date, greater contact with the outside world, preoccupation with external events and a transitory population (Curran and Morrissey, 1989).

For some of those engaging in homosexual relationships, this is their preferred sexual orientation. It is widely said, however, that prison life produces conditions which encourage the establishment of homosexual relationships within the institution, even among those of a usually heterosexual orientation (Aldridge, 1983; Thomas, 1990b). This 'situational homosexuality' has not been quantified. In the study by probation officers (NAPO, 1989) a number of male prisoners serving medium and long term sentences with a hitherto heterosexual background were reported to be engaging in homosexual activity, though the extent of such crossover activity was not known. Thomas (1990b) and Buffum (1971) both quote an American study which estimated that, of those inmates engaging in sexual activity in an American prison, between 5 per cent and 10 per cent had never had any previous homosexual experience and between 25 per cent and 30 per cent had had intermittent, casual previous experience.

There is some debate as to what leads to this situational homosexuality. The more simplistic explanation is that it is an inevitable result of having a single sex group of adults living in close proximity to one another, denied any heterosexual outlet for their sexual frustration. The effects of stress and boredom have also been stated as major factors (NAPO, 1989). Others have suggested that the situation is more complex, as relief from sexual frustration can to some extent be dealt with by masturbation and fantasy. Buffum (1971) suggests sexuality and its expression relate to the social climate in the prison. Prisoners are not only denied sex but are also living in a climate where their needs for autonomy, affection, and durable social relationships are frustrated. Sexual behaviour is one way of trying to satisfy these needs by searching for meaningful relationships that have some durability. Indeed a number of long term prisoners engage in sexual activity as part of stable mutually supportive long term relationships. A second motivation is as a source of validation of masculinity and a symbol of resistance to the prison environment in an atmosphere where individuality is almost non-existent (Buffum, 1971; Newcombe, 1988). This applies especially to those whose primary source of masculine validity outside was sexual success. Such prisoners enter relationships where they are the dominant 'male' partner.

Non-consensual sexual relationships in prison

Though many sexual relationships within prison may be consensual, a number of types of coercive relationship have been described: sexual harassment, sexual intimidation and sexual assault.

A large study of prison sexual behaviour in the US quoted by Lockwood (1983) estimated that 29 per cent of inmates had been propositioned in institutions and two out of 330 had been compelled to perform sexual acts. Another survey showed that 28 per cent of inmates of a New York prison had been the targets of approaches perceived as aggressive (Lockwood, 1983). One man among 76 had been the victim of a sexual assault. Lockwood argues that sexual harassment leads to fights, social isolation, racism, fear, anxiety and crisis.

In one type of coercive relationship, a young, usually socially inadequate inmate makes himself freely available to a number of other inmates as a casual sexual partner in return for small favours such as drugs or money. In a second type, older predatory homosexuals, usually serving long sentences, maintain a sort of harem of one or more younger inmates who are persuaded to engage in sexual activity in return for the offer of protection from competing 'wolves' (Conacher, 1988). The younger inmate is usually seduced by constant companionship, protection and the giving of favours until he is indebted to the older inmate (Buffum, 1971). Conacher argues that in both cases the prisoners involved are helpless and do not really have free choice, though the exploiting partner may be anxious to maintain the illusion that the exploited partner is a willing participant.

Homosexual assaults occur in prisons in the UK and abroad although the exact extent is not known. Offence data on prisoners while in custody in Britain are collected but there is no discrete category of sexual offences, making it difficult to estimate the extent of such assaults. Cotton and Groth (1982) argue that inmate rape, unlike consensual sexual relationships, is not related to deprivation of heterosexual intercourse but is perpetrated for power reasons: to hurt, humiliate, dominate, control and take revenge. It may also be used as a way of expressing racial hostility (Buffum, 1971). Some prison officers in the US have expressed the opinion that sexual threats and prison rapes are the single most prevalent cause of unrest (Rothenberg, 1983) and it has been suggested that homosexual activity is a leading motive for inmate homicide (Lockwood, 1983).

Being the target of unwanted advances can have serious psychological sequelae, depending as much on personal factors as the level of intimidation and force used. Reactions include fearfulness, anger, anxiety and crises which may be accompanied by suicidal thoughts and gestures. It may also affect social functioning, leading to isolation and suspiciousness (Lockwood, 1983). Cotton and Groth (1982) describe the no-win situation in which the victims of sexual assault find themselves. They may try to escape by being placed in protective segregation, thus restricting their own activities, or they may try to escape physically by attempting suicide or acting violently to get moved out. They may try to fight back, often increasing the risk of physical attack from the perpetrator or of facing disciplinary action. They may be forced to continue having sex with one inmate to protect themselves from others or they may endure repeated assaults in silence, refusing to report it. The climate in prisons is not currently such that inmates can easily report sexual assault. The trauma of male rape is similar to that of female rape with potentially serious physical, emotional, cognitive, psychological, social and sexual sequelae.

It can be very difficult to differentiate consensual sex from non-consensual because of the reluctance of prisoners to report harassment, assault or coercion and because there are subtle shades of coercion where the 'predator' is particularly keen to give the appearance of a consensual relationship or the other member of the partnership appears to be consenting but only for a particular gain.

Female sexuality in prison

Female sexuality in prison has received far less attention than male sexuality, partly because of the emphasis on the potential transmission of HIV by male homosexual contact and on male homosexual rape. It has been suggested that, because of prior socialization, women show considerably fewer problems adjusting to sexual deprivation and therefore display less sexual behaviour in prison (Buffum, 1971). This is not backed up by any hard evidence. Buffum suggests that the response of women to the depersonalizing climate of prison is to recreate pseudo-families within the institution with articulated roles of husband and wife to combat the enforced loss of emotionally satisfying, stable relationships. He concedes that sexual relationships may be played out within these families and that the extent is not known. It might be added that the outside relationships were not necessarily emotionally healthy or stable, but there may still be recreation or repetition within the prison. The studies mentioned earlier show that women do engage in sexual activity in prison (Carvell and Hart, 1990; Turnbull et al., 1991). In an American prison a group of female prisoners took part in a series of focus groups exploring attitudes to AIDS education. Many of them stressed the importance of discussing female homosexual activity as it occurred within the prison, and that it is never addressed sufficiently in health education packages (Vadro and Earp, 1991).

Prison and partners outside

Another area that has been little discussed is the effect of separation on sexual relationships with partners outside prison. It is not only the sexuality of prisoners but also that of their partners which is affected by incarceration. Fishman (1988) interviewed a group of prisoners' wives in Vermont, USA. The women described the importance of telephone calls for communicating about intimate matters such as sex, which were difficult to write about. They felt that the exchange of such intimacies on the telephone allowed them to sustain their commitment to the relationships. The wives also discussed the importance of home visits as an opportunity to seek intimacy. Some couples were able to resume sexual intimacy if allowed some privacy. The wives felt that the resumption of sexual intimacy served to reinforce the relationship and alleviate a major pain of separation, the sexual deprivation. A small number of women described how their husbands used the telephone and visits to control their lives jealously (see also Coyle, this volume).

Prisons and HIV

Much of the concern about the potential for spreading HIV in prison stems from the high proportion of high risk individuals in prison, in the form of injecting drug addicts. Harding (1987) found some variation in the HIV prevalence in prisons throughout Europe and concluded that there was an overall seropositivity rate in prisons of member states of the Council of Europe in excess of 10 per cent, with the rate of seropositivity relating closely to the proportion of drug users in custody in each country. In Britain the Home Office has estimated that 0.1 per cent of inmates in British gaols are HIV positive (Thomas, 1990b). It has, however, been argued that this is likely to be a gross underestimate, as it only represents those who have come forward and told the authorities of their status (Harding, 1987; NAPO, 1989; Prison Reform Trust, 1991). HIV status is not routinely screened in Britain. Many conceal their status because of the perceived threat of being treated in segregation. It is likely from the evidence available that drug injecting in prison poses by far the greatest risk of transmission of the virus. Indeed Farmer et al. (1989) found no objective evidence of a high incidence of new cases of any sexually transmitted disease in prison. This is often used as a crude measure of the extent of promiscuous behaviour. Nevertheless, it has been shown that sexual activity of an unprotected orogenital and anogenital kind does occur that could potentially lead to infection (Carvell and Hart, 1990; Turnbull et al., 1992).

Staff attitudes to sexual relationships in prison

Official English policy is that all sexual contact is banned in prison, as the Sexual Offences Act 1967 has been interpreted to mean that homosexuality within a prison is against the law, as nowhere in a prison constitutes a private place (Prison Reform Trust, 1988). There is little systematic evidence regarding how it is managed when it does occur and the literature suggests that responses vary according to the particular penal establishment and according to the individual prison officers (Aldridge, 1983). Aldridge argues that in some cases superhuman self-control is expected of inmates, with the advice being to abstain from all sexual outlets. In other circumstances it is reported that prison officers turn a blind eye to, and occasionally even condone, both consensual and non-consensual sex in order to keep the peace and stabilize difficult inmates (Cotton and Groth, 1982; Farmer et al., 1989; Southwell, 1981).

Future research

Good clinical practice must be informed by sound research information. The discussion so far has demonstrated that there have been few systematic studies of the sexuality of psychiatric inpatients, or their sexual relationships whilst in hospital. Therefore we (Davison, Taylor and Romily) have designed a questionnaire for use with psychiatric inpatients. It is being piloted with male inpatients at a high security hospital and there are plans to pilot a version for women.

It takes the form of a semi-structured interview. It was designed after discussion with the National Addiction Centre at the Institute of Psychiatry who were designing a questionnaire to investigate sexual practices and drug-taking behaviour in prisons. The interview explores actual behaviour as well as attitudes. It collects quantitative and qualitative data. It asks about heterosexual and homosexual behaviour. It covers basic demographic data, sexual orientation and past sexual experience, current sexual relationships, sexual behaviour in hospital and changes between the community and hospital. It asks about involvement in consensual, coerced and paid sex in and out of hospital.

Much thought has to go into the design of such an interview as it needs tact and sensitivity to ask about such intimate areas. From a methodological point of view, given the retrospective nature of the questions, the most accurate quantitative data about behaviour will be about behaviour in the recent past. Patients may, however, fear talking about their recent sexual activities for fear of the consequences on the ward. The interview, therefore, starts with more general questions to put them at their ease and then proceeds to ask about sexual activity ever, sexual activity in the year prior to admission or arrest, sexual activity ever in a psychiatric hospital, and finally focuses in on any sexual relationships or activity during the current admission.

Patients are also asked about their perceptions of what sexual activity takes place in their ward and in the hospital more generally, and about their attitudes towards it and the staff response to it. Although these questions ask about their perceptions and attitudes and do not treat these data about actual behaviour as quantitative for reporting purposes, the answers are useful to compare with the actual behaviour described by the patients for validation purposes. The data can be compared for degree of agreement between estimates of frequency of sexual activity on the ward and also between the sum of the accounts of actual activity and the overall estimates in order to test for direction and degree of bias. This process may also hint at areas the patients do not feel able to discuss in relation to their own behaviour.

Conclusions

Sexuality is a fundamental part of an individual's psychosocial adjustment and institutions cannot afford, perhaps literally, HIV infection or a pregnancy to occur, while either party is resident. Some patients and prisoners will engage in sexual activity even where it is explicitly banned. Staff responses vary, often reflecting their discomfort and training deficits. When considering the sexuality of patients and prisoners, autonomy, freedom of choice and psychosocial rehabilitation needs have to be finely balanced against the need to protect from exploitation, assault, pregnancy, sexually transmitted diseases and emotional distress (Batcup and Thomas, 1994). The needs, feelings and rights of other patients and inmates must also be considered. In addition, such institutions are often in the public eye and may have to contend with adverse publicity. Attention must be paid to homosexual and heterosexual activity in both sexually integrated and supposedly segregated environments.

Differentiation between coercive and exploitative sexuality and consensual relationships can be difficult, and requires a thorough understanding of normal sexuality and of the environmental and psychological factors which can lead to coercion. Protection requires adequate staffing levels and relevant staff skills, coupled with clear policies. In the event of clearly unwarranted attention or assault, legal action must be taken if necessary; good psychological support is essential for the victim, but the duty of care is to both participants and this can easily be forgotten. Preventive measures in prisons include regimes where prisoners have more autonomy, opportunities to express themselves and their gender identity, opportunities to form positive relationships without having to sexualize them (Buffum, 1971; Southwell, 1981) and the creation of a climate where it is acceptable to report harassment and rape. Other things that have been suggested are more home visits (Buffum, 1971; Southwell, 1981), telephone calls and conjugal visits (Conacher, 1988). It is important that the sexuality of patients is acknowledged and that, as in any community, some choose transient relationships. For these and others, however, who do not, elements of practical support for the wider aspects of the relationship are vital.

Practical management of sexual and reproductive health in institutions

Maggie Cole and Pamela J. Taylor

Introduction

All long stay institutions have the potential for compounding certain health problems. Monitoring of sanitation, standards in food hygiene and ventilation systems are among the more familiar tasks if public buildings and their functions are not themselves to become foci of infectious disease. In the UK the lifting (in 1986) of Crown immunity, which had previously had the effect of providing long stay institutions with immunity from prosecution in the event of environmental health hazards such as spread of infections, was an important step forward in this regard.

Psychological health, even in open institutions or hostels, can be impaired in the absence of sufficient stimulation (e.g. Wing, 1990). In prisons and hospitals, measures for the prevention of suicide are vital; suicide rates in UK prisons are again rising. Personal isolation is no longer a tenable proposition in healthy institutions, but with socialization comes the inevitability of other actions that may put health at risk. Some residents will have sexual relations with each other. As the overwhelming majority of secure institutions are exclusively single sex in their residency, homosexual encounters are the most likely. Some residents will share drugs and drug taking equipment. The US National AIDS Committee (1990) even went so far as to say: 'By choosing mass imprisonment as the federal and state governments' response to the use of drugs, we have created a de facto policy of incarcerating more and more people with HIV infection.' A similar claim could be made for the UK, and indeed many other countries.

HIV and hepatitis B infection is particularly likely to occur among intravenous drug users. This generally follows from needle and syringe sharing, although intoxication with any drugs, including alcohol, may increase risk if only by impairing judgement and ability to adopt safe practices with respect to other drugs and sexual intercourse. In general, unprotected sexual activity seems, in the UK and probably other Western countries, to be a less important source of spread, but this is possibly only because the most prevalent strains of virus here seem to transmit less readily in heterosexual intercourse. Sexual transmission is already much more problematic in other parts of the world, such as many African countries. Given the likelihood that a high risk group may continue with, or escalate high risk behaviours in a closed institutional setting, the role of public health and infection control staff is crucial in this area. It is arguable that institutions in which people may be compulsorily detained have an especially strong responsibility to ensure that the health of the residents is at least no worse as a result of the residency. There is also a duty of care to the staff.

Brief history of infection control in prisons and hospitals in the UK

Medical services were appointed to every prison in England and Wales following 'An Act for Preserving the Health of Prisoners in Gaol and Preventing the Gaol Distemper' in 1774. The disease frightening the authorities at that time was typhus, as much for the risk of its spread from prison into the community as within the institution. In 1948, a state funded National Health Service (NHS) was established for the United Kingdom, although the Prison Medical Service (PMS) continued as a separate service. Despite recommendations in a number of official reports to the contrary (e.g. House of Commons, 1986), it has remained so. In 1993, following an efficiency scrutiny by a team drawn from the Home and Health Departments, an 'executive agency' – the Health Care Service for Prisoners – replaced the PMS (HM Prison Service Health Care, 1993). Its brief was to become a body for setting standards for prison medicine, and move toward being a purchaser of care to be provided mainly by the NHS.

The following year, an annual report from the Chief Medical Officer at the Department of Health made recommendations on a number of issues in prisons, including communicable diseases (Acheson, 1994). He recommended that sodium hypochlorite tablets be made available to prisoners for the sterilization of syringes and other equipment that might be used for administering drugs, as was already the practice in Scotland. He welcomed the recommendations of the Joint Committee on Vaccination and Immunisation to offer hepatitis B immunisation to all long term and special risk prisoners. He also recommended that condoms be made available for use by prisoners in England and Wales. Almost simultaneously, the AIDS Advisory Committee to the Home Office made similar recommendations. The recommendations on substance misuse were implemented in September 1995. Denial seems to have prevailed in relation to sexual activity. Ministers merely 'accepted the clinical freedom of prison doctors to prescribe condoms whenever they judge there is a risk of infection' (Wool, 1995).

In hospitals, infection control officers and committees were appointed in all acute hospitals in 1959 after a recommendation from the then Ministry of Health. This followed pandemic staphylococcal infections in the 1950s. An outbreak of salmonella poisoning at the Stanley Royd Hospital in 1984, and the subsequent report, ensured the extension of such services to long stay hospitals, including the special hospitals. It generally changed approaches, which vary now in detail only from one setting to another. By November 1986 there had been the first meeting of an infection control committee in Broadmoor hospital (one of the special hospitals). By 1988 the committee and its work was similar to that to be found in any NHS hospital. It included external specialist representation, and a full time infection control nurse was appointed for the hospital. One of the earliest tasks of the committee was to formulate a policy on HIV and AIDS. It quickly produced a fact sheet for the staff. Consideration was also given to creating an area within the hospital which could be used for isolating patients with HIV/AIDS who might be too disturbed to be nursed in the main wards or hospital infirmary. Such a unit was created, but only ever used for one patient, in full consultation with specialists from a London teaching hospital. A medical centre within the hospital, opened in 1990, allows for the possibility of an isolation suite to be created at short notice for one or two patients with any condition for which barrier nursing might be essential.

Parallel developments outside the UK

The World Health Organization (WHO, 1993) and the Council of Europe (1993) made rather similar recommendations from a public health perspective. These relate to prisons but have application for any institution, particularly any secure institution with a population likely to be sexually active or at risk of drug use. The former opens with a compelling principle:

> 'All prisoners have the right to receive health care, including preventive measures, equivalent to that available in the community without discrimination, in particular with respect to their legal status or nationality.'

The document goes on to include guidance on HIV testing, education for staff and prisoners, confidentiality, care and support of HIV-infected prisoners, women, juvenile and foreign prisoners, community links and release, and research. Of particular importance here are paragraphs 20 and 21:

20. Clear information should be available to prisoners on the types of sexual behaviour that can lead to HIV transmission. The role of condoms in preventing HIV transmission should also be explained. Since penetrative sexual intercourse occurs in prison, even when prohibited, condoms should be made available to prisoners throughout their period of detention. They should also be made available prior to any form of leave or release.
21. Prison authorities are responsible for combating aggressive sexual behaviour such as rape, exploitation of vulnerable prisoners (e.g. transsexual or homosexual prisoners, or mentally disabled prisoners) and all form of prisoner victimization by providing adequate staffing, effective surveillance, disciplinary sanctions, and education, work and leisure programmes. These measures should be applied regardless of the HIV status of the individuals concerned.

Organizations vary in the extent to which such guidance has been applied in practice. It seems likely at the time of writing that only in one Canton in Switzerland have prisons implemented the advice in full. Evaluation of the first year of its being operational should lay to rest one set of anxieties – that supply of materials for health protection will necessarily encourage unwanted or forbidden behaviours. Nelles and Harding (1995) found that in the 'experimental' prison, which housed up to 110 women at any one time, the proportion of prisoners taking heroin or cocaine regularly remained stable throughout the experimental period. Interviews of inmates on four occasions and staff on three confirmed that about 40 per cent of the prisoners continued to use the drugs, about 80 per cent of this group by injection. Before the availability of clean equipment nearly half of the injecting prisoners reported sharing it regularly, but almost no-one during the 12 months. Evaluation of a subsample of the women showed prevalences of 6 per cent for HIV infection, 50 per cent for hepatitis B, and 30 per cent for hepatitis C on entry. There were no seroconversions among these women during imprisonment, no abscesses at injection sites, and no incidents of threatening or aggressive behaviour among the women using the syringes.

There is as yet no report on the relative effectiveness of the different approaches to prevention of spread of hepatitis or HIV infection by contaminated equipment for tattooing or injection. As far as is known, the injection of illicit drugs does not occur in secure hospitals in the UK, but tattooing and body piercing certainly does, with the same attendant risks, so sterilizing equipment should be available for patients.

The supply of contraceptives for home leave applies to prisoners, but not routinely for security hospital patients. Unescorted home leave almost never occurs from high security, but it may from medium security. So far, during imprisonment in English prisons the best compromise that has been reached is that doctors may prescribe condoms. This of all possible solutions would seem the one most likely to imply official sanction for the behaviour, and has the potential for introducing further stresses into anything approaching a normal doctor–patient relationship in these circumstances. Further, the extent to which men or women in such circumstances would feel able to use this route for obtaining this kind of protection from perhaps the only doctor to whom they have access, and the extent to which such doctors would feel able to grant the requests (since none is obliged to act against his or her own conscience) is not at all clear. The WHO injunction to allow prisoners (and we would add compulsorily detained patients) at least the same kind of facility in this regard that they would expect to enjoy in the community seems entirely wise.

Likely extent of the problems

At the beginning of 1996, the prison population for England and Wales was over 52 000, with an estimate of a further rise in daily population of about 15 000 over the next 3 years. By 1992 the number of people known certainly to have active hepatitis B had, after a steady decline, fallen to one fifth the number in 1988/9, while the number of carriers had fallen to just under half the 1988/9 figures. The number of known cases of HIV infection had apparently increased from 112 to 125, with just 19 men and one woman noted as having clinically apparent AIDS (HM Prison Service Health Care, 1993). The slight rise was probably related to better detection rather than any real increase. Sixty per cent of prisoners approached to take part in research carried out by the Public Health Laboratory Service, under Medical Research Council guidance, agreed to anonymous testing. The prevalence of HIV infection was 0.3 per cent, higher than among women presenting to antenatal clinics in London, but not as high as expected (Wool, 1995). Why the high expectation?

In a 1988/9 national sample of sentenced prisoners in England and Wales (Gunn et al., 1991), 10 per cent of the adult men, 2 per cent of male youths and 30 per cent of women were serving sentences for drug (excluding alcohol) crimes. Nine percent of adult men, 3 per cent youths and 1 per cent of women had been sentenced for sex offences. Drug dependency or abuse were the commonest diagnoses regardless of age or sex. Ten per cent of men, 6 per cent of youths and 24 per cent of women were using drugs other than alcohol to an extent to qualify for an ICD-9 (WHO, 1978) diagnosis. The extent of the problem may be even greater in other countries. In 1991, the USA prison population was about 1.22 million at a time when it was about 46 000 in the UK. The proportion of people serving sentences for sex offences was not greatly different between the two countries, (9 : 7 per cent) but three times as many had been jailed for drugs offences in the USA (24 per cent) compared with England and Wales (8 per cent). For these purposes, people had been rated only for their most serious offence (US Department of Justice, 1994).

Once in prison the rate of relevant risk taking behaviours is hard to estimate reliably, but attempts have been made. Drug use and needle sharing is not uncommon and, allegedly, in Scottish prisons is the main source of spread rather than sexual activity (Jolliffe, 1995). Sophie Davison reviews elsewhere in this volume the extent of likely risk from sexual activity.

There is no longer any doubt that spread of HIV has occurred in jail. At some time between January 1 and June 30 1993, 636 inmates were resident in Glenochil prison in Scotland. Of the 378 still available for testing at the time of the study, 227 (60 per cent) came forward for counselling, and 162 opted to be tested for HIV infection (Goldberg, 1995). At the time of testing 12 (7 per cent) were seropositive and 12 in the possible latency period. One-third of those counselled had ever injected drugs, with more than 40 per cent of them maintaining this habit in Glenochil. All the seropositive cases were among those who persisted with injection even in prison, making the prevalence for tested in-prison injectors 44 per cent. Seroconversion data confirmed that eight transmissions definitely occurred in the prison, while viral DNA studies suggested that they all had. There was also a cluster of hepatitis B cases, which Goldberg suggests may be a useful indicator of the practice of high risk behaviours.

The position is, if anything, less well documented among psychiatric patients. Davison (this volume), in reviewing some of the relevant background, also points out that research figures are conspicuous by their absence for current prevalence of sexually transmitted disease among psychiatric patients. Menon *et al.* (1995) suggest that this is misplaced complacency. They studied consecutive psychiatric admissions through 22 months (1989/91) at one hospital and 6 months (1991) at another, both in Philadelphia. Patients over 45 years with mental retardation or dementia were excluded. Of the 239 interviewed, over 40 per cent of the men and 13 per cent of the women reported multiple sex partners. More of the women (11.6 per cent) than the men (2.1 per cent) claimed receptive anal sex during the 6 months before interview. Only half the sexually active said that they had ever used a condom in the 6 months. Use of crack cocaine by the men and mainly other types of cocaine among the women was significantly associated with having sex with a high risk partner.

Even less is known about the prevalence of HIV among patients in secure hospitals, but the presumption is that it is not insignificant. No hospital that we know of has a routine testing policy, but neither has a research sample been studied. Among special hospital patients a substantial minority have misused drugs sufficiently to attract an ICD-10 (WHO, 1992) diagnosis reflecting this, and about 10 per cent have a sexual offence as the principal non-illness reason for admission, but deviant sexual behaviour was additionally involved in some of the more overtly violent offending and the vast majority of people have spent several months at least in prison before admission to the hospital (Taylor *et al.*,

1998). In so far as hepatitis B infection is an indication of particularly high risk for HIV infection in such a population, up to mid 1996 in Broadmoor Hospital only 4 patients had tested positive for hepatitis B and 2 for hepatitis C, but none of these patients had tested positive for HIV and there was no evidence of the suspicious clustering as described by Goldberg (above). Two or three known and clinically symptomatic patients with HIV infection had previously been nursed safely in the special hospitals

Risk of HIV infection and transmission: some frequently encountered problems and prejudices

Uninformed anxieties about HIV infection are still widely prevalent among the general public. Known or suspected sufferers may encounter all kinds of rejection, discrimination and hostility, and those who find their way into prison or hospital are no less vulnerable in this regard. Sensible precautions, including use of gloves when handling body fluids or giving injections and safe disposal of needles and other sharp objects, are in use for everyone. Although the days are largely gone when police or prison service employees and even professional clinicians demanded special protective clothing and to isolate people merely on the grounds of seroconversion, there is still a considerable educational task. Staff may still consciously or unconsciously distance themselves from patients whom they know to be infectious. Patients who have been infected, or think they may be, may become withdrawn, depressed or physically aggressive, expressing the distress or resentment that they feel in the only way that they know, further increasing the invisible barriers and running the risk of reducing the quality of care (Rafferty, 1995). Polk-Walker (1989) describes how even perfectly rational approaches to care can trigger adverse reactions in patients if not fully explained and applied, as far as possible, in an egalitarian fashion. Although staff recognize it as routine, the wearing of gloves for certain procedures, she says, can precipitate delusional or hallucinatory experiences among psychotic patients, predominantly involving feelings of worthlessness, guilt and shame. She suggests that staff should repeat clear and concise explanations every time this has to happen and that patients should be monitored afterwards for any signs of increased anxiety. Specific therapeutic interventions may sometimes be necessary.

Most institutions that could be regarded as at higher than average risk for attracting a clientele who are HIV infected recognize the need for staff training. Some develop their own, others rely on standard packages. The English prison service, for example, has a training video to supplement any local training. Independent charitable trusts with a special interest in the field will also supply literature and training. Much of the literature is intended for potential clientele rather than professional staff. Nevertheless, professional people could do worse than read it. One of the great bonuses is that the material tends to express the issues in terms that patients or prisoners will understand! For examples see the listing under Terrence Higgins Trust (1992–94).

In institutions or regulated communities of other kinds it is also vital to provide general and, for any who want it, personal education for the residents. This is likely to be best supplied as a mixture from people who know the residents well and those who come from entirely without the organization, but who have some special expertise or knowledge. Some may have first hand experience of the disease. The goals of such services include reassurance, assistance to access all services needed (including health, housing, benefits, social support, legal advice as necessary), guidance towards a healthy lifestyle that may extend quality of life or limit the spread of infection if ill, and reduction of future personal risks if not already infected.

Developing policies and procedures for prisons, hospitals and community alternatives

General approach

Good policy development in this area is likely to follow from a group of enthusiastic and informed staff within the organization drawing together advice, which must include expert scientific and technical advice, input from entirely independent sources, lay participation, with particular reference to the more ethical aspects of the work and, as far as possible, contributions from the 'consumers', including those especially at risk. Where there is already experience of practice along lines to be proposed, the policy group will need to take evidence about that, but should not be deterred from breaking new ground if this is defensible according to the present state of knowledge.

Detail will be provided by each part of any organization reflecting special needs for guidance or procedures, but the overarching policy must be clear and precise on key points of principle. Particularly in such a sensitive area as this, any policy must be subject to regular review. While there should perhaps be allowance for emergency adjustment in a crisis, it is important that lasting changes to any policy are made by agreement across interested parties.

Education and training

The raising of knowledge and awareness of a relatively new area of work to be tackled by the staff of institutions is generally an essential preliminary to policy development, an integral part of it, and also a continuing task to be highlighted as an important element of work to follow from policy. It has major resource implications that go beyond the mere provision of seminars or courses, since the majority of staff will expect to attend within their own time. As an example, the Central Prison Health Care Directorate training budget for England and Wales approached £300 000 in 1991/2, and 20 per cent of that was spent specifically on HIV/AIDS training. Not all of this was directed at health care staff, and the figures take no account of local expenditure or staff time (HM Prison Service Health Care, 1993). Staff from the special hospitals have attended national conferences, and in-house training is supplied. A number of nursing staff have gone on to obtain a formal qualification: (English National Board) ENB 934: *The care and management of patients with HIV/AIDS.*

In a hospital setting, it is our impression that probably the majority of patients have very basic sex education needs, and know very little about the specifics of contraception or maintaining health while being sexually active. Staff should not be taken in by the superficial sophistication of some patients in organizing sexual encounters on a personal, or even institutional basis (see also Davison, this volume). In many hospital populations, the prevalence of histories of having been a victim of sexual abuse is high; in secure hospitals it may be exceptionally so, among men as well as women. A few patients may be predatory or coercive, some of them having also been victims. This may mean that educational programmes for patients have to include special elements which would have only a minor place in more general programmes.

While general educational opportunities are important, they are no substitute for individual consultations and help. It is reasonable to expect that such would be available within a hospital setting. Although perhaps more variably so in a prison or community setting, such settings might at least be expected to provide information leaflets for private use and make links, on request, with recognized outside advisory services.

Counselling services

People may need advice about many aspects of their relationships, and some of the other areas are dealt with elsewhere in this volume, e.g. Hodge and Kruppa. Here the focus is predominantly on physical health issues and on the matter of HIV infection in particular. Individual work will fall mainly into three categories.

It is good practice prior to any testing for the possibility of infection, even if the request for a test has been initiated by the patient (or offender), to discuss the test, possible outcomes, and their likely consequences of each eventuality *in advance of testing*. Testing only proceeds on the basis of consent obtained after such an interview. Trained counsellors are available in or to most institutions to help with this, a potentially specialist task in itself. For individuals already under treatment for some other condition, particularly for a psychiatric condition, it is important that the person in charge of that medical care is involved in the decision to counsel and/or test.

In the event of a test being positive, further counselling is likely to be necessary, to ensure that the individual has access to the maximum relevant information about the next medical steps and about any other facilities likely to be needed in the short term; to offer support as requested; to assist as necessary or requested in informing others with a real need to know; and to ensure that the individual is fully appraised on how to limit the spread of infection. It is important to be aware that this is likely to be a long process, both in the first session and in terms of longer term needs. Few people are able to absorb technical medical information in a single session, and this problem is likely to be exaggerated if the information is emotionally charged, as here. Need for support or treatment to come to terms with a positive test finding will vary, and can only be assessed on an individual basis.

Even if the result of a test suggests that the individual has not been infected, some follow up counselling is likely to be advisable. There is an uncertain period of up to 3 months after presumed exposure during which seroconversion may not be evident, but the individual nevertheless may be infected. Re-testing may be necessary. Even when definitely clear, it may be advisable to attempt further individual work in the light of the potential for continuing a high risk lifestyle.

Testing

There is nothing clinically about HIV infection that should distinguish general approaches to management from those for any other serious infection. Assessment and treatment of medical conditions should only ever proceed with the patient's expressed consent and willing continued compliance, except in a few well defined circumstances. These include life saving assessments or treatments for an unconscious patient or, also under common law, in other bona fide emergencies; treatment under the provisions of the Mental Health Act 1983; and treatment supported by specific court order. There is particular sensitivity, however, to testing for HIV infection for two principal reasons – because there remain people even in public service settings who find it difficult to avoid moral judgement of people who may be so infected, to the detriment of their care, and because there remains a possibility of serious social and financial consequences merely from having had a test. For the UK, the General Medical Council (1995) provides essential guidance, including the very rare circumstances in which it may be possible to proceed to testing without explicit consent.

Contrary to a formerly widely held belief, there is almost never any advantage for people in ordinary contact with an HIV positive person to know about their status, nor for those in contact in most clinical settings. It has even been argued that such knowledge can be counter-productive in most clinical settings, since certain basic precautions in handling body fluids or injection equipment should invariably be applied. Knowledge of positive and presumed negative status can lead to the risk of false confidence and slackening of good technique. Some people working in institutions where violent or sexual assault may be a significant risk have pursued the argument for routine testing, but the case for improving policy and practice in limiting these risks of assault is more powerful than the case for singling out an infected individual here or there for ostentatiously different treatment.

The case for exerting pressure on an individual to accept a test would thus be unusual and almost exclusively in his or her own interest. The GMC is also explicit that, even if the testing is to be done as part of an anonymized research or screening programme, explicit consent remains necessary. The GMC guidance enjoins laboratory staff to be as scrupulous in this regard as those in face to face contact with a patient.

With advances in treatment of HIV infection, there is a case to be made that it is of advantage to each affected individual to know as soon as possible, so that they can take appropriate steps to increase the length and quality of their survival. This can, indeed must, be put to the individual as part of the balance of information that he or she needs in order to be able to make a satisfactory decision about the future, but it is not a reason for overriding a decision against testing.

Confidentiality

The principal real difficulties with respect to professional confidentiality are to do with the fact that good, modern health care is almost never provided by a single person and it is arguable that everyone directly involved with the care and treatment of a patient or prisoner should have access to relevant knowledge. Most of the time this is not a problem, because the patient knows all the people concerned, however slightly, and can appreciate the issues. Notwithstanding a laudable wish to bring the principles of assessment and treatment of HIV infection into line with all other clinical conditions, there is probably still a practical case for treating it differently, and most hospitals will have the possibility for varying the storage of data on this condition. In Broadmoor hospital, for example, guidance is that, unless the patient gives consent otherwise, the patient's consultant psychiatrist, the clinical ward manager (a nurse by profession) and the control of infection nurse are the only people other than the patient and the laboratory to know the information and, in so far as they keep records separate from the patient's personal file, these are held under especially secure conditions. In practice, consent to team disclosure has not been a great problem.

Another important issue in relation to offenders and offender patients, is the range of people other than clinicians who have legitimate access to their records, in some cases confidential clinical records. In England and Wales, for example, Mental Health Act Commissioners, only some of whom are clinicians subscribing to a professional code of ethics, may have unfettered access to all hospital records. Although unusual, courts may subpoena records. There is also concern that people may be exceptionally vulnerable to disclosing their status on entry to the criminal justice system, information which is then entered on to data storage systems and transmitted from service to service without their knowledge. Hamilton (1995), for example, cites the problem of people being taken to police stations who may have information on their person in the form of appointment cards or medication which effectively indicates their status, or give the information voluntarily because of a need to continue with essential treatment. This information, it appears, is likely to go on the police national computer. People in this situation may be better served by insisting on access to their chosen medical adviser at the earliest opportunity. Although the police will provide doctors who should subscribe to GMC standards of practice, these doctors are explicitly working for the police.

Environmental precautions

In general, the environmental precautions necessary in psychiatric hospitals, whether secure or not, and in prisons are precisely similar to those in any clinical setting. Universal precautions should be taken to isolate all bodily fluids, to use sterile equipment for any clinical procedure involving breech of usual body boundaries or likely contact with body fluids, and to ensure safe disposal of that equipment. Some of the special worries for staff and general residents in psychiatric or prison facilities lie in the increased risk in these places of self harm, including cutting and blood shed; of assault, which could result in injury to another patient or staff member and mingling of body fluids; and the much more rare but known problem of disinhibited masturbatory activity, with spread of infected semen. Even best policy and practice with respect to the prevention and management of such incidents can only minimize the risk of their occurrence and not prevent them entirely.

Infection of staff in such settings or fellow residents in such circumstances has never been recorded. Fortunately, HIV is a fragile little virus that cannot survive for long outside body fluids. Nevertheless it is good practice to ensure that any surface which has or could have come into contact with such fluids is decontaminated with sodium hypochlorite solution. Staff or fellow residents involved in such incidents may request testing and/or require counselling.

Individual precautions: patients, prisoners and other clientele

Preventive measures against HIV infection must currently depend principally on education and, in institutions, we would argue, the provision of easily accessible protective materials. Immunization against hepatitis B is possible, and should be encouraged. There is a policy within Broadmoor, for example, to try and ensure that as many patients as possible are thus protected, regardless of whether there is any hint of a propensity for high risk behaviours. It may also be important to resume screening for tuberculosis, which has been undergoing a resurgence in the homeless populations of developed countries, especially the USA, and to which HIV infected people are particularly vulnerable.

Once infection with HIV is confirmed, then approaches to the maintenance of general and other aspects of sexual health become proportionately more important. Other venereal infections take on much more serious proportions for the infected individual who is also HIV infected. Women may need additional counselling about the risks of pregnancy.

Individual precautions: staff

Although the first thought of most staff working in such environments may be for their own protection against infection, it is recognized that staff may themselves be HIV positive. Although most clearly acknowledged in professional codes of practice, it is unethical for any person who has paid employment in the care of others to fail to seek appropriate advice about their own clinical state, and to act on it when given. While it should be unlikely that non-clinicians will be carrying out the kind of clinical procedures likely to increase risk of transmission, they will not be immune from other risk activities, and may under some circumstances be even more vulnerable to engaging in inappropriate sexual activities (Dale *et al.*, this volume).

Care and support

As the focus of this book is relatively specific, this is not the place for an extensive treatise on the support, counselling and psychological treatments that may be needed to those who test HIV-positive. There are a number of excellent and more competent reviews of the field than we could provide here, for example Catalan (1997), Miller *et al.* (1991) and Newman *et al.* (1993). As our task is to consider the issues particularly pertinent to couples, suffice to say that there may be special difficulties in these tasks, encouraging an individual to disclose to a casual partner who may otherwise be unaware of the risk to their own health, or even that of others. Where a long standing partner or spouse may have been infected, there may be issues around infidelity and jealousy to be tackled, as well as the potential horror of a fatal disease. When one or both partners have a serious psychiatric illness like schizophrenia, or one or both have a propensity for serious violence, the prospect of deterioration of mental state or escalation to life threatening aggression will also have to be managed.

An important issue for people with a pre-existing psychiatric disorder is that HIV infection may affect their capacity to tolerate psychotropic medication. There are a number of useful reviews on this (Anonymous, 1994; Ayuso, 1994; Fernandez and Levy, 1994; Persico *et al.*, 1991). In brief, in this respect asymptomatic patients are generally unlikely to encounter difficulties which are any different from those of a healthy individual, although tricyclic antidepressants may be less effective and more problematic. People with established illness are likely to be much more sensitive to neuroleptics, with a much higher risk of extrapyramidal symptoms, especially dystonia. Antiparkinsonian agents are likely to cause cerebral impairment and delirium. Tricyclic antidepressants are probably best avoided because of severe anticholinergic effects, and a rather specific risk of dry mouth promoting Candida infections. Serotonin specific re-uptake inhibitors (SSRIs) and even methylphenidate, generally well tolerated, may be acceptable alternatives. Benzodiazepines tend to cause delirium disinhibition and paradoxical reactions. Lithium induces white blood cell production (leucocytosis and neutrophilia) and has even been used for this property, but there are mixed results as to its value in this role or as a psychotropic agent in these circumstances (see Ayuso (1994) review).

Resources

Effective work can be achieved only when the resources are appropriate to the task. Under-staffing, or under-education of the staff, will have a negative influence, but even the most accomplished and well organized staff will be limited in what they can achieve if the means for putting all the educative effort into practice are not available for their clientele. While the limits on staff resource may reasonably be regarded as financial, this appears to be an inadequate explanation for the reluctance to make clean injection equipment and condoms available, particularly when, personal tragedy aside, the costs to public services of the consequences of infection are unequivocally high, often necessitating social care and security benefits as well as medical treatment. It is often national law that is cited as against clinically recommended programmes. Padel (1995) and Costello (1995) discuss the legal realities in the UK, and show that some of the concerns may be exaggerated. Nelles and Harding (1995) demonstrate the extent to which sensitive, evidence based clinical defiance can pay dividends if the timing is right. It is likely, however, to be only the positive experiences of this kind that attract such journal documentation.

Continuity of care between institutions and to the community

One of the problems for part of the population that is particularly at risk is that they may be subject to movement between prison and hospital, and for people in need of high security at any point, it will almost certainly be the case that they will eventually have to move between clinical services. Anxieties about sharing information about HIV infected status will almost certainly re-emerge, and need sensitive re-analysis both in terms of who does need to know to

safeguard maximally the patient/offender's privacy and how to steer the patient/
offender in this matter in his or her best interests. Although in this, as in any
other aspect of their health care, every effort must be made to ensure that there
is continuity of care, the GMC advice is unequivocal that unless failure to
disclose would clearly place the health of another at risk, communication of the
information even among professionals is unethical in the absence of patient
consent. Such situations are truly unusual if there is a good relationship between
doctor and patient, but in cases of doubt, medical staff at least should always
seek guidance specific to the circumstances from the GMC or a medical defence
society.

Opportunities for review of policies and individual work

Policies can only be fully tested in practice, and commonly need revision
accordingly. Happily, too, clinical advances gradually make elements of policy
obsolete, so occasional routine review is as important as review provoked by
circumstance.

Research

If this chapter, indeed this book, has demonstrated nothing else, the need for
research in this field should be obvious. Here the principal issues which could
bear further exploration are the extent to which recommended approaches to
prevention are effective, and whether there are any adverse effects. Opponents
to the provision of condoms for people in secure institutions, for example, fear
prosecution for colluding with illegal acts if all parts of the institution were to
be regarded as public, or fear reinforcement or escalation of promiscuity. If there
were evidence to the contrary, such as the Nelles and Harding evidence on
drugs, then further progress to safer practice might be more rapid.

Contraception

Some of the reasons for avoiding conception while in an institution, and
particularly in a secure institution, seem obvious, but some of the special
problems faced by parents, including pregnant mothers, living in institutions are
explored more fully in Tobin and Taylor (this volume). In prisons almost
everywhere the problem is kept to a minimum by full segregation of prisoners
by sex, although with some integration by sex of staff, this as a sole means of
ensuring 'safety' may gradually erode. Staff are not immune to sexual relationships with their charges, but this may be a prelude to extending integration to
prisoners too. The advantages and difficulties in doing so are rehearsed in
Gordon (this volume).

In hospitals generally, and perhaps in psychiatric and long stay hospitals
in particular, there has always been a small but recognized risk of pregnancy.
It is arguable that in hospitals where women are in the minority and, for a
variety of reasons, perhaps more than averagely susceptible to abuse, and
where the men are more than averagely likely to be predatory, risks may be
even higher. We know of no case of conception within a purpose designed
secure hospital in England or Wales, but suggest that, as patients grasp the

opportunities that they are encouraged to take to lead a lifestyle that will minimize the effects of institutionalization, this risk may increase. We believe that the best safeguards will be to ensure that the women are secure in all senses in their living accommodation, that they have all the protection and supervision that they need in other parts of the unit or hospital, particularly those where they are likely to mix with men, and that they are helped to a sufficient state of health and understanding of their position to be able to make responsible choices for themselves and carry those through in practice. All that said, it would be extremely naive not to concede that there can be lapses of security, but that, perhaps even more importantly, some women will never be able to reach these heights of responsibility, while others at least for substantial parts of their institutional careers will remain truly ambivalent. While being able to acknowledge rationally that a pregnancy could have profoundly adverse consequences for herself or a future child, the woman may nonetheless see her best childbearing years slipping away unfruitfully in the hospital or prison and be faced with an overwhelming desire to reproduce. Or, as a perpetual receiver of care, she may crave the opportunity to have an object on which to bestow her own potential for caring. Or, in a world in which she perceives, perhaps correctly, that no-one loves her, the woman may decide to create for herself a being that she believes undoubtedly will. The possibilities have not been exhausted!

English law takes the position that sexual intercourse is a matter for personal choice except in certain proscribed situations. Thus it is criminal assault or rape to have intercourse with a person who cannot understand what is proposed, or the implications of what is taking place. There are further laws designed more specifically to protect people with a mental disorder from exploitation. Thus, it is a criminal offence for any man who is a manager or employee of a mental nursing home or hospital to have sexual intercourse with a patient there, whether an inpatient or outpatient. Similar provisions exist under mental health legislation to protect women, and men, under guardianship. The difficulties of applying legislation under the Sexual Offences Act 1959 to all circumstances are expanded elsewhere (Gunn, 1987). Protective in many circumstances, however, an automatic bar on developing sexual relationships among peers may place unacceptable limitations on the freedom of some to live a life as close to normal as possible, for example young people with mental retardation. In any event neither law nor hospital policies, however vigilantly applied, will stop sexual intercourse, so consideration of contraception is inescapable.

Once again in institutions there is a fondness for supplying education, but then no means of applying it until after release. Much of what has already been said about the need for the ready availability of condoms applies here too. The provision of contraception for women is in some ways slightly easier than for men in that, if all else fails, there are no clinical indications to the contrary and the woman is consenting, hormonal means can be prescribed under cover of regulating the menstrual cycle. Not all women, however, wish to take this course, and for a few it is contraindicated. Then there are those whose capacity for consent is in doubt. Mental health legislation does not cover contraception, so general principles of consent to treatment still apply even when the reason for being unable to consent is mental incapacity. The test of 'real consent' is quite generous *(Chatterton versus Gerson)* but there are those who nevertheless fall outside it.

There is little precedent in England and Wales on which to base advice, but the case of *re F* is generally cited for guidance, although this referred to contraception in its most extreme and generally irreversible form – sterilization. F was a young woman with mental retardation. The Law Lords were asked to consider whether her sterilization or 'treatment' could or should be given without valid consent. They ruled that it would be lawful to proceed in the absence of consent if the treatment was justified on the principle of necessity. Lord Goff said that to fall within this principle 'not only (1) must there be a necessity to act when it is not practicable to communicate with the assisted person, but also (2) the action taken must be such as a reasonable person would in all circumstances take, acting in the best interests of the assisted person'. In the case of non-therapeutic treatments such as sterilization, it was also indicated that it was highly desirable as a matter of good practice, but not mandatory (one Law Lord dissented) for an application to be made to the court for this to be determined in advance. The Law Commission (1991) consultation paper provides a lengthier discussion of this point and the further issues that it raises. Other jurisdictions have differed in approach – from Canada, where a court refused to authorize sterilization in *re Eve*, to Australia where, in *re 'Jane'*, sterilization was allowed but the court ruled that consent of the Court is always necessary.

Evidence from the USA suggests that even, or perhaps particularly, in developed countries, safeguards against unethical sterilization may be at least as important as protecting against other risks, such as risks to the health of the disabled, for whom a pregnancy could have disastrous consequences. A ruling, however, by a Californian judge that a woman convicted of child abuse must have an implant of a long-acting contraceptive or face several years in jail presented an entirely different situation. It provoked extended critical comment from the American Medical Association (1992). Here the 'treatment' was principally for projected unborn children and not primarily for the woman herself, or even in her interests at all. As such, effectively forcing her to undertake treatment is at best highly questionable. Charo (1992) and Shapiro (1985) have provided a brief and detailed overview respectively of the legal interference in the USA with the reproductive capacities of women. At various times, mainly for political reasons, contraception and abortion have been illegal or, in the case of the former, legally required. The state funding of services in a country where such provision is as a last resort (as in the USA), and thus almost exclusively for women who cannot otherwise afford them, have potential as a potent means of government control. Some observers consider that such control is already happening.

Although in common law jurisdictions the law may provide essential tests, much is explicitly left to clinical judgement, but on the basis that this will rest on a recognized body of opinion. The application of what is general knowledge to an individual case is always fraught with difficulty, but it is essential that this can be as well done in an institutional setting as anywhere else. Overarching policies and acknowledgement of both legislation and institutional rules are needed as much for the safeguard of the individual as the common good.

Cases cited

Re F [1990] 2 Appeal Cases 1; [1970] All ER 545
Re Eve [1986] 2 SCR 388
Re 'Jane' [1988] 85 ALR 409
Chatterton versus Gerson [1981] QB 432

Glossary

All ER	All England Law Reports
ALR	Australian Law Reports
QB	Queen's Bench
SCR	Supreme Court of Canada Reports

9

Pregnancy and early parenting from care or custody

Louise Tobin and Pamela J. Taylor

Facing the realities: basis of a pragmatic approach

When a parent needs care, or is placed in a secure hospital or prison, the relationship with any child inevitably alters, but when there is a dependent child or a minor still in contact with the parent there are care and security issues for the child too. A set of problems which are different again arise when, as occasionally occurs, a woman is pregnant on admission or if a child is conceived in an institution, and the pregnancy must continue while the mother is detained. Further special consideration is necessary if a child is born while the mother remains in that setting. There are three main principles for approaching these eventualities:

First, the needs and welfare of children who have a parent in such circumstances must be paramount;

Second, the need for pragmatism in recognizing the possibility of conception and pregnancy within such settings;

Third, policy, procedures and guidance, and their implementation must be founded in sound principles of good practice, in turn founded, as far as possible, on research findings, and verified information about the individual case.

These three areas involve challenges to established attitudes, habit and routines and require professionals within the secure setting or community to be prepared to work with often unfamiliar external agencies and professionals in an open, pro-active way, perhaps in areas that have previously been resisted.

Much of what follows is a result of 3 years' independent involvement (L.T.) with the special hospitals on patients' relationships, women's services, issues in relation to children and the possibility of pregnancy. Much of the information about the women in special hospitals is anecdotal, from the patients, staff, voluntary organizations and external professionals involved with patients. It is far from exhaustive in coverage, but should further discussion. It is inevitable that much detail will refer to the special hospitals, but much may be helpful elsewhere.

Prison staff have been confronted in practice with the issues of pregnancy and young children for a considerable time.

Much of the emphasis is on women patients. Many male patients are fathers or, in a rare case, an expectant putative father; however, preliminary investigation and the experience of other closed institutions suggest that mothers and their children are more likely to be disadvantaged by admission, not least because it is less likely that the other parent is available. Among prisoners in the USA, for example, with children under the age of 18 years, 90 per cent of the men, but only 25 per cent of the women said that their children were living with the other parent. Women and their children from ethnic minorities were particularly likely to be disadvantaged in this regard (Snell and Morton, 1994).

The children

Those who work with parents in 'made' communities such as prisons or hospitals should be aware there are children in their lives, but are they? Those who are aware also recognize the mixed feelings evoked by consideration of such children, particularly in relation to a parent likely to be detained for many years, perhaps even more so if that parent has a mental disorder. Consideration needs to be given to quality of understanding such children require, and their experiences..

Some children visit, staff see them, in hospitals other patients and their relatives see them, and in prison other prisoners and their families and friends. The visiting areas provide toys, games, books, but often little privacy. Social workers may spend substantial amounts of time dealing with parents' concerns and requests in relation to children. Concerns are raised often by little or no information about a child, or the gradual withering away of contact. Inquiry in one special hospital indicated the importance of professionals within such hospitals, prisons or any other artificial community beginning to accept some responsibility for the interests of the children of such parents, not only on behalf of the parents but for the children too. This work will include not only individual good practices but also effective policy and procedure generated to ensure immediate safety and, as far as possible, longer term well being.

The children of such parents may have been victims of abuse, observed an ill parent, or seen inappropriate or disturbing behaviour; they may never have met their parent except in an institutional setting; they may be cared for by family members who are affected by general public misunderstandings and prejudices in relation to both mental disorder and special hospitals. Some children are likely to be in the care of a local authority. Some may, effectively, lose both parents in the crisis that took one into care or custody. In rare cases one parent may have killed the other (Black and Kaplan, 1988). Very little is known about how such children cope in the longer term, but living within understandably partisan networks of care by traumatized adults, perhaps related to the dead parent, with little therapeutic support, is unlikely to be optimal. A precarious domestic situation may collapse completely in the absence of one parent. Whatever the circumstances, these children are unlikely to be unaffected by the separation or loss of a parent, whether in the reasons for separation or the outcome, and are likely to have special needs.

Following separation of a child from a mentally disordered parent it cannot be assumed that the previous experience of the child or behaviour of the parent prevents a continued relationship. Nor should plans made at an early stage be set in concrete, as a child's needs change over time and will require review and re-assessment, quite apart from any consideration of the effect of a parent's improvement in health or safety.

The Children Act 1989 (implemented England and Wales 1991) significantly changed the balance of rights and responsibilities between children and their parents and between children, their parents and the state. The welfare of any child became explicitly paramount, recognizing both the child's best interests *and wishes* (our italics). Another fundamental principle is that children should be brought up and cared for by their parents wherever possible. The rights and responsibilities of a parent are now encompassed in the concept of parental responsibility. This is an important concept for parents living in a special hospital or prison. Separation from a child, even when this is as a result of the parent's confinement, does not necessarily affect the responsibility conferred on that parent. A parent's duty and responsibility to play an active part in a child's upbringing is not lessened by voluntary agreement or legal intervention, except in the case of an adoption order. All this, and the principle of partnership between parents and the local authority have required substantial changes in attitude as well as practice.

The Children Act requires professionals, who may have statutory responsibility, to take pro-active steps to establish and maintain contact between children and their separated or confined parents as far as it is in the interests of the child. Parents should be involved in planning and decisions for their children, informed of significant events, and consulted if not able to attend reviews of the child's circumstances. This does not exclude situations where a parent is in disagreement or conflict with the local authority.

The UN Convention on the Rights of the Child was adopted, also in 1989, and signed by the UK in 1990. Much of what has become law in the UK was expressed as 'rights' in this document, but two of the 54 articles are particularly pertinent here. Article 2 states that the state is obliged to protect children against all forms of discrimination or punishment

> 'on the basis of the status, activities, expressed opinions or beliefs of the child's parents, legal guardians, or family members.'

Article 9 relates to children's rights to live with their parents, unless this is incompatible with their best interests. The Howard League for Penal Reform (1993) considers that this should mean that the state must take appropriate measures to ensure that children do not suffer punishment because of the action of their parents, as may be the case if their parents are imprisoned. Imprisonment of mothers in particular is seen as often contrary to the best interests of the children.

It is currently unclear how many children of special hospital patients are in care. However, a 'snapshot' in May 1994 of women in one special hospital with children under 18 years old suggests that a high proportion of women who are mothers have children in care. Twelve women in the hospital had 19 children between them and of these, 10 were subject to care orders, three were adopted and six lived with the woman's extended family. Of the 19 children, only eight visited the hospital at all, but the frequency was not clear. Four others had had only exchange of information, maybe photos and letters, while seven children had no contact at all. One 12-year-old living with her father had apparently been told her mother was dead. A 7-year-old living with grandparents visited his mother but was not aware of her relationship to him.

To the best of our knowledge, similar figures are not available for women in lesser security or open hospitals, where separation may be as important if perhaps less geographically difficult or prolonged. In prisons, the size of the problem is particularly worrying. In the UK, the population of women in prison is rising even faster than that of the men. Most of these women are in their childbearing years. In 1967 prison populations were much lower than in the 1990s, but Gibbs (1971) identified 638 women newly received into Holloway prison during the year, representing one quarter of all sentenced or remanded women from the south of England for that year. Two hundred and twenty-three women (35 per cent) had 504 children between them. The Howard League (1993) cites three later surveys of women in English prisons, suggestive of a growing problem. On 15 March 1982 a Prison Department census of 1318 women in prison found 719 (55 per cent) who were mothers, two thirds of the 653 completing the questionnaire having two or more children. In 1986, a similar survey, but focusing on women with children of 5 years or under, found that 340 women in custody that day were mothers to 455 children within that age range. On 1 December 1989, among 1239 women serving prison sentences, 600 (48 per cent) said that they had children under age 18, but nearly 20 per cent of the women declined to answer any questions about this. There may be a bias towards non-response among woman with children, fearful that arrangements they may have made to cover their absence may then be disrupted by official knowledge and interventions (Carlen, 1983). In Scotland the proportion of imprisoned women with children may be even higher. Dobash et al. (1986) found 65 per cent to be mothers. In a 1991 survey of women prisoners in the USA (Snell and Morton, 1994), 25 700 women, more than three-quarters of all women then in prison there, had between them more than 56 000 children under the age of 18, over 70 per cent of them living with their mother at the point of imprisonment. As a result of the imprisonment, grandparents became the commonest carers for the children, just (51 per cent), but nearly 10 per cent were in a foster home, agency or other institution. Nearly 90 per cent of the women maintained contact with their children, although only half had actually seen them, and most relied on phone or mail. Under 20 per cent thus managed daily contact. but about one-third had weekly phone calls or letters; visits rarely happened more than once a month.

It is possible that an advantage of a sick or dangerous parent being 'in care' is that contact with or care of a child that might otherwise have broken down completely may be supported and developed. Lack of contact can be taken up formally either by the patient's social worker or through legal action and the local authority's complaints procedure. It is well established in child care procedures, and reinforced by research and legislation, that contact is in the best interest of children except in a small number of cases. Contact is generally regarded as in the interests of a child's own self knowledge and development but it becomes crucial in the event of a discharge from hospital or prison and the likelihood of a child's return to their parent's care. Currently it is not known how many parents separated from their children by serious illness are reunited and or re-established as primary carers for those children, let alone how many from a secure hospital setting meet their children again. Local authorities cannot decide to end contact without a decision of a court. The local authority would need to be clear about why it would be in the interests of a child. It is a serious step, particularly in light of research from the Dartington Study (Millham *et al.*, 1993):

'Contrary to popular belief 90 per cent of children and adolescents in the care of a Local Authority eventually go home.

Most reunions between children and parents (or wider family) occur regardless of the reasons for separation or length of time children are away. Even young adults, some convicted of serious offences and long separated from home, will rest in the bosom of their families on occasion.'

Whilst this research was looking at children returning home to parents, it indicated that the situations had not necessarily been settled or stable just waiting for re-unification.

An earlier study from the Dartington Unit (Millham *et al.*, 1986) considered simple contact issues in relation to children. A fifth of children in care at the time of the study lost contact with their parents. The reason that contact reduced or withered away was similar to those reasons that parents in special hospitals appear to lose contact with their children: distance, routines, inflexible planning over time, concern about the potential disruption for the child that could be caused by contact with a parent. Further exploration is needed to establish whether the children of parents in special hospitals – or in prisons – are particularly disadvantaged, or whether the guidance provided by the Department of Health (1990) in relation to good practice for child care practitioners is being carried out consistently.

The parents

It is not acceptable for parents to be marginalized due to their own vulnerability.

'Their parenting capacity may be limited temporarily or permanently by poverty, racism, poor housing, unemployment or by personal or marital problems, sensory or physical disability, mental illness or past life experiences. Lack of parenting skills or ability to provide adequate care should not be equated with lack of affection or irresponsibility.'

(Department of Health, 1990)

Placing children's interests first may raise concerns at a professional, clinical and personal level for professionals working with adults. It is rarely, however, a disadvantage for parents to have the needs of their child placed before their own. Focus on this may bring some personal improvement as well as lead to an improvement in the relationship with the child.

It is expected that if children live apart from their parents, each should be given adequate information and support to contribute to the necessary decisions about placement and care. Local authorities are expected to advise and support parents to retain responsibility and remain closely involved in their child's welfare. The importance of the maintenance of links, through visits and other forms of contact is emphasized:

'Both parents are important even if one of them is no longer in the family home. Any sense of continuity no matter how tenuous is to be nurtured.'

(Department of Health, 1990)

Children of one or both parents who have a mental disorder are often still seen as in need of 'rescue' and a new life; mental illness is often regarded as intractable and life long. Responses to people who have been convicted of a criminal offence are generally even less sympathetic or comprehending. As Kennedy writes (Howard League, 1993), of women in prison:

'The response by many is that the women themselves are to blame and that they should have thought of the consequences of their criminality at the time of committing the crime. However, this is no comfort to the grieving child who often wants to be with his or her mother whatever she has done ...

Spending time with her child is rewarding, but also deeply painful for a woman in prison. She is made more conscious of her child's loss. She has to deal with her child's anger with her for leaving and the child's disappointment with her for doing something wrong. With help, confronting those issues can be a very tough and maturing process for the mother. For the children, like any children, the reassurance that THEY are not to blame and that mothers still love them deeply, is an important part of limiting the damage.'

In the special hospitals, parents have the double stigma of mental disorder and, generally, a criminal conviction. Special hospitals also suffer from intrusive interest of the media, and the public has a distorted view of their purpose and activities.

For parents the de-skilling and lack of control imposed by separation, as well as any mental disorder or stigma of crime, is likely to affect their ability to continue to pursue requests for information about or contact with their child. Mental illness itself may, for periods, distort their ability to understand what is likely to be in the interests of their child, as may guilt – whether as part of an illness, consequent on real actions, perceived failings towards the children, or all of these. Staff working with parents will need to consider such problems and work specifically with them. It may be that it is not in the best interests of an individual child to maintain contact with their parent, but professionals should not automatically accept this outcome and should make genuinely objective assessments in each case.

Managing contact between the parent in care or custody and the children

Visiting is a superficial event, contact is a process which must be planned and managed appropriately. Contact with people in long term care, treatment or custody is different from that with a patient in an acute hospital, expected to be home soon. Currently, where visiting occurs, it is inconsistent, dependent on the need for availability of staff for supervision, the state of the parent and numbers involved. In prison it is often the case that the parent must remain seated whilst a young child moves around the visiting area, playing only with toys provided by the institution and confused as to why their parent cannot join them in play with familiar objects.

In order that children and young people experience a worthwhile quality of contact, a structured evaluation of both the supervision and environment might best also be shared by hospital – or prison – management and outside agencies.

There are various practical tasks that parents ordinarily carry out for their children that have both symbolic and emotional significance. Included are the preparation of food, eating together or feeding young children, washing and dressing children, and playing together. Toys can interest and stimulate children, and facilitate interaction between parents and children. Toys are best chosen with the parent with this in mind and the meeting space chosen or, ideally, designed accordingly. Adolescents may be more difficult, but cooking, eating a meal together, washing up, are all actions which allow a normal experience.

Social services departments or voluntary organizations may well have local facilities which lend themselves to family visits. If a patient can leave their secure environment, negotiation of the use of family centres or similar venues during periods of slack use, for example at weekends, may be particularly constructive.

Supervision is not only to prevent breaches of security or to protect children, but can be therapeutic. From hospitals, including secure units more direct involvement of primary nurses or other key professional workers in planning and supervising visits will simultaneously increase safety, and improve the chances of appropriate developments in the relationship. A parent in such circumstances may also simply feel supported by the presence of another trusted, well known adult. Further, using workers with specific child care training and experience may, in the long term, offer additional benefit to each party involved towards some success in outcome.

In the longer term, success may include everything from termination of association or withdrawal from responsibility for parenting, to full restoration of parent–child relationship, providing the resolution is based on mutually and widely informed agreement. In the short term, indicators of success may include increasing privacy in the meetings and a sense of continuity between meetings, for all concerned.

Hospitals – and prisons – should look carefully at reasons if visits are cancelled. Visits from children are not a reward for good behaviour, nor is the cancellation of a visit an appropriate sanction for a breach of discipline. In general, a visit should only be cancelled if it is not in the interests of the child, due to his or her parent's state, or if it poses risk to the child. Staff need to be aware of the impact on a child of cancellation. Just as there is a danger that physical institutions may be run for the sake of the organization rather than for the primary needs of their residents, so the carers of children may have their own agenda about contact, and need support to understand the true benefits to a child. The social workers in a hospital or probation officers in a prison are probably the best placed to initiate and support families or carers, including alerting local social services to the needs of any children and their service responsibilities.

Local authorities have a responsibility to promote contact and act in partnership with parents. It may be necessary in specific cases for them to initiate action in order that children's needs are met and a parent's circumstances are reviewed. Hospitals and prisons, and particularly social workers or probation officers working in them, may well have to accept more responsibility until systems are created which ensure children and parents do not lose contact by default.

Pregnancy

Pregnancy is a natural state, and not itself an illness, although it may have major consequences for the health of the mother and prospective child. There may also be indirect health consequences for others in the prospective family. It presents a woman, and to some extent her family and/or other carers, with choices. If unplanned, these choices may include termination. Even a wanted pregnancy may be terminated if the risks for mother or child are agreed by everyone as greater than continuation. Termination of pregnancy if a mother is not capable of consenting to the procedure is largely untested territory. For England and Wales, in the case of sterilization for a woman incapable of consent, because of, say, her severe mental retardation, the House of Lords, in *re F*, held that the court could grant a declaration that it would be lawful to proceed in the absence of consent if the treatment was justified on the principle of necessity (to preserve the life or health of the patient) *and*, here, in the patient's best interests. The greater difficulty with pregnancy rests in the fact that it is not exclusively the mother's life, health or interests to be considered.

A healthy pregnancy relies on both physical and emotional stability, with women commonly being offered support by family, friends and experienced health professionals who have information available and a wide range of services. Women use these various support systems to make the necessary adaptations both physically and emotionally that pregnancy and motherhood demand. It is important that, however disabled and wherever she is placed, the prospective mother is included in the decisions about assessing and managing a suspected pregnancy. Even when the decisions may finally rest with others, this level of involvement should be attempted.

Women who choose to terminate pregnancy, or through misfortune miscarry their baby, need sensitive support, as the impact of either form of loss can continue for a long period of time. The prospect of carrying a healthy child to term, only to be separated from it at or soon after delivery, is another potentially potent loss. This may be an important consideration for the mother in the question of termination.

Pregnancy and pre-established mental disorder

The relationship between pregnancy and established mental disorder in the mother is of concern both for the impact of the mental disorder on the developing child and for the influence of the pregnancy on the disorder. Mental disorders may have a genetic component but, except for a few, rare syndromes, most usually associated with generalized learning disabilities, specific gene effects are small, with complex developmental interactions with other factors. The latter can generally be discounted in advising the parents and services at this stage. Indirect effects of a mental disorder on the prospective mother's capacity to care for herself adequately during pregnancy are likely to be more important. There may be late attendance for antenatal care, failure to observe a healthy diet or lifestyle, and a probably disproportionately high risk of smoking or use of other non-prescribed drugs, particularly alcohol or cannabis.

A higher than chance risk of foetal abnormalities associated with alcohol consumption during pregnancy has been recognized at least since the 1960s, with tobacco since the 1970s and with most other drugs of potential abuse for rather longer (Brockington and Kumar, 1982). There do appear to be some abnormalities sufficiently specific to most of these drugs to suspect potential for a direct effect in each case, but the situation is complicated by the fact that drug misuse is rarely of a single substance and abusers commonly have lifestyles which are damaged or damaging in other ways too. A comprehensive approach to helping women who smoke, drink, or use illicit drugs through pregnancy is important (Raskin, 1993).

In terms of disease progress, pregnancy itself not uncommonly provides a more stable phase for women with some pre-existing mental disorders. For mothers with bipolar or schizo-affective illness, the disorder may go into remission (Marks et al., 1992). This may be particularly fortunate, because lithium is among therapeutic drugs of concern with respect to foetal abnormality. Although the incidence is less than 5 per cent (Rubin, 1995), the cardiac abnormalities reported are severe (Weinstein and Goldfield, 1975), and the drug best avoided in the first trimester of pregnancy at least. There is similarly little risk of exacerbation of other established affective disorder (e.g. Kumar, 1982), and the risk of suicide appears to be exceptionally low, with a standardized mortality ratio of 0.05 (Appleby, 1991).

In spite of the received wisdom of avoiding as far as possible any drugs during pregnancy, there is little evidence that tricyclic antidepressants harm the foetus although, in common with many other drugs, maternal require-ments may change considerably in the various stages of the pregnancy (Wisner et al., 1993), as the mother's metabolism and clearance changes, particularly with changes in blood circulation. Phenothiazines, like chlorpro-mazine, and butyrophenones, like haloperidol, appear to be safe in terms of foetal development (Slone et al., 1977), although may produce toxic effects in the newborn (O'Connor et al., 1981). Very little is known in this regard about psychotropic medication with which there is shorter experience, including clozapine for schizophrenia and the truly newer antipsychotics, and newer antidepressants including the serotonin specific re-uptake inhibitors (SSRIs). Some drugs for the treatment of epilepsy have a small but definitely increased risk of causing foetal abnormalities, but the risks of damage to the central nervous system can be limited, where counselling of potential mothers and such planning allows, by giving folic acid before conception, and any bleeding disorders averted in the newborn by giving vitamin K immediately after delivery. Occasionally in these circumstances, the new born baby may be liable to withdrawal fits, but these and any irritability, also a form of withdrawal state, are short term problems. *The Prescribers' Journal* has run a useful series of articles on the management of a wide range of physical and psychiatric disorders during pregnancy (starting with Rubin, 1996).

There is little specific knowledge about women with personality disorders during pregnancy. It is true that many of the points about lifestyle, substance misuse and even prescribed medication may apply, but almost all information seems to be about likely associated problems. Eating disorders may worsen

(Fahy and O'Donoghue, 1991) and present problems both at delivery (Fahy and Morrison, 1993) and in looking after the new baby (Stein *et al.*, 1994).

Pregnancy in a security setting

No record has been traced of a pregnancy conceived in a special hospital. There seems little doubt, though, that the Victorians were ready for the arrival of a pregnant woman, if not a conception, on the evidence of the infant's cradle now in the Broadmoor hospital museum. It is certainly realistic to consider that pregnancy may occur, and to recognize that merely forbidding the necessary relationships and supervising meetings between men and women carries no certainty of prevention. Fortunately, with the more open discussions of sexuality and relationships in a special hospital, it is now possible to make contingency plans for the possibility of pregnancy in a constructive way.

Within a special hospital, other secure hospital or prison, the possibility of a pregnancy is properly a matter of concern and anxiety for all involved. Acknowledgement of it makes explicit what is covert, that even within secure institutions there are opportunities for sexual intercourse, whether by consent or assault. Other staff anxieties follow – if sexual activity cannot be prevented, what other, even more serious acts are not preventable, for example a homicide? There are issues of professional and managerial responsibility and disciplinary action which could follow any incident. Staff may be afraid to disclose awareness of an activity if their observations come too late for primary preventive action. If they cannot be reassured in this area, then other important action may not be taken or not taken soon enough. Other concerns involve lack of direction and knowledge about the most appropriate actions. In the absence of informed policies, management, at all levels, can similarly be pressured into actions which are contrary to the health of mother or prospective child.

The media see it as a matter of public interest that a woman could become pregnant in a special hospital. Perhaps such matters should properly be in the public domain, but the manner of presentation should reflect that and that alone, rather than the identity and details of the woman, or indeed the putative father. No discussion of work in this area can or should overlook the nature of interest that may be generated, the possibility of distortion or condemnation from some areas of the outside community, and even Government pressure. Returning to the more personal levels, media involvement can bring at the least hours of extra work for staff. They have to work through the exposure not only with the alleged prospective parents, but also their relatives, who may have just heard the 'news' through a tabloid megaphone.

After the major concerns about security, anxieties among the professional staff focus on other management issues. There is a serious concern that, if established, pregnancy in the hospital could become desirable or 'fashionable'. The attention necessarily paid to the woman, additional services and possible flexibility in care or her transfer elsewhere may be considered as privileges attractive to other patients. The fact of such a pregnancy could exacerbate delusional systems among others with a psychosis, which sometimes include delusions about pregnancy and often bizarre pregnancies; a real pregnancy might also create pathological jealousies, or ordinary envy among women already separated from children or unable to see them? Could it arouse morbid maternal instincts, intensifying the risk of self-harm, assault from others, or both? This list is far from exhaustive. Any woman who becomes pregnant would be entitled to have her circumstances dealt with in the best interests of herself and any child. To take actions only to ensure a deterrent effect on other patients would be unacceptable. If a woman would best moved elsewhere, then that must be a matter for professional judgement in the light of all circumstances. The actual birth would be in a specialist unit in a general obstetric hospital.

The management structure is caught within a not unfamiliar dilemma, the extent to which it must set up a truly specialist service given the rarity of the event. If past history were really the best predictor of future events, a special hospital need not bother at all, and secure units very rarely. Prisons do more commonly receive pregnant women. In England and Wales, approximately 3 per cent of the women in prison are thought to be pregnant at any one time, and during 1995–6, 64 babies were born to women prisoners (Howard League, 1997 report of answer to a Parliamentary question, 28 Feb 1997). The question must arise as to whether, if imprisonment is unavoidable for the mother to be, provision should necessarily be within the regular prison service.

In England and Wales, most pregnant women in prison remain in ordinary locations there and, although the Prison Service is committed to the principle that pregnant prisoners should have access to the same quality of antenatal and other appropriate health care as women in the community, in practice this has not yet been achieved (Department of Health, 1997). Prison protocols, which do not seem to be applied consistently across the country, variously provide for women to have access to local health authority services, antenatal classes, extra milk and/or vitamin rations, relief from certain kinds of duties and shared accommodation (if not already in it) during the final weeks of the pregnancy. Public rows about the shackling of pregnant prisoners when attending local hospitals for antenatal assessments and/or the delivery itself at last seem to have been effective in limiting if not barring the practice altogether.

The Howard League (1997) suggests that imprisonment should be prohibited for pregnant women. Whether or not that is a practical suggestion, they point out that there is a precedent for according pregnant women special legal status. The Sentence to Death (Expectant Mothers) Act 1931 provided that pregnant women convicted of murder (for which the death penalty then applied in England and Wales) had to be sentenced to life imprisonment.

In a secure hospital, additional, immediate areas which must be addressed if a pregnancy is suspected include: competency and consent for the various procedures necessary to safeguard a healthy pregnancy and delivery, more rarely a termination; almost always some adjustment in general treatment measures for mental or other health disorders; pregnancy testing; review of existing medication; optimal placement; the male partner; family outside the hospital; and external agencies (in England, specifically informing the Mental Health Act Commission in the case of a patient compulsorily detained in hospital). In these circumstances, the involvement of the woman's legal advisor is inevitable, and for women in other vulnerable circumstances, such as in prison, it is advisable in view of the issues involved.

Mental disorder and the postnatal period

There is almost nothing to be said about immediate postnatal maternal health that is specific to the position of mothers in security hospitals, partly because the birth of a baby is such a rare event for them during this time. It has not been recorded at all in high security in the UK, and hardly at all in specialist medium secure units. Nevertheless, a brief review of the issues more generally may be of use, and could in any event apply as well to some of the slightly larger group of women who deliver in prison.

For any new mother, lability of mood is usual. Commonly, there is a pattern of crying spells a few hours after the birth, recurring between the third and fifth postpartum day, often with some irritability, but alternating with intense pleasure in the new baby. As a self-limiting, short-lived and very frequent state, it is generally regarded as normal (for a more extended review, see Stein, 1982).

Depression requiring treatment is relatively unusual but, compared with other women of similar age, the risk is elevated for mothers within the first 3 months of delivery, to a prevalence rate of about 10 per cent (Cooper et al., 1988). Adverse social factors seem to have an important but probably complex relationship with this sort of postpartum illness. Lack of a close confiding relationship, major life events and early maternal loss are among these factors combined with uncertainty about the child's future or the prospect of early separation (Stein, 1995). This may mean that women who give birth in an institution may be exceptionally vulnerable to such depressive illness. Beyond the distress of the mother herself, there is special concern for the infant in these circumstances, on two counts. Depressed, morbid thoughts may result in relatively immediate harm to the baby, but also depressive mothers are generally less able to respond to their babies while depressed, and there is evidence that there may be long term delays in the cognitive and/or social development of these children (Kumar and Hipwell, 1994). Obsessional thoughts including recurring, intrusive thoughts of harming the baby are commonly resisted, and therefore relatively harmless to the child in any direct sense. Some, however, may seriously interfere with the mother's capacity to look after the baby (Stein, 1998).

Children under the age of 1 year are nevertheless in the age group, in the UK, at highest risk of dying by homicide, with a rate of 34 per million population compared with an average rate of 12 per million (Home Office, 1987) but in view of apparent risks, it is important to get the role of mental disorder in perspective. Most such children are killed by their mother (Gibson, 1975), but only just over one quarter of these are in association with a mental illness. In his series of 89 women who had killed their child at under 1 year old, d'Orban (1979) found a diagnosis of psychosis in 14 cases, and acute reactive depression or personality disorder with depression in another 10; up to a further 20 had a personality disorder without any evidence of accompanying illness at the time.

Given the institutional context of the discussion here, Stein's (1995) observations about one other group of women are of particular value, and the only other specific reference that we could find to mothers with a personality disorder:

'... pre-existing borderline features which become much more prominent after delivery. The main problems include a poor response to all the anti-depressants, impulsive behaviour in the form of overdoses, occasional child abuse, poor compliance with therapy, and an overdemanding abusive relationship with both spouse and therapists. For some of these women, the stress of looking after their baby seems to provoke hostility and depression, and so an early return to work may prove beneficial. These women often do poorly with medication, and require a high psychotherapeutic input, often from two or more therapists. They enter into repeated emotional and social crises, which the team should anticipate in their care plan.'

Puerperal psychosis is much less common than a non-psychotic depressive illness, with a frequency of about 2 per 1000 deliveries (Meltzer and Kumar, 1985). By contrast with non-psychotic depression, social factors seem to play little part in the aetiology of postpartum psychosis, although caesarean section, death of a baby around the time of delivery and single motherhood are associated with increased risk. There is thought to be some genetic predisposition, and certainly a history of previous psychiatric illness is important (Kendell *et al.*, 1987).

Treatment is principally of the predominant disorder presenting (see Stein, 1998), and the more affective psychoses tend to respond well to antidepressant medication or to ECT. Schizophrenic illness in this context at best tends to take longer to resolve, so decisions about child care may ideally be delayed to take account of this. A relapsing course of the illness, however, bodes ill for the mother–baby relationship. In a 5 to 10 year follow-up study of 17 subjects with a puerperal schizophrenia, two women committed suicide, six others made serious attempts to do so and many of the others were involved in serious child abuse or neglect. Only one of the mothers was still caring for her child and symptom free (Da Silva and Johnstone, 1981).

Mother and baby units

There are only a few highly regarded residential assessment and treatment units for parents (usually mothers) and their children (Royal College of Psychiatrists, 1992). They offer a high level of supervision and a range of specialist professionals. Such units are unknown in security hospitals, and it seems unlikely on present demand that there is a case for developing them. Insofar as it is necessary, however, for a new mother to remain in the security provided by a prison, it may be that consideration should be given to basing mother and baby in a purpose designed unit within or attached to a secure psychiatric hospital setting. There would be good arguments against this too in the absence of any psychiatric disorder on the part of the mother, and we make this observation only in the spirit of recognition that prison facilities in this regard are hardly satisfactory and stimulation of debate is needed about how to improve services for women and their babies if secure confinement of those women is truly unavoidable.

In ordinary psychiatric hospitals mother and baby units are to minimize the need to separate a baby from his or her mother when the mother has a serious psychiatric illness, to allow assessment of the mother–child relationship, and sometimes to assist the women to develop mothering skills that have not been impaired simply by the presence of a mental illness. The first recorded admission of a child to hospital because its mother needed treatment for a mental disorder was as recent as 1948, to the Cassel hospital in Surrey, England (Margison and Brockington, 1982). Specialist hospital inpatient units are needed only rarely, but they have proven to be safe and effective in their short term goals (Margison and Brockington, 1982), although expensive. This last may be a factor in the extreme rarity of such units outside the UK, Canada, Australia and New Zealand (Kumar, 1992). Research which would establish longer term consequences respectively of maintaining mother–child contact, or separating them during the mother's illness, has never been done (Kumar, 1992).

Although few women with a psychotic illness remain in prison, rates of other psychiatric disorders, especially substance abuse, are high among women prisoners (Gunn *et al.*, 1991). Thus, mother and baby units in prisons, which might at first sight be considered as having an entirely different function from those in psychiatric hospitals, should perhaps show some overlap in services.

> 'Pregnant women in prison face unique problems. Stress, environmental and legal restrictions, unhealthy behaviour and reduced or non-existent social support systems – all common among female inmates – have an even greater effect on pregnant inmates.'
>
> (Huft *et al.*, 1992)

The Prison Rules (1964) say that:

> 'The Secretary of State may ... permit a woman prisoner to have her baby with her in prison, and everything necessary for the baby's maintenance and care may be provided there.'
>
> (Rule 9(3))

A Howard League (1995) survey of women's prisons identified four mother and baby units – one at Holloway prison in London, two in closed prisons in the north of England and one in an open prison, near York. Between them they provided for a maximum of 68 places, more than in 1992 (Dillner, 1992), but less than half the estimated need. A 1992 Department of Health inspection of prison facilities for mothers and babies was very critical. The diet was poor, the children were looked after in crèches provided by other prisoners, untrained in child care, and there was no space for the babies to explore. Formal testing of the babies on the Griffiths Mental Development Scale showed that, as a group, those who had been in such a unit for under 4 months fell within normal limits for British babies (Catan, 1989). On comparison with babies of a similar age and background who remained with relatives during their mother's imprisonment, they showed no significant differences. Catan concluded that although there was thus no evidence that either a short stay in a prison nursery or a brief separation was in itself damaging to a pre-lingual child's development, thinking about child care in prisons must move beyond the goals of merely preventing harm and gross deprivation. This is an opportunity for important preventive work with a potentially troubled future generation.

Longer term outcome

The longer term pattern of care for a child born to a woman in hospital would be a matter for child care professionals, working as far as possible in partnership with the woman and any acknowledged putative father, the hospital and within the legal framework for the care and protection of children.

There is a considerable background literature on factors which put the longer term health and social development of children at risk. Longitudinal, prospective studies are the most powerful sources of data in this respect, but their interpretation for practice is difficult. Farrington (1993) reviewed the core group of large, multivariate studies of samples of children or adolescents followed for at least 5 years. They show considerable consistency in the kind of individual (genetic, pregnancy and birth related) factors, and family and wider social problems that are associated, for the groups, with development of delinquent behaviours and other social difficulties.

Rutter (1988) and Rutter and Madge (1976) variously consider the place of such research and of intergenerational carry over of disorder and disadvantage with more additional and specific reference to mental disorder. Mental disorders are heterogeneous in their cause and effect, and individual variations must always be taken into account in practice but, forced to generalize by the space here, one observation seems to stand out particularly – whether the potential disadvantage for the child lies in a parent's mental disorder, social context or both. It is those disorders or problems which directly affect the parent–child relationship rather than the disease or disorder *per se* that are more likely to create problems for the child, and therefore to need some active intervention. This is particularly true where conflict or discord is marked. Early studies showed that children of parents with neurotic, depressive or personality disorders tended to be more at risk for subsequent psychiatric problems of their own than those of a parent with schizophrenia (Rutter, 1966). Rutter *et al.* (1976) and Rutter and Quinton (1984) studied children of parents newly referred for assessment or treatment of psychiatric disorder. While nearly twice as many of the children of parents with disorder showed persistent emotional or behavioural problems compared to age and school matched controls, persistent family discord in this context, including marital conflict, was more important than diagnosis or symptomatology of the parents, especially when hostility or irritability were directed towards the child. Nevertheless, and related to this, there was a tendency for this to be most likely the case when the parental diagnosis was personality disorder.

It is vital to engage the assistance of relevant outside professionals from the earliest possible opportunity. These will include staff from obstetric services, social services, specialist perinatal services and maybe paediatric services. Postnatal care must include adequate contraceptive advice. The legal adviser of the woman patient and any male patient she acknowledges as the putative father should also be involved as far as possible.

It is common practice to accept legal advisors as surrogates or supporters of parents within child care practice, although it is important that they are not seen as substitutes for parents and their professional ethics are consistently recognized as different from those of clinicians. It is likely that the hospital and local authority practitioners would approach working in very different ways, therefore negotiations, openness and mutual recognition and respect are essential when a parent's rights and a child's welfare are involved.

Local authorities have specialist experience in advising women who may be a risk to their children; advising early may inform and support a woman considering termination. In the event a pregnancy continues, the local authority would need to be involved in planning and decisions in order to ensure protection of the child's interests and welfare. Local authorities would expect to work with a woman in order that she was able to carry out her responsibilities to a child as fully as possible. They do, in rare cases, remove a child or children from their mother at birth. This is, however, a distressing and difficult matter and requires thorough assessment and consideration of all possible options available. It is not inevitable in these circumstances that a mother would cease any ongoing relationship with her child.

Avoidance of conflict or distress for parent or child in the short term does not necessarily prevent it later, when it may be complicated by its early avoidance. Contemporaneous and accurate recording of assessments, discussion plans and decisions is essential. The formality of process ensures that roles and responsibilities are clear, as well as assuring later reference points. It would be foolish to ignore the possibility of future enquiry or litigation but, more importantly, the process is of great emotional significance and adjustment for the people involved.

A woman with a mental disorder living in a contained environment is not best placed for a healthy pregnancy. As a pregnancy proceeds the difficulties could be compounded by her knowledge that she would or might not have the care of her child. A woman's ability to make necessary adaptation to pregnancy may well be reduced. Except in the short term, the contained environment is likely to be harmful to her child once born, so residential placement for the child away from the mother is likely to be unavoidable if mother's stay has to continue. It is the ways in which this may best be managed if the mother's – or father's – continuing placement or detention in hospital or prison is unavoidable which needs careful consideration and about which we need greater knowledge.

Policy developments in the event of pregnancy in institutional settings for adults

Policies and procedures are underpinned by implicit principles, which may challenge previous practice, attitudes and prejudices. The following are suggested for discussion in the event of pregnancy but could be the principles which might form the basis of any such policy.

- Prevention of conception within a residential institutional setting is the most important goal. To this end the hostel/hospital/prison will generate policies and procedures which will be well known to residents/patients and staff alike.
- Staff vigilance for developing relationships – impulsive, short or long term – is essential, together with specific counselling for any couple so identified.
- Whatever the qualities of the setting, it is not possible when men and women have any contact at all to ensure that no pregnancy will be conceived.
- There is a basic duty of care to any prospective parent/patient.
- The health, safety and well-being of the potential mother is of primary concern.
- A hostel/hospital/prison has a duty to maintain a regime which meets individual needs while continuing to meet its wider responsibilities.
- The woman's right as far as possible to make informed decisions and give consent must be respected by all professional and non-professional staff working with the woman. To this end she should be involved where possible in all discussions and decisions. Attempts to involve her in these ways should

generally be made even when competence to decide is uncertain. Specialist advice for those with learning difficulty should be sought.

- No assumptions may be made about inevitability of outcome; all decisions should be information based.
- The woman should be encouraged to have early access to a legal advisor and to have that person with her or to represent her at any key meetings.
- All information, decisions and plans must be fully and accurately recorded at the time. As far as possible all relevant information must be verified in advance of each decision.
- The woman's right to confidentiality and privacy in respect of privileged information (medical and social) must be respected according to professional codes. Disclosure of identifiable information to the media or general public without patient/client and organizational agreement should be made a breach of the disciplinary code of the hospital, prison or other institution, regardless of professional status of the disclosing person.
- Until and unless it is established that a suspected pregnancy does not or has ceased to exist, the health and well-being of the expected baby must be taken into account at all time.
- Any named putative father should be offered sensitive support and advice, to include legal advice and specialist counselling if he so wishes.
- Except where a criminal offence may have occurred (rape, assault), if conception occurred within the institution, no disciplinary or punitive action should be taken against either male or female patients thought to be the prospective parents.
- Except where a criminal offence may have occurred, no disciplinary action will be taken against staff in respect of the pregnancy, but in all cases a confidential enquiry will be conducted by the mother's clinical team in conjunction with at least one fully independent, external advisor, and including such other staff as seem relevant. In the event of a criminal offence having occurred, disciplinary action cannot be ruled out.

Conclusions

Legislation will cover some of the actions taken during the progress of a pregnancy and its outcome. For the rest it is important that policies and procedures are set up to cover the major eventualities in advance of a pregnancy having to be managed. They must be subject to occasional routine review and special re-evaluation in the event of any change in law, evidence or experience. It may be necessary to prepare or have contingencies for specialized facilities. Actions based on assumption and prejudice constitute poor or unprofessional practice. Decisions should always be based on information, verified wherever possible, and as far as possible in conjunction with the mother and putative father. One of the areas of risk to good planning is in failing to accept or recognize the possibility of a pregnancy, whether this is failure of recognition on the part of the woman herself, staff or the hospital management.

Child care, whether as a result of a conception in the institutional setting, or more likely of children born prior to residency, must follow similar principles, but here the interests of each child are explicitly and legally paramount. Again, no particular pattern is inevitable, and there is evidence to suggest that, notwithstanding the difficulties and emotional traumas, most children and parents alike are more likely than not to benefit from maintenance of contact. The maintenance, or indeed termination, of such relationships, however, requires expert skills. This work with patients, offenders or offender patients needs much more research, particularly longitudinal research, and training of professionals of all disciplines informed by such work.

It is essential in all of this that the detrimental effects of delay are recognized, whilst not rushing into hasty or ill thought out actions.

10

Couples assessment

Conor Duggan

Preamble

In the preparation of the chapter, I became aware that there is little information available on assessing couples within a custodial setting. For instance, I was unable to find a single reference on the topic from a literature search using the APA Psych Lit program 1974–1994. In the absence of an established literature to guide us, the content of this chapter relies on an adaptation of current practice in non-forensic settings, but having some regard to the special circumstances of the institution (e.g. special hospital or prison) and the client group.

To an outsider, this absence of literature in such an important area must surely appear an anomaly, as an individual's capacity to form a relationship is an important part of a forensic evaluation. I believe that there are three reasons to explain this neglect. First, there is the perception of couples therapy itself. This has been described as the 'poor relation' of the psychotherapies (Ables and Brandsma, 1977), as it lags behind both individual and family therapy in terms of training and research. Second, the practice of successful couples therapy demands the integration of a number of different types of psychotherapy, yet any observer of the contemporary warfare among the psychotherapies cannot but be impressed by their fissiparous nature. Integration of different psychotherapies, then, is not an easy task. Third, there are issues which uniquely face the couples therapist in a forensic setting – issues such as serious aggression, violence, child abuse. Although these issues arise in other settings, they are the exception rather than the rule. Their presence places a heavy burden on a couples therapist in a forensic setting for the eventual welfare of those in the relationship or in the family; hence it is understandable that this is a responsibility which therapists would wish to avoid. There are good reasons, therefore, why this area has been neglected. If this volume results in us facing and discussing some of these difficulties, then perhaps one of the editors' objectives will be met.

Rationale

I have set out above the reasons why couples therapy in a forensic context is difficult; however, there are also some advantages. Although the therapist is now faced with trying to understand not one but *two* individuals and their interaction and while, on the surface, it appears more difficult to grasp the complex dynamics of two individuals, the couples therapist Robin Skynner believes the contrary, namely that '... it is much more difficult to understand and treat the individual in isolation' (Skynner, 1980).

To understand this startling statement, it is first necessary to digress and consider the importance of transference. The best description of transference and its implications that I have come across is that of Stratchey (1969) which is well worth reproducing in full:

'The original conflicts, which lead to the onset of the neurosis began to be re-enacted in relation to the analyst. Now this unexpected event is far from being the misfortune that at first sight it might seem to be. In fact it gives us our great opportunity. Instead of having to deal as best we may with conflicts of the remote past, which are concerned with dead circumstances and mummified personalities, and whose outcome is already determined, we find ourselves involved in an actual and immediate situation in which we and the patient are the principal characters and the development of which is to some extent at least under our control.'

(Stratchey, 1969)

Stratchey's essential point is that the '... actual and immediate situation ...' is not only a re-enactment of the original difficulty, but it also allows an opportunity of some new experiential learning; unfortunately, this 'great opportunity' requires a great deal of time for the development of transference with the analyst. It has been found in couples therapy (and in family therapy) that focusing on the relationship between the individuals rather than on the individuals themselves demonstrates the transferences which are already established between the couple and which can be witnessed acting together rather than through the repetition with the therapist. The result is that the therapy is more rapid and effective than individual work and this is a major consideration where the need is great and resources scarce.

Skynner (1975), however, has identified an additional reason which I believe is of particular interest for those who work with offenders. He writes:

'When one sees members of a couple separately, it is much more difficult to avoid being manipulated and placed in the role of judge, supporter or persecutor. This is partly because it is far more difficult to get at the truth about a real relationship, which is often blatantly obvious after fifteen minutes of watching a couple interact before one's eyes rather than listening to their prepared and carefully edited accounts.'

Working with couples provides us, therefore, with the opportunity of experiencing how two individuals interact with one another *in vivo* rather than being told how this occurs by one of the individuals who is likely to be partisan. Finally, couples therapists believe that this unit (and the same applies to a family) possesses adaptive and self-corrective powers of its own which will do much of the therapy, the therapist acting as a facilitator (see also Hodge and Kruppa, this volume).

Good qualities of relationships

In the assessment of a couple, the therapist(s) will have particular regard to the patterns of interaction within healthy relationships which will act as a comparator. Healthy relationships are personified by a pattern of interaction which is congruent with reality, where communication is clear and direct and where boundaries are sharply drawn and non-invasive. In contrast, poor relationships are characterized by reality being denied, with escape into fantasy, where communication is vague and evasive and where boundaries are blurred (Lewis *et al.*, 1976). The bedrock of a healthy relationship, then, is where there is a secure and well defined identity which allows both separateness and intimacy between the individuals in a couple. Further, in a healthy relationship, there is a strong equally powered parental coalition with clear boundaries between the parents and the children. Thus the task of the therapist is to:

1. Enable the couple to communicate more effectively.
2. Change the structure so that the couple negotiates and resolves conflicts rather than each have their own way through coercion or manipulation.
3. Enable the couple to have a trusting and open relationship rather than one which is based on mistrust and fear.
4. Facilitate growth and differentiation of each individual so that '... they need one another less so that they can enjoy one another more' (Skynner, 1980).

As indicated above, three different psychotherapeutic traditions have contributed to our understanding of the formation of a relationship and its vicissitudes. The important contribution from dynamic therapies (the 'object relations' school in particular) is that marital partners somehow choose one another on the basis of the 'fit' of their projective systems. Thus each partner has a role in supporting the mutual projective and introjective process of the other and avoid its recognition. Research has demonstrated that difficult relationships have as their basis a failure of the couple to outgrow their parental attachments, so that the partner is not seen as how he/she truly is, but as a vehicle for a projected internalized parental image (Dicks, 1985). This explains why it is that vulnerable individuals continue to repeat not only the damaging features of earlier parental relationships in their own choice of a partner, but also why they find it difficult to separate from a non-viable relationship, viz

> 'Sometimes each partner will keep his or her own ghostly persecutor safely contained within the spouse, with inevitable mutual rejection and attack as well as equally inevitable inability to separate.'
>
> (Skynner, 1975).

These 'ghostly persecutors' (in the form of parental images) have a particular resonance for the couples therapist in a forensic context, as the couples' parents' own lives have been blighted by unhappiness, resulting in difficulties in treatment.

> 'No obstacle in the treatment is more powerful than the taboo on accepting happiness denied to (or rejected by) one's parents.'
>
> (Skynner, 1980)

The therapist may have to allow him/herself to be part of the system to the extent that on occasion he/she will be at the end of these projections. This allows for these to be corrected by the therapist, either by interpretation or by modelling a different response to that which is anticipated. One of the difficulties in the assessment is how much attention should one pay to the earlier history in order to gain an understanding of these internalized 'objects'?

A second important strand in treating marital relationships comes from the behavioural tradition, with its emphasis on maladaptive learning (Jacobson and Margolin, 1979; O'Leary and Turkewitz, 1978). This has considerable appeal, with its focus on the immediate here and now behaviour, with some clear guidelines about how change might be effected so that its essentials can be learnt relatively easily by the beginner. An additional advantage is that it attempts to measure its impact and hence is able to assess the efficacy of a particular intervention.

The third important tradition contributing to couples therapy is systems theory, with its origins firmly based in family therapy. The kernel of this approach is that the system whole (i.e. the couple in this discussion) is more than the sum of the individual parts (the individual partners) and that this system has a stability which is difficult to alter by dealing with only one of the components. A very good illustration of how a dysfunctional system is maintained comes from the system therapists Watzlawick *et al.* (1974):

> 'two sailors hanging out of either side of a sailboat in order to steady it: the more the one leans overboard, the more the other has to hang out to compensate for the instability caused by the other's attempts at stabilizing the boat, while the boat itself would be quite steady if not for their acrobatic effort at steadying it. It is not difficult to see that in order to change this absurd situation, at least one of them has to do something quite unreasonable, to 'steady' less and not more, since this will immediately force the other to also do less of the same (unless he wants to finish up in the water), and they may eventually find themselves comfortably back inside a steady boat.'

The importance of this perspective for the couples therapist lies in (1) that a small change in a sensitive area may have significant effects throughout the entire system and (2) an understanding of resistance. Although dealing with resistance is more an issue for later in the therapy rather than for the assessment, nevertheless, it is helpful to view the couple even at the assessment stage as a system with the 'problem', which both causes them to come for help and resists change at one and the same time.

I believe that it is essential that the couples therapist keeps all of these modes of thought in his/her mind in dealing with a couple. The dynamic issue will help an understanding of the 'why' question. The behavioural and systems approach will inform 'how' the difficulty is maintained and what might be done to change it, with the latter being especially effective in dealing with resistance to change within the system.

Principles of assessment

Thus, what I set out hereunder is what a 'couples therapist' would do in making an assessment in an outpatient or office setting, but having regard for some of the issues that would emerge when working with offenders. I am also making the assumption that the individual(s) who are making the assessment will also be conducting the treatment; hence the latter part of the assessment is focused on changing the relationship, and thereby giving the couple early on a sense of achievement and success which will cement the therapeutic alliance. An early intervention at this point may be alarming to some who view the collection of a significant amount of data as essential before attempting to make changes.

An early intervention in couples therapy is important for the following reasons. First, many couples do not persist with the treatment, hence if something needs to be done, it has to be done early. Second, gains in couples therapy are known to occur early in the treatment (Crowe, 1978). Third, an early intervention makes it clear to the couple early on that the responsibility of changing their relationship is theirs and theirs alone, with some secondary help from the therapist. Fourth, and most important, there is an emphasis that many of these interventions are based on conjecture, so that they too are subject to change depending on the subsequent material which emerges. Hence the assessment and the intervention alternate with one another so that, for instance, in the event of an intervention not working, further assessment may be necessary before the next intervention, and so on. This sense of being able to change and adapt as new information becomes available is an important modelling process for the couple to observe.

In the assessment which follows, there is a strong behavioural element. However, there is also some attention to the underlying dynamics of the couple which should inform the therapist's thinking and understanding but which may not necessarily play a large role in the intervention. Finally, although systemic thinking is more part of a later stage of the treatment, it too may have a role in assessment with the use of circular questioning and decentering (see below).

I am aware that I have laid out the assessment process in a rather cook-book fashion, presuming that the person for whom this is written is a beginner without a great deal of experience. If this offends the sensibilities of the more experienced, then I ask for their indulgence. I would strongly recommend Crowe and Ridley's excellent *Therapy with Couples* (1990), which is based on a behavioural systems approach and has been very helpful to my own thinking.

Process of assessment

Source of referral

It is important to realize that the process of assessment begins before the couple are ever seen, given that the couple will often be referred by someone else in the clinical team. Hence, a number of questions will need to be considered by the assessor. First, have the couple been prepared for treatment as a couple? By this I mean, is it acknowledged by the referrer (or those who self-refer) that the couples therapist will see the presentation as a relationship problem rather than primarily the treatment of one member of the couple? Here the pre-therapy of preparing the couple for the assessment is extremely important. It has come as a surprise to me how casual some referrers are in suggesting an alternative or additional psychotherapeutic approach. If the referral is taken seriously by the referrer, then there is a greater chance that the couple too will take it seriously. There is always a considerable amount of ambivalence about being in therapy:

'When couples come in for marital therapy, just as with other types of therapy, they are ambivalent about wanting help. While they may want their problems to disappear magically, they may not want to go through the effort required to make the relationship better.'

(Margolin, 1987)

What the therapist wants is for the couple to feel better after having changed, while the couple want to feel better without having to change. The referrer may well feed into this ambivalence unless the couple are adequately prepared prior to referral.

Further evidence of the importance of the referral comes from research conducted by Crowe (1978). He showed that the source of the referral had an important effect on prognosis, with couples referred by general practitioners doing better than those from psychiatrists. This may have been due to the psychiatrists referring more difficult cases; Crowe (ibid.), however argues that the reasons may have been that the labelling of the problems as psychiatric (by the psychiatrist) made it more difficult for the couple to accept the reframing of the problem as a relationship issue.

Additional history

Many workers in this field (e.g. Crowe and Ridley, 1990) suggest that historical data be gathered *from both partners* in the form of a questionnaire prior to the first assessment. This is done so that the interview can concentrate on the pattern of interaction without being distracted by the need to acquire additional history in the first interview. It also subtly conveys to the couple that they are both coming for treatment, and not the one with the label of being a patient with the problem. This also has the advantage in a custodial setting that the index offence does not become the entire focus of the session. In working with serious offenders again, however, the assessor clearly needs to keep the offence in mind in making the assessment (see below).

Crowe and Ridley (1990) also propose that a hypothesis is formulated before the couple are seen (i.e. on the basis of the referral and response to the questionnaire information), arguing that this gives a focus to the subsequent assessment. Others may feel uncomfortable with this approach, believing that it makes unwarranted assumptions about individuals who are yet unseen. If this approach is adopted, it is essential that it is not taken too rigidly; i.e. one should see the process as essentially speculative – 'I wonder if ...' rather than 'I believe that ...' – so that the hypotheses are subject to iterative change with continuous input from the process of the therapy.

The interview

I believe that it is helpful to consider the initial assessment interview as having the following four stages: (1) initial phase of establishing rapport;(2) detailed examination of the 'problem'; (c) brief details about the couple's past, which is followed by a short break; (d) an initial formulation, which is shared with the couple, followed by discussion of homework for the next session and termination.

The beginning

Here the essential task for the therapist is to develop a positive relationship with *both* the partners, giving each a sense that he/she is being listened to and that one has the interests of both the parties equally at heart. At a later stage in the treatment, it may be desirable to side with one or other partner temporarily to move the more resistant partner on, but this is only after a sense of trust with both parties has been established. At the beginning it is crucial that both parties feel that they are being given equal attention. This is especially difficult if one of them is ostensibly the 'patient' with a problem – e.g. alcoholism, violence – which the other partner wishes the therapist to deal with.

The problem

The next stage of the interview concerns getting details of the complaint and as much information as possible surrounding it. Throughout, the emphasis must be on the members of the couple being responsible for informing the therapist of their difficulty – that is their role. It is essential for the therapist to insist on specific detail and to remain focused on the problem: '... The more such detail is insisted upon, the more the couple must necessarily move from the realm of the imagination, disagreement, argument and mutual blaming to the realm of fact and agreement, since the demand for increasing detail and specific examples makes this inevitable' (Skynner, 1980). This continual focus on the specifics of the problem from both sides needs to continue until some definite pattern of interaction emerges in the assessment.

There is a tendency in much forensic work to focus on the past, and past failures in particular; here, the therapist is advised to 'stay in the present' and examine the current pattern of interaction. Again there is a balance to be reached here between taking the individual's concern seriously and thereby engaging them in the therapy, and trying to direct the focus away from the individual problem and make it an interactional issue.

Initially the interaction will be between each member of the couple and the therapist. After a brief period, however, the therapist must move the focus away from him/herself to the couple so that this becomes a shared problem between the couple rather than between each individual member and the therapist. A number of specific techniques may be used in order to emphasize that what is important is the relationship between the couple. *Decentering* is one technique which facilitates this change. Decentering involves the therapist insisting that the couple talk to one another about the issue rather than to the therapist, so that the therapist becomes an observer. In order for this to be made more manifest, the therapist insists that the couple turn the direction of their chairs toward one another and insists that each one tells the other how he/she construes the problem.

This change of direction enables the therapist to fulfil another important function, namely to observe the pattern of communication between the couple on the premise that the way in which the couple communicate in the session is very much the same way that they communicate outside. One of the assumptions of the therapist is that communication may be impaired – the couples therapist therefore is as interested in 'how' something is said as to 'what' is said. Hence, observation from the very beginning is important. Who takes the lead? Who speaks to whom? When asked to turn their chairs to one another, who takes the lead?, and so on.

Non-verbal exchanges are often very important and may be a real clue as to what is going on. However, as Crowe and Ridley (1990) point out, these observations of non-verbal behaviour are often very unreliable and need to be checked out constantly to see if they are accurate. This has the dual function not only of establishing the veracity of the therapist's conclusion, but as importantly provides an opportunity to model the tentative nature of the understanding for the couple and how important it is to test out one's assumptions with the other partner.

Another technique which helps focus the couple on the relationship is *circular questioning* (Selvini-Palazzoli *et al.*, 1980). The idea here is to ask one of the partners to describe the behaviour of the other during some difficulty – i.e. rather than asking what did you do when X happened, the therapist asks the interviewee to describe the behaviour of the other partner and then in turn asks the latter to describe the behaviour of the first partner, and so on.

The Milan family therapists, the originators of this method, became aware that circular questions were more than a means of gathering information – they were a therapeutic tool in themselves (Slovik and Griffit, 1992). This is another example of how artificial is the distinction between assessment and treatment in this area. Karl Tomm (1987) has extended this work further into what he terms circular and reflective questions. These are designed to enable the individual to be an observer of his/her own behaviour so that his/her links are recognized in the ongoing pattern. A typical example of a circular and reflective question might be: 'What do you do when he feels criticized and withdraws?' Another useful reflective question is the future orientated question, which is designed to help the couple break out of the present-bound monologue so they are projected into the future with the possibility of alternative behaviours for the present. The future orientated question has a particular resonance for a couple because they are confronted by their present unhappiness continuing indefinitely. The idea behind these questions is to mobilize the problem solving skills of the individuals in the couple by the couple reflecting on their current perceptions and behaviour, and to consider new options (Tomm, 1987). Here again, it is more important to concentrate on whether the couple can entertain the possibility of the situation being different rather than the exact content of the answers.

This attempt to talk about the problem between themselves will often recreate the presenting problem established in the therapist's mind, by the same problem of endless and bitter recrimination which is at the kernel of therapist inquiry about the backgrounds of the individuals. There is a fine judgement to be made as to when to intervene at this stage. Too early an intervention will take the responsibility away from the couple and reduce the capacity to see the pattern. Intervening too late may well leave both individuals so upset that they will be unable to engage in anything constructive for the rest of the session.

Details from the couple's past
Some of the steam may be taken out of the session at this point, once the presenting problem has been established in the therapist's mind, by the therapist inquiring into the backgrounds of the individuals. This needs to be kept brief but may be as illuminating about what is omitted as what is declared. Within a forensic context, the therapist will find many individuals who will have been victims themselves of abusive relationships going back to childhood. To what

extent should these experiences be used as mitigating factors in avoiding the commitment to the current relationship?

Having obtained some information about the background of both members of the couple, the therapist requests a break with some time to collect his/her thoughts and perhaps to discuss them with colleagues.

Break in interviewing
Many couple and family therapists use a one-way mirror so that a group not only observes the interaction between the individuals in the couple relationship, but also the interaction between the therapist and the couple. The team may then intervene by telephone during a session and suggest an alternative approach or another area to be explored if it believes that some alteration is required. Options may be evident to the team and not to the therapist because they are not faced directly by the couple and the need to interact with it.

A break in the session therefore provides the therapist with an opportunity of discussing the earlier part of the session with colleagues, share multiple perspectives and attempt to come up with some formulation. The need to resolve these differences, generated by the multiple perspectives on the couple's difficulties by the team, replicates the task of the couple, hence the viability of this exercise.

There has been an interesting recent development which has increased the utility of this exercise whereby the one-way mirror has become a two-way mirror – with the couple or the family now observing the therapist and team discussing their perception of its difficulties. For this to be effective, the ideas of the team should be couched in speculative terms (I wonder if . . . I had a feeling that . . .). The important point is to float possibilities in the knowledge that some of the material may be acceptable to the couple, whereas other material will be rejected. Then the therapy turns back to the couple, who are asked if any of this was useful and the therapy continues with the team again acting as observers (Anderson, 1987).

The idea of having a couple act as a 'fly on the wall' and listen into our discourse about them is novel and perhaps even threatening; in some cases at least, it may be very useful. I took part in a case conference recently where it was clear there was a significant split in the team in their evaluation of a particular patient, with some viewing the patient in a very favourable light, and others seeing her very negatively. The response to those with a negative reaction from the 'opposition' was to explain away her behaviour as either being caused by an understandable response to the constraints of the institution and partly by the lack of understanding by the staff concerned. Conversely, those with a positive view of the patient were believed by the alternative camp to have been duped and credulous. What usually transpires in these situations is that the patient is invited in at the end of the discussion and given the conclusion, whereas what is really important is that she should observe the process so that she becomes aware that she has these two sides. While this discussion was going on, I observed the patient outside the room – it was unclear whether or not she could hear what was going on. What I thought would be valuable was for the patient to sit in on the discussion and hear both sides of her problem. With the clinical team's agreement this was what was done and the debate continued in her presence. The important message for her to hear was that there were these two sides to her and the task for her (and for the clinical team) was to integrate these two parts of herself. Clearly, this needs a great deal of good will and trust on both sides, but it does seem anomalous that on the one hand we expect patients to be completely open with us while, on the other, we need not observe the same obligation on ourselves.

I realize that the provision of a one-way screen on the other side of which is a team with expertise is beyond the scope of many for whom this book is intended, where resources are extremely scarce. However, because of the complex nature of the task of the couples therapist with multiple perspectives, and the possibility of being pulled into one camp or the other however one may fight against it, I believe that to discuss the initial part of the assessment with a colleague during the break is extremely valuable and if both are working with different couples, then each can discuss the other's case. The purpose of the break, then, is to see if one's earlier hypotheses have been confirmed by the assessment interview, to come up with some tentative formulation and to think about setting the first homework task.

Resumption of the assessment interview

There are a number of tasks for the therapist in this second part of the assessment process. First, since many couples will have been demoralized by constant bitter recriminations, it is important to combat this by congratulating the couple for seeking help for their difficulties. Second, a tentative formulation of their problem in terms of difficulties in their relationship may be shared by the therapist. Third, is treatment to be offered and if so, will the couple take it up?

If what is on offer is acceptable, the therapist should immediately move on to the fourth stage, which is the setting of a home work task for the couple. The focus on a particular problem earlier on should lead to the identification of a specific difficulty which, with the therapist's help, the couple should now be encouraged to tackle. This early introduction of homework is important as it will clarify how much motivation the couple has for short-term work. It will also indicate that the responsibility for success rests with them rather than with the therapist. Difficulties that might be anticipated with the homework should be discussed and remedies sought during the session. The time and place for the next session (usually within 1–2 weeks although subsequent sessions can be at longer intervals) should be decided.

Homework

The choice of the homework task will obviously emerge from the earlier assessment and which level of intervention is appropriate. Crowe and Ridley's Alternative Levels of Intervention (ALI) hierarchy is very useful in identifying where the intervention should be made. I will discuss briefly the simplest intervention – reciprocity negotiation, which is often the starting point and concludes the assessment session.

The idea here is that one of the partners makes a request to which the other responds and an agreement is reached after some negotiation. This is followed by the second partner making a request to the first partner and again negotiation takes place. The key to success here is that there should be a focus on a few (or perhaps only one) simple and specific tasks that are observable and achievable. Thus, a member of the couple may make a request that their partner should spend more time talking – usually with her. This would not be an acceptable task as it is too vague, whereas 'I would like my partner to spend 20 minutes discussing what he/she has done during the day on returning from work' would be more satisfactory. Again, the request for more and more detail will demonstrate the resistance on the part of the individual making the request, e.g. 'It's all very well making this request, but I know it won't work'. Comments such as these need to be taken up immediately as they are an opportunity for pointing out some of the difficulties in the relationship. However, instead of blaming the individual concerned, the intervention needs to be framed so that the other individual, if possible, can help the cynical partner to do better.

Summary of the assessment process

1. See the partners conjointly
2. Put the responsibility for informing the therapist firmly with the couple
3. Be specific – this is often very useful in demonstrating resistances
4. Keep the topic of conversation focused on the present or the future
5. Phrase requests in terms of positive change
6. Aim for some change in the pattern of interaction early in the treatment.

Issues special to assessing couples in a secure setting

The assessment process set out above contains nothing that one would not find in an office or outpatient setting, and therefore its relevance to a forensic context may be questioned. Indeed, I have kept the format of this assessment close to the mainstream deliberately, as I wish to make the point that offenders should be assessed as one would assess other couples. However, there are certain issues which are specific to this context and it would be foolish indeed to ignore them although I regard these as additional considerations to those that I have already discussed.

1. The first difficulty is that the contact between the partners may be very limited if one of them is, say, in prison or in a special hospital and the other is outside the secure institution. Hence, issues such as prescribing homework and other tasks which necessitate a degree of sustained contact may seem fanciful. Indeed even the notion of a conjoint assessment may be difficult and expensive if extensive travelling is involved. To counter this, I would argue from the above that a conjoint interview may be especially illuminating and well worth conducting, as it will highlight the need for a subsequent intervention even if this has to be delayed until after the individual is released.

2. The second difficulty arises from the focus within couples therapy on the relationship rather than the problem behaviour in one of the parties. This creates two difficulties:
    (a) It may be difficult to reframe the couple's problem in terms of a relationship issue when the problem behaviour in one of them is objectively so serious. This particularly applies when the boundary between fantasy and reality has been breached, resulting in a killing or sexual exploitation. For instance, a woman with young children wishes to have a relationship with a man who has a history of paedophilia. How much attention should

be given to the relationship rather than to the individual with the problematic history?

(b) The second problem is that it may not be possible to discount the individual behaviour and focus on the relationship if, for example, violence has occurred in the past and is likely to re-occur. The question, therefore, is how much attention should be given to the problem behaviour? Not to discuss it at all would seem wilfully avoidant. Conversely, to make that the only issue of the couple's current difficulty may lead one to miss out on some very important relationship issues. Judging where the middle ground lies between these two alternatives is not easy. Murray Cox (1974) gave the following very sound advice in dealing with this difficulty: 'It is an equal mistake for the offender never to talk about their crime as it is to talk *only* about their crime'.

An additional issue to consider here is to what extent should the various parties have knowledge of the other individual's offences? To what degree is the therapist obliged to take these into account? How does the therapist cope with this information? A child-like female patient becomes engaged to another patient with a history of paedophilia. He does not disclose this background information and she does not inquire. How does the therapist deal with this dilemma?

3. The third difficulty is caused by taking a circular rather than a linear explanation for the problem (as advocated by the systems theorists) and applying it to a forensic context. This focuses on complementarity and on the reciprocal elements which exist in a relationship and assumes that everyone participates in a mutual causal pattern of behaviour which resulted perhaps in the violent episode (Hoffman *et al.*, 1990). Hence there is a de-emphasis on power, and feminists in particular vociferously object to this when it is applied to the relationship between men and women, claiming that this view ignores the power of men, who are physically stronger, and the vulnerability of women. The same argument would apply to adults who physically abuse or sexually exploit children. One advantage of the systems approach, however, in such cases is that the 'system' can be extended to encompass other agencies as necessary so that within this larger 'system' sufficient safeguards may be built in, especially if there is evidence of violence or concern about the welfare of the children.

The other issue which may create additional concerns for the couples therapist working within a forensic context is that unlike many other settings, a therapist seeing a couple in this context can anticipate that reports on the progress of the treatment will be required by outside agencies and that these reports may have a considerable bearing on whether a relationship is permitted at all. The therapist will have to consider then to what extent he/she is an agent of the authority (or is seen to be so by those in therapy), the mechanism of reporting and who will have access to the reports.

At the present state of knowledge in treating couples in a custodial setting, it is clear that it is easier to raise these questions rather than provide answers. I believe that the foundations have been laid in non-custodial settings to allow us to take those basic ideas and move forward. However, it is also clear that the application of these ideas in a custodial setting will require their development and that this will only come from practitioners who have direct experience in dealing with couples in custody. In as much as many of these questions also trouble the therapist in non-custodial settings, I believe that the therapist in a forensic setting will have a great deal to teach their colleagues who practice with clients in less adverse circumstances.

11

Managing relationships

Tom Swan and Pamela J. Taylor

Climate

The leading article in the May 1992 edition of *The Chronicle*, the magazine written for patients by patients at Broadmoor Hospital, was entitled 'Can I kiss you?'. The discussion outlined within this article was not, as may have been expected, about the question of whether or not patients within the walls of Broadmoor should be allowed to develop intimate sexual encounters. Rather, the author asserted that sexual activity takes place with frequent regularity within its confines, that this is 'usually undetected', and that 'no one sees it take place so no one is offended'. There is an interesting parallel here with the report from Valkenberg Hospital in South Africa (Kaliski *et al.*, 1994), in which staff and patients had claimed that sexual activities between male patients were widely prevalent there, *but* the vast majority had never observed it for themselves and only a minority believed it occurred on their own wards. The real prevalence of sexual behaviour and erotic attachments in institutions remains a mystery.

The Chronicle article was nevertheless important, mainly for challenging the management of Broadmoor, and indeed any other hospital, to take a more responsible role with regard to relationships. The author further cemented this proposal by asking, 'is it not time that such relationships should be expressed in the open without fear of ridicule or disciplinary action?'

At worst, there can be quite a strong moral repugnance attached to the idea of people who are sick even being interested in the notion of sexual or emotional enjoyment. At best, staff tend to take on the role of restrictive parents, infantilizing patients, with the notion that people suffering from a mental health problem are necessarily sexually 'innocent'. Fears and affronted morality are compounded if the individuals concerned have been dangerous in the past, particularly if this danger has been expressed in relation to their emotional or sexual attachments. There is thought to be quite a strong resistance among the general public and even some health professionals to the notion that such a person should have access to anything nice, particularly something as nice as someone who is fond of them, someone to cuddle, or indeed someone to have sex with. An apparent need to punish these individuals and prevent them from having ordinary pleasures can place a tremendous amount of pressure on the management of any institution wishing to develop safe and responsible policies.

Opinions and influences external to hospitals – and to prisons – cannot be ignored in developing policies. Some require damage limitation exercises, some might usefully inform policy. The mass media, including newspapers, radio and television can be wonderful educational tools – in this area too (e.g. O'Sullivan, 1992). Informed discussion in this context can also be constructive. The ability to present complex concepts simply is undoubtedly a skill, and one that can perhaps be best learned from good journalists. Other tasks, like choice of time and journalist for disclosure of innovative policy or its orchestrated defence, may be more serendipitous.

In less positive mode, irresponsible people close to the services may meet with or inform sensationalist writers, and thus set up distractions to the process of providing safe services. Hospital staff time has to be spent managing false stories and half truths, trying to restore protection to patients whose confidentiality has been breached. This sort of media intrusion is probably more common in relation to special hospitals, or perhaps high security prisons, but still it is worth recognizing the effort that may be required to diffuse unnecessary resultant anxieties raised among a range of people who may, in these circumstances, include patients' relatives, but also the general public, health service professionals and, for high security hospitals, even government officials.

Whether in the positive informing or defending against malign gossip, media management (or perhaps more accurately self-management in relation to the media) is an essential skill and component of work in this field. It is not straightforward. If a patient has been named, even when a story is completely untrue, public refutation may not be helpful. Denial implies at the least acknowledging officially that the person named is indeed a patient. Then, while it may be possible to deny absolutely an allegation, say, that a pregnancy has occurred, or that there has been any sexual consummation of a relationship, there may be a relationship (which is a private matter), and the fact that there may come a point when denials are no longer possible should perhaps give pause to starting such a process. Time must be spent discussing the implications of any intrusion or disclosure with the individual(s) concerned, but some may not be fully competent to assist in the media management discussions.

Other organized external influences include patients' or prisoners' voluntary organizations and pressure groups. The highly partisan nature of most such organizations must be recognized, but they have viewpoints which must be heard. In turn, most of the organizations are prepared to spend time advising on developments and supporting individual residents. In the course of work on understanding and managing relationships in the special hospitals, particularly challenging but constructive relationships between organizations were set up with Women in Special Hospital (WISH), the National Association for the Care and Resettlement of Offenders (NACRO), MIND, and other individuals. These were able to make representations which assisted in clarifying and guiding strategy to best support the needs and views of service users with service developers. Arbitration in these discussions and identification of middle ground was often difficult; however, issues that had previously been left without acknowledgement were aired, leading to a new openness between parties.

Fostering openness about sexuality and relationships

'If sexuality is part of being a human being, every day and in every way, then it must be linked with health. If people feel well, they have the energy to invest in life and in relationships, and they feel positive about themselves. They give an impression of health and vigour to other people who then see them as attractive and worthwhile. Self esteem is reinforced as we live our lives with other people.'

(Webb, 1987)

Acceptance of this philosophy means that it is important for clinicians who are dedicated to improving the health and welfare of those in their care to understanding sexuality in their patients and, where appropriate, provide for its expression. The latter part of this objective is not invariably achievable, but it is not unreasonable to expect clinicians to recognize these needs when planning care, and make management decisions explicit, whatever they may be.

As clinicians, we need to free ourselves from the use of euphemisms in order to communicate effectively and sensitively on this subject. It is probably necessary to consider and be comfortable with our own sexuality and sexual attitudes before effective progress can be made (Gunner, 1988). Vandereycken (1993) cites Strauss et al. (1988) as finding that, when responding to a survey of attitudes and experiences in relation to inpatients, psychiatric staff from a range of disciplines who themselves lived with a partner were more likely than the others to rate the sexuality of patients as important. If staff are uncomfortable with sexuality, it seems likely that one of two prevailing approaches is likely to persist unchecked – denial or 'the blind eye' or, when recognition of eroticized relationships is unavoidable, routine imposition of blocks on contact or activity. Whereas the first strategy is inexcusable because it takes no account of the possibilities of abuse or harm as highlighted by Feinmann (1988), the second may well have some justification. In effect, however, it may also be a variant of denial. Anecdotal evidence from patients in hospitals, whether secure or not, indicates that even when restrictions are in place they are neither consistently applied nor necessarily adopted as part of an explicit individual care plan.

Open assessment of sexuality in an accepting if not necessarily permissive atmosphere may provide the clinician with new routes to understanding behaviour more generally, and/or raise new therapeutic possibilities. It may encourage many patients to develop their own self assessment and support systems, for example women's groups, gay groups, or disabled groups.

Planning facilities

Gender integration or segregation?

Along with the move from asylum care, the emphasis in general and forensic mental health settings has been towards the creation of therapeutic environments which include the provision of facilities which are fully gender integrated. The high security hospitals have generally maintained segregation of living accommodation for men and women, but encouraged patients to share education, work and social activities, regardless of sex.

Desegregation or integration and the introduction of mixed gender accommodation first began to occur in general psychiatry in the early 1960s and was part of an emerging trend towards less restrictive and more humane forms of care. By the mid 1970s gender mixing of both staff and patients in most psychiatric hospitals in Britain was the accepted policy and practice, but had never been without its opponents. Lack of privacy was stressed as a problem. The role of the male nurse in relation to female patients was questioned, while male patients tended to be regarded as likely abusers of women, and the older ones also potential predators on young men.

In 1978 the Council of the Royal College of Nursing accepted that in some caring situations mixed sex units can have a positive therapeutic value in that they provide for a more normal lifestyle for the patients, e.g. in psychiatric and geriatric care. Nevertheless, it was also recommended that mixed sex units should not be established indiscriminately, that they should be purpose designed and that in any event those due for admission to hospital should be offered the free choice of admission into a single or mixed sex ward.

Instances of confirmed sexual abuse of one patient by another have been recorded in general psychiatric hospitals or units, and a number of psychiatrists in these settings have begun to raise awareness of the issue (Gath, 1989; Subotsky, 1991; Tonks, 1992). Subotsky (1993) offers some principles for the management of both the risk of abuse and its actuality. Urging steps to prevent or divert consenting sexual activity from an acute hospital setting, she sets out the rights of patients to be both safe and free from harassment, and points to the need for attention to factors in the physical environment as well as patient problems and vulnerabilities as relevant to securing these rights. In the event of alleged or apparent assault, she emphasizes that the safety of each party must be re-secured as a first priority, and then the process of systematic information collection started in conjunction with any immediate treatment needs. A decision has to be taken as to whether to involve police or not, when, where and the nature of continuing hospital staff attendance needed. Longer term considerations, for example testing for pregnancy or sexually transmitted diseases and for providing for needs for counselling or other support, require following through.

The Butler Report (Home Office, DHSS, 1975) framed the development of regional secure hospital units. From the outset, these units were planned to be integrated by sex (staff and patients) allowing for their therapeutic environments to be similar to, albeit more secure than, the parent hospital of which they were usually a part. In practice, the tiny minority of women who become patients in such a unit have often been without a real peer group and, while guaranteed a room of her own, a woman may not, essentially on economic grounds, be guaranteed any other entirely separate facilities, even bathroom facilities. Separate, but supra-regional units for women are now under consideration as a result.

Advice about the suitability of gender integrated facilities within a high security hospital setting has, over the years, been conflicting. The 1975 report by the NHS Health Advisory Service (HAS) into Broadmoor Hospital recommended the need to pilot more integrated treatment areas and wards. Later, however, the Boynton inquiry into Rampton Hospital (Department of Health and Social Security, 1980) placed no central emphasis on the need to integrate. The second report of the Hospital Advisory Service on Broadmoor Hospital (National Health Service, HAS, DHSS Social Services Inspectorate, 1988), however, reiterated as one of its recommendations the need to reconsider the extension of integrated facilities.

When the first ward for men and women patients within the special hospitals opened its doors in 1985, many were sceptical about its viability and chances of survival. Over 10 years later that ward is still functioning and has made an established and successful contribution to the service. It has explored new territory and encountered a range of problems; some anticipated, some not.

When this facility was planned, it was argued that:

1. Often mentally disordered offenders have difficulties in forming and maintaining relationships with others; these problems can contribute to their offending behaviour and their ongoing psychopathology.
2. The problems of assessment and, therefore, prediction of future dangerousness can be less clear if such individuals are placed in sexually segregated units.
3. Residence in sexually segregated units may even foster the development of further forms of deviant behaviour and place new or additional barriers in the way of the rehabilitative process.
4. The principles of normalization, seen as both therapeutically and ethically desirable, require that gender integration be introduced to mirror conditions in society outside the institution (Mogallapu et al., 1988).

There was, however, clear recognition of some of the problems that might be encountered. Foremost, for some, was an expectation that patients could not be sexually continent. For others the risks that may be posed by placing sexually and/or otherwise physically assaultive men with previously victimized women were considered paramount.

In practice, patients were carefully selected for this facility on the basis that they were well advanced in their treatment and rehabilitation, and each patient, having been assessed as suitable for the unit and visited it, made the final decision about going there, albeit sometimes after considerable encouragement. Whatever the offence that had brought a man or woman into the hospital, each was considered safe for and likely to benefit from the unit.

An analysis of the characteristics of the patients resident during the first 6 years of the unit's operation, including their index offences, showed that less than one third of the men had been convicted of a sexual offence (Swan, 1994). Other data from the study showed clear benefit for the patient. After both 2 and 5 years of residence, assessed separately, marked reductions in the amount of major tranquillizers used by patients could be demonstrated when compared with the amounts they had used elsewhere in the hospital. Comparisons were also made into the number and length of seclusion periods and number and nature of self injurious behaviours recorded prior to and following residence on this ward. In each case significant reduction in frequency and seriousness was observed (Swan, 1993).

Notwithstanding the success of the specialist unit just described, there will be a number of people for whom integration is not a viable option because of personal preference, cultural or religious background, when it is not clinically indicated or considered too dangerous. Among secure hospital patients and prisoners, the ratio of men to women overall means that integration cannot be achieved for everyone, even if it were seen as essential. Consequently, services must develop flexible and comprehensive facilities which cater for all individual needs wherever it is practicable. The right of individuals to choice of placement should be paramount wherever possible, but in the mid 1990s this remains an ideal. Free choice can only be an option when a full range of facilities is available.

Specialist facilities for recognized couples?

As described in the first chapter, the number of people recognized as being in an exclusive or special relationship in any hospital, let alone a special hospital, is small. Numbers are perhaps rather greater in a prison setting, but even here, people who have stable relationships tend to be in a minority. As such, they hardly constitute an effective lobbying group, so the moral duty incumbent on management to provide appropriate facilities for them is, perhaps, particularly high. In ordinary hospitals, surroundings are rarely if ever ideal for satisfying social meetings, but a not wholly unreasonable response is that stay is likely to be short for an acute condition, and for most other states a patient is likely to have opportunities for leaving the confines of the ward or even the hospital buildings altogether, allowing a little more privacy in any contacts, and rather more natural surroundings. For those with chronic disabling physical conditions as well as those who may need a measure of confinement because of their mental state, there is a case for special facilities. The core criteria that most patients immediately highlight for such facilities, if asked, are a degree of privacy, domestic scale and style surroundings and the opportunity to entertain their guests – generally entailing nothing more complicated than the possibility of making and sharing a cup of coffee or tea or a meal with them. Most services fall short of these very basic provisions, but security services – in hospitals and prisons both – tend to fall very far short. There is generally insistence on communal visiting areas, where each couple or family is as conspicuous to each other as to monitoring staff, and even the content of conversations can rarely be wholly private. In hospitals at least, there is a case to be made that even security would be improved by encouraging patients to take visits in their home unit, among staff who know them well and can make a more individualized judgement of what may or may not be feasible in each individual case. It is striking that a few patients will argue against such a proposal on grounds that they think they may have more freedoms under the anomie of the communal system.

The case for fully private visiting for couples, that would allow but not necessarily be followed by sexual intercourse, is more complex. It is not generally available in open hospitals for voluntary patients. Commonly, there are valid arguments that while the members of a couple continue to require security in their care and treatment, to allow them total privacy might carry unacceptable dangers. There are undoubtedly some cases for whom, as a couple, the danger argument can be sustained and some for whom it cannot; each may still pose a risk of harm to others, but not to each other. Management of a flexible system always seems, however, to pose more difficulties for staff than management of a system which has one set of rules for all. A formal comparison between flexible and rigid systems has to our knowledge never been done. Outcome measures might include ward/institutional atmosphere, resolving challenges to or complaints about policies and procedures and, for staff, job satisfaction. A sense of safety and efficiency in held rules may be misplaced. Prisons in the UK officially put the emphasis on couples sustaining relationships through weekend leave, earned for 'good behaviour' on the part of the prisoner. This is seen as more 'normalizing'; in practice there is little of it granted. Further, although the 'leave as reward' approach is understandable, the ethics of treating a relationship as entirely contingent on relationship-unrelated behaviour of one of the partners may not have been fully thought through. In this, as in all other situations, almost no specific thought is given to the needs of the healthy or 'innocent' partner. There may be some checking of this person's willingness to receive the offender/patient, but little or no encouragement to express wishes for and views about the relationship more generally.

Most established couples, as well as any new ones, would benefit from the less tangible facility of having the option to discuss how their situation – be that their illness, its treatment, their hospitalization, their crime or their incarceration – is likely to affect their relationship, and what they can do to minimize the damage. If that is to be done successfully, it is almost certain that there will need to be specific training made available for the staff, covering couples interviewing and basic counselling skills, accurate knowledge of the treatments used and of the system, and ways of canvassing for individual needs.

General principles of supporting couples

The speciality field of caring for individuals with learning disabilities provides guidance which could largely apply to other mental health services too. Craft (1987) suggests six rights pertaining to sexuality:

- the right to grow up, i.e. to be treated with the respect and dignity accorded to adults
- the right to know, i.e. to have access to as much information about themselves and their bodies and those of other people, their emotions, appropriate sexual behaviour, etc. as they can assimilate
- the right to be sexual and to make and break relationships
- the right not to be at the mercy of the individual sexual attitudes of different care-givers
- the right not to be sexually abused
- the right to humane and dignified environments.

The human rights philosophy which is fundamental to these assertions can easily be translated into other fields. However, service providers need to be aware that many service users will require considerable support and guidance if they are to be able to exercise these and other rights effectively and within acceptable risks. Further, it is important to consider and plan for any continuing need once an individual has moved on from the first assessing and managing service.

Beyond a secure institution

For those people who have been in secure institutions, and indeed for many who have not, the problems do not end with the end of their stay. The special hospitals are illustrative of the particular difficulties in this area, compounded by their national service/tertiary referral centre position. Given the nature of public health and social services funding in the UK, the matter would be much less problematic if patients would fall in love with partners from the same geographical area, and with a similar date for transfer from that service. This would make after-care provision so much easier as, in theory, strategies could be developed with other service providers at a very early stage, safe in the knowledge that both parties would be moving on at roughly the same time and to similar parts of the country, with their funding guaranteed. In any event, patients are not so organized in their passions. A telephone survey of the offices of all Heads of Social Service and Chief Officers of Probation in 1992 confirmed that there was no known facility prepared to take recovered or recovering patients as a couple in the community (Cameron, personal communication).

The Effra trust is an independent charity working in partnership with London and Quadrant housing trusts to provide homes and support services for ex-offenders, usually leaving prison or a security hospital, in South East London. It was established in 1974 to provide long-term support and accommodation for such men who also suffered from epilepsy, and expanded its service in 1980 to ex-offenders with mental or physical illness and other disabilities. The Effra trust is, where needed, a home for life. A 'couples' project was set up within this framework with six bed spaces. The trust was prepared to accept referrals in relation to heterosexual, homosexual, lesbian couples or couples who had established a long term platonic relationship. Paradoxically, this community service set up to respond to documented need from the special hospitals at least, was forced to vary its provision because of no take-up for the facility offered. As this was an imaginative and innovative development that could be reinstated, it will be described in more detail.

The building itself provided sufficient flexibility that at any one time a couple could choose to link their bed-sitting rooms by a communicating door, or maintain their privacy through restoring individual bed-sitters. Further, a formal arrangement had been negotiated with an independent hostel scheme for women such that, should a male/female or female/female relationship deteriorate to a point where greater separation became advisable, an emergency bed would be made available for the woman. Breakdown of a male/male relationship would have been similarly accommodated within the network of Effra trust hostels. Experienced staff attended the hostel daily, and were available on call at other times. Supported occupational and recreational activities are available within the trust's network and would have been open to the residents of this hostel.

The building still exists, but in the absence of clients referred as couples, the trust has accepted appropriate single men needing accommodation. It remains prepared to consider any application on behalf of a couple, provided that the clients and their clinical teams or other referring agency consider the fostering and maintenance of the relationship as being therapeutically advantageous or in the best interest of both parties in their rehabilitation.

Recognition and assessment of important relationships

Conor Duggan's chapter has already dealt with most of the important issues preparatory to treating a couple as a couple. In this chapter, much of the emphasis is on maintaining the immediate safety of the environment and any couples within it, managing the tension between public and private needs in a communal setting and enabling treatment, where appropriate, for a couple as well as individuals and groups. Thus there is generally common ground in the approach to assessment, but perhaps some shift in emphasis here, given these management tasks.

Accurate assessment is the genesis of effective management, and at the heart of assessment is focused, objective observation and reliable historical information. Multi-disciplinary work on this is most likely to be productive. Table 11.1 summarizes some principal areas that staff and patients as a group see as important elements in assessment. The potential for important losses and gains along these lines apply to any relationships, including those of supposedly healthy people, but may simply be more exaggerated here. The list is far from exhaustive, nor does every risk or benefit apply to every couple, but here is a framework for beginning the process. It is critical that risks and benefits are regularly monitored, as relationships change over time. A relationship which one day may be beneficial in making a patient feel wanted and attractive could, following some apparently trivial disagreement, leave the same individual feeling rejected, despairing and possibly suicidal.

Often it is not immediately apparent where an element fits on the risk/benefit spectrum. As discussed earlier, many patients have been the victims of extensive abuse in previous intimate relationships and have expressed their anger in various forms of self and other abuse. A new intimate relationship in an environment such as a special hospital or prison can present the risk of more abuse. It is very important as far as possible to protect individuals from this risk. The resurgence of powerful, negative emotions may, however, occur in new non-abusive relationships, as any closeness may be coloured with perceived abusive or potentially genuine abusive qualities. With careful and sensitive supervision, such painful developments can be converted into benefit, enabling the patient, perhaps for the first time, to disclose earlier abuse and begin the process of working through its consequences. This was an early lesson experienced by the staff on the integrated ward at Ashworth hospital. Staff had been prepared to recognize and, where appropriate, intervene in physical approaches between patients. However, perhaps surprisingly, few opportunities arose for staff to call upon their prepared skills. What was unexpected, and called for a new direction in skill acquisition, was the flow of people coming forward for the first time to reveal earlier otherwise undisclosed abuse.

Relationship assessment is likely to be most useful if it explores the risk/benefit differential in each of the social, psychological and health domains.

Table 11.1 Patient relationships: a risk : benefit analysis of becoming a couple

Benefits	Risks
Self preoccupation	Individual identity
Personal isolation	Avoidance of personal reflection
Self esteem	Attention to real deficits/needs
Concern for another/others	Blame others for problems (blames relationship)
Opportunity to develop capacity for caring (used to being cared for)	Denial personal problems in concern for another's
Chosen personal support	Personal stress/relapse of disorder during relationship crises
Harmful practices with mutual support	Harmful habit sharing, e.g. drug misuse
Pleasure/contentment in satisfying relationship	Re-experience of previous traumatic/abusive relationships
Genuine maturation	'Flight into normality'; repetition of maladaptive/ dangerous relationship style
Respect from peers	Envy and hostility from unpaired peers; aggressive competition for partners
Range and quality of relationships more generally	Tension in already fragile family relationships

Table 11.1 largely confines itself to the former. Even if, within a physical institution such as a hospital, full physical expression of the relationship is denied or discouraged, the risk of such progression anyway must be assessed, and evaluation of contraceptive need or other physical protection completed (see Cole and Taylor, this volume). This is likely to be useful, too, for the longer term.

Management plan

Accurate observation is as important in the successful management of relationships as it is to precise assessment. Effective management needs a continuous evaluation, modification and re-evaluation cycle. This should include a formal note of the process and, in any given situation, of what people say and do, and the circumstances of that situation.

Anxiety about relationship formation and the potential for sexual expression is so general that staff may be as enthusiastic as patients that such relationships remain covert. Staff often feel unprepared for the complexity of judgements and interventions that may need to be made over time. They tend to lack any formal training in this complicated area, they feel unsupported in a vacuum of policy and procedure and, as a consequence, some feel confident only in an atmosphere which manufactures a complete bar on any overt physicality. Concerns about criticism from others regarding perceived failure to take affirmative action, and claims of negligence and dereliction of duty from managers when preliminaries were not seen or consummation not foreseen, collaborate to reinforce inadvertently an atmosphere of denial. This is an important issue for the multidisciplinary team. An effective team is likely to recognize the potential for splitting within the team over a potentially contentious area such as this, but to manage it and to allow a coherent plan to emerge which gives each person tasks or roles in which they can feel informed and supported. Such management of anxiety is fundamental.

There is a risk of mistaken emphasis in what need and need not be recognized. Staff may correctly assess a relationship as being transitory in nature; this does not however, carry an automatic implication that it can be ignored. In institutions as elsewhere, some risks, including unprotected sexual intercourse, are at their highest within transient relationships. In terms of management planning, each phase of a relationship – its making, maintenance and end – is likely to need attention. Transient relationships simply have fewer maintenance needs.

Staff need to develop an awareness that facilitation and tolerance do not equate to abdication and abandonment; that support and encouragement are precisely that. J. F. Kennedy once said, 'There are costs and risks to a programme of action, but they are far less than the long range risks and costs of comfortable inaction.' Management is directed at promoting the benefits and minimizing the risks.

During planning discussions a number of very practical issues can be raised, for example the problem of communication between the couple. If they reside apart from each other, or in separate units within an institution, they may need help in arranging phone calls or the writing and receiving of letters. When the couple meet together, transport, escorting and supervision may all present problems.

Planning for the maintenance of a relationship may involve more input than merely offering opportunities to communicate. It may be seen to be in the couples interest to acquire a greater level of understanding and knowledge of relationships. They may have educational needs, including access to sex education, health promotion and sexual health, contraception and family planning, as well as more specifically directed work on how this applies to their own situation.

The expertise required by staff to be effective within this perplexing and sometimes worrying emotional domain ranges from modest skills of observation, listening and simple support to the more complex and advanced skills of couple and marital counselling and couple and family therapy (see Hodge and Kruppa, and Dale *et al.*, this volume). It is important not to overlook the sense of vulnerability described by staff working in this area. Some can be picked up under general support and supervision arrangements, but for others specific training will be required (see also Cole and Taylor, and Hodge and Kruppa, this volume).

Assisting separation

It can, on occasion, become apparent that a management plan is needed to assist in the termination of the relationship, for example in the interest of physical safety. This objective may need to be achieved against the wishes of one or both parties and may occur against a backdrop of resentment and hostility. Not uncommonly, however, one or both parties want to terminate a relationship without knowing how, or do so in a way that is unnecessarily painful or destructive. Enforcing or assisting separation from a perceived counter-therapeutic relationship is never simple.

Managing the issues around a viable relationship can be difficult if it should happen that both parties are being cared for or treated by the same staff or clinical team. It is generally worthwhile giving some consideration whether, in these circumstances, it may be more constructive for one partner to be under the care of a different team. This is not invariably necessary for the safeguard of individual care and treatment, or even constructive, but the potential for bias in the event of separation has to be acknowledged. In one case known to us, a man had moved rapidly to sexualize a relationship with a younger man, both of whom were cared for by the same clinical team. The younger man had previously been a victim of sexual assaults and, having initially encouraged the relationship, began to construe his place as a victim again, initially indicating his vulnerability with a number of episodes of self harm. Following a tendency to sympathize with the more obviously wounded, other patients and staff both initially accepted the implication that the older man was necessarily a predator. The staff were saved from an inappropriately partisan and restrictive, if not punitive approach towards the older man principally by an urgent need to protect him from the more overtly and aggressively disapproving actions of his patient peers. In this case, temporary transfer of the older man to another clinical team assisted the process of establishing a more realistic appraisal of the situation. Great care has to be taken, however, even over such a temporary arrangement, as the person moved can perceive the move in itself as punitive or counter-therapeutic.

Other therapeutic tensions may arise if the partners are at different stages of their treatment and/or rehabilitation. They may not be able to leave the hospital (or, more rarely, prison) together and at least temporary separation must be accommodated. Patients will need special support both of an emotional and practical kind in these circumstances. A commitment to facilitating visits is vital, but the patients will nevertheless fear, and may well be justified in this, that their relationship will not survive such a strain.

As indicated, on occasion the clinical team may be urged by one of the parties involved to enable separation. This can present the team with a number of problems. If patients wish and/or are allowed to take on the responsibility of making relationships, it is arguable that they must accept the responsibility for breaking them – or at least telling the partner in person of their decision. In practice, people who are still inpatients are usually, by definition, ill and less able than healthy people to manage the difficult and painful aspects of relationships. Occasionally staff may have to convey the new reality, or a message, but every attempt should be made to encourage each patient to take as much responsibility as possible, as part of their habilitation or rehabilitation. If s/he cannot meet his/her partner, then a letter or a phone call might be encouraged. A meeting might be facilitated if each person felt supported by his/her key worker. One form or occasion of such communications is unlikely to be enough for satisfactory termination of the relationship and staff might prepare the patient(s) for a more-or-less fixed package of communications, tailored to best fit for the individuals or circumstances. A series of joint interviews with an experienced counsellor might be best for some, an exchange of letters the most others could achieve, while still others might follow a combined approach. The implications of satisfactory termination go beyond the immediate event. The ability to end an unhappy or unsatisfying relationship without self-harming behaviour or violence to the departing partner may be among the most important skills that patients – or prisoners – can learn in relation to their longer term safety and social adjustment.

Staff-enforced separation in the context of a perception of high risk is perhaps the most difficult of all tasks. Although there is evidence that clinicians have better than chance outcome in rating the risk of violence by men (Lidz *et al.*, 1993), risk assessment it is not among their best honed skills. Assessment of risk of violence by women is poor, with a tendency to under-estimate risk. Although not to our knowledge tested specifically within relationships, our impression is that prediction of risk of violence to others may be at its most accurate in this context. People who form risky relationships appear very likely to repeat the nature and quality of those relationships. People are often not candid with each other about their past behaviours and any risks, even if they recognize them. There seems a readily renewable faith at each new relationship that 'this time it will be different'. The clinical team and other professionals with responsibility to a patient have a primary duty of confidentiality to that patient which can be ethically breached only if serious harm appears imminent. Where both partners in a couple are patients, the problems in maintaining confidentiality may be one of the arguments for separate teams for each. A case example may serve best to illustrate some of the issues in process and management:

Steve is a man with a severe personality disorder who is detained under Section 37/41 of the Mental Health Act 1983 and has a history of violent assault towards his female partners. Steve's first wife divorced him after a marriage of 3 years which had been punctuated by violent physical assaults. Steve's second wife died following a beating administered by Steve after a heavy drinking bout.

Steve had been receiving weekly visits from a woman, Mary, who was a voluntary visitor, and after a period of a few months announced to his clinical team that they had agreed a date for marriage.

The clinical team were aware that there was little that they could do legally to prevent this union (see Fitzgerald and Harbour, this volume). However, they were deeply concerned about the risk of violence to Mary. Steve still viewed his treatment of his former wives as largely justified, and simply regarded Mary as 'different'. Fuelling their anxieties, the team recognized that the establishment of an apparently stable relationship with a presumed healthy partner can be used as a powerful argument in itself for discharge. Further, the new spouse becomes the nearest relative and can personally advocate to a tribunal for discharge.

A key dilemma facing the man's clinical team centred on the questions: Does Mary know about Steve's previous offences, particularly the ones related to his previous partners? Based upon an accurate understanding of those facts is she now able to make an informed choice? A third question inevitably follows: If Mary does not have all the facts, should she be told, whether or not Steve consents?

Steve's consultant psychiatrist, with Steve's knowledge, arranged a meeting with Mary on her own to ask about the relationship and test her level of knowledge with regard to Steve and his past offending behaviour. This interview left the doctor in no doubt that Steve had withheld important information from Mary.

The psychiatrist returned to Steve. He told Steve of his impression that Mary knew almost nothing of his violence in previous relationships, and that he thought disclosure was essential if the relationship were to continue. He gave Steve a deadline of 8 weeks from the time of their interview to inform Mary fully, in his own way, or terminate the relationship. He offered to help Steve explain and/or support him in finishing the relationship, but stressed that, with or without Steve he (the psychiatrist) would do so at that time.

Steve eventually decided with some belated maturity to speak to Mary during her next visit. Mary was taken aback with what she heard. She was clearly upset and left saying that she needed time to think things through but she would be in touch.

It was some time before Steve heard from Mary again despite his efforts to make contact. Communication, when it did finally arrive, came in the form of a short letter in which Mary severed their relationship.

Steve felt that he had been betrayed and unjustly treated and as a consequence there followed several weeks of unpredictable behaviour from Steve. Steve and Mary have not seen each other since their relationship ended. Steve remains an inpatient in a secure hospital.

For a second couple the importance of disclosure emerged in a different way:

Jack and Judy were both patients in a security hospital, each with a history of several relationships which had ended in violence. They nevertheless expressed an intention to marry, and each insisted they had been candid with the other about the past. It was similarly apparent to each clinical team that this was not so. Each had indeed been truthful in telling the other that their actions had resulted in homicide, but each had varied the motive. The clinical teams, however, while advising each patient to disclose in full, decided that as each was likely to be many years from discharge and had had other intense relationships in the hospital which had naturally ended after a month or two, they would simply maintain a watching brief.

Another patient, jealous of the relationship, told Judy that Jack's girlfriend had not, as he claimed, died in a suicide pact which he had miraculously survived. She produced an old newspaper cutting describing multiple stabbings by Jack in a jealous rage.

Judy refused to see, speak or write to Jack again. When he sought to make explanations and amends, she issued threats against him. Strict separation of the couple was maintained thereafter.

Relationship development

It is difficult to make relationships in care or custody; it is even more difficult to maintain them. The following case vignette, however, shows relationships may, when given support and encouragement, not only flourish but significantly increase the likelihood of successful return into ordinary society:

When Harold was admitted to a special hospital after having been found guilty of killing his next door neighbour, he lost much more than his liberty.

On admission Harold was 36 years old. He had left at home his wife, Maud, and his 5-year-old daughter, Marie. Prior to the onset of his illness Harold had worked as a fitter with a central heating firm and, although money was tight, the family got by and had a great deal to look forward to.

Admission to hospital did not immediately have an effect upon Harold's condition. His behaviour was disruptive. He was extremely angry, continuously arguing with other patients and regularly involved in fights with others. His belief that his neighbour had been spreading malicious rumours about him and seeking to drive him out of his house expanded to incorporate everyone, including Maud. His distrust of her grew to such a degree that he would refuse to see her when she visited.

For 2 years Maud nevertheless visited regularly and tolerated Harold's anger, hostility, accusations, threats, and rejection. She then began to feel that she had lost her husband, and she needed to devote her energies to Marie. Communications between Maud and Harold dwindled, and they divorced a few weeks after Marie's 9th birthday.

Years later Harold confirms that the end of his marriage became a turning point for him. He felt 'that he had reached the bottom of a pit' and so he could sink no lower. He began a slow improvement.

Aged 47 years, Harold had been in hospital for 11 years. He had became comfortable with institutional life; everything was predictable and, as a consequence, safe. He then began to receive letters from his daughter Marie. She was now 16, and had for some time wanted to re-establish contact with her father. Communications between the two gained in frequency, and, with support from hospital staff, Marie began to visit her father. She learned that he was very lonely and carried an enormous burden of guilt for the way he had treated his wife. Marie, was aware that Maud's feelings were similar. She became determined to reintroduce her parents.

Maud and Harold's relationship was rekindled. Two years later Harold and Maud enjoyed their second wedding. Some 2 years later still he returned home to Maud. The family has remained together and content.

Harold's case is unusual. Although his daughter was the catalyst for change, both community and hospital staff responded first to her, and then to provide practical and emotional support for the couple as they started to visit and rebuild their life. For the first time, each was able to come to terms with the tragedy of his violence, the nature of his mental disorder and to learn together how to live with the guilt of the offence and manage and reduce the risk of recurrence of his illness.

Summary

There are potential risks attached to any relationship that develops when one or both parties are ill and/or violent, and in hospital, but there are potential advantages too. Relationships will happen. One of the greatest difficulties in writing this chapter is recognition that, because of a tendency on the part of clinicians and custodians alike to ignore or deny relationships, there is little knowledge of their true prevalence, and even less of the effect of current policy and practice on their outcome.

It is no longer acceptable to turn a blind eye to what goes on. This is the most dangerous route of all. As students, each of us can recall wise senior clinicians advising the planners of any interventions on the premise that they should meet the standards we would wish and expect for ourselves or our families. There seem two key elements in this – a sympathetic and humane approach, perhaps the warm, positive, unconditional regard for the person advocated by Rogers (1961), and information based practice. Much more systematic information, including testing of management approaches, is needed to fulfil the second part of this ideal.

12

Relationships – A case for intervention
Why treat the couple rather than the individual?

John E. Hodge and Ilona Kruppa

Introduction

In the previous chapter the discussion focused on the business of little more than accommodation or limitation of relationships in an artificial and/or secure community. The core tasks of management are to ensure safety and, as far as possible, harmony with the minimum restrictions possible in the circumstances. Successful management in certain cases allows for specific treatment, a task with a goal of achieving fundamental beneficial changes in a relationship.

Treating couples in care or custody, like the other tasks, is complicated and difficult and requires a great deal of commitment, tact and perseverance. It causes problems for staff. They often, for example, find themselves caught up if conflicts develop in relationships. They may have personal views and attitudes which are at odds with the type of relationship they are faced with (e.g. homosexual). Emotional issues stemming from patients' relationships may considerably add to their problems of managing individual patients.

Such treatments also cause problems for the institution. Procedures, rules and indeed most treatments focus on individuals rather than couples. Issues which, in the community, are relatively straightforward can pose major problems within an institution. For example, allowing couples to spend time together, enabling communication between them, and setting boundaries about acceptable behaviour can all be difficult and problematic, especially if the institution is designated secure.

Becoming a couple in a managed or secure community causes special problems for the couple themselves. It is rare to have opportunities for privacy, to learn the skills of living together, even to spend a significant amount of time together. Institutional and staff indifference or outright antipathy to the relationship can place considerable strain on it. Attempts to support and help resolve problems can create considerable strain if intervention is handled badly or insensitively, and on occasion even when it is handled well.

It is little wonder that there is very little literature to be found about the institutional management and/or treatment of relationships. For most institutional staff, the size and complexity of the problem leads to choosing the course of least resistance and 'turning a blind eye'. In some cases, it can lead to relationships being actively discouraged, a course which is rarely preceded by adequate assessment of the value and risks of the relationship to the participants, although it is almost always justified as being in one or other partner's 'best interests'.

Why are relationships important?

For most people the relationships they have with others are the major influence on their emotional state and long term well-being. Relationships, and the social interaction that they engender, influence people's self esteem and self confidence. They have been shown to be particularly important in maintaining the well-being of people with psychological and psychiatric disturbances. The stability and depth of a patient's social network is now well recognized to be a major factor in the maintenance of mentally ill patients discharged into the community (Cook and Hoffschmidt, 1993; Woodside, 1985) and the quality of interactions which occur within a family setting are now a well-established factor in the prediction of relapse in patients with a variety of psychiatric diagnoses (schizophrenia, bipolar affective disorder, depression; see Kavanagh, 1992). Interventions aimed at improving relationships within families, either by improving the whole family's social problem solving (Faloon *et al.*, 1982) or by developing the patient's social skills and social interactions (Liberman, *et al.*, 1987), have been shown to reduce the likelihood of relapse among people with schizophrenia.

Good quality relationships can constantly provide individuals with feedback supporting a positive view of themselves and each other. The opportunity to discuss mistakes and problems with partners and friends helps put them into context, and the support offered in times of crisis can often be crucial to effective coping. In contrast, poor quality relationships can consistently undermine self esteem and self confidence, and exacerbate the effects of life crises when they occur. This may be particularly true where people are vulnerable to mental illness. Cognitive behaviour therapists such as Fowler *et al.* (1995) have recently highlighted the importance of tackling dysfunctional beliefs about the self, given the evidence that a sense of self worth may be very important to the long term outcome of mental disorder.

Relationships and mental disorder

An aspect of the quality of relationships in families of patients with mental illness which has received particular attention is *expressed emotion* (EE). Brown *et al.* (1972) found that where families display high levels of criticism, hostility or emotional over-involvement (*high EE*) the likelihood of relapse of schizophrenia increases, as compared to those patients whose families do not display these characteristics (*low EE*). Vaughn and Leff (1976) even named *high EE* as a causative factor. Although the work has not gone unchallenged (MacMillan *et al.*, 1986; McCreadie and Phillips, 1988), there is some independent and objective support from psychological evidence (Tarrier *et al.*, 1988) and a general acceptance of its continued relevance (see Kavanagh 1992 for a fuller review; see also Heads, this volume). This research is consistent with the vulnerability–stress (diathesis–stress) model of psychotic illness, in which it is hypothesized that vulnerability factors (biological/developmental) interact with situational (precipitant) factors producing psychotic breakdown. A similar model has been proposed recently as underlying violent episodes in offenders with personality disorder (Blackburn, 1993).

It is important to understand that the vulnerability–stress models do not necessarily imply causality for any particular factor. Essentially they suggest that the individual's vulnerability itself, together with his/her reaction to concomitant environmental factors, can come together to create a crisis. This in turn leads to further reactions on the part of the individual and further inter-actions within the environment, producing a continuously interactive cyclical effect. A dysfunctional relationship can contribute to this cycle, and while it is not the relationship itself which causes the breakdown, successful intervention or appropriate support focused on the relationship can change the matrix and may help break the cycle of crises.

While most of the research on the quality of relationships has been under-taken on patients and their families using a sophisticated structured interview incorporating behavioural observations, recent research has shown a strong and significant correlation between this measure and a measure of marital distress – the Dyadic Adjustment Scale (Hooley and Halweg, 1986). With depressed patients, Hooley and Teasdale (cited in Hooley, 1987) found that marital satisfaction ratings of patients and EE levels of spouses were equally successful in predicting the likelihood of relapse over a 9-month period. The quality of the relationship was important to the maintenance of treatment gain. In the case of couples within institutional settings, this would lead to a hypothesis that quality of relationships could be a strong influence on institutional progress and suitability for discharge.

It seems very unlikely that such a powerful influence on emotional well-being in open community settings will have no influence within more artificial institutional settings. Indeed, in secure institutions, given the confinement and lack of regular interaction with family, it may be that constructive personal relationships formed within the institution are even more essential. Attending to these relationships is particularly important with mentally disordered offenders for two reasons. Firstly, there is the duty of care towards the emotional well-being of the patient, client or prisoner but, in addition, there is the issue of risk. A vast majority of violent offences are perpetrated within the context of relation-ships, with the partner being the most frequent victim, and this holds for people with a mental disorder as well as those without.

Relationships in care and custody: strength of a holistic approach

Psychiatry in the first half of the 20th century tended to focus more or less exclusively on the presenting patient and his or her mental state. From a more holistic perspective it is only possible to have a full understanding of patients having taken into account their developmental, current social and other environ-mental factors. This applies as much to institutions and therapeutically derived communities as to communities of origin.

Patient relationships in hospital create a valuable opportunity not only to obtain important clinical information directly, but also to intervene in what may be a crucial aspect of the patient's life directly relevant to their major problems. In secure settings, behaviour patterns relevant to risk assessment, much of which can only be guessed at otherwise, can become available for direct observation and intervention. For example, interpersonal tensions generated within relationships provide a forum for assessing coping and self-management skills; offence triggers (e.g. termination of relationships, infidelity) can be monitored within a 'safe' environment; development of adaptive interpersonal skills (e.g. problem solving, sharing and conflict resolution) can be monitored and encouraged; risk behaviours such as abuse, bullying, interpersonal violence, manipulation and exploitation can be identified and addressed with suitable intervention packages.

Ethical predicaments

Ethical predicaments arise when a relationship involves two patients and one is seen to be more vulnerable or more at risk that than the other, in other words the balance of power in the relationship is grossly unequal from the outset. Clinically, a relationship which may provide useful information and opportunities for intervention with respect to one partner may not be so clinically advantageous to the other partner, who may be put at risk by the relationship. Clinical considerations apart, clearly there is also an issue about what right the organization has to intervene in a consenting relationship between adults, and by how much. This dilemma may be at its most acute where one partner has a history of predatory sexual offending, and the other of being a victim of violent sexual abuse. We have chosen this type of relationship to exemplify the process of assessment and treatment which such a relationship may require and the challenges it is likely to present to the participants, the professionals and the institution. It is important to emphasize that, while we have focused on a heterosexual relationship, many of the issues would be equally relevant to a homosexual relationship.

The relationship and process we describe below is a fictitious and highly idealized one. It is a composite of issues which have arisen in a number of situations encountered in clinical work. We have attempted to highlight some of the major problems and suggest solutions based on good clinical practice.

Unfortunately, in many real situations, the behaviour of clinical teams is not well coordinated or considered as described below. In the real world, cooperation both within and between teams is not always ideal, communications do not work efficiently and team decisions are not always carried out as intended. When this happens, it is almost always to the detriment of the patients involved. In any situation where clinical teams become involved with a couple, there is a real tendency for staff attitudes to polarize, and for staff to 'blame' the other party when problems arise. If only one team is involved with both patients, problems are likely to arise as factions develop within the team. These problems can be compounded if more than one team is involved. It is very important to emphasize that unless there is an extreme and immediate risk to one member of the relationship, both parties have an equal right to full support from all staff involved. *It is essential to establish as early as possible that where one team is managing both patients each member has a responsibility to each patient, and where there are two teams both teams have responsibilities* to *both* patients. This can help to ensure an equitable perspective is taken which disadvantages neither participant at the expense of the other. Such a perspective can also help the team(s) to focus on the interactions between the two participants, where help is often needed. However, the teams should be aware that they need to adopt different perspectives at different times. When taking into account the needs of the couple, they must not lose sight of the needs of the individual patients.

Problems and solutions: a relationship modelled in practice

'David' and 'Debbie'

David has a history of increasingly serious sexual assaults on young women, culminating in two serious rapes, within a few weeks of each other. His victims were usually strangers, met in pubs or clubs. There was some evidence of acceptable attempts to initiate relationships, but these were rapidly replaced by assault if rebuffed. There was no history of successful or sustained heterosexual relationships.

On admission to secure hospital 5 years previously, he was assessed to have poor interpersonal skills, particularly with women. He reports a belief that he has a strong sex drive which must be released or he will come to harm. Soon after admission he was reported to be threatening to women at the hospital's social functions. There were then some attempts at homosexual relationships, during which he was exploited by more able patients. He stopped attending social functions and became quiet and withdrawn, and reports of his threatening behaviour ceased.

David had engaged in a number of modules of a sex offender treatment programme. He was developing some insights, but staff considered it unlikely that he could yet use these.

Debbie had a history of 'random' violence and was admitted after stabbing a man outside a public house. The man was a stranger and the assault appeared motiveless. She gave a history of long term sexual abuse, initially from her father. After being put into care, she was further abused and when she ran away she became a prostitute for a time under the control of a pimp who was very violent to her. She ran away from him, but continued as a prostitute, cohabiting with a number of men in succession. On two occasions she was violent. Just prior to the index offence, she had heard that the violent pimp was looking for her.

She was admitted to secure hospital 3 years previously. Treatment focused on intrusive trauma-related symptoms. Some work was also done to improve her assertiveness towards men, but she remains confused about them – attracted to an ideal of affection, but repelled by their sexual advances.

Their relationship begins

The two met when Debbie started attending the same education sessions as David. Education staff reported that the first moves appeared to have been made by Debbie, David being rather withdrawn. Over a period of 2 weeks they began to sit together and David appeared to become less withdrawn and more cheerful, and then it was reported that they had attended a social function together. David had not attended these for some years. In Debbie's case there was little behavioural change, but concern was expressed by her clinical team at David's background and offence history.

Initial clinical responses

Reaction of the staff in the two clinical teams was different. In David's team, it was thought that this relationship would provide the opportunity to assess David's progress, especially in his social behaviour towards women. Even if the relationship did not last long, it would enable them to gather some information to plan the next stages of David's treatment and to update their assessment of his risk towards women. There was a belief that David now had better interpersonal skills for dealing with women, and that he was now much less of a risk than he had been. They were also pleased that David had become more responsive to staff approaches and were hopeful that this might continue long enough to re-engage him in a more active treatment programme.

In the case of Debbie's team, there was real concern that she was not yet 'ready' for a relationship, and a belief that she needed to acquire more skills to protect herself from exploitation and further abuse. It was thought that exposure to coercion or sexual demands at this time would undo all the progress she had made since admission. They were also particularly concerned about what they knew of David and his history of sexual assault and rape. While they were aware that they could not tell Debbie about David's background, some members were already strongly advocating that she should be 'counselled out' of the relationship, and protected from David. Their concerns were taken by their nursing team leader to David's team leader, who explained the very different objectives and expectations of David's team. It was recognized that a meeting involving both clinical teams was needed. Due to the numbers of people involved this took some time to arrange.

Observed behaviour alone can mislead

While this meeting was being arranged, David and Debbie continued to see each other regularly and more frequently at education sessions and social functions. David's behaviour on the ward became noticeably more confident, indeed some members of the clinical team were concerned that he was becoming over-confident. Debbie, on the other hand, was becoming more withdrawn, and resisted attempts by staff to discuss her relationship with David. On one or two occasions she had been quite irritable with little provocation. Her sleep had become disturbed. Education and social function staff reported that there was increasing physical contact between the two, usually initiated by David, but they had not observed any sexual contact. All staff in close daily contact with them wanted clinical team guidance on how to respond to the couple and how to react if their behaviour did become more sexual.

Just before the meeting of the clinical teams, Debbie became very disturbed and aggressive on the ward, trying to attack members of staff. When she calmed down she became very tearful and admitted that she had been having nightmares about her previous experiences of abuse. She told staff that she had also experienced these during the day while she was still awake – she would see her father's face very vividly, and this was making her very frightened and afraid to go to sleep. Asked about her relationship with David, she said that she was very fond of David and wanted it to continue, but was very afraid of the demands he was now beginning to make about sex. She had tried to explain to him about what had happened to her, but David had just got jealous about the other men and could not understand why she could not offer him the same. He had told her he didn't believe that sex could hurt anybody.

Staff observations were accurate in indicating the presence of problems, but not their nature. Assumed knowledge of risks from David could have been very misleading at this stage.

Enabling the clinical teams to function therapeutically
At the meeting of the clinical teams, it was obvious that there was some polarization of staff attitudes. Staff on Debbie's team thought she should end the relationship because of the stress it was placing on her. They had already suggested several times to Debbie that she should stop seeing David, and restrictions on her attending social functions had been attempted. Most of her team saw David as a typical sex offender and a risk to Debbie. In David's team, views ranged from concern that the ending of the relationship would lead to David becoming withdrawn again, to concern that he had not acquired enough empathy skills to realize when he should reduce his demands for sexual contact. They recognized that he was still inappropriate in his sexual demands but that he had moved a long way from his previous behaviour of responding to rebuff by committing sexual assault. In their attempts to help the relationship survive, David had had a number of 'man-to-man' talks with staff attempting to help him see the need to reduce his sexual demands on Debbie for the present.

David's team, then, tended to minimize any risk to Debbie, while Debbie's team emphasized this. They also pointed out that Debbie was becoming a management problem on the ward, and disrupting other patients. To overcome this polarization, a number of strategies were adopted:

- It was explained that a decision to intervene directly to end the relationship against the wishes of David and Debbie could only be justified if there was an extreme or immediate risk to one of them.
- Both teams were given some time on their own within the meeting to examine the problems of the other team and come up with some suggested solutions.
- When this was accomplished, each team was asked to recognize that while they may have primary responsibility for one patient, in fact they also had responsibility for both patients in that any decision affecting the one would inevitably affect the other.

It was recognized that it was very important to involve Debbie and David as soon as possible so that they could participate fully in any decisions made. However, there were concerns about confidentiality. Involving both carried the risk that issues could come out which one partner had not divulged to the other. The main issue discussed concerned David's convictions for sex offences, and the effect that this might have on the relationship if David left it too long to disclose these. Staff on both teams were fairly sure that he had not yet told Debbie about his history. Debbie's team argued that this was a major and urgent issue since they believed that, once she was aware of David's background, she might not wish anything more to do with him.

It was agreed that if both Debbie and David wished help to develop their relationship, the teams needed to establish the areas of confidentiality on both sides. However, there was general agreement that each patient should be counselled to disclose their offending and offered any help needed to do this by his or her own team. Additional specialist support was to be provided for Debbie to help her understand her recent experiences and to help her overcome her distressing intrusions. Otherwise there was agreement to respond to requests for advice from either Debbie or David with empathy and non-directive counselling.

Management of disclosure between patients

The rationale for persuading both to disclose their offence backgrounds was based on a value concept of openness in relationships. Some staff were uncomfortable that David and Debbie may not necessarily share these 'middle class' values. However, there was the possibility that other patients may know of one or other's background and either inadvertently or deliberately tell the partner. Both teams also took the view that they needed to be fully aware of the risks involved in this relationship. There was also a view that if the relationship survived the disclosures, then the two clinical teams involved would be in a much better position to plan a joint approach to rehabilitation for the couple.

David was very reluctant to tell Debbie of his background, believing that she would end the relationship. The risk of other people telling her eventually persuaded him, and he admitted she had been asking him to tell her what he had done to be admitted to hospital. So far he had only admitted that he had lost his temper and assaulted some people. Once he had decided, David rehearsed with his primary worker how he was going to tell Debbie, until he was confident that he could do so sensitively. The consequences of disclosure were fully discussed with David, including the very real risk that Debbie might wish not to see him again.

The couple asked that their respective primary workers supported their disclosures and a meeting was set up to offer them plenty of time to talk through the issues if this were necessary.

Relationship survival

David was relatively unaffected by Debbie's disclosure. Debbie, on the other hand, became very upset. She indicated she wanted nothing more to do with David and broke off contact with him. David's initial reaction was one of anger, directed at the clinical team for encouraging him to disclose. He became withdrawn, and refused support from his team. He was viewed as a serious suicide risk for some time. There was no contact between the two for several weeks, Debbie having stopped attending education and social functions.

David's hostility to his clinical team gradually waned, but he remained withdrawn. Debbie, on the other hand, was receiving a lot of support in the form of non-directive counselling, mainly from her primary worker. Over time, she admitted during counselling sessions that she was missing David, and that although he had been making sexual demands of her, he had never been aggressive towards her. At this point it was agreed that it was important that Debbie was made fully aware of her rights in relationships, and particularly her right to say no. Her background of sexual abuse had led to her being considerably confused on this issue. This input helped her to clarify exactly what kind of physical contact she was prepared to accept.

The clinical teams became aware that contact had been re-established between the two, probably via mutual friends. Both teams agreed that there should be no further intervention in the relationship, beyond discreet monitoring, until requested by either party. Both partners appeared very tentative at first, but gradually began to spend more time together again.

Attaining treatment as a couple
Debbie made the next approach to her primary worker, complaining that David was persistent in attempting sexual contact beyond what she was prepared to accept. When David became aware of this he complained to his own primary worker that Debbie was unreasonable and inconsistent in her objections to sexual contact. Both clinical teams met and agreed to offer joint counselling sessions, led by the two primary nurses and supervised by an experienced relationship counsellor.

David was reluctant at first, because of what had happened when staff had advised him to disclose his offence background to Debbie. However, Debbie persuaded him that they needed help to deal with the current problem. Each was offered an individual session with their primary nurse to ensure that they each understood the purpose of joint counselling and to clarify their individual objectives. Both parties initially viewed this process as a way of persuading the other to do what s/he wanted. It took some time to persuade both that the purpose was to help them jointly solve their own problems and come to a reasonable compromise.

Over time, counselling enabled the two to develop an agreed contract about acceptable limits of physical contact. This success encouraged the couple to continue in joint counselling to tackle other communication problems. They were guided during sessions to discuss their individual treatment needs to safeguard the long term success of their relationship. Their motivation for their individual treatment programmes improved.

The two clinical teams agreed that while this relationship continued and was clearly of central importance to both patients, that a joint approach to rehabilitation would be established and that the needs of each partner would be considered in future decisions. Plans were formulated to raise the couple's awareness about the very real difficulties they might encounter if their relationship survived into their discharge back into the community, e.g. close monitoring by social services, likely police attention, stigma. While these issues are relevant to the release of any mentally disordered offender, they might also create additional and unacceptable pressures on their relationship.

Extracting the principles and scope for further work

The above is an idealized vignette aggregated from a number of cases, aimed at illustrating some of the major problems and possible 'good practice' solutions, not yet typical of overall current practice in the experience of either author. In reality, relationship difficulties in institutions are rarely successfully resolved. The institutional environment, along with the attitudes of peers and staff, often create too many hurdles for patients to cope with.

In the idealized summary above, both parties agreed to disclose their offence background. In practice, resistance to disclosure may not be as easily resolved, and a very real dilemma arises when one or other patient refuses to disclose. The issue is not only one of a possible conflict of class values as suggested in the text, but also of the risk to either or both parties of non-disclosure. Where this risk is perceived to be high, it is our experience that clinical teams may place considerable pressure on patients to disclose. Such pressure often results in the ending of the relationship anyway, since these circumstances are rarely conducive to allowing adequate preparation to undertake this highly sensitive task properly. We would suggest that this outcome is most likely when there is poor communication between the clinical teams involved and no agreement about acceptance of joint responsibility for both patients.

Timing of disclosures can also be a contentious issue. Ideally, disclosure should not come too early or too late in the development of a relationship. When this 'window' occurs will obviously vary from relationship to relationship. In practice, the timing is often determined by one or other party asking the other, or by clinical teams becoming concerned when the couple make a public commitment, such as getting engaged to be married. If this stage is reached, it can often be the case that one party has been deliberately misled by the other about their background, creating even more resistance to honest disclosure. Good practice would suggest that the primary worker should emphasize the importance of honest disclosure early in the relationship, without any undue pressure, to allow the patient as much control as possible over the timing and strategy for disclosure. Where possible, clinical teams should also offer advice about timing and presentation.

The vignette suggested considerable monitoring and involvement in the relationship by staff as an example of good practice. A word of caution needs to be introduced here. There is a tendency for staff to become over-involved and over-controlling in the relationship, excusing this as their professional role. It may be unavoidable that their involvement in the relationship is initiated by the staff themselves, but this may be indicative of staff problems in accepting developing relationships and/or of greater risk of poor longer-term management. In any event, the manner of staff engagement in the process is worthy of consideration as part of assessment. Staff over-involvement parallels the behaviour, in other contexts, of relatives scoring high in 'expressed emotion', and is likely to have the same effect, i.e. an increase in distress and symptomatology of the patients. As in the community, this may well be interpreted as a deterioration in mental state and trigger even further involvement of staff, leading to further deterioration. It is very important to emphasize to all members of the clinical team that, except on issues where clinical team intervention may be necessary to reduce risk, direct staff involvement should be at the invitation of the couple. When this occurs, it should also be founded in pertinent skills and, generally, on-going supervision, however experienced the primary worker.

The individual work which may parallel couple counselling needs to address a range of topics. Apart from the work necessary to reduce the risk of reoffending, and to provide effective rehabilitation, many interpersonal skill deficits may become highlighted by the relationship. The most likely problem areas are empathy, assertiveness and problem solving.

Empathy is often the most complex issue when dealing with offenders. It is a multi-dimensional concept (Davis, 1983; Marshall et al., 1995), covering areas such as the individual's ability to perceive and accurately recognize emotion in others, to respond appropriately, and cope with another person's distress. Individual offenders may present with generalized deficits in their ability to empathize with others, or with specific deficits in their ability to empathize with particular groups (e.g. women or children). These deficits may arise from distorted beliefs about sexuality and sexual rights. Treatment needs to be based on detailed assessment and tailored to the individual (Hanson, 1997). Both partners in a relationship may have assertiveness problems, but these may be quite different in nature, requiring individual intervention, possibly later supplemented with joint work (Goldstein and Keller, 1987; Hollin and Trower, 1986).

Problem solving is likely to be essential to the long term survival of any relationship in which the participants have little or no prior experience of relationships. If the couple are to avoid becoming dependent on staff support and solutions to their problems, they have to develop their own style of resolving contentious issues.

Conclusions

This chapter has addressed some of the complex issues faced when dealing and 'treating' relationships in institutional settings. While we have largely focused on the problems of heterosexual couples, many of the same considerations apply to homosexual couples, although here there may be even more complicating factors (e.g. institutional homophobia, issues of 'coming out' to family and friends). Space does not permit a full account of the huge range of issues involved. We have argued that a considered response to relationships is extremely important for a number of reasons. The couple has the right that their relationship be recognized by the organization. The relationship is likely to be a major source of their emotional well-being or distress. Both over- and under-involvement of staff can create risks and tensions. Intervention which recognizes the couple's rights and which is largely at their own invitation usually minimizes the risk of damage to either the individuals concerned or the couple. Where direct intervention is necessary, it should be done sensitively, with support being provided for both parties.

13

Professional, contractual and volunteer relationships
Maintenance of strengths, and prevention and management of breach

Colin Dale, Eithne V. Wallis and Pamela J. Taylor

Nature of professional relationships

Professional values

A profession is defined not only by its body of expertise, but also its values and ethics. Medical ethics codes are among the oldest recorded professional codes. Consistent throughout them are the principles that the health of the patient will be the first consideration, that human dignity will always be respected, and concepts of dedication to the service of humanity generally. Such codes and concepts include care of the profession and fellow professionals, in the senses of being honest and committed to furthering knowledge and its application in the field. The corollary is that intentional harm to those seeking help from physicians, lack of respect for them as people, or action in unnecessary ignorance are all unacceptable, and breaches of the professional code. (For a selection of ethical codes as applied to medicine and psychiatry over time and between nations, see: Bloch and Chodoff, 1991; Taylor and Gunn, 1993.) Within health services, trained personnel other than doctors have generally now adopted similar codes and formed professions too. Within the criminal justice system, lawyers have long had such professional standing, but other disciplines, for example the probation service, are now also joining these ranks. The clergy constitutes the other important professional body in this field. Many others enter into formal, contractual relationships with individuals. When they do so in conjunction with health, social or criminal justice services, their standards in this respect ought to be similar. In addition, these are services that depend considerably on voluntary workers who, for safe and effective practice, will also need to consider and embrace such principles.

The earliest of the recorded medical professional codes, enshrined in the Hippocratic oath, recognized the potential perils of the eroticization of the doctor–patient relationship:

> 'Whatever houses I may visit, I will come for the benefit of the sick, remaining free of all intentional injustice, of all mischief and in particular of sexual relations with both male and female persons, be they free or slaves.'

It follows that anyone in a similarly confiding, intimate and relatively exclusive service relationship with another individual may be similarly at risk of taking advantage of the vulnerability of his or her patient/client and, where other professional codes exist as indicated, they reflect this. It is something of a surprise, therefore, that training programmes for many of these professional groups do not invariably incorporate education in these matters. Gartrell *et al.* (1995), for example, among nearly 200 questionnaires returned by physicians in the USA, found that 56 per cent reported that physician–patient sexual contact had never been addressed during medical school or residency.

We could find no such figures for other disciplines, but have no reason to believe that it is likely to be any better. At the heart of probation service work too, for example, is the establishment of a connection between offender and worker sufficient to facilitate communication and cooperation, and a delicate balance of care and control so that attitudes and offending behaviours can be challenged and positively changed. In 1983, Willis studied 30 male probationers; 80 per cent said that probation gave them an opportunity to talk to a patient and sympathetic listener. Twenty-two young adult offenders told Bailey and Ward (1992) much the same thing, valuing also practical help. Merrington (1995), after interviewing 16 offenders, found much the same image:

> 'The probation officer qualities needed for a successful relationship were: being a good listener, relating to people, not imposing solutions, honesty and accepting people for what they are ... A bad officer would be one with no interest or time to give.'

As part of preparing this chapter, one of us (E.V.W.), interviewed managers and practitioners in one English probation service. They too emphasized the value of 'the relationship', linking job satisfaction directly to its quality.

As in health services, both practitioners and offenders thus bring high expectations to this relationship, which may continue over a long period of time. For those serving lengthy prison sentences, for example, probation service contact can be the single continuous thread enduring after other relationships have fallen away. My (E.V.W.) reading of case files over 13 years, both as a practitioner and for service inspections, reveals that, commonly, offenders' other relationships have been short term and characterized by intimidation, dishonesty, abuse, collusion or violence. They may have been victim, perpetrator or both, but show high levels of personal and social inadequacy, feelings of isolation, hopelessness and low self esteem. One study of young offenders (Association of Chief Officers of Probation, 1993) reported that over 60 per cent had left home by the time they were 16, generally because of abuse, deprivation and poor relationships with parents. Another, commissioned research project (Akhurst *et al.*, 1995) revealed that around one in three reported attempting suicide or self harm.

Thus offenders often bring to their relationship with any worker high levels of emotional need and vulnerability and the experience of abuse and manipulation. Previous dysfunctional relationships add to the proclivity to distort and misinterpret the behaviour and signals given out by others. Most offenders are prepared to trust and reveal personal feelings and experiences, in this context, but may expect an equal investment on the part of the worker.

It is easy to see the potential for role boundaries to slide should the worker lose focus and concentration, when daily walking the tightrope of care and control. All staff interviewed as part of my (E.V.W.) survey for this chapter referred to these dangers and their experience of offenders 'pulling' the relationship in some inappropriate way, either knowingly or inadvertently. All saw the eroticized or sexualized relationship as 'unprofessional'. All expected that the disciplinary process should apply, with at least the certainty of a formal warning if the case were established, and the possibility of dismissal depending on circumstances.

Among a random 25 per cent sample of 59 probation officers newly appointed to one service, however, it appeared that preparation for the task was scant in this respect.

- All but one acknowledged that s/he had received a copy of the service's *Code of Conduct* or had access to it. Three said they had read it carefully. None reported having it drawn to his/her attention or explicitly working through it in induction or supervision.
- None of these officers had experienced his/her own supervisor making offender–worker relationships an explicit item in work or training.
- Six of the probation officers said they would find it difficult, and nine impossible, to raise their own fears and experiences in supervision.

Can a professional relationship cease for these purposes?

The Task Force on Sexual Abuse of Patients (1991), set up by the College of Physicians and Surgeons of Ontario, provides, as a result of its inquiries and among other recommendations, a useful framework for changes in education that could be adapted for other professional disciplines too.

If professional codes are clear about the incompatibility of coterminous professional and private relationships, they are less so on sequencing, although the American Psychiatric Association code (APA, 1989) states:

'Sexual involvement with one's former patient generally exploits emotions deriving from treatment and therefore almost always is unethical.'

Some other codes refer to such relationships as unethical only if the physician (American Medical Association) or psychologist (American Psychological Association) exploit their position or knowledge from the earlier professional relationship in the later personal one. A survey of psychotherapists (Conte *et al.*, 1989) found that less than one third of respondents were against a personal relationship becoming sexual after 'proper' termination of therapy. While there are those that view the therapist–patient relationship as analogous to the parent–child relationship, and therefore something that can never include sexual intimacy, for most commentators the issue here is how to ensure adequate safeguards for a patient beyond as well as during a relationship in which the qualities have genuinely changed. While some call for demonstration of real change in those qualities, for example that the patient should no longer be emotionally dependent on the therapist, others require recognized procedure, for example that the patient should be referred to another therapist, and perhaps too that the therapist should enter treatment.

Passage of time after termination of the professional relationship is the central issue for many. Appelbaum and Jorgenson (1991) cite the American Association for Marriage and Family Therapy as having amended its ethics code in 1988 to prohibit sexual contact with former patients for 2 years after termination. Appelbaum and Jorgenson's experience of over 100 cases of sexual contact between therapists and patients or former patients yielded only one case in which sexual contact with a former patient began more than 1 year after termination of the treatment. They also cite Schoener's experience of more than 2000 such cases, among whom fewer than 1 per cent of such relationships had begun more than 1 year after termination (see also Schoener *et al.*, 1989). These data are suggestive that, providing patients are protected during and for up to a year after therapy, then the chances of a sexualized relationship occurring are very small. The risk is principally of immediate or early infatuation. A proposal from Appelbaum and Jorgenson, on this basis, that prohibition might be lifted a year after termination, produced a response to the correspondence column of the *American Journal of Psychiatry* (1992) that was 'by far the most vigorous and extensive the Journal has seen in many years'. Although most published letters applauded the opening of the debate, few were supportive of the proposal and some very hostile. The editors felt compelled, indeed had been asked by some, to justify their editorial policy in publishing such an article, and further to state 'disagreement with its basic ethical conclusions'. In this, as in most areas of the business of managing erotic and sexual relationships in 'made situations', there is little consensus, much that is well reasoned and even supported by some evidence, and as yet no absolutely right answers. Where it can be shown that there is a high risk of harm following from a particular course of action, as in sexualizing a professional relationship, then it is indefensible to do so. Where it cannot be proven that no harm follows, then it is almost certainly wise to maintain the most conservative ethic. The position may evolve as more evidence accrues one way or the other, but those points may serve as guiding principles.

Other boundary confusions

Most of what has been said so far takes the professional relationship as the starting point. It is possible, however, that the starting point for an unethical relationship lay in the personal and private, but extended into the professional. This is one of the most difficult areas of all because the threshold between right and wrong – what is acceptable and not acceptable – is so much less clear. In relation to some trained or professional skills, this is not uncommon and widely accepted. Doctors may prescribe drugs within the family on occasion, for example an antibiotic to save a trip to the busy local practitioner. It may not be very good practice, but it is neither illegal nor unethical. At extremes, spouses, lovers and parents, whether from a professional background or not, may be called upon to do the most intimate of semi-professional tasks, for example toileting the physically disabled, or even life saving, technically skilled procedures, such as haemodialysis. There is recognition that these mixings of qualities in relationships can be destructive, but it suits service and national budgets, so, far from showing disapprobation towards such role confusion, it tends to be encouraged.

This is true within mental health practice, and more covertly in criminal justice system practice too. This is despite the fact that it is recognized that violence by people with a mental illness is most commonly acted out within families, perhaps particularly commonly towards parents who may be attempting to limit the disabilities and threat from their offspring at the time. Those few with a major mental disorder and a spouse have also been highlighted as at special risk in this respect (e.g. Häfner and Böker, 1973; Planansky and

Johnston, 1977). When the issue is discussed, solutions offered seem to focus on trying to separate the people rather than the roles.

Distinction between office based and community workers?

There is no distinction in terms of requirements in professional commitment between workers according to the place of work, but the environment in which people meet undoubtedly has some impact on the way in which they relate. The rather formal setting of an office, a hospital ward, or a prison cell perhaps enhances formality in relationships, and there are certain safeguards in that. For various good reasons in health, social and probation services, there is considerable emphasis on wider community activities and assessment at home. Accurate assessment of progress and abilities or of risk is an essential part of service planning, and commonly people are at their most revealing at home. Some may not attend offices, or at least not consistently, and home visits become essential to maintain supervision, support or treatment. More often than not, the worker is alone with the patient, client or offender on home visits. Services are primarily dependent on the worker's case record for knowledge of what took place in the work session. As much of the work is not directly observed, there is a high level of practitioner autonomy, and trust by employers and society alike that s/he will not cross that fine line which separates professional behaviour from the personal and self-interested. Practitioners do increasingly receive advice and support about managing potentially violent situations in the course of their community work. It is advisable that they are also prepared for emotional risks. These may lie in the early signs that something more than a professional relationship is developing, but may also lie simply in misperceptions on the part of a lonely person, or even entrapment on the part of that person. Just as shared visiting, or call checking arrangements may be good safety measures in preventing or diffusing violence, so they may usefully be applied to other potential relationship problems.

Hidden dangers in 'equality' and 'liberalization' in practice?

White coats, immaculate suits, uniforms and formal terms of address were never proof against the eroticization of professional relationships. They may even have encouraged some of it. Nevertheless, casual dress and first name communications are introduced explicitly to break down barriers between practitioners and clientele, and, within physical institutions like hospitals, to lower the risk of institutionalization. It may be difficult for staff to determine constructive and safe limits in this process, but it is frankly confusing for many of the clientele. Particularly working with men who are primarily offenders, generally a surprisingly conservative group, relaxation of dress and address codes has sometimes had a paradoxical effect. Decisions about staff uniforms are almost invariably management decisions, with some reference to staff wishes in more liberal institutions or settings, but little or none to those of the clientele.

A study of children is quite telling in this regard. Barrett and Booth (1994) found that they perceived a formally dressed paediatrician as competent while not friendly, but a casually dressed doctor as friendly but not competent. Gledhill *et al.* (1997) specifically enquired among psychiatric inpatients for their preferences. Male and female, white and non-white, and a full range of social classes and ages from 17 to 78 were represented. Jeans were associated with lack of competence without enhancing other attributes. A doctor wearing a smart dress was considered most friendly and easy to talk to, and a doctor in a white coat 'most understanding'. Most patients preferred to be called by their first name, while retaining title and surname for the doctors. Sparrow (1991) and Franzoi (1988) advanced not dissimilar findings in relation to nurses' uniforms, but related to short term care. A study (Brennan *et al.*, 1995) was conducted of small samples of patients and staff on each of two wards in a secure hospital after nurses had been out of uniforms for 3 months. Patients and staff were almost equally divided in many of their views about casual dress, but with some clearly preferential comments, for example:

- Felt 'them and us' factor would be lessened – 82 per cent patients
- Thought uniform to be an outmoded concept – 75 per cent staff.

Probably the best safeguard for practitioner and clientele alike is that the practitioner should be very secure in conception of his or her role, and in the confidence to act in it. Evolving practice within disciplines calls for this, but so too does multidisciplinary work, when conventional disciplinary boundaries may regularly be crossed. The advantage of working in such a team is that role variations can be discussed, planned openly, agreed, made explicit and monitored. This is also true of professional partnerships and supervision arrangements within and between disciplines, for example a nurse specialist supervising the counselling sessions between a regular nurse and a patient, or a psychiatrist and probation officer working with a client within the framework of a probation order with a condition of treatment.

Other employed carers

Heterogeneity of background and aims

Health, social and criminal justice services each employ a large number and range of non-professional lay workers. Some, while not having a health or social services professional qualification, bring specific, relevant skills directly to the clientele, for example occupational skills. Others are brought in precisely because they are volunteers and may befriend, or have the capacity to link back to the relevant local community in a way that the professional is unable to do. Such arrangements, however, still do not give licence to the development of a relationship of any kind, although it is here that boundaries are most blurred and all parties potentially most vulnerable.

We know of no systematic research of the backgrounds of people who take unqualified and generally relatively poorly paid or voluntary work with sick, disabled, disadvantaged and even dangerous people. Within our experience they are a very mixed group of people who include: the truly altruistic; those with generally relevant social skills but no specific experience or skill in the field; those with considerable specific skills, experience and long-standing interest in the work, but unqualified because their financial or social circumstances had never permitted that; those who are motivated and experienced, but unlikely to be able to complete the more academic demands of a full professional training; people with a much more personal agenda, sometimes declared, sometimes not, fed perhaps by some early experience, for example to help people who have suffered childhood abuse because they did; and people who have been patients or clients of a system and want to use their particularly specialist kind of knowledge to help others now going through it. Few, if any, of these people will have a professional code, some may not even recognize anything of the kind, and others will hold to a set of ethics in their practice which may be consciously and expressly in conflict with traditional professional ethics. Of considerably more concern, some may unconsciously and/or covertly follow a different code. Perhaps a couple of case examples will best illustrate some of the problems and benefits that may accrue.

Enid was a nursing assistant in her late twenties. She had no professional qualifications, but 8 years of such experience. She was well liked, regarded as reliable and had never been involved in any disciplinary proceedings.

Danny was a patient with a long history of psychotic illness who had been admitted to a secure ward in a hospital after conviction for a very serious attack on his mother. His hallucinations and delusions had responded well to antipsychotic medication, but he remained aloof from all the staff and patients on the ward, refusing to take part in any therapy or activities.

Enid had grown up in a very similar community to Danny's, and had had similar pressures through childhood and adolescence, feeling something of an outsider much of the time. She began to build a special relationship with him. Initially her colleagues saw this as further evidence of her special sensitivity with patients. She then began to explain his behaviours on the ward in terms only of failures of understanding and empathy on the part of others. This perhaps should have rung alarm bells for the qualified staff but, as a sensitive group themselves, they thought that she could be right. He would only engage in activities if she were there. Occasionally, on her own initiative, she brought small, harmless items in for him to enhance his projects. She took his part more and more on the ward, and started to become irritable with colleagues if they made any negative observations about him at all. He started to have occasional leave from the hospital, escorted by the staff. After several uneventful occasions, he ran away. As soon as Enid heard the news, she asked to see the senior nurse, and burst into tears.

Enid confessed that, as part of befriending Danny, she had given him her home phone number, so that he could ring her out of hours if he needed her. Then, when she had had a few days off, he had persuaded her to give him her home address, so that he could also write to her. As her birthday drew near, he had insisted that he should come to her party. He had absconded the day before it.

Some of the other staff arranged to be at her party too. Danny turned up as expected. He was surprised, but compliant with the insistence on immediate return to the hospital.

Enid had never made any physical overtures to Danny, nor had she made any direct suggestions to him that she should become his girlfriend. After the crisis, however, she admitted that she had begun to feel very differently about him than about all the other patients; she conceded that she was lonely too. He was convinced that she was his girlfriend. As he became more pressing for personal information about her, and then rather threatening, she got increasingly scared both of him and of telling other staff about her plight.

Enid could not be said to be 'unprofessional'. She had had little specialist training and no professional background. Her naivety and the failure of the qualified staff to recognize the developments at an earlier stage contributed to serious problems for everyone involved. The patient's leave was cancelled and his progress apparently set back by some months, although it is arguable that this fortuitous demonstration of his capacity to pose threat was important for more complete resolution of his problems. She lost much of her confidence in work that she had enjoyed. She had to work elsewhere in the hospital, but with intensive support and supervision did manage to continue working. Hospital staff from another unit interviewed her colleagues to consider whether policies, practice and procedure might have failed Danny and Enid, and how they might be improved.

Polly was a 52-year-old schoolteacher, and had been living on her own for a year since her partner had died from breast cancer. With a good deal of spare time, and a lot of caring experience, she decided she would like to befriend someone with a chronic illness but that, in the circumstances, she would probably cope best with the effects of a mental illness.

Elizabeth was in her early forties, recovering from a schizophrenic illness that had cut her off from her family. When very ill she had threatened to kill various family members. She had been forced to leave the family home as a result, but stayed in the area. One night she returned home with a knife and slashed or gouged most items in the house. The family rejected her completely.

Elizabeth spent several years in a secure hospital after this episode, her symptoms and consequent hostility to her family hardly touched by medication. She made no friends in the hospital, she had very little in common with any of the other patients in terms of her educational level and interests or her premorbid social experiences. Staff sought an outside befriender for her.

Polly started visiting Elizabeth, who clearly enjoyed the visits. She became generally more sociable on the ward, and often talked to her primary nurse about what the two of them had discussed. After about 6 months, Polly suggested that Elizabeth might visit her at home.

With Elizabeth's consent, staff told Polly a lot more about her story, and the concerns about her risk of violence towards those she became close to. Polly was still content for the visit to take place. Hospital staff accompanied Elizabeth. The visit was a great success; more followed, and, after a change in medication, Elizabeth made such good progress generally that the time came for her to move on from the hospital.

Not yet ready to live independently, this meant that she had to get to know a new group of health workers. The move was very stressful but eased by the fact that one constant was Polly, who had discussed the situation both with the hospital staff and with Elizabeth and resolved to stay in touch. When some 18 months later Elizabeth moved into her own flat, the women had established a firm friendship which each saw as very satisfying.

An important feature of this relationship was that both women allowed and maintained an openness throughout with professionals working with Elizabeth. No steps were taken in the relationship without consultation and consideration of the issues. It was of value to both women but most particularly to Elizabeth, who otherwise had little prospect of developing a satisfying friendship.

Replacing code with contract

For people who are employed in health, social or criminal justice services who have no professional training or code of practice, it may be wise to incorporate explicit guidance on the limits to relationships with patients or offenders in such circumstances in their contract of employment, or a letter of appointment which may accompany such contract. What is perhaps more commonly done in the health service at least is formal job review, perhaps annually, with an explicit note about expectations and formal supervision sessions for untrained as well as trained staff. Another helpful and wise approach, that need not be mutually exclusive, is the generation of a hospital or service policy on such relationships. Adequate information and guidance is then available to everyone working in the organization, and it is clear what behaviour would constitute a disciplinary matter.

In the USA, even subscribing to a professional code is not necessarily seen as an adequate safeguard. At least seven states (California, Colorado, Florida, Maine, Minnesota, North Dakota and Wisconsin) have criminal statute law prohibiting psychotherapist–patient sexual contact, while others have extended basic civil rights into civil cause of action statutes (Appelbaum and Jorgenson, 1991)

Frequency of boundary breaches

Gartrell and colleagues (1995) concluded from a review of seven studies between 1973 and 1988, three of them their own, that a consistent estimate of the order of the problem among psychiatrists was that 5–8 per cent acknowledged sex with their patients. The psychiatrists were usually male and the patients female, but all combinations had occurred. In their survey of physicians, they found 9 per cent reported such contact, some several times, with a similar heavy preponderance of male physician–female patient relationships. What is perhaps most remarkable is that two thirds of the respondents, *including 38 per cent of the involved clinicians*, indicated that such relationships were always harmful. For clinical psychologists, similar proportions of sexual relationships have been reported – 5.5 per cent for men and 0.6 per cent for women (Holroyd and Brodsky, 1977). Gottlieb (1990) reported more than a 275 per cent increase in complaints by patients of such abuse, but Pope (1990) was more optimistic. Reviewing only peer evaluated publications, he asserted a steady decline in self-reported rates of abuse, suggesting that a combination of professional efforts at prevention and multi-million malpractice awards may be having some impact.

Most reviewers, though (e.g. Gartrell *et al.*, 1995; Pope, 1990; Schoener 1989) are explicit about some of the problems in researching such matters. In the Gartrell physician survey, for example, questionnaires and a one page letter explaining the procedures for establishing complete confidentiality and anonymity were sent to 10 000 physicians. Nineteen per cent (1891) replied. The biases in such reporting can only be guessed at. It is arguable that physicians who had had sexual contact with their patients, particularly those in a state where such behaviour is against the criminal law, would be least likely to respond to such a questionnaire. About 23 per cent of the respondents indicated that they had at least one patient who had told them of sexual contact with another physician, which the authors take as evidence that their figure is likely to be a considerable underestimate of the real size of the problem. It is possible to argue also, however, that for those who are engaging in such behaviour, the confessional opportunity of an anonymous questionnaire is irresistible, thus leading to an overestimate. Wilbers *et al.* (1992), with a 74 per cent response rate from gynaecologists and ENT specialists, found 4 per cent had had actual sexual contact with patients; not a very different figure from other surveys. Beyond the problem of sampling, a further question arises as to the value of self report in such matters.

One of us (E.V.W.) attempted to investigate the issue in the probation service by a range of approaches. This served to emphasize further the barriers, both to assuring good clinical practice, and to research. First, a general observation: in reading hundreds of case files over a period of 13 years, no record of a consummated probation officer–client relationship has been found. Staff record approaches by an offender and how they dealt with it, but no record of an officer approach has been found. Even when a case has been removed from an officer for quality of relationship reasons, the officer factors will not be noted in the offender's file. There is no agreed protocol on how staff records are kept, this hardly being an issue that is exclusive to any one probation service. A preliminary review in one service confirmed these as an unlikely source of reliable information on this particular issue. Consequently, neither offender nor standard staff files were pursued as a source of frequency information.

Staff disciplinary records seemed to offer the best prospect of finding real and reliable evidence. Probation services work to codes of conduct and disciplinary procedures. In a sample of such disciplinary records in eight probation services, all included personal and sexual relationships in the misconduct or gross misconduct category. There is an expectation that any known or alleged sexual or personal relationship will be investigated within these procedures.

In 1987, the Association of Chief Officers of Probation (for England and Wales) produced a confidential, intra-service *Digest of Disciplinary Matters*. Fifty-five chief probation officers were invited to submit details of cases dealt with at chief officer or probation committee level in the previous three and a half years. Forty-eight services responded and, of these, 17 had no cases to return. The remaining 31 services yielded 65 cases, of which 13 concerned 'unprofessional relationships with clients, including sexual relationships'. This exercise has not yet been repeated, but on checking records in one of the larger services included in the original returns, only four cases were found, suggesting that the rate is unlikely to have changed substantially.

The 13 cited behaviours were:

- Experienced male officer exposed his penis to offender.
- Male officer working with one probation service engaged in sexual relationship with woman offender supervised from another.
- Female officer admitted personal relationship with life sentenced prisoner
- Female officer admitted sexual relationship with a client of the service who had previously been supervised by her.
- Probation officer had a sexual relationship with a client.
- Wife of a prisoner due for parole claimed that a male probation officer had been making advances to her, e.g. holding hands with her, visiting her at home frequently, and getting her to sit on his lap.
- Female probation officer reported to have had sexual relationship with an 18-year-old male supervisee of the service while supervising a group of offenders at an outdoor pursuits centre.

- Probation officer became personally involved with the new partner of one party in a divorce where access to the children was in dispute.
- Male deputy warden of a hostel committed acts of gross indecency with a resident under 21.
- Female officer developed a personal relationship with a male offender.
- Female officer formed relationship with a male parolee.
- Community service supervisor, on visiting one of his female clients at home, kissed her three times against her wishes.
- Residential hostel worker had off-duty personal relationships with residents.

In each case the 'defence to the charge' gives some indication of the needs that were being met. On the basis of self report, sexual attraction was the predominant ingredient, while one probation officer said that she had looked for friendship. Three linked the behaviours to stress at work and/or in their own domestic circumstances. Three stated that they had been trying to help the offender, and that their actions had been misinterpreted. One denied the allegations altogether, although the case was proven, while another did not see anything improper in establishing personal relationships with offenders under supervision.

Two instances were established from the range of inquiries of the probation officer/worker and supervisee becoming established as a couple.

Perhaps one of the most important things to emphasize is that this trawl from a majority of probation services in England and Wales suggests that the development of personal intimacy, whether sexual or otherwise, between probation officers and those under their supervision is very rare indeed. In just one of the years covered by this official review, 1994, the courts in England and Wales placed 112 000 individuals under the statutory supervision of probation services, while 34 000 prisoners also began a period of statutory supervision. As might be expected, in other professions a discrepancy between estimates from self report studies and those from formally investigated cases has been demonstrated (Gartrell et al., 1983). At first sight, the suggestion in these probation figures that the incidence of inappropriately intimate relationships between officer and offender is so much lower than that in other comparable professional situations (about one in ten physicians, psychiatrists or psychotherapists (see above); about 13 per cent of clergy (Church of Christ, 1986, cited in Fortune, 1995)) might be explained away on this basis. Fortune, as many before her and since, speculates that such relationships primarily reflect the balance of power between the sexes and wider sexual abuse and exploitation by men of women in the general population. If there is anything in this assumption, it may be a better explanation than mere data inadequacy as to why probation service breaches appear so much lower. Men form the majority of the offender group, and the majority of the workers in the 1990s have been women. The power in the worker role is thus more commonly vested in women.

One further approach to data collection was attempted. Over a few weeks towards the end of 1995, ten officers in one large probation service, who had held more than 5 years' management and supervisory responsibilities, were asked about their experiences in this regard. All 'knew of' such cases, but felt that they were rare. Three spoke of 'suspicions', one of experience of a staff member becoming 'directly involved' with a supervisee. Eight field probation officers chosen at random for interview all saw drifting into a personal relationship with an offender as a potential occupational hazard. All the officers felt safer discussing the general issues rather than specific cases or direct experience. Discovery draws the supervisor and the senior manager into a protracted investigation of the most demanding and sensitive kind, whilst facing anger and denial by the worker. For the latter, it carries professional disgrace and disciplinary action. For the agency itself, inquiry is a resource intensive process which, if it becomes public, can undermine and discredit the whole service. No more reliable data on frequency were elicited by this additional survey; only information about attitudes and worries.

Consequences of varying professional boundaries

A case for benefit?

As formality in relationships in society generally has lessened, so it has in professional relationships. It is now commonplace, for example, although not invariable, for a professional and a patient or offender to be on first name terms with each other. There is talk of such informality as breaking down barriers to therapy but, in spite of this testable hypothesis, there is no research evidence for such an effect, and none which explores the possibility of adverse 'side effects', for example increased risk of abuse. If a manoeuvre even as apparently simple as varying the form of address is as powerful in a positive direction as suggested, it is unlikely that it has no negative effects. Then, there is little evidence of any consistent attempt to treat this matter as part of the clinical process. The decision to use first names is generally applied across the board, or occasionally not, and for any individual is thus commonly a decision by default, not one based on perceived individual needs. The same arguments apply to breach of recognized styles of dress, whether designated uniform or a kind of dress style that becomes almost a surrogate for it although here, as described above, a little more is known about the limited benefits of informality.

Schoener (1995a) reviews some of the confusion that has reigned over the case for more intimacy, up to and including sexual relations. Some of the pioneers of psychotherapy are cited as having crossed this final boundary with one or more of their patients, but rarely as claiming any therapeutic advantage for it. The advent of 'sex therapy' in the 1970s brought tantalizing talk of 'sexual surrogates' as an acceptable approach to the therapy of sexual difficulties, but again there was no evidence in favour of this. Schoener notes that among the leaders of the sex therapy movement, Masters and Johnson rather drew attention to the numbers of their clients who had reported sexual encounters with previous therapists, by implication a contributing factor to their need for treatment.

One of the most challenging variations in personal boundaries to be advocated that we know of in relation to offender patients was at the high security hospital, Oak Ridge at Penetanguishene in Ontario, Canada. 'Defence-disrupting' therapy was advocated through an extraordinary mixture of powerful psychoactive drugs, including barbiturates, amphetamines and LSD and nude encounter groups in an isolation capsule. The treatment was compulsory (Barker and McLaughlin, 1977; Barker et al., 1969). There was no suggestion that sexual activity between the participants would be beneficial, and no record of whether that occurred. The treatment was described rather than researched, and the evidence of benefit slight.

Case for harm to the patient or client

Harm accruing to patients or clients from sexual encounters with professional people attending them may vary from perceptions of being exploited or betrayed, through impaired treatment, care or supervision as objectivity is impaired, to post-traumatic stress disorders. All have been documented, sometimes all problems within one person. Damage may extend, too, beyond the immediate patient or client to his or her family (College of Physicians and Surgeons of Ontario, 1991). The majority of psychiatrists who later treat such patients report that the sexual contact was harmful, and at least one of the reasons for the patient being in the new treatment (Gartrell *et al.*, 1987). The rating of harm, however, was related to their own probity. Among those who had assaulted patients in this way on more than one occasion, only 39 per cent rated therapist–patient contact as invariably harmful, compared with 70 per cent of one-time offenders and 88 per cent of those who had never assaulted patients. A particularly disturbing problem is that, within psychotherapeutic relationships, a person may have sought the therapy in part because of a previous experience of abuse, only to find it compounded by repetition in the therapy. Bouhoutsos *et al.* (1983) sent questionnaires to all 4385 licensed psychologists in California. Only 704 returned, but 318 of these provided accounts of 559 patients under treatment at the time who had been intimate with previous therapists. Ninety per cent of the patients were reported to have suffered ill effects, including increased depression, loss of motivation, increased drug or alcohol use, deterioration in other intimate relationships, interference with therapy and attitudes to therapists. Eleven per cent of the patients had to be admitted to hospital and 1 per cent committed suicide. Durre (1980) similarly concluded that therapist erotic or sexual attachment was 'detrimental if not devastating to the client'.

Again, a case example perhaps best brings bald statistics to life.

Mick was 19 and had had a chaotic life almost from the moment of conception. His mother was beaten by her partner throughout her pregnancy until she ran away. After his premature birth, she sought refuge with one man after another, but each was abusive. Mick was often beaten too by a succession of 'uncles' and stepfathers, but during his mother's longest relationship punitive harshness was replaced by sexual abuse. Whenever his mother was out, Mick, by then aged 10, was expected to engage in mutual fondling with this father figure. After the first month he was regularly buggered. When he was 12, he ran away from home and, in between periods in children's homes, lived by his wits on the streets.

Living by his wits included theft of various kinds, including cars, substance misuse, and damage to property. Increasingly he got into fights, and violent convictions. After attacking a drinking acquaintance with a broken bottle, he was remanded to prison to await trial.

He survived 2 months on remand without major incident, but he frequently demanded medical services for trivial complaints. The doctor arranged regular appointments for him, insisting on full physical examinations each time. He then started fondling Mick's genitals. A month later Mick was found hanging in his cell during a routine patrol. He had stopped breathing and was blue, but was resuscitated.

The story of the progression to sexual abuse on the part of a person that Mick had initially responded to as a caring person in an otherwise tough regime only came to light at that point. Mick's story was consistent with independent accounts of similar experiences from other prisoners in that jail, which only came to light when the service had been alerted in this way. Confronted with the evidence, the doctor confessed to his problems. Mick was admitted to a psychiatric hospital.

Harm to the professional, semi-professional or voluntary carer

Perhaps embarrassed by early tendencies to warn against the threat posed to male therapists, carers and clergy by disordered, hysterical and predatory women, there has been a tendency to presume the patient or client necessarily takes a passive role in the development of any relationship. Sometimes this is true, perhaps most commonly, although there are no satisfactory data on this point, but sometimes the patient/offender is active in promoting the relationship. Collusion or erotic responsiveness to this is nonetheless likely to be damaging to the patient or offender, but real threat, usually in career terms, can accrue to the clinician, carer, or supervisor. Recognition of such potential is not to justify inappropriate responses on their part, but rather to acknowledge a real problem and better prepare such people for preventive action.

Occasionally, eroticization of a relationship can be more directly physically and/or emotionally damaging to the practitioner.

Erotomania is a disorder of loving, and invokes debate as to whether it is a primary disorder, or invariably a part of a more generalized psychotic process (Taylor et al., 1993). There is probably a heterogeneity of presentations and prognosis; Rudden et al. (1990), for example, found that about one quarter of their sample had a monodelusional presentation (i.e. the feature in isolation). The rest, whose symptoms seemed to be part of a schizophrenic illness, tended to have the poorer longer term outcome. Presentations may range between an exaggerated sentimental attachment to the more classically described delusional state, in which the patient/sufferer believes that a relatively remote, powerful or distinguished person loves him/her. Initially this may be a source of comfort or pleasure, but it commonly leads to resentment, distress and anger. Sometimes the love object may be fanatically pursued and, more rarely, attacked. The importance of raising this condition here is that the object of love is not uncommonly a doctor, other health care worker, social worker, probation officer or a lawyer who, until the condition becomes manifest, may have had only the most marginal contact with the sufferer.

In the care and supervision of offenders, the role of a mental disorder in disordered attachments may be less obvious. The case of a man who was well advanced in the process of resettling in the community illustrates the dangers that can arise when the blurring of professional boundaries coincide with an offender's repetitive disorder in relationships and his disordered sexuality.

Luke, at the age of 30, was on parole as part of a 10-year prison sentence for rape. It was not his first sexual offence. During his imprisonment he started to pursue one of the qualified nurses, Ann, in the infirmary there. She had treated him several times for minor ailments. She developed an affection for him. She began to realize that the relationship was going beyond professional bounds and, wanting to continue it, she left the service. He was transferred to an open prison as the planning of his prison career was implemented. She became a regular visitor for him, and made a home for him to come to when he left. His parole may well have been brought forward because of this arrangement. Information about her former status had not transferred with him and his prison files.

Once out of prison, he told his partner that he wanted her support in protecting his privacy, since his imprisonment had made him sick of intrusive professionals, whom he generally regarded as useless anyway. He told her and his probation officer that he was so determined to find work that he was prepared to travel the country to do so. They were impressed. The probation officer decided to work closely with his partner and to trust her, in effect, to do some of the supervision, because she had reported that she had had substantial experience as a psychiatric nurse, only leaving for a job with better pay. The probation officer had checked this account and found it to be broadly true; she was not told and did not find out about the brief period for which the nurse worked in the prison service, nor the circumstances of her client's meeting.

Luke was away from home a lot during the week, but was in fact using his time to be with a new girlfriend. He told her that he was in the Territorial Army and would be away most weekends on exercises. This covered his time with Ann. As financial problems grew in both partnerships, he 'confessed' to Ann and his probation officer that he had lost his job, had not been working for some time, but had been too afraid to tell them in case his licence should be revoked. Sympathetic, his probation officer arranged for him to attend a voluntary project.

Sue was a voluntary worker there while waiting to go to university. She knew that he had committed an offence, but no details of it. Luke found her very attractive, and she agreed to go for a drink with him on a couple of occasions. As he increased pressure on her, however, to become his girlfriend, she realized what was happening, and tried to distance herself. He persuaded her not to tell the probation officer supervising the project of the situation between them, saying she would be the cause of his recall to prison if she did. With the complexities in his relationships growing, he became more and more anxious and irritable. He kept checking with Sue that she had not told anyone about them, until in desperation she said that she would have to do so if he did not leave her alone. That night he insisted, by way of atonement, on walking her home from the project, in a deprived inner city area. He killed her.

Professional staff are naturally reluctant to supply information about people with a mental disorder, or who have been offenders beyond the bounds of a professional group involved with an individual. Here the natural caution in sharing information, and advice on how to seek help in the event of problems, was compounded by the expectation that the placement in the project was a very temporary expedient, pending resumption of paid employment. The tragedy for Sue and her family touched all those who had been trying to help Luke, as the professionals involved each had a sense of great personal responsibility for what had happened and, further, an independent inquiry into events inevitably followed.

Prevention of damage

It is important to recognize that there is no policy or procedure that can entirely eliminate risk of unwanted or harmful event or practice. Good practice involves a certain amount of risk taking, but calculated, shared or agreed and documented risks with in-built systems for monitoring each step, giving the opportunity to change management at an early stage if necessary. The idea is prevention of harm in the first place, but if this has not been achieved, harm limitation and prevention of repetition are vital, if again, not always achievable, goals. Accidental risk taking, or risk taking by default is generally poor practice.

There is much that can be done to minimize the risks of harmful practice, and, indeed, risk of harm through generally good practice. This includes clear service policies and, often, procedures and accurate implementation of these. They must incorporate general principles about the limits to relationships, but also guidance on appropriate basic training for staff and workers on recognition and management of problems, on supervision and support for them, and on their access to confidential advice. Less often appreciated is the importance of staff recruitment, selection and allocation. Not everyone is suited to this sort of work, and training cannot solve all personal skill deficiencies. At one extreme, some people may be frankly dangerous if, for example, they are known to have a propensity for over-stepping personal boundaries; appointment to posts in which people will be working with children, for example, should generally include a criminal records screen for offences against children. Then, on occasion, someone who is eminently suited in terms of personal qualities may not be suited because of the mix of workers required. It is unlikely to be appropriate, for example, for all members of a work or volunteer force to be men when the clientele are all women, or vice versa.

Staff recruitment and selection

Identification of the right workers for a task is still more art than science when this is extended beyond a requirement for specific skills. The service must be clear about the range and nature of the tasks to be done, and have an ability to convey the essence of these to prospective employees. Then an attempt to specify not only the professional qualifications and/or skills required, but also some of the more personal qualities, is likely to be helpful in the process of selection. Table 13.1 offers one possible practical approach, albeit still open to a good deal of subjectivity. It is important never to appoint a person to a post or task simply because that person is the only one available. In many parts of the mental health and criminal justice services this can be a very great temptation because of the shortage of people with appropriate motivation, aptitude and specialist skills.

Schoener (1995b) discusses administrative risk management and employer liability, also with particular reference to selection of staff. The importance of checking previous employment records, references and licence status is emphasized. His checklist of safeguards goes on to include the existence of up-to-date and pertinent policies, an established 'complaints' procedure, staff education about policies and disciplinary matters, supervision and support and the nature of information for patients or clients.

Recognition of risk – the need for and creation of the organizational climate

Reference has already been made to how poorly staff in many caring services are prepared for these risks. By the same token, it becomes generally 'unsafe' for discussion of such problems in an explicit, personal way and the organization

Table 13.1 Framework for self and other assessment of ability to work in a close professional or contractual relationship with people who need care, treatment and/or custody

Quality or skill	Indicators that might be tested
Capacity for self-awareness	Reflective statements/practice Identification of own interactive strengths/weaknesses Strengths/weaknesses in relevant knowledge base Triggers to defensive responses Ability to challenge practice of others Awareness of own attitudes to presenting problem(s) of patient/offender
Perception of role	Clarity about primary purpose of relationship
General planning abilities	Make judgements based only on observations and knowledge List achievable short term goals in the relationship List longer term goals
Ability to communicate	Ability to listen Ability to observe Awareness of non-verbal forms of communication in self and in patient/offender Unambiguous verbal communication with patients Unambiguous verbal communication with colleagues Accurate and concise written communications Ability to work as part of a team and/or supervision

Empathetic approach to patients/ supervisees	Recognition of the *patient's* perceptions of:
	  being in the service
	  any maladaptive behaviour(s)
	  any illness/disorder
	  need for treatment, care and/or control

Negotiation of relationship boundaries	Patient/client centred approach Genuineness, warmth and positive regard of the person Ability to create and maintain trust Ability in this context to maintain awareness of disorder and risk of harm to self or others Understanding of dynamics in relationships Willingness/ability to challenge others and to be challenged Evidence of appropriate limit setting Ability to evaluate boundary practice to be evaluated
Reality based risk taking	Shared decision making with patient/offender Constructive non-coercive use of influence/role modelling
Achievement motivation	Setting the environment in which the patient/offender can achieve

Sense of humour	Appropriate use of humour to:
	  create rapport
	  lower tension

Supportive evidence of ability to:	recognize anxiety in self and colleagues express concerns, at an early stage share care, control tasks and/or treatment obtain appropriate support and supervision for self support others

can become trapped in a vicious circle where practitioners are afraid, and supervisors too insecure in their own experience, to tackle such issues voluntarily.

An organizational approach which openly acknowledges the considerable potential within cases for a slide towards intimacy between worker and supervisee seems preferable. Within this framework, risk would be seen as naturally occurring because of the patient or offender profile and the nature of the task, rather than incompetence or immorality in the worker. The service could work to create a professional environment within which it is safe to recognize and disclose the fact that inappropriate involvement with a patient or offender is a risk, or is beginning to happen, and then tackle it objectively at an early stage before damage is done to either party.

If it is to be accepted as an organizational as well as an individual responsibility, the process needs to begin at the worker's induction stage. Awareness and skills must be developed through training, and then continuously supported and reinforced in supervision. Practitioners need to be aware of, and able to recognize, the indicators that relationship distortion is happening. and to have practised and rehearsed tackling this directly with the patient or offender and bringing it into supervision. A great deal of inappropriate supervisee behaviour could also be prevented by 'setting the case up' properly. This would mean the practitioner being very clear with the patient or offender from the outset about the purpose and likely content of work sessions, the nature of the professional relationship and the ground rules which apply.

Similar awareness and skill is needed in the supervisor of the worker, both in supporting and developing the worker in this field and in recognizing and handling the situation should it appear that appropriate boundaries are threatened.

One of the great benefits for the practitioner in involving a supervisor is that the latter can be more objective about what is happening, suggest alternative approaches or, occasionally, transfer the case if the risk otherwise is too high. This model can be applied with benefit even when the practitioner is senior and experienced in the field. Then, case review may be with a peer, may be less frequent, but is still an important safeguard for patient/offender and practitioner alike.

Where this is insufficient as a primary prevention, and a personal relationship does develop, there should still be an incentive to disclose. The organization could transfer the case, or move the worker, whilst giving him/her a period of time within which to consider and receive objective help in exploring the cost or benefits of sustaining the relationship. If a worker refused to comply, or there were evidence of continuing or widespread intimacy with supervisees, the service would still have recourse to its disciplinary procedures.

This same framework is needed for volunteers. Services which use volunteers have a responsibility for their care of the patient or offender – and indeed the safety and well-being of the volunteer. The prescribed duties of volunteers are much narrower and more finely circumscribed than those of trained professional staff but, in part because of this, the vulnerabilities are potentially greater. The purpose of intervention and ground rules for behaviour must be established clearly through induction, training and supervision appropriate to the task. Volunteers must be helped to set appropriate boundaries with patients or offenders and both recognize and feel supported to involve the supervisor if these are threatened in any way. It then becomes the supervisor's responsibility to decide whether it is appropriate to keep the volunteer involvement or use professional staff only. One added dilemma in volunteer involvement, however, is the greater ease with which a person in that role can switch from 'official' volunteer to unofficial befriender, with the consequent shedding of many opportunities for limit setting.

Importance of practice framework and accurate and timely records

Evidence suggests boundary violations frequently accompany or precede sexual misconduct, but the violations themselves do not always constitute malpractice or misconduct or even bad technique. As Gutheil and Gabbard (1993) point out, however, clinicians should be aware of three principles that govern relationships: boundary crossings; boundary violations (a harmful crossing) and sexual misconduct. Boundaries for these purposes cover the following:

1. Role
Many of the issues here have already been covered, but it cannot be emphasized too often that it is useful for professional and lay workers alike to clarify their role with the patient/offender and record it.

2. Time
An interesting prejudice about violating the boundaries of time has evolved in sexual misconduct cases in the health service. The clinician interested in having a sexual relationship with the patient might well schedule that patient for the last hour of the day. Another risk may arise if sessions frequently run over time or are scheduled for longer than 45–60 minutes. In the fog of uncertainty surrounding sexual misconduct, usually a conflict of credibilities without witnesses, practitioners should be aware of the possibility of time delinquencies as an indicator of potential problems and, where there is a good case for deviance from common practice, discuss it with colleagues and/or record it.

3. Place and space
Privacy is an essential component of most individual therapy sessions. Reference has already been made to the increasingly common situation of the practitioner seeing the person – whether patient or probationer – in his or her own home. Transporting the individual in the practitioner's car is also quite common. For psychotherapists, the position is not uncommonly reversed, with the office an integral part of the therapist's home. Again, ground-rules for structuring the sessions, and for systems' awareness of them, should be explicit.

4. Money, gifts, services and related matters
In the UK, where public health and social services are the norm, it is relatively unusual for it to be necessary for money or goods to change hands between patients or offenders and their workers. Psychotherapy and some forms of counselling may form the exception, and here practitioners would argue that if the process of money exchange is handled properly, this in itself may be a useful way of clarifying boundaries. The place of gifts is much more difficult. Small gifts may well be an important way of a patient or client saying a more personal and natural 'thank you', and a refusal of such a gift is churlish at best and

counter-therapeutic at worst. Nevertheless, even small gifts can be an intrusion on acceptable relationship boundaries, and are rarely appropriate until the therapy or supervision is complete.

5. Clothing
Revealing or frankly seductive clothing worn by practitioners may be construed by patients or offenders as provocative in all sorts of ways. Unconventional dress may raise personal curiosity in a way that deflects from the therapeutic or supervisory task in hand, the curiosity not necessarily about matters sexual at all in the first instance. One of us had an interesting experience when nursing staff first came out of uniform in one English teaching hospital. There was a vogue at the time for military style clothing, and several staff tended to appear on duty in camouflage type battle dress. They may well have felt beleaguered, but interpretations aside, one or two patients attending a forensic psychiatry clinic were quick to see this as an invitation to engage in battle games, and one had already begun to act out some of his more sadistic fantasies before the new staff dress 'code' was questioned and modified.

6. Language
Forms of address from practitioner to patient/offender and vice versa have already been discussed. There are few hard and fast rules about what is acceptable, but again a good general rule is that naming should not be simply a process that happens by default.

7. Self-disclosure
This is another complex issue. Staff may occasionally and usefully use a neutral example from their own lives to illustrate a point. Sharing the impact of a patient's behaviour may also be useful. The attempt at empathy through sharing personal experience is more dangerous ground. Some people who have been abused, for example, find it difficult to work on that experience with anyone who has not also been through it, on grounds that they see the therapist as a voyeur. There is little evidence either way on sharing such experiences *per se* in therapy, but until an irrefutably positive case can be made for it, the general principle of being there only for the problems of the patient or offender is wise. The therapist's self revelation in any other sense, of personal fantasies or dreams or of social, sexual and financial details of special holiday plans or of expected births or deaths in the family, is generally inappropriate.

8. Physical contact
Some staff argue that some benign physical contact can be positive, particularly when working through a difficult and painful episode with a patient. If employed, it must be clear and open and preferably documented to prevent any misconstruction of this.

Gutheil and Gabbard suggest that sexual misconduct usually begins with relatively minor boundary crossings, which may crescendo into a pattern of increasing intrusion into a supervisee's space. The shift from talking to intercourse is rare. A number of authors have suggested a common pathway lies in transition from last name to first name, then personal conversation intruding into the clinical work, then body contact from a touch on the shoulder, massages, progressing to hugs, increasing closeness, and finally sexual intercourse. Such a pattern would give plenty of opportunity for cessation or intervention, but seems rather too neat compared with our experience of accounts. Useful guidance for self monitoring was suggested to us by Feldbrugge (see also Acknowledgements). If, as a clinician, one develops a sense of not wanting to share a particular aspect of a patient/offender relationship with others in the clinical team or supervisory structure, then that may be exactly the time to do so. Epstein and Simon (1990) offer a simple self-assessment questionnaire for therapists which may serve as an early self-warning of potential boundary violations.

Not all boundary crossings or even boundary violations, however, lead to sexual misconduct. Further, a clear boundary violation from one clinical perspective may be standard professional practice from another. Bad training, sloppy practice, lapses of judgement, idiosyncratic treatment philosophies, regional variations and social and cultural conditioning may variously be reflected in behaviour that appears to violate boundaries, but may not necessarily be harmful or deviate from the relevant standards of care. A transparent framework for practice reduces the chance of misunderstanding.

Despite the complexity of meaning of boundary transitions, disciplinary committees or professional conduct committees tend to believe that boundary violation or crossing is presumptive evidence or corroboration of allegations of sexual misconduct. In an area where the extremes between rigid professionalism and sexual exploitation are obvious, proper intermediate thresholds are far from clear and still evolving. The best advice must be to test practice constantly within one's peer group, and to record in writing all key events and decisions in a relationship. This becomes particularly important if any activity has taken place or is about to take place that the body of the profession or peer group would regard as unusual.

Education and training

It follows from all we have said that we would favour incorporation of a training module, however brief, in this area for all professional health and criminal justice staff who will be working in close contact with patients or clients, or who will be supervising those who are. This would include an understanding of the principles of relationships in this context – that there are expectations of trust on the part of the patient/client and society alike, that there are unusual power dynamics in such relationships and that breach of trust almost invariably has a harmful effect. It would also include teaching about transference and counter-transference and their development, attention to the possibility that many of the clientele may have suffered sexual or physical abuse or both, awareness of personal feelings, beliefs and attitudes to human relationships and sexuality, and acknowledgement of the possibility that professional workers and their patient/clients may be vulnerable to non-professional developments in those relationships. They may also be vulnerable simply to allegations that this has happened.

In the 1990s the Family Planning Association developed courses in the UK and an array of practically based materials which were designed for group activity to facilitate the exploration of key problems in this area in institutional care, particularly for people with learning disability (e.g. McCormick and Shevlin, 1997). These materials allowed staff to debate perceived problems in a safe setting. They were expected to get in touch with their own attitudes and prejudices towards sexuality, in particular among those with disability, illness or needing to live in an institution. Staff groups using such material need some expert facilitation and the opportunity for all staff who work in any given unit, irrespective of their position within the hierarchy, to share their views and perceptions. Such sessions could be a precursor for policy formation based on a shared understanding of the issues. The work of Wolfensberger (1972) is also useful here.

General principles of staff support and supervision

An essential part of professional training involves learning how to deal with the emotional by-products of treating and supervising patients and clients. Cognitive understanding is not enough to deal adequately with these problems; support and introspection are also necessary. Good supervision contains some basic elements, regardless of detail in the model. Norman (1987) suggests that first the supervisee (here referring to the professional/volunteer) and supervisor should have a supervisory contract, by which she means an agreed time and frequency of meetings, and some agreement about the work to be done and the expectations each has of the other. Secondly, the supervisor should acknowledge that s/he is to supervise not only the supervisee's case(s), but the supervisee as well, and recognize that the relationship is a therapeutic alliance. The supervisee must accept this too. The supervisor is there to help develop the supervisee's diagnostic and treatment skills and aid in the supervisee's professional growth. Supervision is the arena in which to deal with transference and counter-transference issues. The supervisee should be able to depend on the supervisor and use him or her on a crisis basis when needed. Finally, the supervisee should be emotionally supported by the supervisor. These elements make supervision an optimum learning and development tool in the mental health field.

As for other disciplines, supervision has emerged as a critical issue for nursing. The latter was particularly striking during the early 1990s with the United Kingdom Central Council for Nurses, Midwives and Health Visitors (1995) making a statement in this regard. This suggested an advantage in separating supervision from line management. This view is supported by Powell *et al.* (1990), who state that 'good supervision gets to the heart of the work in a way that single focus in line management cannot'. Not only does supervision provide for more accountable decision making, but it gives support to carers as they wrestle with their own uncertainties. Powell and co-workers go on to suggest that a core curriculum for training supervision would contribute towards a greater consistency of supervision received by trainees, in turn providing for safer practice. The core curriculum recommended includes:

1. *Negotiation.* Supervisors need to be aware of possible areas for negotiation in supervision and possible barriers for success in this, for example relative status/role in the organization; relative experience in other matters. These areas might include: amount of supervision; timing and frequency; agenda; modes of supervision; special interest; who supervises.

2. *Giving and receiving feedback.* Elements here may include: how to give positive feedback; how to give negative feedback; how to receive feedback;

how to give feedback on the way feedback is given or received; and how to enable the other person to give you feedback.

3. *Assessment of supervisee's work*. Issues here may involve: what to assess and how to record it; how to manage the different emphasis of supervision and assessment; how to enable the supervisee to manage the supervision and assessment; how to assess jointly the effect of any supervision session and the overall progress of supervision.

4. *Dealing with difficult issues within supervision*. Powell *et al.* (1990) suggest there are four basic assumptions in supervision. The first is that trust will develop between supervisor and supervisee. The second is that boundaries will be protected in relation to time and space allocated to the supervision sessions. Thirdly, all aspects of the supervisor's behaviour and attitudes may be seen as contributing to the modelling of good practice for the supervisee, i.e. punctuality, reliability, respect for privacy at the supervision sessions. The final basic assumption asserts that supervision is a process of continual development with application throughout a person's professional life.

Whilst clearly emphasizing that good supervision is important for staff working closely with people on their personal problems in relationship counselling, it is not without difficulties. Sarnat (1992) suggested that 'despite recent developments in our thinking about psycho-analytic supervision, controversy persists as to whether a supervisor can safely and appropriately engage a supervisee in exploring the conflicts and relationship problems that emerge in their work with patients'.

Mollon (1989) said, 'there is nothing in conventional psychology and clinical psychology to provide any intellectual structure for understanding and emotionally preparing for the fact that the patient may be hostile in a way which is genuinely damaging to the mental state of the therapist. This means that the psychologist is highly vulnerable to the sadistic or perverse patient and bewildered when their well intentioned applications of scientifically respectable techniques are not appreciated by their client'. Mollon points out that patients who have suffered very damaging early interactions with parents are often compelled unconsciously to recreate these in the transference. This underscores the need for sound supervisory sessions. Mollon describes one student's experience as, 'following this supervision, the supervisee felt more in control of the next session. She described the effect of the supervision in terms of helping her to feel less sucked in as she put it and to recover her own boundaries and her sense of objectivity'. Other supervisees describe the supervision sessions as having a temporary effect, one indication of the importance of regular, continuing supervision. It is part of the supervisor's task to empathize accurately with the experiences of both the patient and the therapist, and to follow up needs accordingly. He or she has responsibilities to both, to function as a third party mediating and giving perspective to the therapeutic dyad. The crucial task in the supervisory session is to create a setting in which uncertainty, ignorance and feelings of incompetence can be tolerated and discussed, a culture quite different from the usual professional practitioner expectation of 'being supposed to know'.

Greben (1991) goes so far as to suggest that, in training supervision, there may be some advantage in having access to more than one supervisor. In practice, there are generally and perhaps should be limitations to the range of supervision available. Multiple supervision offering an extensive range of opinion is all very fine in an unpressured training situation, but in busy practice is unlikely to be an option, and if it were, quite likely to be confusing. One very practical model is offered by Relate, the marriage guidance counselling service in the UK. This comprises a parallel system of personal supervision and group support. The regional tutor sees individual counsellors on a one to one basis, usually at 2-weekly intervals for a session of 1 hour. During these sessions the counsellor and supervisor focus in turn on each of the cases in the counsellor's caseload, and refer to the files. An important element of these sessions is always to consider the feelings of the counsellor towards the individuals or couples seen. On a weekly basis, each counsellor also takes part in a 1-hour, facilitated group. Individual counsellors ask for time for cases which may be giving them particular concern, and seek the advice of fellow counsellors on how to progress.

In the Probation Service one to one supervision between practitioners and manager continues to be the bedrock of professional development. Increasingly, however, regular team support meetings provide additional challenge and support, and service-wide practice forums or learning sets play a major role in the development of practice.

Management of allegations of sexual misconduct

Allegations of violations of professional boundaries, and/or sexual misconduct may arise in a number of ways. On the whole patients and offenders find them difficult to make. In common with people who have been victimized in other ways, people who have become involved sexually with a supervisor or therapist feel guilt and shame about what has happened, regardless of the balance of responsibilities. In addition, they have good reason to question whether the system is trustworthy enough to handle any complaint fairly. Betrayed by one professional, they have little ground for optimism that another will believe them or, in cases where their liberty may be at stake, to be confident that they will not merely be punished for presumption in challenging an authority figure.

One of the most likely ways for such an allegation to emerge, therefore, even in what many professionals would now regard as a 'complaints culture', is during individual or group therapy with another professional, possibly not even employed by the same service or authority. In this situation, the prime task is the management of the problems with which the patient/offender is seeking help, but there is an inescapable issue as to whether the current professional has a duty to pass on information about the alleged abuser, or at least to encourage the complainant to make a formal complaint to the relevant authority. It is unlikely to be appropriate for the new therapist or supervisor to act without the patient/ offender's consent in this matter. Any allegation or complaint of such seriousness would lead to investigation and involve the patient/offender in questioning and probably confrontation by their former abuser and/or at the very least their legal representative.

Any complaint may be to the employing authority, the alleged abuser's professional body, or both. At some stage there may also be a question of civil litigation. In the UK, unlike some states in the USA, professional–patient/client sexual or eroticized relationships *per se* do not constitute a criminal offence but if related matters, such as evidence of coercion, or relationships with a person under the age for sexual consent, could be established then these would be independent grounds for criminal prosecution over and above any disciplinary, professional or civil case.

In the UK it is probable that the first place of complaint about such matters, or the repository of first suspicions that anything irregular is happening, is the professional's employing authority. Effective employers will have clear policies for the management of complaints in general and specifically for complaints of distorted, unprofessional relationships, whether these are between staff and patients or supervisees, or to do with staff allegations of sexual harassment. It is probably not uncommon for the two things to go together. People who show disrespect for their colleagues are unlikely to show greater respect for their clientele.

It is crucial for both the complainant and the complained against that the procedure for dealing with the complaint is transparent and fair and, as far as possible, speedy. It is known for false and unproven allegations of this kind to have been made against professionals (Sederer and Libby, 1995) so, notwithstanding the balance in favour of complainants on evidence to date (e.g. Schoener and Milgrom, 1989), there must be no presumption of guilt. This is particularly difficult in practice when suspension of the employee may be unavoidable, pending enquiries. Equally, even a complainant known to have made previous false, exaggerated or, rarely, psychotic accusations must be taken seriously. Both complainant and complained against must be supported through the period of enquiry, and in so far as the treatment or supervision of the patient/ offender is affected by the withdrawal of the complained against, then a substitute may have to be made available. In addition, the needs of other patients or offenders in the professional's caseload must be considered. It is unlikely that many, if any, will remain in ignorance of the situation, and it is probably best that each receives a simple factual statement of the circumstances. For some it may be essential to arrange an immediate replacement worker/therapist, if only on an interim basis.

The situation may be complicated in relation to a more serious complaint, in the UK at least, by the variety of routes by which it may be pursued simultaneously (outlined above) and it is important that, as far as possible, one system does not interfere with another. An internal organizational investigation and/or disciplinary hearing need not and should not be in conflict with criminal proceedings and, further, in the event of the latter, need not and probably should not be suspended. There has, in some organizations, been a tendency to assume that investigation of allegations of abuse is better handed over in its entirety to the police, and/or that a simultaneous investigation by the employing organization might prejudice a criminal case. In fact the two systems tend to be interested in rather different aspects of the alleged behaviour. Also, the standards of proof required for establishment of breach of employment contract or professional disciplinary matters are different from (lower than) those for criminal convictions.

For an employing authority or its agents, clear documentation of all aspects of the case is an essential first step – including existing documentation, statements from the immediate protagonists, observation from others who know the patient/

offender and therapist/supervisor well, and/or the qualities in their relationship. Evidence from other patients/offenders may be important.

In the event of a complaint being upheld, the organizational response will depend on the nature of the behaviour and how it arose. The case of the nursing assistant who had given her personal details to a patient, described above, was dealt with as being as much an organizational problem as a personal problem for her and for the patient. True, the patient's security had to be re-established and her position in the hospital changed, but also it was imperative for the hospital to get clarity in its contractual arrangements with staff on these matters and to introduce training for them, most particularly for those who had no professional code.

In cases of clear personal responsibility, responses may vary from relocation of the employee, often with a formal warning, to dismissal. Whatever the outcome in these terms, established misconduct results in loss of reputation and professional credibility. For those retained in employment, promotion prospects are affected. While the details of proceedings are confidential, and records may even be expunged with the passage of time, the oral tradition ensures that these cases live long in the organizational memory. We suspect that few cases of misconduct in professional and other caring relationships were calculated, but in so far as warnings are relevant it appears that the gratification from such liaisons is short lived, but the workers pay a high price over a long time. Gartrell *et al.* (1995) for example, observed that between physicians and patients the duration of sexual involvement ranged from one encounter to more than 5 years, but in about two thirds of cases it was well under a year. Almost all professionals, of whatever discipline, expect and believe disciplinary action is appropriate.

Management of eroticized staff–patient/offender relationship

Where the principal tasks in the management of complaints are to try and establish truth and restore discipline, in the management of the relationship itself, the main goals are to re-establish the well-being of the patient/offender, of the staff person, and sometimes of the organization itself. Attention to each of these may be necessary even if no grounds for a complaint have been established. The patient/offender may feel doubly damaged or abused by a system which s/he may still perceive as abusive; even if vindicated, the process of examination is likely to have been extremely traumatic to the accused party, and in these circumstances other staff are likely to start engaging in defensive practices and/or to be less cooperative with primarily institutional tasks. Negative media interest in an organization or person has never depended on establishment of adverse facts. Nevertheless, most of the following discussion will apply to the assumption that wrongdoing was established.

Focus on the patient or offender

It is a problem in this as in so much else in this field, that there is almost no evidence on which to base advice. Much of the following is attractive for its common sense, but has little more than this face validity. Pioneers in the field have carefully documented each approach, described people who have come to them for help, and something of the outcomes, including personal testimony, for those who have completed their programmes, but approaches have not been formally tested.

At the heart of most work is the recognition that exploitation in a previous professional or caring relationship may have created new and serious needs that may need immediate attention. Suicidal and other self-harming behaviours may have become acute. The impact and meaning of the abuse itself will then need further exploration, before turning to the nature and extent of the problems for which therapy was originally sought or supervision ordered.

Small group therapy has been advanced as potentially the most helpful approach for abused clientele. Milgrom (1989a), one of the first to set up such a group, met with some curious responses from her professional peers, some considering that her announcement of the group was little more than a warning for other professionals not to get so involved. She argues that having a co-facilitator in such a group is almost necessary, both for the therapists in supporting each other in very difficult and demanding work, and also for the patient/offenders who may, in the circumstances, find it less intimidating to meet with two group leaders than one. She also suggested that these leaders/facilitators should be experienced clinicians because of the wide range of problems presenting, including depression and suicidal potential. The women who attended felt helped by the reduction in isolation they experienced when recognizing that others also had been trapped in unsafe therapy, and the relief in being able to channel their distress into the sessions and concentrate better on other issues through the rest of the week. While Milgrom's work was open ended, Luepker (1989, same volume) set up a time limited group programme, again relying on small groups, but primarily only to complete the task of becoming free from the exploitation and its effects, so that they would be able to clarify any continuing need to re-open work on the problems for which they had originally sought help and resume that, as appropriate. Disch (1989, same volume) set up 1-day workshops for ventilation of the therapist abuse and action on it, incorporating guided imagery techniques.

Acknowledgement is also given (Milgrom, 1989b) to the need to assist associates of the victims – the so-called secondary victims. One of us (P.J.T.) who has worked with such a situation would reinforce this point in yet another way, as being as important to the continuing development of the primary victim as the secondary. In one particularly difficult case, treated on an individual basis, a young, very beautiful but quite severely learning disabled woman had been raped by a care worker in her team. Very slowly she was able to describe what had happened to her in the primary incident and ventilate her distress about that. Two subsequent problems had, however, she said, distressed her even more. The first was that criminal proceedings had been taken against the care worker, and his barrister had attempted to demolish her testimony in court, attempting to portray her as incapable of appreciating the truth or without capacity to observe or recall events accurately. On the contrary she had no capacity for dissembling, and was perfectly capable of accuracy with respect to major incidents, but she found this challenge to her integrity immensely painful. (In another case, witness ability in similar circumstances was called into question on grounds of suggestibility, and formal testing was devised to assist the court with such competence issues (Gudjonsson and Gunn, 1982)). The other problem was more difficult to resolve. Her mother, who had just begun to acknowledge that her daughter was emerging into adult womanhood, was unable to continue to allow her the freedoms to travel and see friends that she had just begun to master and still wanted. The fact that no harm had come to her on such occasions, but rather only when in official care, was not something that her mother could acknowledge. Listening was the main direct work with the daughter; a structured programme of increasing independence in activities, although ostensibly focused on her, was in fact fulfilling her mother's need for reassurance and a gradual return to the previous gains.

Counselling or treatment for the staff person

As for the victim, the perpetrator of abuse is likely to need assessment and probably help at a number of different levels. Isolation is likely to be an early problem, and even risk factor for self-harm or suicidal behaviours. Isolation may arise as the individual has perhaps been asked not to discuss his or her situation with others, but more likely because of avoidance behaviours on all sides as allegations are assimilated. At this stage the individual is likely to be most needy of support and practical advice, including legal advice. Many for whom the allegations of abuse are substantiated are likely to need treatment, although it is unclear how many accept it. Among those who do have sexual contact with their patients or clients, serial contacts appear likely and suggest profound problems. Gartrell *et al.* (1995), for example, found that 42 per cent of physicians who reported sexual contact with patients claimed multiple contacts.

Gonsiorek (1989) describes a model for approaching therapy for this group. He points out that it is particularly difficult for those attempting to assess or treat such therapists (or supervisors or counsellors) to remain in an objective role and to avoid the punitive, even abusive position themselves. He distinguishes between work with those people who may have the possibility of resuming responsible or therapeutic work with others and those who will not. The goals and expectations for therapy should always be as explicit as possible, and discussion of the actual likelihood of a return to work must be included in this exercise. Even for those for whom no ban is ultimately imposed, or who retain or have licence to practice restored, resumption of work as they previously knew it is often not realistic. In Gonsoriek's view therapy can proceed only when there is agreement on realistic goals.

Conclusions

Close personal attachment to a person is probably incompatible with having that person in therapy or supervision on grounds of illness or antisocial behaviour. A frankly eroticized or sexual relationship in these circumstances is unacceptable, being almost invariably harmful to the patient or offender and commonly so to the therapist or supervisor. Depending on the status of the latter the behaviour is likely to be unprofessional and/or against employment contract, liable to civil suit and in some cases open to criminal prosecution. As the risks of such breaches of professional or contracted relationships seem high and the actual breach not negligible, it is essential that organizations employing people for this work ensure that the matter is not taboo, but that staff have training open to them and clear policies to work by. People who work in singleton practice may need to take active steps to avoid professional or practice isolation.

14

International perspectives on relationships and sexuality in secure institutions

Harvey Gordon

Across the world, a range of factors contribute to policies and procedures intended to safeguard people in the context of relationship and sexual needs if they become prisoners or patients. Often the effect is to deny them. Indeed, such relationships may be among the first civil rights that these groups lose (Gochros, 1972). Some of these factors are remarkably consistent between countries and cultures. Although most of the common ground is discussed elsewhere in this volume, a brief summary of the main points will serve to set the scene.

Factors influencing policies on relationships and sexuality

Moral factors

In the past, psychiatric patients were segregated by gender. This allowed for a relatively simplistic, moralistic and negativistic approach by society and by staff in psychiatric hospitals to their romantic or sexual partnerships. Philippe Pinel, in eighteenth/early nineteenth century France, inaugurated the release of psychiatric patients from physical restraint, and instituted in its place a form of moral treatment. In this construct, in an asylum as a place of rest, social and sexual intercourse was largely forbidden between the sexes and, further, neither masturbation nor homosexuality was permitted (Bourgeois, 1975).

A growing problem with the growth in elderly institutionalized populations is the prejudice against the notion that elderly people, elsewhere even healthy elderly people, might enjoy sex. Many nursing homes have no shared accommodation for married couples (Brown 1989; see also Taylor, this volume).

Religious influences

In societies influenced by strict orthodox religious communities, profound conflict may occur in psychiatric hospitals, not only in regard to policies on sexuality but even in relation to whether mixed wards should be allowed (Greenberg, 1993). In Israel, Greenberg and Witztum (1991) have recommended guidelines for working with religious psychiatric patients, whose beliefs may tend to preclude them from participation in secular life, whether in hospital or in the community. Religious issues are not always, however, paramount in considering issues of sexuality. Termination of pregnancy, for example is viewed very differently in Italy and Spain compared with Ireland, where it is illegal and socially disapproved – and yet all are predominantly Roman Catholic countries (Ester *et al.*, 1993).

Moral and religious issues overlap, and religion can be used as a rationalization for particularly stringent strictures, for example with regard to homosexuality (Chaimowitz, 1991; Leviticus, 18.3–18.22; Rose, 1994; Union of Liberal and Progressive Synagogues, 1990). Although Western countries and many others have relaxed laws against homosexuality, commonly some discrimination remains, for example in age of consent. Attitudes too have improved, but still public demonstrations of affection between couples of the same sex may be poorly tolerated even in many liberal Judeo-Christian societies.

Clinical factors

Disordered relationships and sexual behaviour are known to occur among the mentally ill (see e.g. Taylor, Davison, this volume), but this is not a consistent picture. Indeed, it is not even clear whether such disorder is more likely than among the well. Secure psychiatric hospitals, however, do hold a substantial number of patients who have been admitted following serious violence within partnerships or conviction for sex offences (Dell and Parker, 1979; Tennent *et al.*, 1980), or for sexually motivated offences, including murder (MacCulloch *et al.*, 1983; Podolsky, 1965). In prisons and secure psychiatric hospitals, therefore, are those who may be physically dangerous in established relationships, and sexually dangerous, often more randomly, but who require programmes of assessment and treatment to address these aspects of pathology. For these groups, as they recover, development of healthier relationships and expression of appropriate sexuality are important parts of psychosocial development and rehabilitation.

Role of psychoanalysis

Psychoanalysis has, from its beginnings, concerned itself with the centrality of sexuality in the human condition (Rozan *et al.*, 1971). Erikson (1959) wrote: 'psychoanalysis has emphasized genitality as one of the chief signs of a healthy personality'. The repression of romantic relationships and sexuality in secure institutions may thereby serve to stagnate or distort human development and compromise the achievement of full mental recovery. The developmental stage in this regard poses particular problems in delivering safe and effective management and is probably particularly acute for adolescents (see also Mason, this volume).

Effects of gender integration of services

The introduction of mixed wards began to occur all over the word from the late 1950s including Britain (Ortega, 1962), Canada (Costello and Gazan, 1962), the USA (Gligor and Tryon, 1973), France (Eiguer *et al.*, 1974) and the former Soviet Union (Voronou and Lisovenko, 1984).

Concurrently, greater availability of effective means of contraception allowed for any man or woman to engage in sexual intimacy without the risk of unwanted pregnancy. It was thought, therefore, that the need to segregate people with a mental disorder to prevent childbirth or hereditary transmission of disorder was reduced (Bourgeois, 1975). While there is evidence that patients may not be able to use such measures effectively (e.g. Abernathy *et al.*, 1975; Baillard-Lapresle, 1975; Kelly *et al.*, 1992; Menon *et al.*, 1994), sex education programmes for psychiatric patients have been shown to be effective in such respects as well as in creating awareness of sexuality in relationships as a more positive aspect of their life (Dincin and Wise, 1979; Rozensky and Berman, 1984).

Clinical staff in psychiatric hospitals often have feelings of personal discomfort when dealing with sexuality (Meier, 1975; Payne, 1993; Withersty, 1976), and managers fear a sexual incident or, worse, a pregnancy becoming public, and for these reasons developing relationships between patients may be variously ignored or made difficult. Indeed, the manner in which the media portrays psychiatric hospitals may significantly affect the polices adopted and the public's perception of mental illness (Kaye, 1994; Philo, 1994; Scott, 1994). People with a mental disorder may want to express their sexuality, but for them, as well as anyone else, this is not the only reason for tender relationships.

Venereal disease

Gender integration was blamed for transmission of venereal disease among psychiatric patients in France (Maleville *et al.*, 1975). They acknowledged that the problem rested with a tiny minority of patients who were promiscuous, and that this created an adverse atmosphere within the hospital even though the infections were easy to treat. Prostitution in hospitals has been acknowledged (e.g. Gabbai and Degos in 1975, cited by Bourgeois, 1975). One of the editors once had the costs – usually in quantities of cigarettes – explained to her by an elderly male patient resident in an old-fashioned mental hospital and making use of the 'services' apparently readily available from some other patients.

Since the 1980s the concern has been of an entirely different order because of the emergence of the human immunodeficiency virus (HIV) and the acquired immune deficiency syndrome (AIDS). This has had a profound impact on the rest of society (Pinching *et al.*, 1988), and is regarded as a major public health priority (e.g. USA: Seidman and Rieder, 1994). There is concern that people with chronic mental illness may be at particular risk because of poor judgement and limited understanding of counselling (Rector and Seeman, 1992). Not only may their impulse control be poor, but they may engage in high-risk sexual behaviour as a covert form of self-destructive or suicidal behaviour, or even of homicidal impulses (Seidman and Rieder, 1994) (for further discussion and management strategies see Cole and Taylor, this volume).

Legal factors

In the United States, almost three-quarters of a million women are held in institutions, prisons and jails and the State has been involved in regulation of their decisions over marriage, conjugal and sexual rights, pregnancy and childbirth (Stefan, 1994). In the United States the eugenics movement to sterilize the unfit only began to slow in the 1940s, having become discredited by knowledge of practices in Nazi Germany where thousands of mentally ill patients were systematically killed even before the subsequent Holocaust (Meyer-Lindenberg, 1991). Recent resurgence of eugenic practice has been reported in China (Pearson, 1995).

In a landmark judgment in the United States in 1983, *Foy*, a court recognized institutionalized patients as human beings whose right to privacy protected their voluntary sexual activities without diminishing the institution's obligation to protect them from sexual assault. It also recognized the institution's duty to maximize a woman's choice by providing her with counselling and offering her contraceptives. It affirmed a woman's right to choose to be pregnant and to carry her pregnancy to term, and expressed doubt about abortion as the presumptive response to an institutionalized woman's pregnancy. However, despite extensive legislation relating to a Patient's Bill of Rights, few states in the United States have adopted standards guaranteeing the right of patients to engage in consensual heterosexual activity (Lyon, 1982; Perlin, 1993). (Fitzgerald and Harbour, this volume, deals with European rights.)

Risk of rape and other involuntary sexual activity in psychiatric hospitals and prisons

Concern has been expressed about episodes of sexual harassment, abduction, assault and rape of female patients by male patients, staff or uninvited visitors in Britain (Altounyan, 1993; Copperman, 1991; Feinmann, 1988; Tonks, 1992). The Royal College of Psychiatrists (1996) has issued guidance on this matter. In the USA there have been similar concerns (Stefan, 1994), and it is acknowledged that when the State holds a woman in custody, there is an obligation to provide for her reasonable protection from foreseeable harm.

Homosexual rape has also been recorded in psychiatric hospitals (Holbrook, 1989) and in prisons (Nacci and Kane, 1984). The United States Department of Justice (1995) has issued guidance on a sexual assault prevention or intervention programme for the protection of prisoners. Some assaultive behaviour, or even homicide, may be a direct consequence of homosexual liaisons in prisons or secure psychiatric hospitals (Grounds *et al.*, 1993; Rowe Report, 1991).

Institutional bias

Almost by definition, institutions, whether open or closed, for people with mental disorder or convicted of crime, have behaviour control as a major goal, and that generally includes sexual behaviours and other relationships (Grounds *et al.*, 1993). The major risks in not doing so have been touched on here, and taken up more fully elsewhere in this volume. Expressed managerial concerns and policies are generally, however, about heterosexual activity (Wignall and Meredith, 1968). My enquiries indicate that in prisons and secure psychiatric hospitals worldwide, homosexual activity occurs whether or not it is allowed officially; it is a matter of record in France (Andrieux, 1995), the USA (Wettstein, 1995) and Sweden (Ullman, 1995). The American Psychiatric Association (1993) has issued a position statement calling on all appropriate organizations to seek to reduce the stigma related to homosexuality, wherever it may occur. The ability to recognize it, and offer safeguards for homosexual and heterosexual couples alike, seems important.

Social change and economic factors

In Europe and North America studies have shown significant changes in sexual mores, including increases in the rate of divorce and proportion of births outside marriage. Marriage itself remains popular, but with true monogamy replaced by 'serial marriage'. The nuclear family also remains the major source of intimacy and childcare, but single parents are no longer generally regarded as outcast (Ashford and Timms, 1992; Ester *et al.*, 1993; Inglehart, 1990). Such social changes might possibly have facilitated the acceptance by the community of relationships between psychiatric patients, but there is little evidence of this. In Western societies, people with psychiatric illnesses are too readily viewed as a burden on society, and marriage potentially as extending this burden. In Hong Kong, where there is full employment, even the majority of people with schizophrenia are in work. In the pre-1997 climate this enabled many of them to attract wife, generally healthy, from across the Chinese border with the prospect of positive rehabilitative effects (Leff, personal communication).

Shifts in social attitudes towards homosexuality have also been detected by the surveys mentioned in the previous paragraph. In European societies, Holland followed by Denmark were found to be the most liberal in attitude to same sex couples. The United States was found to be very much less so, though improving (NORC, 1987). Some countries, both in the old and new world, retain a strongly negative attitude towards homosexuality (Ester *et al.*, 1993; Inglehart, 1990).

Country-specific developments

Throughout the world, with only a few exceptions, secure psychiatric hospitals and prisons tend to discourage close intimate relationships between patients or prisoners, and even between patients or prisoners and established partners still living in the community. The latter may be more by poor provision than design, but still it is the case. Physical sexual relations are generally forbidden. It is impossible to capture a full picture, and in the general spirit of this book, I would welcome information from places with innovative and successful approaches that I am not aware of. The following comments, however, are illustrative of some of the variation. If they appear to emphasize sexuality at the expense of wider partnership qualities, that is because of the way organizational polices and commentaries seem to be. Sexual relationships are important, but there are many other aspects to relationships which are potentially harmed in artificial communities but which may be helped by management sensitivity.

Europe

France

France may be connected in English minds with more liberal attitudes to sexual activity, but there is no sexual autonomy for psychiatric patients. Andrieux (1995), a forensic psychiatrist in a maximum security hospital near Paris, acknowledges that, although sexual contact between patients is not officially allowed, homosexual liaisons do occur. There is no provision for conjugal visits in hospitals or penal settings, and all visits are supervised in one central facility. Contraceptives are not generally available.

Germany

In Germany, relatives of patients are forbidden to enter wards at all in psychiatric hospitals, on grounds of confidentiality and security (Kobbe, 1988). Hence if privacy were to be provided, it would have to be in some other location, and it is felt that patients may feel embarrassed at requesting access (Kobbe, 1991). Kobbe, a sociologist working in a maximum security hospital in Lippstadt, expresses concern that sexuality tends to be ignored in the rehabilitation process and that such institutions should address the sexual needs of patients.

Holland

In the Netherlands a change in attitudes towards custodial care occurred after the Second World War, possibly as a result of the imprisonment of influential Dutch citizens during Nazi occupation (Koenraadt, 1992). The necessity for prisoners' rights were stressed and emphasis on greater attention to individual needs (Leaute, 1959; Moedikdo, 1976). Further, shorter custodial sentences were generally applied, although more recently there have been some reverse trends.

Forensic psychiatric inpatient clinics in Holland tend to be units with about 70 patients, mostly men who suffer from personality disorder, though a growing minority may have a psychosis. There is one high security hospital (the Van Mesdag Clinic in Groningen). Several of the clinics have flats and rooms provided for overnight stays for patients and their partners (Edmond and Kaye, 1997).

Philipse (1995) confirms that privacy may be offered, in the expectation that sexual activity may occur, between patients and visitors at the Pompe Clinic, Nijmegen. A visit may be in the patient's own room for up to 12 hours. Alternatively, there are two small flats in the clinic building which may be used by the patient, his partner, and children if there are any. There must be agreement between clinicians, including a family therapist, before a private visit can take place. Clinical staff must have access to the flat at all times. These arrangements apply to both heterosexual and homosexual relationships and are not contingent on the partners being married. Since the emergence of HIV and AIDS, condoms are distributed in machines in the unit's toilets or telephone booths. Staff intervene in such visits only if someone is subject to force by another, or where the relationship is showing features linked with the index offence. A further, more recent development being piloted is the use of surrogate partners for psychosexual education, with the debate ongoing about indications for this and for the safety of the visitor. Previously, by agreement, certain patients had been allowed access to prostitutes, but a surrogate partner known to clinical staff came to be regarded as preferable. Practice is evolving and there is no research data on its benefits or adverse effects.

The Van der Hoeven Clinic in Utrecht has been described by Feldbrugge (1991) and by Feldbrugge and Haverkamp (1993). This is the only forensic psychiatric hospital in Holland where men and women are resident as patients in the same facility. The men outnumber the women by 9 : 1. It recognizes that relationships for patients in all their aspects, including sex, are to be seen as facts of life. Through the human interaction involved, treatment is aimed to address both the rewards of the relationship and its problems. It is thought preferable that this work be done while the patient remains in hospital, rather than such problems revealing themselves after discharge when problems may be much less identifiable, manageable or treatable. In the 36 years between 1955 and 1991, 92 women had been admitted to the clinic; thirteen 'clinic' babies were born in that time. The father had usually been a patient in the clinic too, but in a few cases the father was a visitor living in the community. When a baby is born it is allowed to stay with its mother until it is 2 years old, after which it must go to a foster family. This, however, has never been necessary as each female patient involved has always become ready for discharge by then. Patients and partners can use contraception. In one case where staff at the clinic considered that a pregnancy should be prevented, a court refused to allow depot contraceptives to be administered without the woman's consent. The clinic requested her transfer to another hospital.

In deciding about conjugal or relational visits, whether or not the patient and partner are married, the key issue in assessment is that of risk to the patient, the partner, or to children should there be any. Visits are therefore not granted automatically, even to married couples. An assessment of the visitor by a hospital family therapist is always undertaken as part of the evaluation of the visitor's level of knowledge and understanding about the patient, and level of stability. Once visits are authorized, ongoing evaluation is undertaken of the effects of the relationship. Usually authorization is not given to casual relationships or access to prostitutes. If a patient who is married develops a relationship with a new partner, the patient him/herself is expected to inform the spouse, as it is understood that staff will not deceive visitors. A further important issue is that the clinic recognizes that jealousies among patients may and do develop. In order to offset this, information about relationships must be shared with other patients in the unit. Relationships have also rarely developed between a patient and a member of staff, but where this has occurred, the staff member must leave the clinic if, after counselling, he or she wishes to continue with the relationship. Feldbrugge and colleagues take the view that a fundamental requirement for improving forensic psychiatric units depends on staff being allowed to learn from experience, which includes making mistakes. Such mistakes, however, must occur only on the background of a clear policy framework and documented team agreement on a particular course of action.

Denmark

In all Scandinavian countries, criminal activity is low and duration of imprisonment amongst the lowest in the world (Hoyer, 1988). In most prisons there are small sections or purpose designed suites for receiving approved external visitors in privacy.

Herstedvester is a prison on the outskirts of Cophenhagen with a long history in the treatment of 'criminal psychopaths' (Stürup, 1968). In the past it undertook programmes of voluntary castration for sex offenders (Ortmann, 1980). Nowadays the prison operates a system of psychiatric evaluation and psychotherapeutic treatment for offenders with personality disorders who may require such an approach. A small number of female prisoners are now also accommodated (Hansen, 1991). Prisoners may have visitors and, depending on their level of stability, these may be either supervised or not. Conjugal and relational visits, therefore, do occur and are seen as a natural part of a prisoner's life.

In Denmark, there is also one maximum security psychiatric unit at Nykøping. This unit has 30 beds for male patients only and is situated within the grounds of a general psychiatric hospital which has about 200 beds for men and women. Conjugal and relational visits are allowed within the context of an established relationship, subject to clinical evaluation of safety, and occur in a private room near the ward (Haugen, 1991). This applies whether both partners are resident in hospital, or only one.

In May 1989, in Denmark, a new law allowed for 'registered partnerships' between people of the same sex. The first such couple to make use of that law had cohabited together for 41 years. Such couples are allowed almost the same rights as a heterosexual couple, except that they are not allowed to adopt children.

Sweden

In Sweden there are a range of forensic psychiatric units, which, as elsewhere, house a preponderance of men (Dernevik, 1995; Ullman, 1995). Conjugal and relational visits are allowed with spouses or partners from outside the hospitals. Sexual relations between patients within the units are not allowed, regardless of whether the partnership is heterosexual or same sex.

Norway

In secure psychiatric units in Norway, gender segregated wards are seen as anti-therapeutic with regard to the rehabilitative process. Within such units, however, close relationships, whether heterosexual or homosexual, are not encouraged. For psychotic patients, intimate relationships are actively prevented. It is thought such patients may not be able to cope with such intimacy and there is concern about the practical consequences. Social interaction is, however, encouraged. Secure units, in which the majority of patients have a psychotic illness, report few relationships and low levels of sexual interest and activity by patients. In units with a majority of patients with personality disorder, relationships and the challenges they pose are more frequent.

Former Soviet Union

In the states of the former Soviet Union, and in countries of Central and Eastern Europe formerly under its influence, there is generally quite a progressive approach to relationships established before imprisonment. Perhaps partly dictated by some of the very considerable distances commonly involved between home community and prison, these distances in turn tend to mean that the principles work less well in practice. Two types of visit are available. Short visits, which may last up to 4 hours, are closely comparable to those which occur widely in Western Europe. In addition, long visits, lasting up to 72 hours, may be allowed two or three times a year. In most prisons these would take place in a small flat, specially designated for the purpose. Visitors may be parents, spouse, children or other closer relatives (Coyle, personal communication).

North America

United States

Presentation of the situation in the USA is complicated by the fact that there are three levels of provision – federal, state and county prisons and/or city jails. Although there is some common ground in their management, there are also many differences. As standard, however, sexual relations of any kind between inmates, whether consenting or not, are not allowed (Moritsugu, 1995).

Conjugal visits are not allowed widely, but there are some family visiting programmes similar to those described (below) for Canada. Home leave or furloughs to renew family ties are authorized depending on custody level, severity of offence, time left to serve sentence and level of adjustment and conduct. This is very similar to the situation in England. For England and Wales, in the National Prison Survey (1991) for which 4000 prisoners were interviewed, the most often requested change in regime was for conjugal visits (30 per cent).

Each USA institution has a separate sexual assault prevention and intervention programme (US Department of Justice, Federal Bureau of Prisons, 1995). There has been a return to mixed prisons in the United States since 1971. In the 19th century, penal reformers campaigned vigorously for women to have separate prisons, as mixed prisons had previously been the norm, and some concern has again been expressed that, as women prisoners are in a minority, their interests may be subordinated to those of the men (SchWeber, 1984). At the time of her writing there were three federal and ten co-correctional/co-ed prisons for adults. The minority status for women was common but not invariable, e.g. Clinton, New Jersey. As with almost any unit structure of any kind the mixed environment can work, but only providing there are staff with adequate skills and in appropriate numbers of men and women. Research assessments of mixed units have employed both objective measures, such as programme participation rates and disciplinary infractions, and satisfaction scales. On all aspects, inclusive even of post-prison recidivism rates, Almy et al. (1980) found an advantage for the co-educational prison at Framingham, Massachusetts. Cavior and Cohen (1980), however, in evaluating an attitudinal scale in two settings (Lexington and Pleasanton, both federal prisons) were struck by a reversal in expected views. In general, they suggested, staff had a more positive view than inmates of the prison as an institution. Prisoners of both sexes, however, were invariably more positive than staff about a co-ed regime, and female staff more positive than male staff.

Although most interest has been directed at integration in the US scene, the ratio of men to women corrections officers is at least 2 : 1. Whilst there is acknowledgement that the majority of staff behave appropriately, some do not and a prison is a particularly difficult place in which, as a prisoner, to bring a complaint of sexual harassment or worse (Human Rights Watch Women's Rights Project, 1996; see also Dale et al., this volume). SchWeber (1984) recommends a 'coordinate model' – administratively separate prisons for men and women but geographically close enough to be able to share programmes and services.

In forensic psychiatric hospitals in the United States, patients are not allowed conjugal visits and sexual contact between patients is not allowed (Gutheil, 1995; Wettstein 1995).

Canada

In the Canadian Correctional Service, private family visiting programmes were introduced in 1980 and have been found to be beneficial (Champagne, 1992). Prisoners are eligible to participate if they have served a minimum of 6 months with good conduct and have not, within the last 6 months, been transferred to an institution of higher security. Visitors must be assessed by Correctional Service staff before authorization is given. Visits are conducted in a special family visit unit, with a recreation area provided also for children. Such family visits can be suspended in the event of visitors bringing in alcohol or illegal drugs or implements for the purpose of violence or to assist escape (Correctional Service of Canada, 1988; Fowler, 1995).

Psychiatric hospitals in Canada generally do not allow conjugal visits or afford privacy for patients with each other. An exception to this is Riverview Hospital, a general psychiatric hospital in British Columbia (Welch and Clements, 1996). Its policy statement on patients' sexuality is based on the principles that patients in the hospital have a right to sexual intimacy in a private and dignified setting regardless of sexual orientation or marital status, hospital administrators have a duty to protect patients, and a policy should reduce the risk of contracting sexually transmitted diseases. Contraception, sex education and counselling are also all made available. Detained patients may also have conjugal visits, subject to there being no medical or psychiatric contraindication whereby he or she is either incapable of consenting to sexual intimacy or engaging in responsible sexual behaviour. (See also Appendix, pp. 201–202.)

The difficulties facing secure psychiatric hospitals in Canada are, however, illustrated by that of the maximum secure hospital, Oak Ridge, at Penetanguishene in Ontario, where security concerns have tended to take precedence over therapeutic considerations (Grounds *et al.*, 1993; Rice and Harris, 1993). A recommendation made in an official report (Hucker, 1986) for a number of changes, including a conjugal visiting programme, has not been implemented due to staff concerns over issues of security.

Middle America

Mexico

In Mexico, in common with many South American countries, prisoners tend to be housed in large 'patios' or communal areas. Families are not excluded from these areas during the visiting hours. By the same token, conjugal visits are not excluded (Gochros, 1972).

West Indies

According to Edwardes (1995), the psychiatric hospital in Trinidad does not allow for conjugal visits or authorized sexual encounters between patients.

Similarly, in Jamaica, at Bellevue Hospital, sexual activity between patients is officially forbidden, but is known to occur and causes concern to staff. Long stay hospital patients not uncommonly become pregnant, and a local obstetric hospital provides antenatal and delivery care. The mental hospital provides a special ward for such patients and the infants can remain for several months before arrangements are made for adoption. Preventative measures, however, are regarded as a priority and the hospital runs a contraceptive clinic (Hickling, 1993).

Australia

In the prison system in Australia, residential visits may be permitted whereby a prisoner may receive a visit from his family, including near relatives and any other person with whom he or she may have a long standing relationship (Office of Correction, Victoria, 1992). Proof of family relationship may be required and the prisoner must not have been found guilty of a prison offence, especially where illegal drugs or alcohol were involved.

The forensic psychiatric units have no such provision. Patient relationships would be monitored for sexual contact, which is not permitted. Nevertheless, some units are pragmatic and provide condoms (Mullen, 1995; O'Brien, 1995).

South Africa

The issue of sexuality may be especially relevant in parts of central and southern Africa, where AIDS is almost epidemic (Pinching et al., 1988). In prisons and psychiatric facilities in South Africa and in Zimbabwe, beyond brief, supervised, prearranged visits that the prisoner or patient chooses, there is no provision for conjugal visits or sexual contact between prisoners or patients (Vermeulen, 1995; Zondo, 1995). In South Africa, Kaliski et al. (1994) conducted a survey of staff and patient beliefs about and observations of sexual activity in an all male hospital unit, where the belief in activity levels seemed far greater than the actuality (see also Swan and Taylor, this volume).

Summary and overview

Internationally, various factors have contributed to the evolution of policies for the support and maintenance of established relationships, and development in attitudes towards new ones. Moral, religious, clinical, legal, institutional, social and risk of harm parameters all interact in different societies to produce varying trends in approach, and crystallize out particularly in relation to explicitly sexual activities. The most liberal practices in secure facilities occur in some of the countries with recent experience of alien and oppressive occupation, such as Holland and Denmark. In most other countries of the world, secure psychiatric hospitals do not sanction close sexual encounters, although they almost certainly happen anyway. Perhaps more worrying is the apparently sparse consideration given to the wider aspects of relationship care. Some prison systems are better at this. Canada, for example, has well developed family programmes in some prisons.

In most countries, for couples, home leave or furloughs are preferred, explicitly because this provides for more normal relations, but perhaps also because it relieves the institution of a significant management role in this respect. In no country is the approach to homosexuality the same as that to heterosexuality, although in Holland the differences are at a minimum. The discrepancies in practice across the world are perhaps most illustrative of the complexity of the issues, but also the place of institutions and their residents in wider society. What happens to residents of institutions and societies and other made communities, whether liberal or moralistic, anxious or punitive, still tends to depend on popular beliefs and practice rather than evidence.

Case cited

Foy Foy versus Greenblott, 190 Cal. Rptr. 84 (Cal. Ct. App. 1983)

Glossary

Cal. Rptr   California Reporter
Cal. Ct. App.   California Court of Appeal

Appendix

Towards practical policies

> Whatever I do in this place I feel that I cannot win. If I sit in a group with other patients, the nurses think we are plotting something. If I keep myself to myself I am seen to be a loner. When I make what I feel to be a reasonable request for some private time with my girlfriend when she visits, I am told no policy exists. Why? I mean, it can't be the first time that this question is being posed.
>
> Secure hospital patient

> Whilst accompanying a patient on a home visit, as part of a detailed pre-discharge programme, my patient asked me if I could make myself scarce while he and his wife had some private time together. I had received no guidance about this in my briefing prior to leaving the hospital, and was frankly in a quandary. What if this was a ruse to create time to abscond? What if an assault took place? I felt totally unprepared for this request, and yet felt a degree of empathy for the situation. Feeling intensely pressurised, isolated and unsupported I made a decision based on instinct and intuition and kept my fingers crossed for the remainder of the trip.
>
> Forensic mental health nurse from a secure hospital

> Should psychiatric patients be allowed to engage in sexual activities? When many psychiatrists are asked this question, they respond, 'Not in my hospital!' and cite potential liability risks ... If psychiatrists wish to deter patients from sexual interaction to reduce liability risk, do they have an *unlimited* right to do so?
>
> Mossman *et al.* (1997)

Policies and procedures offer a number of protections to service users and providers. They support a systematic approach to assessment and management and fairness in service delivery. They can be misused, for example in limiting appropriate flexibility in care or treatment, but at best they provide a vehicle for developing and driving good practice. The latter is particularly true of policies under regular review, as far as possible informed by evidence, and, where not, subjected to research and/or audit.

Lack of space precludes much reproduction of policies currently in use. Buckley and Hyde (1997) found a majority of 86 hospitals in 10 US states had a policy of some kind. This seems exceptional. Perhaps reflecting common presumptions about the risks of relationships in such communities, those polices that we have been able to trace focus more or less exclusively on some aspect of sexual, particularly genital activity. While one of us (TS) has worked mainly in a high security hospital setting, the other (PJT) has had experience overseas and in a wide range of general and forensic psychiatric settings from community to security, and with probation and prison services too. A secure hospital, with its long stay population, is the one place where patient/client relationships cannot be entirely ignored in their wider qualities. The need to recognize positive aspects of relationships for general well being and safety as well as being realistic about risks, is, however, far from unique to such settings. For all other psychiatric services and hostels and for criminal justice settings it is important to consider ordinary visiting arrangements, including such matters as privacy for all sorts of reasons, and not simply the sexual act. For secure hospitals it is simply more of a challenge to set minimum limits on privacy without compromising the safety of either partner in the couple, other contacts or the institution. While the Special Hospitals' Service Authority existed between 1990 and 1996, we worked with the Advisory Group on Patient Relationships and other external advisors (see acknowledgements), to draft a preliminary policy for all the special hospitals. Each hospital has now developed its own from these primitive beginnings, and we have chosen to reproduce a substantial part of the Rampton Hospital policy as being the one that has best retained this principle of emphasizing the relationship as a whole before progressing to its more sexual aspects. We would like to commend this philosophy to people developing a relationships policy for any setting.

The Rampton Hospital policy on patient relationships is also useful for its layout. For each matter considered, there is a brief and clear statement of policy; this is followed by a short set of notes, defining any terms, circumstances or qualifiers; and guidelines toward more detailed procedures are then added. The aim, principles, objectives, definition and scope are given in full, together with two full sample sections – those on security and risk and patient–patient relationships. While recognizing that some of the marital issues apply only to compulsorily detained hospital patients, we have nevertheless offered that document's appendix in full, because the extent of disclosure of otherwise confidential medical information and the extent of responsibility that one spouse has for the other in these circumstances is potentially so great. For all the other items we have reproduced the statement of policy only.

Policies about sexual activities involving psychiatric patients have more features than not in common. They acknowledge a likelihood of some sexual activity and a duty to safeguard patients. Two from North America which have been published in professional journals go on to specify 'rights' to sexual activity.

Riverview Hospital, Port Coquitlan, British Columbia

- Patients have a right to sexual intimacy; hospital administrators have a duty to protect patients.
- A policy on patient sexuality should balance these rights and duties.
- A policy should reduce the risk of contracting sexually transmitted disease.

Welch and Clements (1996)

One of the principal concerns of Welch and Clements about this Canadian policy is that it may be too conservative. The policy had been approved for implementation among chronic psychiatric in-patients at Riverview Hospital at the time of these authors writing, on a presumption that those patients exercising such a right would be competent to consent to the activity. They recommend using the policy in conjunction with a checklist for evaluating capacity 'for these purposes' (Freedman *et al.*, 1991; Alexander, 1988).

Again presenting a 'model policy' rather than one yet in use, Mossman and colleagues (1997) from the USA assert:

> Human beings have an innate need and desire for emotional and sexual intimacy. This model policy offers psychiatric facilities guidelines to balance the rights and needs of patients with health and safety concerns ...
>
> Competent patients who reside in intermediate and long-term care facilities should not be prevented from engaging in consensual sexual relations.
>
> All mental health facilities should offer patients sex education and contraceptive counseling services, and should make contraceptive devices reasonably accessible to their patients ...
>
> Upon admission, all patients will:
> ... receive a written copy of this policy ...

Psychiatric patients, in other words, in North American long-stay hospital services should be in no doubt from the point of entry to hospital about their rights to sexual intercourse if competent, with an onus on the hospital to demonstrate incompetence as necessary.

Europe does appear to take a more cautious view. Even though in some countries in-patient and/or residential treatment facilities may support responsible sexual activity, there is no acknowledged right to it. In the UK, even in open psychiatric hospital facilities policy is generally to prevent sexual activities involving patients in the hospital, while acknowledging the importance of providing contraceptive advice and protection and, as far as possible, protective measures for safer sex if it should occur. The Bethlem Royal and Maudsley NHS Trust, in London, provides psychiatric services, including extensive in-patient services on two sites, mainly for voluntary patients. The Trust's policy, which like the Rampton Hospital policy is in current use, is reproduced in full.

Few other psychiatric hospitals in England were able to offer such a policy, although our enquiries were limited. Staff at the Edenfield Regional Secure Unit in the Salford NHS Trust, in the North of England, provided full guidelines for patients' sexuality while resident there. In addition to familiar headings (alleged or apparent sexual assault; intimacy/privacy; condoms; staff/patient relationships) this policy included a section on proposed guidance for use of pornography and sex aids. While the USA model policy makes no mention of this, the Canadian policy tends to confirm our impression that use of pornography and sexual aids is likely to be an issue for any patient group (indeed any human group), and not just offender patients. The special hospitals have long followed the principles common to those policies that raise such matters – that patients are allowed erotic pictures, books or videos so long as they are legal, available to the general public and held entirely privately to the person who has acquired them. In Broadmoor Hospital, for example, such materials are routinely screened by staff before a patient may have them; further, some other home made videotapes, brought in by visitors may ostensibly be of a football match or other non-sexual pursuits, but include unacceptable, pornographic sequences, so these are screened too.

Cambridge and McCarthy (1997) tackle the issue of sexual activity outside hospital but in community residential settings. Their model policy was drawn up after extensive consultation with professional staff and hostel workers, patient/ service users and their relatives, particularly with people with clinically impor- tant learning disability in mind, but much would appear to be appropriate for other community residential settings – at least for those with other mental disorders or for the elderly. Among their potentially valuable contributions was development both of an educational programme and a booklet which allow for the difficulty of conveying ideas and models for behaviour when learning difficulties (or other mental disorders) are disabling. The booklet, for example, on the issue of masturbation offers words and a picture:

- touching yourself sexually is a good and normal thing to do in private (with a picture of a young man masturbating in bed under a sheet).

The educational discussions are set to convey such ideas as:

- bad sex was when you didn't want to have sex [or] a person said 'no', or when sex hurt;
- good sex was when both people wanted to have sex and liked it;
- if you had a boyfriend or girlfriend you didn't have to have sex with each other if you didn't want to;
- two men, two women or a man and a woman can have sex with each other.

Few policies in any sphere of health or social services are subjected to formal or scientific evaluation. The extracts, near full and full policy presented here are no exceptions. Perhaps since this is such a difficult and contentious area, such testing should be attempted. The Dutch have acknowledged that their liberal policies on the TBS units (see Gordon, this volume) have been associated with some pregnancies. It is known that with explicitly prohibitive policies, HIV has been transmitted between prisoners elsewhere (see Cole and Taylor, this volume), although perhaps needle sharing contributed to this. These are, though, only the grossest and rarest potential outcomes of sexual activity in such settings; more subtle measures of safety, of patient/service user satisfaction, of staff perceptions and of success in longer-term habilitation or rehabilitation are needed. While acknowledging such ideals, a sharing of information about how such policies work in practice would surely be of value. We hope to hear from readers.

RAMPTON HOSPITAL AUTHORITY PATIENT RELATIONSHIPS POLICY

POLICY [Extracts]

1.   **AIM**

1.1   To provide a Policy for the management of patient relationships in Rampton Hospital.

2.   **PRINCIPLES**

2.1   Forming relationships is a perfectly normal human activity and patients should not be discouraged from this while they are in Hospital. However, many patients have a history of relationships that have caused harm to themselves or others. Furthermore, by its nature, the Hospital environment imposes restrictions on privacy, on time together and on the availability of appropriate partners. For these reasons, and particularly for the safety and security of patients, staff and visitors, the importance of relationships must be recognized and they must be managed.

2.2   In order to manage relationships without discouraging them, it is essential that the issues raised by intimate relationships and the sexual feelings of patients are not avoided, but openly and sensitively addressed so that patients and staff can be offered reassurance, protection, guidance and support. To achieve this, staff must be consistent in their approach to relationships and must be made aware (by Managers) of the dangers of expressing inappropriate moral or ethical opinions or beliefs towards patients inconsistent with Hospital Policy. This Policy applies to both heterosexual and homosexual relationships.

2.3   Staff who work closely with a patient, and particularly those in the clinical team for a patient, must take responsibility for early awareness of a developing relationship and its full assessment. Plans for the management, and if necessary treatment of the relationship should be clearly documented in the care and treatment plan. The clinical team for each must ensure that each patient understands as fully as possible the boundaries for their behaviour in the relationship. Staff who are required to work with patients in relationships must have access to relevant and effective supervision.

3.   **OBJECTIVES**

The objectives of this policy are to:

- Preserve the personal safety of patients and staff and the security of the Hospital.
- Promote a consistent approach by staff.
- Ensure that the Hospital fulfils its responsibilities to patients.
- Clarify what behaviour is defined as acceptable or unacceptable and the rules and procedures by which that is determined.

- Provide a framework of management accountability which ensures that direct care staff feel supported in working to the Hospital Policy.

4.   <u>DEFINITION</u>

4.1   The relationships addressed by this Policy are defined as attachments between two adult persons of the same or opposite gender that may or may not include the following qualities: feelings of love, specialness, caring, exclusivity, romance, sexual attraction, secretiveness. These may be unevenly shared between the two parties, but must be expressed to some degree by each.

5.   <u>SCOPE OF THE POLICY</u>

5.1   This Policy is intended to address issues that may result from relationships between patients and staff, between patients and visitors, as well as relationships between patients.

6.   <u>SECURITY AND RISK</u>

Policy

6.1.1   The security and safety of all parties concerned are of paramount priority.

Notes

6.2.1   All parties mean all patients, staff, voluntary agencies, visitors and the community at large.

6.2.2   Security and safety reflect both immediate and long-term concerns.

Procedure

6.3.1   Clinical Risk Assessment will take any relationship into account and will be updated whenever there is a change in relationship status.

6.3.2   Clinical Risk Assessment will identify the potential for abusive and/or exploitative elements in the relationship including history of violence, abuse, hostage taking, and victimization.

6.3.3   Clinical Risk Assessment must include possible risk to all parties including access to children.

6.3.4   Clinical Risk Assessment will lead to a risk management/risk reduction strategy that should be recorded in the patient's multidisciplinary treatment plan and updated as relationships develop and change.

7.   Staff–Patient Relationships

7.1.1   While some degree of relationship between staff and patients is necessary for therapeutic progress, no member of staff will form a close personal friendship or intimate relationship with a patient or a member of a patient's immediate family. (Notes etc. omitted here, except for 9.)

8.   Patient−Visitor Relationships

8.1.1   It is recognized that there may be, or may become, an emotional attachment between the patient and a visitor. The Hospital's response will be based on an assessment in each individual case and undertaken by the patient's multidisciplinary team (MDT), of the implications of the friendship for safety and/or security and for the clinical needs of the patient.

9.   Patient−Patient Relationships

Policy

9.1.1   In general, relationships between patients should not be discouraged subject to considerations of safety, security and any clinical risk a relationship may create for a patient.

Notes

9.2.1   This Policy applies to all established relationships, whether heterosexual or homosexual.

Procedure

9.3.1   Once a relationship is recognized by staff, risk assessment and management Procedures (as described under Section 6, "Security and Risk") should be initiated by the Multi-Disciplinary Team (MDT).

9.3.2   Direct care staff should be encouraged to adopt a consistent approach to all relationships and required to avoid expressing personal moral or ethical opinions or beliefs inconsistent with Hospital Policy.

9.3.3   If patients from more than one MDT are involved, it is essential that there is good communication and liaison between the teams on matters pertinent to the relationship, up to and including the option of a joint meeting between the teams to establish a consistent approach.

9.3.4   Managers must ensure that direct care staff are familiar with Hospital Policy on relationships and ensure that staff comply with the Policy and are supported in doing so.

9.3.5   Where necessary, relationship counselling should be made available to patients (as described in Section 18, "Relationship Counselling").

9.3.6   Patients must be sensitively encouraged to conform to the guidelines on appropriate behaviour expected within the Hospital (as described in Section 10, "Appropriate Conduct").

10.   Acceptable Conduct

10.1.1   Since patients are not allowed to be with other patients unless under observation at all times by staff, patients must be encouraged to behave in a way which reflects this i.e. hugging or kissing is acceptable, whereas intimate contact with others, including sexual intercourse, is not acceptable.

10.1.2   Masturbation is viewed as a normal outlet for sexual feelings, provided it is discretely conducted in the <u>relative</u> privacy of the patient's own room. In any other context it would be viewed as unacceptable.

11.   Marriage Ceremonies taking place within Rampton Hospital

11.1.1   Patients in the Hospital are legally entitled to apply to get married and the Hospital will ensure that any marriage is undertaken in a managed and planned fashion.

12.   Married Patients

12.1   Rampton Hospital accords no special privileges to married patients. Hospital Policy does not allow for sexual behaviour between patients, so marriages cannot be consummated.

13.   Pregnancy

13.1.1   In the case of a pregnant woman patient requiring care in the Hospital, a full assessment will be undertaken to determine both the risks to and the needs of mother and unborn child. From this assessment, appropriate staffing, accommodation and plan of care will be determined.

14.   Safe Sex

14.1.1   Intimate contact and sexual intercourse between patients or between patients and other persons is prohibited (Section 10.2.1) and the Authority will expect staff to take all reasonable steps to prevent this taking place. However, since it is still possible that some patients may engage in sexual intercourse, condoms, the most practical protection against HIV and other sexually transmitted diseases, will be made available to patients along with sex and health education programmes.

15.   Exploitative and Abusive Relationships

15.1.1   The Hospital has a responsibility to protect patients who may become involved in exploitative or abusive relationships.

16.   Media and Public Communications

16.1.1   The Hospital will seek to ensure that any general information about patients' relationships is presented in such a way as to emphasize the importance of relationships in maintaining the patients' quality of life and also in supporting their long term rehabilitation. Patients' entitlement to confidentiality extends to any information about their relationships.

17.   Confidentiality and Disclosure

17.1.1   The confidentiality of patient information must be respected. However where patients form close relationships with another patient or a visitor, the Clinical Teams will liaise on the advisability of disclosure of information about their offences or other personal information and counsel patients on the appropriateness and extent of disclosure, taking into consideration the risks involved.

18.   **Relationship Counselling**

18.1.1   Management should ensure that counselling is available to patients and that trained staff are available to provide appropriate counselling to couples as well as individuals.

APPENDIX 1   (To Rampton Hospital Patient relationship policy)

PRE-MARITAL COUNSELLING

General Guidelines
It is vitally important that patients are fully aware of all the implications of marriage *before* the marriage ceremony. Many patients have a history of failed and sometimes abusive relationships and can have a very idealistic perception of marriage. Others may not be aware of some of the legal implications of the married state or alternatively may view it casually and expect to be easily able to annul the marriage since it will not be consummated while either patient remains in the hospital. It is very important that the patients proceed into marriage fully informed of what their rights will and will not be.

Specific Issues
1.   Next of Kin Status

Patients need to know that by becoming 'next of kin' they acquire rights to have access to each other's health records. The advice in Section 17 of the Policy is pertinent here. Ideally patients should be counselled to discuss their reasons for being in a High Secure Hospital with each other before marriage. This particularly applies where the male partner's crime involved violence or sexual violence.

2.   Rights and privileges

Patients contemplating marriage must be made aware that the hospital accords no special privileges to married patients. They will have no 'rights' of extra time together, telephone calls or opportunities to consummate the marriage (Section 12).

3.   Non-consummation

Some patients believe that since their marriage will not be consummated in hospital, it will easily be annulled if it doesn't work out to their satisfaction. However, our legal advice is that *if they know* that the marriage will not be consummated *before* they enter the marriage contract then non-consummation ceases to be grounds for voiding the marriage. They will have to go through full divorce proceedings if they wish to terminate the marriage.

4.   Pregnancy

While sexual intercourse is prohibited, women patients may believe that becoming pregnant may offer a short cut to discharge from hospital. It should be carefully explained to them that this would not be so and that discharge decisions and arrangements will be made exclusively on the multidisciplinary team's estimate of their risk and clinical state (and, if necessary, Home Office approval).

Other Relevant Sections

Patients' attention should particularly be drawn to Sections 10, 15, 16, and 18 of the Policy. These sections are designed to provide as much protection as possible for patients and particularly apply to married couples.

Recording pre-marital counselling
It is important that the advice given to couples is recognized as part of the clinical service of the Hospital and is recorded in detail in their clinical notes. Such a record may be necessary to protect both patients and the Hospital if the relationship breaks down in the future.

Relationship Issues
While it is very important that patients are fully informed before committing themselves to marriage, it is equally, if not more important that both patients have as much opportunity to discuss their expectations, worries, concerns both jointly and individually with someone they trust. If they choose to do this with a member of the MDT who has little previous experience of pre-marital counselling, this person should be given proper support and supervision from other members of the team. Patients who express doubts or reservations should be encouraged to take as much time as they need before setting a date. Obviously staff should be on the lookout for any coercion of one partner by the other and should act to protect the more vulnerable partner, and to ensure that they are not being coerced into a decision. Specialist relationship counsellors are available to clinical teams should this be seen as necessary.

BETHLEM AND MAUDSLEY NHS TRUST

GUIDELINES ON SEXUAL ACTIVITIES INVOLVING PATIENTS

Introduction and background

In these guidelines which are specific to the care of adults, it is acknowledged that most patients need to have a degree of privacy and some unstructured and unsupervised time. In such circumstances, sexual activities between patients sometimes occur.

The Government has made HIV/AIDS and Sexual Health a key area in the Health of the Nation strategy. In the key area handbook, it is stated:

> Rewarding personal and sexual relationships promote health and well-being. However, sexual activity can also have undesired results such as unwanted pregnancies and the transmission of Human Immunodeficiency Virus (HIV) and other sexually transmitted diseases (STDs).

Among the general objectives identified in this document are:

- to reduce the incidence of HIV infection
- to reduce the incidence of other sexually transmitted diseases
- to reduce the number of unwanted pregnancies
- to ensure the provision of effective family planning services for those people who want them.

With these concerns in mind, issues around sexual health are required to be considered as part of any individual's plan of care. Indeed, many people with mental health problems may not previously have received information relating to HIV and sexual health problems which is appropriate to their needs and level of functioning. However, it is acknowledged that a number of factors may influence when, or whether, such issues are raised with some patients. These include the nature of a patient's illness, their age, cultural and religious beliefs and their length of stay in hospital.

Individual clinical units may wish to meet to discuss local policies pertinent to their particular client group and care environment.

1 Sexual activities

As a general principle, patients' rights to make their own decisions are respected, although due consideration must be given to the nature of a patient's mental health problems and whether they are detained under a Section as this may indicate they are unable to make informed judgements. However, sexual activities between in-patients are not acceptable if in any way these are judged likely to adversely affect a patient's health or social well-being.

If staff become aware that sexual activities between in-patients are occurring, management and care decisions need to be based upon an individual assessment which aims to ensure that informed consent is forthcoming from both parties and that there are no legal or treatment issues which prohibit the activities taking place. Regard should be given to the following factors:

(i)   whether there is any evidence or history of coercive, exploitative or threatening behaviour in relation to the sexual activities;

(ii)   whether, by nature of their mental health problems, patients are not in complete control of their sexual behaviour;

(iii)   whether the patients involved are aware of, and able to understand, any potential risk of unwanted pregnancy or sexually transmitted disease (including Hepatitis B and HIV);

(iv)   whether there are any relevant legal issues pertaining to the activities;

(v)   the context within which the activities are taking place and whether this may interfere with the treatment, care and recovery of the patients involved, other patients on the ward or significant others.

If the assessment identifies concerns related to any of the above factors, it is the responsibility of staff to act with discretion and sensitivity. Staff will act in the best interests of the patients involved. This may include taking steps to prevent the continuation of the activities.

It is envisaged that the management and care decisions will be taken by the multidisciplinary care team. The Senior Nurse/Responsible Medical Officer should be informed. Any actions taken must be accurately recorded and communicated whilst respecting issues of confidentiality.

2   Sex education, counselling and support for patients

Whenever appropriate, issues around sexual health need to be dealt with proactively as part of the assessment and induction procedure.

The aims of this are:

(i)   to facilitate the assessment and exploration of any issues around sexual health relevant to the patient's care;

(ii)   to identify patients who may be vulnerable and enable precautions to be taken;

(iii)   to identify needs such as information about contraception and safer sex practices and the development of skills and attributes necessary to link this knowledge with behaviour;

(iv)   to inform patients of the policy of the Trust regarding sexual activities between patients;

(v)   wherever possible, to enable patients to take responsibility for their actions if they do engage in sexual activities.

These issues may also be incorporated into health education groups or discussions. The Lecturer/Practitioner (HIV) is available to facilitate sessions on a group or individual basis. Arrangements should be made for women to be able to attend or have advice from a family planning nurse or doctor.

3   Provision of condoms

When sexual activity occurs within the hospital between patients it is desirable that such individuals have access to barrier contraception, such as condoms, in order to reduce or minimize the risk of HIV or other sexually transmitted diseases and to reduce unwanted pregnancies. To this end consideration may be given to the provision of condoms.

If this course of action is decided upon, discussion would need to take place within the care team to reach agreement about where and how the patient may obtain condoms.

4 Confidentiality

The general principle of confidentiality continues to be maintained. That is, all information regarding a patient is treated as privileged and divulged only in the context of professional activities such as those of the multidisciplinary team.

In general, the patient must consent to any divulging of confidential information to a third party. If a patient's consent is to be set aside, it is desirable that this is a multiprofessional decision which is based upon legal advice.

5 Same sex – sexual activities between patients

The trust has a commitment to ensuring that patients should not be discriminated against on the basis of their sexual orientation.

Sexual activities between patients of the same sex should be addressed according to the criteria laid out in this policy for assessing all sexual activities. Particular legal requirements for same sex activities (e.g., the age of consent for men having sex with men is currently 18) must be observed.

6 Sexual harassment, sexual assault, sexual abuse and rape

In the event of any of these occurring, the relevant management and procedures are detailed in separate Bethlem and Maudsley policies which should be followed. The titles of the appropriate policies are *Policy for dealing with allegations of sexual assault, sexual abuse and rape* and *Sexual discrimination and sexual harassment policy: a code for practice for all staff.*

7 Sexual activities within the trust between an in-patient and a partner who is not a patient

This will need to be addressed with particular discretion and each situation individually assessed in accordance with the criteria detailed in this policy for managing sexual activities between in-patients.

Those wards where patients may have prolonged stays in hospital, along with limited opportunities for leave, may wish to consider the provision of facilities for patients to spend time in complete privacy with their spouse or partners.

If such a facility was provided, the care team would need to assess the appropriateness of its use in each case, in conjunction with the patient and their spouse or partner.

8 Sexual activities between staff and patients

Sexual activity between staff and patients is unacceptable. This is a serious disciplinary offence that would usually lead to dismissal.

9   Staff mix

It is recognized that patients have the right to request to discuss issues around sexuality with a member of staff of either sex.

Consideration needs to be given to the provision of an adequate mix of female and male staff on each ward and shift. Wherever possible, patients should be offered the choice of being cared for by same sex staff.

10   Training for staff

It is recognized that addressing issues around sexuality with patients, relatives and significant others can be a particularly difficult area of practice.

Staff training needs in this area need to be identified and provision made for them being met. If the necessary skills do not exist in the ward team, at least one permanent member of staff should attend education and training seminars addressing this subject. The Lecturer/Practitioner (HIV) can provide information and training in this area.

November 1994

References

Abernethy, V. (1974) Sexual, knowledge, attitudes and practices of young female psychiatric patients. *Archives of General Psychiatry*, **30**: 180–2.

Abernethy, V., Robbins, D., Abernethy, G., Grunebaum, H. and Weiss, J. (1975) Identification of women at risk of unwanted pregnancy. *American Journal of Psychiatry*, **132**: 1027–31.

Ables, B. S. and Brandsma, J. M. (1977) *Therapy for Couples*. Jossey-Bass, San Francisco.

Acheson, D. (1994) *Commentary of the Health Advisory Committee on the Second Annual Report of the Director of Health Care Services for Prisoners*. Department of Public Health and Policy, 24 March 1994.

Addad, M., Benezech, M., Bourgeois, M. and Yesavage J. (1981) Criminal acts among schizophrenics in French mental hospitals. *Journal of Nervous and Mental Disease*, **169**: 2892–93.

Ainsworth, M. D. S., Blehar, M. C., Waters, E. and Wall, S. (1978) *Patterns of Attachment: A Psychological Study of the Strange Situation*. Erlbaum Associates, Hillsdale, NJ.

Ainsworth, M. D. S. (1991) Attachments and other affectional bonds across the life cycle. In *Attachments Across the Life Cycle* (C. M. Parkes, J. Stevenson-Hinde and P. Marris, eds). Routledge, London, pp. 33–51.

Akhtar, S., Crocker, E., Dickey, N. *et al.* (1977) Overt sexual behaviour among psychiatric inpatients. *Archives of General Psychiatry*, **30**: 180–2.

Akhtar, S. and Thompson, J. A. (1980) Schizophrenia and sexuality; a review and a report of twelve unusual cases – Part I. *Journal of Clinical Psychiatry*, **41**: 134–42.

Akhurst, M., Brown, I. and Wessely, S. (1995) *Dying for Help: Offenders at Risk of Suicide?* West Yorkshire Probation Service, West Yorkshire Health Authority, Association of Chief Officers of Probation: Cliff Hill House, Sandy Walk, Wakefield WF1 2DJ, UK.

Aldridge, R. G. (1983) Sexuality and Incarceration. *Corrective and Social Psychiatry and Journal of Behavioural Techniques*, Methods and Therapy, **29**: 74–77.

Alexander, M. (1988) Clinical determination of mental competence. *Archives of Neurology*, **45**: 23–26.

Almy, L., Bravo, V., Bird, L., Chin, P., Cohan, L., Galls, F. *et al.* (1980) A study of a coeducation correctional facility. In J. O. Smykla (ed.) *Coed Prison*. Human Sciences Press, New York, pp. 120–49.

Altounyan, B. (1993) Sex on the ward. *Nursing Standard*, **7**(24): 20–1.

Altschul, A. T. (1978) A system approach to the nursing process. *Journal of Advanced Nursing*, **34**: 333–40.

American Journal of Psychiatry (1992) Letters to editor. *American Journal of Psychiatry*, **149**: 979–89.

American Medical Association (1992) Diagnostic and treatment guidelines on domestic violence. *Archives of Family Medicine*, **1**: 39–47.

American Medical Association Board of Trustees (1992) Requirements or incentives by government for the use of long-acting contraceptives. *Journal of the American Association*, **267**: 1812–21.

American Psychiatric Association (1993) Position statement on homosexuality. *American Journal of Psychiatry*, **150**: 4.

American Psychiatric Association (1989) *The Principles of Medical Ethics with Annotations Especially Applicable to Psychiatry*. American Psychiatric Association, Washington, DC.

American Psychiatric Association (1994) *Diagnostical and Statistical Manual of Mental Disorders*, 4th edn (DSM-IV). American Psychiatric Association, Washington, DC.

Anderson, T. (1987) The reflecting team: Dialogue and meta-dialogue in clinical work. *Family Process*, **26**: 415–28.

Andrau, R. (1969) Sexualite et institution. *Evolution Psychiatrique*, **32**: 503–24.

Andrieux, D. (1995) Psychiatrist, Centre Hôpitalier Specialise De Villejuif, 54 Avenue de la Republique, 94806 Villejuif Cedex, France. Personal communication.

Anonymous (1988) Sexual drive of patients in psychiatric hospitals. Letter. *BMJ*, **297**: 561.

Anonymous (1994) HIV infection may modify psychotropic drug choice. *Drugs and Therapy Perspectives*, **4**: 10–12.

Appelbaum, P. S. and Jorgenson, L. (1991) Psychiatrist–patient sexual contact after termination: an analysis and a proposal. *American Journal of Psychiatry*, **148**: 1466–73.

Appleby, L. (1991) Suicide during pregnancy and during the first postnatal year. *British Medical Journal*, **301**: 137–40.

Apter, T. (1986) *Loose Relations. Your In-Laws and You*. Macmillan.

Ashford, S. and Timms, N. (1992) *What Europe Thinks: A Study of Western European Values*. Dartmouth, Aldershot, Hants.

Association of Chief Officers of Probation (1993) *Social Circumstances of Young Offenders*. Association of Cheif Officers of Probation, London E1 1BJ, UK.

Averbruch, I. E. and Lichtenberg, P. (1992) Mixed psychiatric wards. Letter. *BMJ*, **305**: 479.

Ayuso, J. L. (1994) Use of psychotropic drugs in patients with HIV infection. *Drugs*, **47**: 599–610.

Bach-y-Rita, G and Veno, A. (1974) Habitual violence: a profile of 62 men. *American Journal of Psychiatry*, **131**: 1015–17.

Bailey, S. and Higginbotham, N. (1994) *Young Women in Secure and Intensive Care. Margins to Mainstream*. Conference proceedings, Resource Network for Adolescents.

Bailey, R. and Ward, D. (1992) *Probation Supervision: Attitudes to Formalising Helping*. Centre for Social Action, University of Nottingham.

Baillard-Lapresle, A. (1975) *Vie Sexuelle et Contraception des Malades Mentale d'un Hôpital Psychiatrique*. Thèse Medicine. Bordeux No. 162.

Bancroft, J. (1989) *Human Sexuality and its Problems*, 2nd edn. Churchill Livingstone, pp. 148–53.

Barker, E. T. and McLaughlin, A. J. (1977) The total encounter capsule. *Canadian Psychiatric Association Journal*, **22**: 355–60.

Barker, E. T., Mason, M. H. and Wilson, V. (1969) Defense-disrupting therapy. *Canadian Psychiatric Association Journal*, **14**: 355–9.

Barker, P. (1992) *Basic Family Therapy*, 3rd edn. Blackwell Scientific Publications, Oxford.

Barlow, D. H. (1977) Assessment of sexual behavior. In *Handbook of Behavioral Assessment* (R. A. Ciminero, K. S. Calhoun and H. E. Adams, eds). Wiley, New York.

Barrett, T. G. and Booth, J. W. (1994) Sartorial eloquence: does it exist in the paediatrician–patient relationship? *British Medical Journal*, **309**: 1710–12.

Bartholomew, K. (1993) From childhood to adult relationships: Attachment theory and research. In *Learning About Relationships*. Understanding Relationship Processes Series, Vol. 2 (S. Duck, ed.). SAGE Publications, pp. 30–62.

Batcup, D. (1994) *Mixed Sex Wards. Recognising and Responding to Gender Issues in Mental Health Settings and Evaluating their Safety for Women*. Bethlem and Maudsley Trust.

Batcup, D. and Thomas, B. (1994) Mixing the genders, an ethical dilemma: How nursing theory has dealt with sexuality and gender. *Nursing Ethics*, **1**: 43–52.

Bates, A. (1942) Parental roles in courtship. *Social Forces*, **20**: 483–6.

Beels, C. C. (1979) Social networks and schizophrenia. *Psychiatric Quarterly*, **51**: 209–15.

Belsky, J. and Pensky, E. (1988) Developmental history, personality, and family relationships: toward an emergent family system. In *Relationships within Families. Mutual Influences.* (R. A. Hinde and J. Stevenson-Hinde, eds). Clarendon Press, Oxford, pp. 193–217.

Berry J. M. and Shapiro A. (1975) Married mentally handicapped patients in the community. *Proceedings of the Royal Society of Medicine*, **68**: 795–8.

Binder, R. L. (1985) Sex between psychiatric inpatients. *Psychiatric Quarterly*, **57**: 121–6.

Birtchnell, J. and Kennard, J. (1983) Marriage and mental illness. *British Journal of Psychiatry*, **142**: 193–8.

Blackburn, R. (1993) Psychopathy, personality disorder, and aggression: a cognitive–interpersonal analysis. In *Proceedings of the Fourth Symposium on Violence and Aggression* (L. Klose, ed.). University of Saskatchewan, Saskatoon, pp. 29–52.

Bloch, S. and Chodoff, P. (eds) (1991) *Psychiatric Ethics*, 2nd edn. Oxford University Press, Oxford.

Blochk, S., Hafner, J., Harari, E. and Szmuklerg, I. (1994) *The Family and Clinical Psychiatry*. Oxford University Press, Oxford.

Blumethal, R., Kreisman, D., and O'Connor, P. (1982) Return to the family and its consequence for rehospitalization among recently discharged mental patients. *Psychological Medicine*, **12**: 141–7.

Boszormenyi-Nagy, I. and Spark, G. M. (1973) *Invisible Loyalties: Reciprocity in Intergenerational Family Therapy*. Harper and Row, London.

Bouhoutsos, J., Holroyd, J., Lerman, H., Forer, B. and Greenberg, M. (1983) Sexual intimacy between psychotherapists and patients. *Professional Psychology Research and Practice*, **14**: 185–96.

Bourgeois, M. (1975) Sexualité et institution psychiatrique. *Evolution Psychiatrique*, **40**: 551–73.

Bowen, M. (1978) *Family Therapy in Clinical Practice*. Jason Aronson.

Bowlby, J. (1969) *Attachment and Loss*, Vol. 1: *Attachment*. Basic Books.

Bowlby, J. (1973) *Attachment and Loss*, Vol. 2: *Separation: Anxiety and Anger*. Basic Books.

Bowlby, J. (1979) *The Making and Breaking of Affectional Bonds*. Tavistock.

Bowlby, J. (1980) *Attachment and Loss*, Vol. 3: *Loss: Sadness and Depression*. Basic Books.

Brennan, P. A., Mednick, S. A., and Jacobson, B. (1996) Assessing the role of genetics in crime using adoption cohorts. In *Genetics of Criminal and Antisocial Behaviour* (G. R. Bock and J. A. Goode, eds). Ciba Foundation Symposium 194. Wiley, Chichester:

Brennan, W., Scully, W., Tarbuck, P. and Young, C. (1995) Nurses' attire in a special hospital: perceptions of patients and staff. *Nursing Standard*, **9**: 35–38.

Bretschnieider, J. G. and McCoy, N. L. (1988) Sexual interest and behavior in healthy 80 to 102 year-olds. *Archives of Sexual Behaviour*, **17**: 109–29.

Britton, R. (1981) Re-enactment as an unwitting professional response to family dynamics. In *Psychotherapy with Families* (S. Box, B. Copley, J. Magagna and E. Moustaki, eds). Routledge and Kegan Paul, pp. 48–58.

Brockington, I. F. and Kumar, R. (1982) Drug addiction and psychotropic drug treatment during pregnancy and lactation. In *Motherhood and Mental Illness* (I. F. Brockington and R. Kumar, eds). Academic Press, London, pp. 239–55.

Brown, G. W., Birley, J. L. T. and Wing, J. K. (1972) The influence of family life on the course of schizophrenic disorders; a replication. *British Journal of Psychiatry*, **121**: 241–58.

Brown, G. W. and Harris, T. (1978) *Social Origins of Depression*. Tavistock Publications.

Brown, G. W., Monck, E. M., Carstairs, G. M. and Wing, J. K. (1962) The influence of family life on the course of schizophrenic illness. *British Journal of Preventative and Social Medicine*, **16**: 58–68.

Brown, L. (1989) Is there sexual freedom for our ageing population in longterm care institutions? *Journal of Gerontological Social Work*, **13**(3/4): 75–93.

Bruce, T. (1982) Family work in a secure unit. In *Family Therapy. Complementary Frameworks of Theory and Practice*, Vol. 2. (A. Bentovim, G. G. Barnes, and A. Cooklin, eds). London Academic Press, London, pp. 497–514.

Brugha, T. S. (1989) Social support and social networks. *Current Opinion in Psychiatry*, **2**: 278–82.

Brugha, T. S. (1990) Social networks and support. *Current Opinion in Psychiatry*, **3**: 264–8.

Brugha, T. S., Wing, J. K., Brewin, C. R. *et al.* (1993) The relationship of social network deficits with deficits in social functioning in long-term psychiatric disorders. *Social Psychiatry and Psychiatric Epidemiology*, **28**: 218–24.

Buckley, P. F. and Hyde, J. L. (1997) State hospitals' responses to the sexual behavior of psychiatric inpatients. *Psychiatric Services*, **48**: 398–9

Buffum, P. C. (1971) *Homosexuality in Prisons*. The Pennsylvania Prison Society.

Bullock, R., Little, M. and Millham, S. (1994) *The Care Careers of Extremely Difficult and*

Disturbed Young People. An Introduction. Dartington Social Research Unit, Dartington, Devon.

Bullock, R., Little, M. and Millham, S. (1994) *The Experience of YTC Look-Alikes Sheltered in Other Secure Settings.* Dartington Social Research Unit, Darington, Devon.

Bullock, R., Little, M. and Millham, S. (1994) *The Part Played by Career, Individual Circumstance and Treatment Interventions in the Outcomes of Leavers from the Youth Treatment Centres.* Dartington Social Research Unit, Dartington, Devon.

Bullock, R., Little, M. and Millham, S. (1994) *The Characteristics of Young People in Youth Treatment Centres.* Dartington Social Research Unit, Dartington, Devon.

Bullock, R., Little, M. and Millham, S. (1994) Alternative care careers: The experience of very difficult adolescents outside Youth Treatment Centre provision. Dartington Social Research Unit, Dartington, Devon.

Cambridge, P. and McCarthy, M. (1997) Developing and implementing sexuality policy for a learning disability provider service. *Health and Social Care in the Community,* **5**: 227–236.

Capp, B. (1996) Serial killers in 17th-century England. *History Today,* **46**: 21–26.

Carvell, A. L. M. and Hart, G. J. (1990) Risk behaviours for HIV infection among drug users in prison. *British Medical Journal,* **300**: 1383–4.

Cassel C. K. (1995) Sex, lies, and social science: another exchange. *The New York Review of Books,* **XLII**: 55.

Catalan, J. (1997) The psychiatry of HIV infection. *Advances in Psychiatric Treatment,* **3**: 17–24.

Catan, L. (1989) *The Development of Young Children in Prison Mother and Baby Units.* Research Bulletin No. 26, Home Office Research and Planning Unit. Home Office: London.

Cavior, H. E. and Cohen, S. H. (1980) The development of a scale to assess inmate and staff attitudes toward co-corrections. In *Coed Prison* (J. O. Smykla, ed.). Human Sciences Press, New York:, pp. 181–202.

Chaimowitz, G. A. (1991) Homophobia among psychiatric residents, family practice residents and psychiatric faculty. *Canadian Journal of Psychiatry,* **36**: 206–9.

Champagne, D. (1992) *Alternative Family Forms: A Study of the Penitentiary and Offender Management in Canada.* School of Social Work, Carlton University, Carlton, Canada.

Chandler, R. (1950) Goldfish. *In Trouble is my Business.* Penguin books, Harmondsworth. (Also as single story in 1995 edn.).

Charo, R. A. (1992) Mandatory contraception. *Lancet,* **339**: 1104–5.

Clarke, L. (1989) *Children's Changing Circumstances: Recent Trends and Future Prospects.* Centre for Population Studies, London School of Hygiene and Tropical Medicine Research Paper, London, pp. 89–94.

Coleman, J. C. and Hendry, L. (1990) *The Nature of Adolescence,* 2nd edn. Routledge, London, pp. 140–161.

College of Physicians and Surgeons of Ontario, Task Force on Sexual Abuse of Patients. (1991) *Final Report.* College of Physicians and Surgeons of Ontario, Toronto, Ontario.

Collins, A. C. and Kellner, R. (1986) Neuroleptics and sexual functioning. *Integrative Psychiatry,* **4**: 96–108.

Collins, N. L. and Read, S. J. (1990) Adult attachment, working models, and relationship quality in dating couples. *Journal of Personality and Social Psychology,* **38**: 644–63.

Committee on the Family, Group for the Advancement of Psychiatry (1995) A model for the classification and diagnosis of relational disorder. *Psychiatric Services,* **46**: 926–31.

Commons, M. L., Bohn, J. T., Godon, L. T. *et al.* (1992) Professionals' attitudes towards sex between institutionalised patients. *American Journal of Psychotherapy,* **XLVI**: 571–80.

Conacher, G. N. (1988) AIDS, condoms and prisons (letter). *Lancet,* July 2, pp. 41–2.

Conte, H., Plutchik, R., Picard, S., Karasu, T. B. (1989) Ethics in the practice of psychotherapy: a survey. *American Journal of Psychotherapy,* **43**: 32–42.

Cook, J. A. and Hoffschmidt, S. J. (1993) *Comprehensive Models of Psychosocial Rehabilitation.* In *Psychiatric Rehabilitation in Practice* (R. W. Flexer and P. L. Solomon, eds). Andover, pp. 81–97.

Cooper, P. J., Campbell, E. A., Kennerley, H. and Bond, A. (1988) Non psychotic disorders after childbirth: a prospective study of prevalence, incidence, course and nature. *British Journal of Psychiatry,* **152**: 799–806.

Copperman, J. and Burrows, F. (1992) Reducing the risk of assault. *Nursing Times*, **88**: 64–5.

Copperman, J. (1991) No refuge from rape? *Open Mind*, **51**: June/July, p. 4.

Correctional Service of Canada (1988) *Private Family Visiting Programme*. Minister of Supply and Services, Canada.

Costello, C. G. and Gazan, M. (1962) Desegregation in a psychiatric unit. *Canadian Nurse*, **58**: 1098–9.

Costello, T. (1995) Legal structures and responsibilities of voluntary organisations. In *AIDS: A Guide to the Law* (R. Haigh and D. Harris, eds). Routledge, London.

Cotton, D. J. and Groth, A. N. (1982) Inmate rape: prevention and intervention. *Journal of Prison and Jail Health*, **2**: 47–57.

Council of Europe (1993) Recommendation No. R(93)6 of the Ministers of Member States. Council of Europe, Strasbourg.

Cournos, F., Empfield, M., Horwath, E. and Kramer, M. (1989) The management of HIV infection in state psychiatric hospitals. *Hospital and Community Psychiatry*, **40**: 153–7.

Cox, M. (1974) Dynamic psychotherapy with sex-offenders. In *Sexual Deviation*, 3rd edn. (I. Rosen, ed.). Oxford University Press, Oxford, pp. 300–35.

Craft, A. and Craft, M. (1979) *Handicapped Married Couples*. Routledge and Kegan Paul, London.

Craft, A. (1987) Mental handicap & sexuality: issues for individuals with a mental handicap, their parents & professionals. In *Mental Handicap and Sexuality: Issues & Perspectives* (A. Craft, ed.) Costello, Tunbridge Wells.

Craft, A. (1994) *Practice Issues in Sexuality and Learning Disabilities*. Routledge, London.

Crowe, M. (1978) Conjoint marital therapy: a controlled outcome study. *Psychological Medicine*, **8**: 623–36.

Crowe, M. and Ridley, J. (1990) *Therapy with Couples. A Behavioural-Systems Approach to Marital and Sexual Problems*. Blackwell, Oxford.

Curle, C. (1989) Unpublished PhD Thesis, London University.

Curran, L. and Morrissey, C. (1989) *AIDS/HIV Risk Behaviour in Prison, an Exploratory Study at HMP Wormwood Scrubs*. Summary report.

Daly, M. and Wilson, M. I. (1996) Violence against stepchildren. *Current Directory of Psychological Science*, **5**: 77–81.

Da Silva, L. and Johnstone, E. C. (1981) A follow up study of severe puerperal psychiatric illness. *British Journal of Psychiatry*, **139**: 346–54.

Davis, M. H. (1983) Measuring individual differences in empathy: evidence for a multidimensional approach. *Journal of Personality and Social Psychology*, **44**: 113–26.

Dell, S. and Parker, E. (1979) *Special Hospitals Case Register. Triennial Statistics 1972–74*. In Special Hospitals' Case Register: Special Hospitals Research Report No. 15, London.

Department of Health Personal Social Services Local Authority Statistics (1995) *Children and Young People on Child Protection Registers Year Ending 31 March 1995 England*. Government Statistical Service A/F 95/13.

Department of Health and Social Security (1980) *Report of the Committee of Inquiry into Rampton Hospital*. Cmnd 8073. HMSO, London.

Department of Health (1990) *The Care of Children: Principles and Practice in Regulations and Guidance*. HMSO, London.

Department of Health (1992) *The Health of the Nation: A Strategy for Health in England*. Cm. 1523.

Department of Health (1992) *Inspection of Facilities for Mothers and Babies in Prison*. Department of Health, London.

Department of Health (1993) *Health of a Nation: Key Area Handbook HIV/AIDS and Sexual Health*. DoH, London.

Department of Health (1994) *Clinical Supervision for the Nursing and Health Visiting Professions*. CNO Professional Letter 1994(5), Department of Health, London.

Department of Health (1997) *Inspection of Facilities for Mothers and Babies in Prison, Third Multi-Disciplinary Inspection by the Department of Health*. Department of Health, London.

Dernevik, M. (1995) Chartered Clinical Psychologist, Rättspsykiatriska regionkliniken, Birgittas sjukhus, Klosterledsgatan 35. 59281 Vadstena, Sweden. Personal communication.

Dickens, C. (1852) *American Notes*. Now available in Penguin, Harmondsworth.

Dicks, H. (1967) *Marital Tensions*. Routledge and Kegan Paul, London.

Dicks, H. V. (1985) *Marital Tensions*. Maresfield Press, London.

Dillner, L. (1992) Keeping babies in prison. *British Medical Journal*, **304**: 932–3.

Dincin, J. and Wise, S. (1979) Sexual attitude reassessment for psychiatric patients. *Rehabilitation Literature*, **40**: 233–9.

Disch, E. (1989) One day workshops for female survivors of sexual abuse by psychotherapists. In *Psychotherapists' Involvement with Clients* (G. Schoener *et al.*, eds). Intervention and Prevention Walk-in Counseling Center, Minneapolis, MN, pp. 209–13.

Dobash, R. P., Dobash, R. E. and Guttridge, S. (1986) *The Imprisonment of Women*. Basil Blackwell, Oxford.

Dolan, K. A. (1990) Drug injecting and syringe sharing in custody and in the community: an exploratory survey of HIV risk behaviour. *The Howard Journal*, **29**: 177–86.

d'Orban, P. (1979) Women who kill their children. *British Journal of Psychiatry*, **134**: 560–71.

Driscoll, R., Davis, K. E. and Lipetz, M. E. (1972) Parental interference and romantic love: The Romeo and Juliet effect. *Journal of Personality and Social Psychology*, **24**: 1–10.

Dunn, M., O'Driscoll, C., Dayson, D. *et al.* (1990) The TAPS project. 4: An observational study of the social life of long-stay patients. *British Journal of Psychiatry*, **157**: 842–8.

Durre, L. (1980) Comparing romantic and therapeutic relationships. In *On Love and Loving. Psychological Perspectives on the Nature and Experience of Romantic Love* (K. S. Pope, ed.) Jessey Bass, San Fransisco, CA. 228–43.

Easson, W. M. and Kan, T. (1967) Adolescent inpatients in love, a therapeutic contradiction. *Archives of General Psychiatry*, **16**: 758–63.

Edmond, D. and Kaye, C. (1991) Study Tour of Forensic Psychiatric Services for Offenders in the Netherlands. April 1991. Unpublished. Special Hospitals Service Authority, London. (Available from C. Kaye, Broadmoor Hospital, Crowthorne, Berkshire. RG47 7EG).

Edwardes, W. (1995) Formerly Consultant Psychiatrist, St. Anne's Hospital, Trinidad, now Consultant Psychiatrist, Yarmouth Regional Hospital, Psychiatric Unit, 60 Vancouver Street, Yarmouth, Nova Scotia B5A 2PS, Canada. Personal communication.

Eiguer, A., Litousky de Eiguer, D. and Chapuis, F. (1974) Contribution à l'étude de la mixité et de la formation des couples en milieu psychiatrique. *Information Psychiatrique*, **50**: 915–29.

Epstein, R. S. and Simon, R. I. (1990) An early warning indicator of boundary violations in psychotherapy. *Bulletin of the Meriger Clinic*, **54**: 450–65.

Erikson, E. H. (1959) Identity and the life cycle. In *Psychological Issues*, (G.S. Klein, ed.), Monograph 1, International University Press, New York.

Ester, P., Halman, L. and de Moor, R. (1993) *The Individualising Society: Value Change in Europe and North America*. Tilburg University Press, Tilburg, The Netherlands.

Estroff, S. E., Zimmer, C., Lachicotte, W. S. and Benoit, J. (1994) The influence of social networks and social support on violence by persons with serious mental illness. *Hospital and Community Psychiatry*, **45**: 669–79.

Evans *et al.* (1990) Reducing AIDS anxiety on the unit with preventative infection control. *Journal of Psychosocial Nursing*, **28**: 1–36.

Fahy, T. A. and O'Donoghue, G. (1991) Eating disorders in pregnancy. *Psychological Medicine*, **21**: 577–80.

Fahy, T. and Fisher, N. (1992) Sexual contact between doctors and patients, almost always harmful. *British Medical Journal*, **304**: 1519–20.

Fahy, T. A. and Morrison, J. J. (1993) The clinical significance of eating disorders in obstetrics. *British Journal of Obstetrics and Gynaecology*, **100**: 708–10.

Fairbairn, W. R. D. (1952) *An Object–Relations Theory of the Personality*. Basic Books, New York.

Falloon, I. R. H., Boyd, J. L., McGill, C. W., Razani, J., Moss, H. B. and Gilderman, A. M. (1982) Family management in the prevention of exacerbations of schizophrenia. *New England Journal of Medicine*, **306**: 1437–40.

Falloon, I. R. H., Boyd, J. L., McGill, C. W. *et al.* (1985) Family versus individual management in the prevention of morbidity of schizophrenia: I. Clinical outcome of a two year controlled study. *Archives of General Psychiatry*, **42**: 887–96.

Farmer, R., Preston, D., Emami, J. and Barker, M. (1989) *The Transmission of HIV Within Prisons and its Likely Effect on the Growth of the Epidemic in the General Population.* North Thames Regional Health Authority, London.

Farrington, D. P. (1993) The psychosocial milieu of the offender. In *Forensic Psychiatry. Clinical, Legal and Ethical Issues* (J. Gunn and P. J. Taylor, eds). Butterworth–Heinemann, Oxford, pp. 252–85.

Feeney, J. A. and Noller, P. (1990) Attachment style as a predictor of adult romantic relationships. *Journal of Personality and Social Psychology,* **58**: 281–91.

Feinmann, J. (1988) Corridors of fear. *Nursing Times,* **84**: 16–17.

Feldbrugge, J. T. T. M. (1991) Partner relationships in a forensic mental hospital: seen as part of life, with benefits and costs. An empirical report. *XVIIth Congress on Law and Mental Health,* Leuven, 26–30 May, 1991.

Feldbrugge, J. T. T. M. and Haverkamp, A. D. (1993) Identity and development: the Dr. Henri van der Hoeven Kliniek in the nineties. *International Journal of Law and Psychiatry,* **16**: 241–6.

Felmlee, D., Sprecher, S. and Bassin, E. (1990) The dissolution of intimate relationships: a hazard model. *Social Psychology Quarterly,* **53**: 13–30.

Fernandez, F. and Levy, J. K. (1994) Psychopharmacology in HIV spectrum disorders. *Psychiatric Clinics of North America,* **17**: 135–48.

Ferraro, D., Kennedy, M., Leese, M. and Taylor P. J. Rehabilitation of special hospital patients: Are national principles and the care programme approach likely to be enough? (Submitted for publication.) (Institute of Psychiatry, London SE5 8AF).

Fiore, J., Becker, J. and Coppel, D. B. (1983) Social network interaction: a buffer or a stress. *American Journal of Community Psychology,* **11**: 423–39.

Fishman, L. T. (1988) Prisoners and their wives: marital and domestic effects of telephone contacts and home visits. *International Journal of Offender Therapy and Comparative Criminology,* **32**: 55–66.

Fortune, M. M. (1995) When sex invades the pastoral relationship. In *Breach of Trust* (J. C. Gonsiorek, ed.) Sage, Thousand Oaks, CA, pp. 29–40.

Fowler, R. C. and Tsuang, M. C. (1975) Spouses of schizophrenics. *Comprehensive Psychiatry,* **16**: 339–42.

Fowler, D., Garety, P. and Kuipers, E. (1995) *Cognitive Behaviour Therapy for Psychosis: Theory and Practice.* John Wiley, Chichester.

Fowler, J. (1995) Coordinator Case Management. Correctional Service of Canada. Regional Treatment Centre, PO Box 22, Kingston, Ontario K7L 4V7, Canada. Personal communication.

Framo, J. L. (1981) The integration of marital therapy with sessions with family of origin. In *Handbook of Family Therapy* (A. S. Gurman and D. P. Kniskern, eds). Brunner/Mazel, New York, pp. 133–58.

Franzoi, S. L. (1988) A picture of competence. *American Journal of Nursing,* **88**: 1109.

Freedman M., Stuss, D. and Gordon, M. (1991) Assessment of competency: the role of neurobehavioral deficits. *Annals of Internal Medicine,* **115**: 203–208.

Gabbai, P. and Degos, D. (1975) Notes sur la sexualité des handicappes mentaux. (Observations et experiences à la Fondation John Bost à la Force) Symposium sur la sexualité des débiles. 28–29 avril, à paraitre. (Quoted in Bourgeois, M. 1975.)

Gartrell, N., Herman, J., Olarte, S. *et al.* (1986) Psychiatrist–patient sexual contact: results of a national survey. I: Prevalence. *American Journal of Psychiatry,* **143**: 1126–31.

Gartrell, N. K., Milliken, N., Goodson, W. H., Thiemann, S. and Lo, B. (1995) Physician–patient sexual contact. In *Breach of Trust* (J. C. Gonsiorek, ed.) Sage, Thousand Oaks, CA.

Gartrell, N., Herman, J., Olarte, S., Feldstein, M. and Localio, R (1987) Reporting practices of psychiatrists who knew of sexual misconduct by colleagues. *American Journal of Orthopsychiatry,* **57**: 287–95.

General Medical Council. (1995) *HIV and AIDS: The Ethical Considerations.* General Medical Council, 1780202, Great Portland Street, London WIN 6JE.

George, C., Kaplan, N. and Main, M. (1985) An adult attachment interview: interview protocol. Unpublished manuscript. University of California, Berkeley.

Ghosh, C. (1995) Personal communication. Consultant Psychiatrist, Broadmoor Hospital Authority,

Crowthorne, Berkshire RG45 7EG, UK.

Gibbens T. C. N. (1958) Sane and insane homicide. *Journal of Criminal Law*, Criminology and Police Service, **49**: 110–15.

Gibbs, C. (1971) The effect of the imprisonment of women on their children. *British Journal of Criminology*, **11**: 113–30.

Gibson, E. (1975) *Homicide in England & Wales 1967–1971*. Home Office Research Study No. 31. HMSO, London.

Gitlin, M. J. H. (1994) Psychotropic medication and their effects on sexual function: diagnosis, biology, and treatment approaches. *Journal of Clinical Psychiatry*, **55**: 406–13.

Gledhill, J. A., Warner, J. P. and King, M. (1997) Psychiatrists and their patients: views on forms of dress and address. *British Journal of Psychiatry*, **171**: 228–32.

Gligor, A. and Tryon, W. (1973) An evaluation of the integration of male and female patients in a psychiatric hospital. *Newsletter for Research in Mental Health and Behavioural Sciences*, **15**: 18–19.

Gochros, H. L. (1972) The sexually oppressed. *Social Work*, March 16–23.

Goldstein, A. P. and Keller, H. (1987) *Aggressive Behaviour: Assessment and Treatment*. Pergamon Press.

Goldstein, J. M. (1988) Gender differences in the course of schizophrenia. *American Journal of Psychiatry*, **145**: 684–89.

Goldstein, J. M. and Caton, C. L. M. (1983) The effects of the community environment on chronic psychiatric patients. *Psychological Medicine*, **13**: 193–9.

Gonsiorek, J. C. (ed.) *(1989) Breach of Trust*. Sage, Thousand Oaks, CA.

Gottlieb, M. C. (1990) Accusation of sexual misconduct: assisting in the complaint process. *Professional Psychology: Research and Practice*, **21**: 451–61.

Greben, S. E. (1991) Interpersonal aspects of the supervision of individual psychotherapy. *American Journal of Psychotherapy*, **XLV**: 306–16.

Greenberg, D. (1993) Israel. In: Payne A (1993) Sexual activity among psychiatric inpatients: international perspectives. *Journal of Forensic Psychiatry*, **4**: 109–29.

Greenberg, D. (1993) International perspectives: Israel. In: Sexual activity among psychiatric inpatients (A. Payne, ed.) *Journal of Forensic Psychiatry*, **4**: 115–17.

Greenberg, D. and Witztum, E. (1991) Problems in the treatment of religious patients. *American Journal of Psychotherapy*, **45**: 554–65.

Grounds, A., Gunn, J., Mullen, P. and Taylor, P. J. (1993) Secure institutions: their characteristics and problems. In *Forensic Psychiatry: Clinical, Legal and Ethical Issues* (J. Gunn and P. J. Taylor, eds). Butterworth–Heinemann, Oxford, pp. 794–825.

Gudjonsson, G. H. and Gunn, J. (1982) The competence and reliability of a witness in the criminal court: a case report. *British Journal of Psychiatry*, **141**: 624–7.

Gunn, J., Maden, A. and Swinton, M. (1991) Treatment needs of prisoners with psychiatric disorders. *British Medical Journal*, **303**: 338–40.

Gunn, J., Robertson, G., Dell, S. and Way, C. (1978) *Psychiatric Aspects of Imprisonment*. London: Academic Press.

Gunn M. J. (1987) Sexual right of the mentally handicapped. In *Issues in Criminological and Legal Psychology* No. 10. *Mental Handicap and the Law* (E. Alves, ed.).

Gunner, A. (1988) Are we handicapped by our sexual preferences? *The Professional Nurse*, **3**: 436–8.

Gutheil, T. G. (1995) Psychiatrist, Massachusetts Mental Health Center, 74 Fenwood Road, Boston, Massachusetts 02115, USA. Personal communication.

Gutheil, T. G. and Gabbard, G. O. (1993) The concept of boundaries in clinical practice: theoretical and risk-management dimensions. *American Journal of Psychiatry*, **150**: 180–96.

Häfner, H. and Böker, W. (1973) (translated by H. Marshall, 1982) *Crimes of Violence by Mentally Abnormal Offenders*. Cambridge University Press, Cambridge.

Hagnell, O. and Kreitman, N., with Duffy, J. (1974) Mental illness in married pairs in a total population. *British Journal of Psychiatry*, **125**: 293–302.

Hamilton, A. (1995) The criminal law and HIV infection. In *AIDS: A Guide to the Law* (R. Haigh and D. Harris, eds). London: Routledge, pp. 21–37.

Hammer, M., Makiesky-Barrow, S. and Gutwirth, L. (1978) Social networks and schizophrenia.

Schizophrenia Bulletin, **4**: 522–45.

Hansen, H. (1991) Medical Director, Herstedvester Prison. Anstalten ved Hertedvester, Holsbjervej 20, DK-2620 Albertslund, Denmark. Personal communication.

Hanson, R. K. (1997) Invoking sympathy: The assessment and treatment of empathy deficits among sexual offenders. In *The Sex Offender: New Insights, Treatment Innovations and Legal Developments. (Volume 2).* (B. K. Schwartz and H. R. Cellini, eds). Civic Research Institute, Kingston, NJ, pp. 1–12.

Harding, T. (1987) AIDS in prison. *Lancet*, **ii**: 1260–63.

Harticollis, P. (1964) Hospital Romances: some vicissitudes of the transference. *Bulletin of the Meninger Clinic*, **28**: 62–71.

Hartup, W. H. and Rubin, Z. (eds) (1986) *Relationships and Development*. Lawrence Erlbaum Associates.

Haugen, T. (1991) Medical Director. Ampshospitalet, Nykøbing. Egebjergvej 106, 4500 Nykfbing Sjaelland, Denmark. Personal communication.

Havel, V. (1990) *Letters to Olga*. Faber and Faber, London.

Hazan, C. and Shaver, P. R. (1987) Romantic love conceptualised as an attachment process. *Journal of Personality and Social Psychology*, **52**: 511–24.

Heads, T. C., Taylor, P. J. and Leese, M. (1887) Childhood experiences of patient with schizophrenia and a history of violence: a special hospital sample. *Criminal Behaviour and Mental Health*, **7**: 117–30.

Henderson, S. (1980) A development in social psychiatry. The systematic study of social bonds. *Journal of Nervous and Mental Disease*, **168**: 63–9.

Henderson, S., Duncan-Jones, P., McAuley, H. and Ritchie, K. (1978) The patient's primary group. *British Journal of Psychiatry*, **132**: 74–86.

Herman, J. and Hirschman, L. (1981) Families at risk for father/daughter incest. *American Journal of Psychiatry*, **138**: 967–70.

Heston, L. L. (1966) Psychiatric disasters in foster home-ʳ ʼared children of schizophrenic mothers. *British Journal of Psychiatry*, **112**: 819–25.

Hickling, F. (1993) International perspectives: Jamaica. In *Sexual activity among psychiatric inpatients* (A. Payne, ed.) *Journal of Forensic Psychiatry*, **4**: 121–3.

Hinde, R. A. and Stevenson-Hinde, J. (1988) *Relationships within Families. Mutual Influences.* Clarendon Press, Oxford.

HM Prison Service Health Care (1993) *First Report of the Director of Health Care for Prisoners*. Home Office, London.

HM Prison Service (1995) *Prison Service Annual Report and Accounts April 1993–March 1994.* HMSO, London.

HM Inspectorate of Probation (1995) *Dealing with Dangerous People: The Probation Service and Public Protection Report of a Thematic Inspection.* Home Office, London.

Hoffman, L. (1990) Constructing realities: an art of lenses. *Family Process*, **20**: 1–13.

Hoggett, B. (1990) *Mental Health Law*, 3rd edn. Sweet and Maxwell, London.

Holbrook, T. (1989) Policing sexuality in a modern state hospital. *Hospital and Community Psychiatry*, **40**: 75–9.

Hollin, C. R. and Trower, P. (1986) *Handbook of Social Skills Training*, Vols 1 and 2. Pergamon Press, Oxford.

Holmes, J. (1993) *John Bowlby and Attachment Theory*. Routledge, London.

Holmes-Eber, P. and Riger, S. (1990) Hospitalization and the composition of mental patients' social networks. *Schizophrenia Bulletin*, **16**: 157–64.

Holroyd, J. C. and Brodsky, A. (1977) Psychologists' attitudes and practices regarding erotic and non-erotic physical contact with patients. *American Psychologist*, **32**: 843–9.

Home Office, Department of Health and Social Security (1975) *Report of the Committee on Mentally Abnormal Offenders (The Butler Report)*. Cmnd. 6244 HMSO, London.

Home Office (1987) *Criminal Statistics England and Wales 1986*, Supplementary Vols 1 and 2. HMSO, London.

Home Office (1995) *Domestic Violence Fact Sheet*. Home Office, London.

Hooley, J. M. (1987) The nature and origins of expressed emotion. In *Understanding Major Mental*

Disorder: The Contribution of Family Interaction Research. (K. Hahlweg and M. J. Goldstein, eds). Family Process Press, pp. 176–94.

Hooley, J. M. and Hahlweg, K. (1986) Interaction patterns of depressed patients and their spouses: comparing high and low EE diads. In *Treatment of Schizophrenia: Family Assessment and Intervention* (M. J. Goldstein, I. Hand and K. Hahlweg, eds). Springer–Verlag, Berlin.

House of Commons (1975) *Report from the Select Committee on Violence in Marriage* (HC 553). HMSO, London.

House of Commons (1986) *Third Report from the Social Services Committee, Session 1985–6.* Prison Medical Services. HMSO, London.

Howard League for Penal Reform (1993) *The Voice of a Child.* The Impact on Children of their Mothers' Imprisonment. Howard League, London.

Howard League for Penal Reform (1995) *Prison Mother and Baby Units.* Information leaflet compiled and circulated by the Howard League, London N19 3NL, UK.

Howard League for Penal Reform (1997) *Pregnant and in Prison.* Information leaflet compiled and circulated by the Howard League, London N19 3NL, UK.

Howell, J. R. (1987) Assessment of sexual function, interest and activity in depressed men. *Journal of Affective Disorders,* **13**: 61–6.

Hoyer, G. (1988) Management of mentally ill offenders in Scandinavia. *International Journal of Law and Psychiatry,* **11**: 317–27.

Hucker, S.J., Arnup, J., Busse, E.W. *et al.* (1986) *Oak Ridge: A Review and an Alternative.* Ontario Ministry of Health: Toronto, Canada. (Unpublished – private circulation).

Huft, A., Fawkes L. S. and Lawson Jnr, W. T. (1992) Care of the pregnant offender. *Federal Prisons Journal.*

Hughes T. (1997) *Tales from Ovid.* Faber and Faber, London, p. 246.

Human Rights Watch Women's Rights Project (1996) All Too Familiar: Sexual Abuse of Women in US State Prisons. Human Rights Watch, New York.

Inglehart, R. (1990) *Culture Shift in Advanced Industrial Society.* Princeton University Press, New Jersey.

Inner London Probation Service (ILPS) (1995) *Identification and Management of Risk and Dangerousness.* Unpublished document for the Service available from ILPS 73–5 Great Peter Street, London SW1P 2BN.

Jacobson, N. S. and Margolin, G. (1979) *Marital Therapy.* Brunner/Mazel, New York.

Johnson, M. P. and Milardo, R. M. (1984) Network interference in pair relationships: A social psychological recasting of Slater's theory of social regression. *Journal of Marriage and the Family,* **46**: 893–9.

Johnson, M. P. and Leslie, L. (1982) Couple involvement and network structure: A test of the dyadic withdrawal hypothesis. *Social Psychology Quarterly,* **45**: 34–43.

Kaiser, F. E. (1991) Sexuality and impotence in aging men. *Clinical Geriatric Medicine,* **7**: 63–72.

Kaliski, S., Twiggs, J., Jedaar, A. and Lay, S. (1994) Sexual behaviour between male in-patients in a forensic unit. Poster presentation at the Biennial Congress of the Society of Psychiatrists of South Africa, and available from Sean Kaliski, Valkenberg Hospital, Observatory, 7935, South Africa.

Kavanagh, D. J. (1992) Recent developments in expressed emotion and schizophrenia. *British Journal of Psychiatry,* **160**: 601–20.

Kaye, C. (1994) Prurience and public interest. *Health Service Journal* Open Space, 7 April, p. 15.

Keitner, G. I., Baldwin, L. M. and McKendall, M. J. (1986) Copatient relationships on a short-term psychiatric unit. *Hospital and Community Psychiatry,* **37**: 166–70.

Keitner, G. and Grof, P. (1981) Sexual and emotional intimacy between psychiatric inpatients: formulating a policy. *Hospital and Community Psychiatry,* **32**: 188–93.

Kelly, J.A., Murphy, D.A., Bahr, R. *et al.* (1992) AIDS/HIV risk behaviour among the chronically mentally ill. *American Journal of Psychiatry,* **140**: 886–9.

Kempe C. H., Silverman F. N., Steel B. S., Droegemeuller, W. and Silver, H. K. (1962) The battered child syndrome. *Journal of the American Medical Association,* **181**: 17–24.

Kendell, R. E., Chalmers, J. C. and Platz, C. (1987) Epidemiology of puerperal psychosis. *British Journal of Psychiatry,* **150**: 662–73.

Kobak, R. R. and Hazan, C. (1991) Attachment in marriage: effects of security and accuracy of working models. *Journal of Personality and Social Psychology*, **60**: 861–9.

Kobbe, U. (1988) Uber die Sexualatrophie psychiatrischer Patienten – Ein essayistischer Uberblick. *Psychiatrische Praxis*. Georg Threme Verlag, Stuttgart, New York, pp. 192–201.

Kobbe, U. (1991) Sexualitat: Pro und Kontra: Interview mit B. Dimmek Lippstadt, Germany Heft 3/4. 5 Jahrgang Dezember 1991.

Koenraadt, F. (1992) The individualising function of forensic multidisciplinary assessment in a Dutch residential setting. The Pieter Baan experience. *International Journal of Law and Psychiatry*, **15**: 195–203.

Kreitman, N. (1968) Married couples admitted to mental hospital. *British Journal of Psychiatry*, **114**: 699–718.

Kretz, H. (1969) Sozialpsychiatrische Einrichtungen mit oder ohne Trennung der Geschlechter? *Nervenartz*, **4**: 176–83.

Kuipers, L., Leff, J. and Lam, D. (1992) *Family Work for Schizophrenia. A Practical Guide.* Gaskell.

Kumar, R. (1982) Neurotic disorders in childbearing women. In *Motherhood and Mental Illness* (I. F. Brockington and R. Kumar, eds). Academic Press, London, pp. 71–118.

Kumar, R. (1992) Mentally ill mothers and their babies: what are the benefits and risks of joint hospital admission? In *Practical Problems in Clinical Psychiatry* (K. Hawton and P. J. Cowen, eds). Oxford University Press, Oxford, pp. 184–96.

Kumar, R. and Hipwell, A. (1994) Implications for the infant of maternal puerperal psychiatric disorders. In *Child and Adolescent Psychiatry* (M. Rutter, L. Hersov and E. Taylor, eds). Blackwell, Oxford, pp. 759–75.

Laing, R. D. and Esterson, A. (1964) *Sanity, Madness and the Family.* Tavistock, London.

Lam, D. H. (1991) Psychosocial family intervention in schizophrenia: a review of empirical studies. *Psychological Medicine*, **21**: 423–41.

Lancet (1991) HIV in prisons. Letter. *Lancet*, **337**: 546.

Laumann, E. O., Gagnon, J. H., Michael, R. T. and Michaels, S. (1994) *The Social Organization of Sexuality: Sexual Practices in the United States.* University of Chicago Press, Chicago.

Law Commission (1991) *Mentally Incapacitated Adults and Decision-Making: An Overview.* Consultation Paper No. 119. HMSO, London.

Leaute, J. (1959) *Une Nouvelle École de Science Criminelle, L'École d'Utrecht.* Cujas, Paris.

Leff, J. Director of Social and Community Psychiatry, Social Psychiatry Section, Institute of Psychiatry, De Crespigny Park, London, SE5 8AF. Personal communication.

Leff, J., Kuipers, L., Berkowitz, R. *et al.* (1982) A controlled trial of social intervention in the families of schizophrenic patients. *British Journal of Psychiatry*, **141**: 121–34.

Leff, J., Kuipers, L., Berkowitz, R. and Sturgeon, D. (1985) A controlled trial of social intervention in the families of schizophrenic patients: Two year follow-up. *British Journal of Psychiatry*, **146**: 594–600.

Leff, J., Berkowitz, R., Shavit, N. *et al.* (1990a) A trial of family therapy versus a relatives' group for schizophrenia. *British Journal of Psychiatry*, **157**: 571–7.

Leff, J., O'Driscoll, C., Dayson, D. *et al.* (1990b) The TAPS Project. 5: The structure of social-network data obtained from long-stay patients. *British Journal of Psychiatry*, **157**: 848–52.

Leslie, L. A., Huston, T. L. and Johnson, M. P. (1986) Parental reactions to dating relationships: Do they make a difference? *Journal of Marriage and the Family*, **48**: 57–66.

Lewis, J. M., Beavers, W. R., Gossett, J. T. and Phillips, V. A. (1976) *No Single Thread: Psychological Health in Family Systems.* Brunner/Mazel, New York.

Lewis, R. A. (1973) Social reaction and the formation of dyads: an interactionist approach to mate selection. *Sociometry*, **36**: 409–18.

Lewontin, R. C. (1995) Sex, lies and social science. *New York Review of Books*, **XLII**: 24–9.

Lexington, M. A., Lexington Books, Stacey W. A., Hazlewood L. R. and Shupe A. (1994) *The Violent Couple.* Praeger, Westport, CON.

Liberman, R. P., Jacobs, H. E., Boone, S. E. *et al.* (1987) Skills training for the community adaptation of schizophrenics. In *Psychosocial Treatments of Schizophrenia* (J. S. Strauss, W. Boker and H. D. Brenner, eds). Hans Huber, Toronto.

Lockwood, D. (1983) Issues in prison sexual violence. *Prison Journal*, pp. 73–9.

Loeber, R. and Stouthamer-Loeber, M. (1986) Family factors as correlates and predictors of juvenile conduct problems and delinquency. In *Crime and Justice: An Annual Review of Research*, Vol. VII (M. Tonry and N. Morris, eds) University of Chicago Press, Chicago, pp. 29–149.

Loza, N. and Zaki, B. (1993) Egypt. In Payne, A. (1993) Sexual activity among psychiatric inpatients: international perspectives. *Journal of Forensic Psychiatry*, **4**: 109–29.

Luckianowicz, N. (1963) Sexual drive and its gratification in schizophrenia. *International Journal of Social Psychiatry*, **9**: 250–8.

Luepker, E. T. (1989) Time limited treatment/support groups for clients who have been sexually exploited by therapists: a nine year perspective. In *Psychotherapists' Involvement with Clients: Intervention and Prevention* (G. R. Schoener *et al.*, eds). Walk-in Counseling Center, Minneapolis, MN.

Lyon, M., Levine, M. and Zusman, J. (1982) Patients' bills of rights: a survey of state statutes. *Mental Disability Law Reporter*, **6**: 178–202.

MacCulloch, M. J., Snowden, P. R., Wood, P. J. W. and Mills, H. E. (1983) Sadistic fantasy, sadistic behaviour and offending. *British Journal of Psychiatry*, **143**: 20–9.

MacMillan J.F., Gold, A., Crow, T.J., Johnston, A.L. and Johnstone, E.C. (1986) Expressed emotion and relapse. *British Journal of Psychiatry*, **148**: 133–43.

Maleville, G., Gauthier, O., Vermande-Bourgeois, M. and Texier, L. (1975) Aspects actuels de venerologie en milieu psychiatrique. *Communication à La Réunion de La Ligue Contre Le Perilvenerien Les Tréponematoses*. Malte 13–18 Avril.

Marce, L. V. (1858) *Traite de La Folie des Femmes Inceintes, des Nouvelles Acouchees et des Nourrices*. Bailliere, Paris.

Margison, F. and Brockington, I. F. (1982) Psychiatric mother and baby units. In *Motherhood and Mental Illness* (I. F. Brockington and R. Kumar, eds). Academic Press, London, pp. 223–38.

Margolin, G. (1987) Marital therapy: a cognitive–behavioral–affective approach. In *Psychotherapists in Clinical Practice* (N. Jacobson, ed.) The Guilford Press, London.

Marks, M. N., Wiek, A., Checkley, S. A. and Kumar, R. (1992) Contribution of psychological and social factors to psychotic and non-psychotic relapse after childbirth in women with previous histories of affective disorder. *Journal of the Affective Disorders*, **29**: 253–64.

Marshall, W. L., Hudson, S. M., Jones, R. and Fernandez, Y. M. (1995) Empathy in sex offenders. *Clinical Psychology Review*, **15**, 99–113.

Martin J. J. (1978) *Violence in the Family*. Wiley, Chichester.

Matthews, J. (1983) *Forgotten Victims. How Prison Affects the Family*. National Association for the Care and Resettlement of Offenders, London.

Mattinson, J. (1970) *Marriage and Mental Handicap*. Duckworth, London.

McCann, G. (1991) Involving the family. *Nursing Times*, **87**: 67–8.

McCann, G. (1993) Relatives' support groups in a special hospital: an evaluation study. *Journal of Advanced Nursing*, **18**: 1883–8.

MccGuire S. (1994) *Women Who Love Men Who Kill*. Virgin Publishing, London.

McConaghy, N. (1993) *Sexual Behaviour, Problems and Management*. Plenum Press, pp. 52–78.

McCormick, G. and Shevlin, M. (1997) *Exploring Sexuality and Disability: 'Walk You Talk'*. Family Planning Association, London.

McCreadie, R.G. and Phillips, K. (1988) The Nithsdale Schizophrenia Survey: VII. Does relatives' high expressed emotion predict relapse? *British Journal of Psychiatry*, **152**: 477–81.

McGoldrick, M. (1989) The joining of families through marriage: The new couple. In *The Changing Family Life Cycle* (B. Carter and M. McGoldrick, eds). Allyn and Bacon, pp. 209–33.

Mednick, S. A., and Schulsinger, F. (1965) A longitudinal study of children with a high risk for schizophrenia: A preliminary report. In *Methods and Goals in Human Behavior Genetics* (S. Vandenberg. ed.) Academic Press, New York.

Meier, G. (1975) A health orientated programme for emotionally disturbed women. *Social Casework*, **56**: 411–7.

Meltzer, E. S. and Kumar, R. S. (1985) Puerperal mental illness, clinical features and classification: a study of 142 mother-and-baby admissions. *British Journal of Psychiatry*, **147**: 647–54.

Menon, A. S., Pomerantz, S., Horowitz, S. *et al.* (1994) The high prevalence of unsafe sexual behaviours among acute psychiatric inpatients: implications for AIDS prevention. *Journal of Nervous and Mental Diseases*, **182**: 661–6.

Merinkangas (1982) Assortive mating for psychiatric disorders and psychological traits. *Archives of General Psychiatry*, **39**: 173–80.

Merrington, S. (1995) *Offenders on Probation: A Qualitative Study of Offenders' Views on their Probation Orders*. Unpublished document from Cambridgeshire Probation Service, Godwin House, Castle Park, Cambridge, CB3 ORA.

Meyer-Lindenberg, J. (1991) The Holocaust and German psychiatry. *British Journal of Psychiatry*, **159**: 7–12.

Michael, R. T., Gagnon, J. H., Laumann, E. O. and Kolata, G. (1994) *Sex in America: A Definitive Survey*. Little, Brown, Boston, MA.

Milardo, R. M. (1982) Friendship networks in developing relationships: converging and diverging social environments. *Social Psychology Quarterly*, **45**: 162–72.

Milardo, R. M., Johnson, M. P. and Huston, T. L. (1983) Developing close relationships: changing patterns of interaction between pair members and social networks. *Journal of Personality and Social Psychology*, **44**: 964–76.

Milgrom (1989a) The first group for clients sexually exploited by their therapists: a twelve-year retrospective. In *Psychotherapists' Involvement with Clients: Intervention and Prevention* (G. R. Schoener et al., eds). Walk-in Counseling Center, Minneapolis, MN.

Milgrom (1989b) Secondary victims of sexual exploitation by counselors and therapists: some observations Ibid, 235–40.

Miller L. J. and Finnerty M. (1996) Sexuality, pregnancy, and child rearing among women with schizophrenia–spectrum disorders. *Psychiatric Services*, **47**: 502–6.

Miller, R. R., Scher, I. and Salt, H. (1991) The practice of counselling HIV/AIDS clients. *British Journal of Guidance and Counselling*, **19**: 129–38.

Millham, S., Bullock, R., Hosie, K. and Little, M. (1986) *Lost in Care. The Problems of Separation Experienced by Children in Care*. Dartington Social Research Unit. Gower, London.

Millham, S., Bullock, R. and Little, M. (1993) *The Return of Children Separated From Their Families*. Dartington Social Research Unit, Dartmouth.

Minuchin, S. (1974) *Families and Family Therapy*. Harvard University Press, Harvard, MA.

Mirrless-Black, C. (1995) Estimating the extent of domestic violence: findings from the 1992 BCS. *Home Office Research and Statistical Department Research Bulletin* No. **37**. Home Office, London.

Modestin, J. (1981) Patterns of overt sexual interaction among acute psychiatric inpatients. *Acta Psychiatrica Scandinavica*, **64**: 446–59.

Moedikdo, P. (1976) De Utrechste School van Pompë, Baan en Kempe. In *Recht, Macht en Manipulatie* (C. Kelk, ed.) Spectrum, Utrecht and Antwerpen, pp. 90–149.

Moffitt, T. (1997) MRC Genetics Unit, Institute of Psychiatry, London, SE5 7AF, UK. Personal communication.

Mogallapu, H., Flower, B., Jackson, H. and Ashcroft J. B. (1988) *Eiders Ward, An Experiment in the Sexual Integration of Patients*. Unpublished report available from the first author at Ashworth Hospital, Merseyside, L31 1HW.

Mollon, P. (1989) Anxiety, supervision and a space for thinking: some narcissistic perils for clinical psychologists in learning psychotherapy. *British Journal of Medical Psychology*, **62**: 113–22.

Monahan, J. and Klassen, D. (1982) Situational approaches to understanding and predicting individual violent behaviour. In *Criminal Violence* (M. E. Wolfgang and N. A. Weiner, eds). SAGE Publications, Newbury Park, CA, pp. 292–319.

Moore, E., Ball, R. A. and Kuipers, L. (1992) Expressed emotion in staff working with the long-term adult mentally ill. *British Journal of Psychiatry*, **161**: 802–8.

Morgan, R. and Rogers, J. (1971) Some results of the policy of integrating men and women in a mental hospital. *Social Psychiatry*, **6**: 113–16.

Moritsugu, K. P. (1995) Assistant Surgeon General and Medical Director, US Department of Justice, Federal Bureau of Prisons, Washington, DC 20534, USA. Personal communication.

Morris, P., (1964) *Prisoners and Their Families*. George Allen and Unwin, London.

Mossman, D., Perlin, M. L. and Dorfman, D. A. (1997) Sex on the wards: conundra for clinicians.

Journal of the American Academy of Psychiatry and the Law, **25**: 441–460.

Mrazek, P. and Mrazek, D. (1981) The effects of child sexual abuse: methodological considerations. In *Sexually Abused Children and their Families* (P. Mrazek and C. Kempe, eds). Pergamon Press, Oxford, pp. 235–45.

Mullen, P. (1995) Professor and Director, Forensic Health Service, Rosanna Forensic Psychiatry Center, Waiora Road, Macleod 3085, Rosanna 3084, Australia. Personal communication.

Mullen, P. E. and Maack, L. H. (1985) Jealousy, pathological jealousy, and aggression. In *Aggression and Dangerousness* (D. P. Farrington and J. Gunn, eds). Wiley, Chichester, UK, pp. 103–26.

Mullen, P. E., Martin, J. L. Anderson, J. C. *et al.* (1993a) Childhood sexual abuse and mental health in adult life. *British Journal of Psychiatry*, **163**: 721–32.

Mullen, P. E., Taylor, P. J. and Wessely, S. (1993b) Psychosis, violence and crime. In *Forensic Psychiatry. Clinical, Legal and Ethical Issues* (J. Gunn and P. J. Taylor, eds). Butterworth–Heinemann, Oxford, pp. 329–72.

Mulligan T. and Moss C. R. (1991) Sexuality and aging in in-mate veterans: a cross-sectional study of interest, ability and activity. *Archives of Sexual Behavior*, **20**: 17–25.

Nacci, P. L. and Kane, T. R. (1984) Sex and sexual aggression in federal prisons: inmate involvement and employee impact. *Federal Probation*, **40**: 46–53.

NACRO'S National Policy Committee on Resettlement (1995) *Opening the Doors: Prisoners' Families*. NACRO, London.

NAPO (1989) *Prisons, Risks and HIV.* National Association of Probation Officers, London.

National Health Service Health Advisory Service (1975) *Report on Broadmoor Hospital, Crowthorne, Berks*. Health Advisory Service (unpublished report).

National Health Service Health Advisory Service, Department of Health and Social Services Inspectorate (1988) *Report on Services Provided by Broadmoor Hospital*. Department of Health and Social Security, London.

NORC (1987) *General Social Surveys 1972–1987. Cumulative Codebook*. Storrs. Conn: Roper Centre.

Nelles, J. and Harding, T. (1995) Preventing HIV transmission in prison: a tale of medical disobedience and Swiss pragmatism. *Lancet*, **346**: 1507–8.

Newcombe, R. (1988) *Preventing and Responding to the Spread of HIV Infection in Prisons*. Health Promotion Department, Mersey Regional Health Authority.

Newman, S., Durrance, P. and Fel, M. (1993) Counselling in HIV and AIDS. *British Journal of Clinical Psychology*, **32**: 117–19.

Nibert, D., Cooper, S. and Crossmaker, M. (1989) Assaults against residents of a psychiatric institution. *Journal of Interpersonal Violence*, **4**: 342–9.

Norman, J. S. (1987) Supervision: the affective process. *Journal of Contemporary Social Work*, 374–9.

O'Brien, K. P. (1995) Director. Forensic Services, Hillcrest Hospital, South Australia. Fosters Road, Gilles Plains, PO Box 233, Greenacres, South Australia 5086. Personal communication.

O'Connor, A. (1987) Female sex offenders. *British Journal of Psychiatry*, **150**: 615–20.

O'Connor M., Johnson, G. H. and James, D. (1981) Intrauterine effects of phenothiazines. *Medical Journal of Australia*, **1**: 416–17.

Office of Corrections (1992) *Director General's Rules*. Prisons Division, Victoria, Australia.

Office of Population Censuses and Surveys (1993) 1991 *Census Communal Establishments Great Britain*, Vols 1 and 2. HMSO, London.

Office of Population Censuses and Surveys (1994) 1991 *Census Household and Family Composition (10 per cent) Great Britain*. HMSO, London.

Office of Population Censuses and Surveys, Social Survey Division (1995) *1993 General Household Survey*. HMSO, London.

O'Leary, K. D. and Turkewitz, J. (1978) Marital therapy from a behavioural perspective. In *Marriage and Marital Therapy* (T. J. Paolino and B. S. McGrady, eds). Brunner/Mazel, New York.

Ortega, M. J. (1962) Open-ward management of disturbed mental patients of both sexes. *Mental Hygiene*, **46**: 48–58.

Ortmann, J. (1980) The treatment of sexual offenders. *International Journal of Law and Psychiatry*, **3**: 443–51.

Packman, J. (1986) *Who Needs Care? Social-Work Decisions About Children*. Blackwell, Oxford.

Padel, U. and Stevenson, P. (1988) *Insiders: Women's Experience of Prison*. Virago, London.

Padel, U. (1995) HIV, prisons and prisoners' rights. In *AIDS: A Guide to the Law* (R Haigh and D. Harris, eds). Routledge, London, pp. 131–8.

Pagel, M. D., Erdly, W. W. and Becker, J. (1987) Social networks: We get by with (and in spite of) a little help from our friends. *Journal of Personality and Social Psychology*, **53**: 793–804.

Parker, G. Tupling, H. and Brown, L. (1979) A parental bonding instrument. *British Journal of Medical Psychology*, **52**: 1–10.

Parkes, C. M., Stevenson-Hinde, J. and Marris, P. (1991) *Attachment Across the Life Cycle*. Tavistock/Routledge.

Parkin, W. and Green, L., (1994) Sexuality and Residential Care. Research in Progress. British Sociological Association Annual Conference: *Sexualities in Context*.

Parkin, W. (1989) Private experiences in the public domain: sexuality and residential care organisations. In *The Sexuality of Organisation* (J. Hearn, D. L. Sheppard, P. Tancrad-Sheriff and G. Burrell, eds). Sage, pp. 110–124.

Parkinson, M. and Bateman, N. (1994) Disorders of sexual function caused by drugs. *Prescribers' Journal*, **34**: 183–90.

Parks, M. R., Stan, C. M. and Eggert, L. L. (1983) Romantic involvement and social network involvement. *Social Psychology Quarterly*, **46**: 116–31.

Parnas, J. (1985) Mates of schizophrenic mothers; a study of assortative mating from the American–Danish High Risk Project. *British Journal of Psychiatry*, **146**: 490–7.

Patrick, M., Hobson, R. P., Castle, D. *et al.* (1994) Personality disorder and the mental representation of early social experience. *Development and Psychopathology*, **6**: 375–88.

Pattison, E. M. and Pattison, M. L. (1981) Analysis of a schizophrenic psychosocial network. *Schizophrenia Bulletin*, **7**: 135–43.

Payne, A. (1993) Sexual activity among psychiatric inpatients: international perspectives. *Journal of Forensic Psychiatry*, **4**: 109–29.

Pearson, V. (1995) Population policy and eugenics in China. *British Journal of Psychiatry*, **167**: 1–4.

Perlin, M. (1993) International perspectives: the United States In Sexual activity among psychiatric inpatients (A. Payne, ed.) *Journal of Forensic Psychiatry*, **44**: 109–115.

Persico, A. M., di Giannantonio, M., Mattioni, T., Lestingi, L., Zeppatelli, E. and Tempesta, E. (1994) AIDS and psychiatric disorders: guidelines for psychopharmacological treatment. *Journal of Sex Education and Therapy*, **17**: 167–84.

Pfeiffer, E., Verwoerdt, A. and Wang, H. S. (1969) The natural history of sexual behavior in a biologically advantaged group of aged individuals. *Journal of Gerontology*, **24**: 193–8.

Philipse, M. (1995) Research psychologist, Pompekliniek, Weg door Jonkerbos 55, 6532 CN, Nijmegen, The Netherlands. Personal communication.

Philo, G. (1994) Media images and popular beliefs. *Psychiatric Bulletin*, **18**: 173–4.

Pilgrim, D. (1988) Psychotherapy in British special hospitals. A case of failure to thrive. *Free Associations*, **11**: 58–72.

Pinching, A. J., Weiss, R. A. and Miller, D. (1988) AIDS and HIV infection: the wider perspective. *British Medical Bulletin*, **44**(1): 1–19.

Pinderhughes, C. A., Grace, E. B. and Reyna, L. J. (1972) Psychiatric disorders and sexual functioning. *American Journal of Psychiatry*, **128**: 1276–83.

Pistole, M. C. (1989) Attachment in adult romantic relationships: style of conflict resolution and relationship satisfaction. *Journal of Social and Personal Relationships*, **6**: 505–10.

Planansky, K. and Johnston, R. (1977) Homicidal aggression in schizophrenic men. *Acta Psychiatrica Scandinavica*, **55**: 65–73.

Podolsky, E. (1965) The lust murderer. *Medico-Legal Journal*, **33**: 174–8.

Polk-Walker, G. C. (1989) Treatment of AIDS in a psychiatric setting. *Perspectives in Psychiatric Care*, **25**: 9–13.

Pope K. S. (1990) Therapist–patient sexual involvement: a review of the research. *Clinical Psychology Review*, **10**: 477–90.

Powell, M., Leyden, G. and Osborne, E. (1990) A curriculum for training in supervision. *Educational and Child Psychology*, **7**: 44–52.

Power, K. G., Markova, I., Rowlands, A. *et al.* (1991) Sexual behaviour in Scottish prisons. *British Medical Journal*, **302**: 1507–8.

Prison Reform Trust (1991) *HIV, AIDS and Prisons: Update*. Prison Reform Trust, London.

Prison Reform Trust (1988) *HIV, AIDS and Prisons*. Prison Reform Trust, London.

Quinton, D., Rutter, M. and Rowlands, O. (1976) An evaluation of an interview assessment of marriage. *Psychological Medicine*, **6**: 577–84.

Rafferty, D. (1995) Putting sexuality on the agenda. *Nursing Times*, **91**: 17–28.

Raskin, V. D. (1993) Psychiatric aspects of substance use disorders in childbearing populations. In *Psychiatric Clinics of North America: Recent Advances in Addictive Studies* (N. S. Miller, ed.), **16**: 157–65.

Rector, N. A. and Seeman, M. V. (1992) Schizophrenia and AIDS (letter). *Hospital and Community Psychiatry*, **43**: 181.

Registrar General (1971) *Statistical Review of England and Wales for Year 1967*. Part III Commentary. HMSO, London.

Report of the Committee of Inquiry into Complaints about Ashworth Hospital, Vol. 1. (1992) Cm 2028-1. HMSO, London.

Rice, M. E. and Harris, G. T. (1993) Ontario's maximum security hospital at Penetanguishene: past, present and future. *International Journal of Law and Psychiatry*, **16**: 195–215.

Richards, M., McWilliams, B., Allcock L., Enterkin J., Owens, P. and Woodrow, J. (1994) The family ties of English prisoners. *Centre for Family Research Occasional Papers*, No. **2**. Cambridge.

Ridley, C. A. and Avery, A. W. (1979) Social network influence on the dyadic relationship. In *Social Exchange in Developing Relationships* (R. L. Burgess and T. L. Huston, eds). Academic Press, pp. 223–46.

Robins, L. N. (1978) Sturdy childhood predictors of adult antisocial behaviour: Replications from longitudinal studies. *Psychological Medicine*, **8**: 611–22.

Robinson, S., Vivian-Byrne, S., Driscoll, R. and Cordess, C. (1991) Family work with victims and offenders in a secure unit. *Journal of Family Therapy*, **13**: 105–16.

Rook, K. (1984) The negative side of social interaction: impact on psychological well-being. *Journal of Personality and Social Psychology*, **46**: 1097–108.

Rose, L. (1994) Homophobia among doctors. *British Medical Journal*, **308**: 586–7.

Rose, M. (1990) *Healing Hurt Minds, The Peper Harow Experience*. Routledge, London, pp. 176–82.

Rosenthal, D. (1974) The concept of sub-schizophrenic disorders. In *Genetics, Environment and Psychopathology* (S. A. Mednick *et al.*, eds). American Elsevier, New York, pp. 167–76.

Rothenberg, D. (1983) Sexual behaviour in an abnormal setting. *Corrective and Social Psychiatry and Journal of Behaviour Techniques, Methods and Therapy*, **29**: 78–81.

Rowe, J. J. (Chairman of Inquiry) *(1991) Report of the Independent Inquiry into the Death of Derek Anthony Williams who Died on 19 November 1990 in Forster Ward, Ashworth Hospital (North)*. Ashworth Hospital, Liverpool.

Rowland, D. L., Greenleaf, W. J., Dorfman, L. J. *et al.* (1993) Aging and sexual function in men. *Archives of Sexual Behavior*, **19**: 753–8.

Royal College of Nursing Statement (1978) *Mixed Sex Wards*.

Royal College of Psychiatrists (1992) Report of the general psychiatry section working party on postnatal illness. *Psychiatric Bulletin*, **16**: 519–22.

Royal College of Psychiatrists (1996) Sexual Abuse and Harassment in Psychiatric Settings. Council Report 52. Royal College of Psychiatrists, London SW1X 8PG.

Rozan, G. Tuchin, T and Kurland, M. (1971) Some implications of sexual activity for mental illness. *Mental Hygiene*, **55**: 318–23.

Rozensky, R. H. and Berman, C. (1984) Sexual knowledge, attitudes and experiences of chronic psychiatric patients. *Psychosocial Rehabilitation Journal*, **8**: 21–7.

Rubin, P. C. (1996) Management of pre-existing disorders in pregnancy: principles of prescribing. *Prescribers' Journal*, **36**: 21–7.

Rudden, M., Sweeney, J. and Allen, F. (1990) Diagnosis and clinical course of erotomanic and other delusional patients. *American Journal of Psychiatry*, **147**: 625–8.

Rutter, M. L. (1966) *Children of Sick Parents: An Environmental and Psychiatric Study.* Maudsley Monograph No. 16. Oxford University Press, Oxford.

Rutter, M. (ed.) (1988) *Studies of Psychosocial Risk: The Power of Longitudinal Data.* Cambridge University Press, Cambridge.

Rutter, M. (1988) Functions and consequences of relationships: some psychopathological considerations. In *Relationships within Families. Mutual Influences* (R. A. Hinde and J. Stevenson-Hinde, eds). Clarendon Press, Oxford, pp. 332–53.

Rutter, M., Graham, P., Chadwick, O. F. D. and Yule, W. (1976) Adolescent turmoil: fact or fiction? *Journal of Child Psychology and Psychiatry,* **17**: 35–56.

Rutter, M. and Madge, N. (1976) *Cycles of Disadvantage.* Heinemann, London.

Rutter, M. and Quinton, D. (1984) Parental psychiatric disorders: effects on the children. *Psychological Medicine,* **14**: 853–80.

Rutter, M., Quinton, D. and Yule, B. A. (1976) *Family Pathology and Disorder in the Children.* John Wiley, Chichester.

Rutter, M. and Smith, D. J. (Eds) *(1995) Psychosocial Disorders in Young People. Time Trends and their Causes.* John Wiley, Chichester, UK.

Ryder, R. G., Kafka, J. S. and Olson, D. H. (1971) Separating and joining influences in courtship and early marriage. *American Journal of Orthopsychiatry,* **41**: 450–64.

Salokangas, R. K. R. (1983) Prognostic implications of the sex of schizophrenic patients. *British Journal of Psychiatry,* **142**: 145–51.

Sarnat, J. E. (1992) Supervision in relationships: resolving the teach–treat controversy in psychoanalytic supervision. *Psychoanalytic Psychology,* **9**: 387–403.

Save The Children (1992) *Scottish Prisoners and their Families.* Centre for the Study of the Child and Society, University of Glasgow, Glasgow.

Schneider, P.-B., Abraham, G. and Panayotopoulos, D. (1964) Quelques aspects de la vie sexuelle des psychotiques: enquete sur 84 cas hospitalises. *Evolution Psychiatrique,* **29**: 45–73.

Schoener, G. R. (1989) A look at the literature. In *Psychotherapists' Sexual Involvement with Clients: Intervention and Prevention* (G. R. Schoener et al., eds). Walk-in Counseling Center, Minneapolis, MN.

Schoener, G. R. and Milgrom, J. H. (1989) False or misleading complaints. In *Psychotherapists' Sexual Involvement with Clients: Intervention and Prevention* (G. R. Schoener et al., eds). Walk-in Counseling Center, Minneapolis, MN, pp. 147–55.

Schoener, G. R. (1995a) Historical overview. In *Breach of Trust* (J. C. Gonsiorek, ed.) Sage, Thousand Oaks, CA, pp. 3–17.

Schoener, G. R. (1995b) Employer/supervisor liability and risk management: An administrator's view. Ibid, 300–16.

SchWeber, C. (1984) Beauty marks and blemishes: the coed prison as a microcosm of integrated society. *Prison Journal,* **64**: 3–14.

Scott, J. (1994) What the papers say. *Psychiatric Bulletin,* 489–91.

Sederer, L. I. and Libby, M. (1995) False allegations of sexual misconduct: clinical and institutional considerations. *Psychiatric Services,* **46**: 160–63.

Seidman, S. N. and Rieder, R. O. (1994) A review of sexual behaviour in the United States. *American Journal of Psychiatry,* **151**: 330–41.

Selvini-Palazzoli, M., Boscolo, L., Cechin, G. and Prata, G. (1980) Hypothesising–circularity–neutrality: three guidelines for the conductor of the session. *Family Process,* **19**: 3–12.

Senchak, M. and Leonard, K. E. (1992) Attachment styles and marital adjustment among newlywed couples. *Journal of Social and Personal Relationships,* **9**: 51–64.

Shanks, J. and Atkins, P. (1985) Psychiatric patients who marry each other. *Psychological Medicine,* **15**: 377–82.

Shapiro, T. (1985) *Population Control Politics: Women, Sterilisation and Reproductive Choices.* Temple University Press, Philadelphia.

Shaw, J. A., Applegate, B., Perez, D. et al., (1993) Young boys who commit serious sexual offences: demographics, psychometrics and phenomenology. *Bulletin of the American Academy of Psychiatry and Law,* **21**: 399–408.

Shupe, A., Stacey, W. A. and Hazlewood, L. R. 1987) *Violent Men, Violent Couples: The Dynamics* of Domestic Violence. Lexington Books, Lexington, MA.

Sirkin, M., Maxey, J., Ryan, M., French, C. and Clements, O. (1988) Gender awareness group therapy. Exploring gender-related issues in a day-treatment population. International Journal of Partial Hospitalisation, 5: 263–72.

Skynner, R. (1975) Marital problems and their treatment. Proceedings of the Royal Society of Medicine 68, July 1975, and reprinted in Schlapobersky, J. R. (ed.) (1987) Explorations of Families – Group Analysis and Family Therapy. Collected papers of Robin Skynner. Methuen, London.

Skynner, R. (1980) Recent developments in marital therapy. Journal of Family Therapy, 2: 271–96.

Slater, P. E. (1963) On social regression. American Sociological Review, 28: 339–64.

Slone, D., Siskind, V., Heinonen, O. P., et al. (1977) Antenatal exposure to the phenothiazines in relation to congenital malformations, perinatal mortality rate, birth weight, and intelligence quotient score. American Journal of Obstetrics and Gynaecology, 128: 486–88.

Slovik, L.S. and Griffit, J.L. (1992) The current face of family therapy. In Psychotherapy for the 1990s (J. Scott Rutan, ed.). Guilford Press, New York.

Smith, L. J. F. (1989) Domestic Violence: An Overview of the Literature. Home Office Research Study No. 107. HMSO, London.

Snell, T. L. and Morton, D. C. (1994) Women in Prison. Survey of State Prison Inmates, 1991. US Department of Justice, Washington, DC.

Southwell, M. (1981) Counselling the young prison prostitute. JPNMHS, 19: 25–26.

Sparrow, S. (1991) An exploration of the role of nurses' uniform through a period of non-uniform wear on an acute medical ward. Journal of Advanced Nursing, 16: 116–22.

Sprecher, S. and Felmlee, D. (1992) The influence of parents and friends on the quality and stability of romantic relationships: a three-wave longitudinal investigation. Journal of Marriage and the Family, 54: 888–900.

Stacey, W. A. and Shupe, A. (1983) The Family Secret: Domestic Violence in America. Beacon Press, Boston.

Stefan, S. (1989) Whose egg is it anyway? Nova Law Review, 13: 405–56.

Stein, A. S., Woolley, H., Cooper, S. D. and Fairburn, C. G. (1994) An observational study of mothers with eating disorders and their infants. Journal of Child Psychology and Psychiatry, 35: 733–48.

Stein, G. S. (1982) The maternity blues. In Motherhood and Mental Illness (I. F. Brockington and R. Kumar, eds). Academic Press, London, pp. 119–54.

Stein, G. S. (1995) Postpartum and related disorders. In College Seminars in Adult Psychiatry (G. S. Stein and G. Wilkinson, eds). Gaskell, London.

Stein, G. S. (1998) Postpartum and related disorders. In Seminars in General Adult Psychiatry, vol. 2 (G. S. Stein and G. Wilkinson, eds). Gaskell, London.

Steinberg, D. (1987) Basic Adolescent Psychiatry. Blackwell Scientific Publications, Oxford, pp. 1–16.

Stevens, B. C. (1969) Marriage and Fertility of Women Suffering from Schizophrenia or Affective Disorders. Maudsley Monograph No. 19. Oxford University Press, London.

Stewart, J. and Stewart, J. (1993) Social Circumstances of Young Offenders. Association of Chief Officers of Probation, 212 Whitechapel Road, London E1 BJ.

Strang, J. (1993) Sexual and injecting behaviours in prisons: from disciplinary problem to public health conundrum. Criminal Behaviour and Mental Health, 3: 393–402.

Stratchey, J. (1969) The nature and the therapeutic action of psychoanalysis. Journal of Psycho-analysis, 50: 275–92.

Strauss, B., Pager, H., Appelt, H. and Gross, J. (1988) Der Stellen wert der Sexualität im psychia-trischen Klinikalltag: Ergebmisse einer Personalbefragung. Psychiatrische Praxis, 15: 202–8.

Stürup, G. K. (1968) Treating the Untreatable: Chronic Criminals in Herstedvester. John Hopkins Press, Baltimore.

Sussman, M. B. (1953) Parental participation in mate selection and its effect upon family continuity. Social Forces, 32: 76–81.

Swan, T. (l992) Integration of the Sexes within the Special Hospitals: An Analysis of the Current Situation. Unpublished report prepared for the SHSA.

Swan, T. (1993) An unpublished paper presented to the 20th Quadrennial Congress of the ICN, Madrid, Spain. Text available from the author, Ashworth Hospital.

Swan, T. (1994) Living together. *Nursing Times*, **90**(2): 34–36.

Swanson, J. W., Holzer, C. E., Ganju, V. K. and Jono, R. T. (1990) Violence and psychiatric disorder in the community: evidence from the epidemiologic catchment area surveys. *Hospital and Community Psychiatry*, **41**: 761–70.

Swanson, J. W. (1994) Mental disorder, substance abuse, and community violence: an epidemiological approach. In *Violence and Mental Disorder. Developments in Risk Assessment* (J. Monahan and H. J. Steadman, eds.) University of Chicago Press, Chicago, pp. 101–36.

Tarrier, N., Barrowclough, C., Porceddu, K. and Watts, S. (1988) The assessment of psychophysiological reactivity to the expressed emotion of the relatives of schizophrenic patients. *British Journal of Psychiatry*, **152**: 618–24.

Task Force on Sexual Abuse of Patients (1991) *The Final Report*. The College of Physicians and Surgeons of Ontario, Canada.

Taylor, P. J. (1993) Schizophrenia and crime: distinctive patterns in association. In *Mental Disorder and Crime* (S. Hodgins, ed.) Sage, Newbury Park, CA, pp. 63–85.

Taylor, P. J. and Gunn J. C. (1993) *Forensic Psychiatry: Clinical, Legal and Ethical Issues*. Butterworth–Heinemann, Oxford, pp. 1015–24.

Taylor, P. J. and Parrott, J. M. (1988) Elderly offenders: a study of age-related factors among custodially remanded prisoners. *British Journal of Psychiatry*, **152**: 340–6.

Taylor, P. J., Lees, M., Williams, D., Butwell, M., Daly, R. and Larkin, E. (1998) Mental disorder and violence. *British Journal of Psychiatry*, **172**: 218–26.

Taylor, P. J., Mullen, P. and Wessely, S. (1993) Psychosis, violence and crime. In *Forensic Psychiatry. Clinical, Legal and Ethical Issues* (J. Gunn and P. J. Taylor, eds). Butterworth–Heinemann, Oxford, pp. 329–72.

Tennent, G., Parker, E., McGrath, P. and Street, D. (1980) Male admissions to the English Special Hospitals 1961–65: a demographic survey. *British Journal of Psychiatry*, **136**: 181–90.

Terrence Higgins Trust (1992) *HIV and AIDS. Information for Lesbians*. Terrence Higgins Trust, 52–54 Grays Inn Road, London WC1X 8JU.

Terrence Higgins Trust (1993) *The Housing Leaflet*.

Terrence Higgins Trust (1994, April) *Understanding HIV Infection and AIDS*.

Terrence Higgins Trust (1994, June) *Preventing HIV Infection. A Booklet about Transmission*.

Terrence Higgins Trust (1994, November) *Information About Mothers and Babies with HIV Infection*.

Test, M. A., Burke, S. S. and Wallischls, (1990) Gender differences of young adults with schizophrenic disorders in community care. *Schizophrenia Bulletin*, **16**: 331–44.

The Alternative Service Book (1980) Cambridge University Press, Cambridge.

The Chronical (1992) Newsletter for patients at Broadmoor hospital.

Thomas, B. (1990) Working out sexuality. *Nursing Times*, January 3, **86**(1): 41–43.

Thomas, P. A. (1990) HIV/AIDS in prisons. *The Howard Journal*, **29**: 1–13.

Thompson, S. C. and Sobolow-Shubin, A. (1993) Overprotective relationships: A nonsupportive side of social networks. *Basic and Applied Psychology*, **14**: 363–83.

Thornicroft, G. and Breakey, W. R. (1991) The COSTAR programme. 1: Improving social networks of the long-term mentally ill. *British Journal of Psychiatry*, **159**: 245–9.

Tidmarsh, D. (1997) Risk assessment among prisoners: a view from a parole board member. *International Review of Psychiatry*, **9**: 273–81.

Tomm, K. (1987) Interventive interviewing: Part 11. Reflexive questioning as a means of establishing self-healing. *Family Process*, **26**: 1967–83.

Tonks, A. (1992) Women patients vulnerable on psychiatric wards. *British Medical Journal*, **304**: 1331.

Turnbull, P. J., Stimson, G. V. and Dolan, K. A. (1992) Prisons, HIV and AIDS: risks and experiences in custodial care. Horsham, AVERT.

Ullman, E. (1995) Psychiatrist, Region Psykiatriska Kliniken, Box 1223, S-351 12, VSxjs, Sweden. Personal communication.

Union of Liberal and Progressive Synagogues (1990) *On Homosexuality*. Union of Liberal and

Progressive Synagogues, London.

United Kingdom Central Council for Nurses, Midwives and Health Visitors (UKCC) *(1995) Clinical Supervision*. Registrar's letter 4/1995. UKCC, London.

United States Department of Justice, Federal Bureau of Prisons (1995) *Sexual Assault Prevention and Intervention Programmes, Inmates*. May.

US Department of Justice (1994) *Profiles of Inmates in the United States and in England and Wales, 1991*. US Department of Justice, Washington, DC.

US National Commission on AIDS (1990) Report: *HIV Disease in Correctional Facilities*. National Institutes of Justice, Washington, DC.

Vadro, C. I. and Earp, J. A. (1991) AIDS education and incarcerated women: a neglected opportunity. *Women and Health*, **1**: 105–17.

Vandereycken, W. (1993) Shrinking sexuality: the half-known sex life of psychiatric patients. *Therapeutic Communities*, **14**: 143–9.

Vartiainen, H. (1993) Finland. In Sexual activity among psychiatric inpatients: international perspectives (A. Payne, ed.) *Journal of Forensic Psychiatry*, **4**: 109–29.

Vaughan, P. (1980) Letters and visits to long-stay Broadmoor patients. *British Journal of Social Work*, **10**: 471–81.

Vaughan, P. (1981) Special hospital patients have families too . . . *Mind Out*, (February): 16–18.

Vaughn C. E. and Leff J. P. (1976) The influence of family and social factors on the course of psychiatric patients. *British Journal of Psychiatry*, **129**: 125–37.

Vermeulen, J. (1995) formerly Psychiatrist, Zimbabwe, now Broadmoor Hospital Authority, Crowthorne, Berkshire, RG45 7EG. Personal communication.

Voronou, G. L. and Lisovenko, V. L. (1984) Pressing questions concerning the organisation of treatment divisions of modern psychiatric hospitals. *Zhurnal Nevropatologii Psikhiatrii im SS Korakova*, **84**: 1354–7.

Walmsley, R., Howard L. and White, S. (1992) *National Prison Survey 1991, Main Findings*. Home Office Research Study 128. Home Office, London.

Warton, E. (1920) *The Age of Innocence*. Dent, London.

Webb, C. (l987) Sexuality. *Nursing Times* **83**(32).

Weinstein, M. R. and Goldfield, M. D. (1975) Cardiovascular malformations with lithium use during pregnancy. *American Journal of Psychiatry*, **132**: 529–31.

Weiss, R. S. (1991) The attachment bond in childhood and adulthood. In *Attachment Across the Life Cycle* (C. M. Parkes, J. Stevenson-Hinde and P. Marris, eds). Tavistock/Routledge, pp. 66–76.

Welch, S. J. and Clements, G. W. (1996) Development of a policy on sexuality for hospitalized chronic psychiatric patients. *Canadian Journal of Psychiatry*, **41**: 273–9.

West, D. J. and Farrington, D. P. (1977) *The Delinquent Way of Life*. Heinemann, London.

Wettstein, R. M. (1995) Psychiatrist, University of Pittsburgh and Western Psychiatric Institute. 3811 O'Hara Street, Pittsburgh, Philadelphia 15213–2593. USA Personal communication.

White G. L. and Mullen P. E. (1989) *Jealousy. Theory, Research, and Clinical Strategies*. The Guilford Press, London/New York.

Widom, C. S. and White, H. R. (1997) Problem behaviours in abused and neglected children grown up: prevalence and co-occurrence of substance abuse, crime and violence. *Criminal Behaviour and Mental Health*, **7**: 287–310.

Wignall, C. M. and Meredith, C. E. (1968) Illegitimate pregnancies in state institutions. *Archives of General Psychiatry*, **18**: 580–3.

Wilbers, D., Veenstra, G., van de Weil, H. B. M. and Weijmar Schultz, W. C. M. (1992) Sexual contact in the doctor–patient relationship in the Netherlands. *British Medical Journal*, **304**: 1531–4.

Wilkinson, T. R. (1983) *Child and Adolescent Psychiatric Nursing*. Blackwell Scientific Publications, Oxford.

Willis, A. (1983) The balance between care and control in probation; a research note. *British Journal of Social Work*, **13**: 339–46.

Wing, J. K. (1990) The functions of asylum. *British Medical Journal*, **157**: 822–7.

Winnicott, D. W. (1990) *The Maturational Process and the Facilitating Environment*. H. Karnac, (Books) Ltd, London, pp. 242–8.

Wisner, K. L., Perel, J. M. and Wheeler, S. B. (1993) Tricyclic dose requirements across pregnancy. *American Journal of Psychiatry*, **150**: 1541–2.

Withersty, D. J. (1976) Sexual attitudes of hospital personnel: a model for continuing education. *American Journal of Psychiatry*, **133**: 573–5.

Wolfensberger, W. (1972) *The Principal of Normalisation in Human Services*. National Institute in Retardation, York University, Ontario.

Wolfgag, M. E. (1958) *Patterns in Criminal Homicide*. University of Pennsylvania Press, Philadelphia.

Woodside, H. (1985) The day centre and its role as a social network. *Hospital and Community Psychiatry*, **36**(2): 177–80.

World Health Organization (WHO). *(1978) Mental Disorders: Glossary and Guide to their Classification in Accordance with the Ninth Revision of the International Classification of Diseases*. WHO, Geneva.

World Health Organization (1993) *WHO Guidelines on HIV Infection and AIDS in Prisons*. WHO, Geneva.

World Health Organization (1992) *The ICD-10 Classification of Mental and Behavioural Disorders*. WHO, Geneva.

Zelnik, M. and Katner, J. F. (1980) Sexual activity, contraceptive use and pregnancy among metropolitan-area teenagers: 1971–1979. *Family Planning Perspectives*, **12**: 230–7.

Zondo, J. G. (1995) Superintendent, Mlondolozi Mental Institution, PO Box 2094, Bulawayo, Zimbabwe. Personal communication.

Zubenko, G. S., George, A. W., Soloff, P. H. and Schulz, P. (1987) Sexual practices among patients with borderline personality disorder. *American Journal of Psychiatry*, **144**: 748–52.

Index

LANGUAGE AND MINOR

This new edition of Stephen May's benchmark volume in the field of language rights and language policy is a timely and useful revision of its core arguments and examples. The provocative and groundbreaking first edition, an outstanding interdisciplinary analysis of the questions and issues concerning minority language rights in modern nation-states, is now regarded as a key benchmark in the field of language rights and language policy. The second edition addresses new theoretical and empirical developments since its initial publication, including the burgeoning influence of globalization and the relentless rise of English as the current world language. May's broad position, however, remains largely unchanged. He argues that the causes of many of the language-based conflicts in the world today still lie with the nation-state and its preoccupation with establishing a 'common' language and culture via mass education. The solution, he suggests, is to rethink nation-states in more culturally and linguistically plural ways while avoiding, at the same time, essentializing the language–identity link.

This second edition, like the first, adopts a wide interdisciplinary framework, drawing on sociolinguistics, applied linguistics, sociology, political theory, education and law. This edition also presents new discussions of cosmopolitanism, globalization, the role of English, and language and mobility, as well as updated discussions of a wide range of contexts where language rights are an issue, including Ireland, France, Quebec, the 'English Only movement' in the USA, Wales, Catalonia, and New Zealand.

Language and Minority Rights is essential reading for students, teachers, and researchers in the sociology of language, sociolinguistics, applied linguistics, language policy and planning, sociology, politics, and education.

Stephen May is Professor of Education in the School of Critical Studies in Education, University of Auckland, New Zealand. He is Editor of the interdisciplinary journal *Ethnicities* and Associate Editor of the journal *Language Policy*.

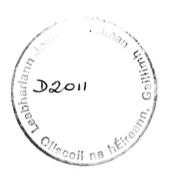

LANGUAGE AND MINORITY RIGHTS

ETHNICITY, NATIONALISM AND THE POLITICS OF LANGUAGE

Second Edition

STEPHEN MAY

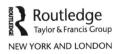
Routledge
Taylor & Francis Group

NEW YORK AND LONDON

First published 2012
by Routledge
711 Third Avenue, New York, NY 10017

Simultaneously published in the UK
by Routledge
2 Park Square, Milton Park, Abingdon, Oxon OX14 4RN

Routledge is an imprint of the Taylor & Francis Group, an informa business

© 2012 Taylor & Francis

Library of Congress Cataloging in Publication Data
May, Stephen, 1962–
   Language and minority rights : ethnicity, nationalism and the
   politics of language / Stephen May. –2nd ed.
        p. cm.
   Includes bibliographical references and index.
   1. Language and languages--Political aspects. 2. Linguistic
   minorities. 3. Ethnicity. 4. Nationalism. 5. Sociolinguistics.
   6. Language and education. I. Title.
   P119.3.M39 2011
   306.44´9--dc23   2011023100

ISBN13: 978-0-8058-6307-9 (hbk)
ISBN13: 978-0-8058-6306-2 (pbk)
ISBN13: 978-0-203-83254-7 (ebk)

Typeset in Bembo
by HWA Text and Data Management, London

To Ella, Grace, Tomas and Luke

Ki aku piki kotuku

... those who seek to defend a threatened [language] ... are obliged to wage a total struggle. (Bourdieu, 1991: 57)

The language of the conqueror in the mouth of the conquered is ever the language of the slave. (Tacitus)

CONTENTS

PREFACE TO THE SECOND EDITION

I must confess that I've always been somewhat skeptical about second editions, especially if you've actually read the original. What added value is there exactly in a few updated references here and there, if the arguments are basically the same? Not much, I always thought, and so passed resolutely by yet another second edition on the bookshelves. Little wonder that first editions still predominate in my library.

This perhaps helps to explain why it has taken me so long to produce a second edition of *Language and Minority Rights*. It also helps to explain what I have attempted to do in (re)writing it. The first edition of *Language and Minority Rights* was published toward the end of 2000 but I began the book in 1994. The intervening period thus seems a decent enough amount of time to warrant revisiting it. In doing so, I still stand by the arguments that I developed in the original edition and I believe the majority of them have survived the test of time (the two aren't always the same). The many positive reviews and comments on the book's significant contribution to, and influence on the field of language rights, and sociolinguistics more generally, have also contributed to me turning once again to its core arguments.

But there is a major difference between re-engagement and mere rehearsal. Given my own diffidence toward second editions, I could not simply revisit the arguments after all this time and leave them largely unattended, or only nominally changed. Instead, I've embarked on an extensive re-engagement with the interdisciplinary debates in sociolinguistics, applied linguistics, sociological theory, political theory, international law and education that underpinned the first edition. Developments in critical sociolinguistics, in particular, pose significant questions about how we view languages. Indeed, such developments increasingly question the validity of talking about languages as distinct, enumerable entities in the first place. Meanwhile, sociological debates about the constructedness of ethnicity, language and culture have continued unabated, as have political theory debates on the merits of individual versus group-based rights. And then, of course, there are the various supranational, national and regional contexts wherein debates about language rights (or the lack thereof) are played out. Much has obviously happened in each of these arenas in the interim as well.

Accordingly, what I have attempted to do in this second edition is undertake a substantial and substantive rewriting of the book. All chapters are thoroughly updated, both in terms of theoretical debates, as well as the examples discussed. The Introduction addresses briefly the key critiques of language rights that have arisen over the last decade and (re)situates the wider arguments in the book in relation to them. Chapters 1 and 2 incorporate significant new material from the ongoing theoretical debates on ethnicity and nationalism. Chapter 3 introduces a new section, examining the influential contribution of the late Brian Barry to political theory debates on rights, most notably via his polemical critique of multiculturalism, *Culture and Equality* (2001). Chapter 4 updates discussions on language and identity, and revisits in greater detail the sociolinguistic critiques of language rights over the last decade. The language contexts in Ireland and France are also brought into the present. Chapter 5 re-examines the role of language and education, along with recent developments in international law.

Chapter 6 provides a substantive new discussion of globalization and cosmopolitanism, including an examination of their links with English as the current world language. In this regard, the work of Abram de Swaan and Daniele Archibugi are introduced and critically appraised. The chapter also addresses arguments that link English ineluctably to social and economic mobility, as well as the wider normative influence of monolingualism. Developments over the last decade are incorporated into the examination of the English Only Movement in the USA. Chapter 7 updates the language contexts of Quebec, Catalonia, and Wales to the present day. Chapter 8 updates developments in indigenous language and education rights, including the significant ratification of the United Nations Declaration on the Rights of Indigenous Peoples (UNDRIP) in 2007. Discussion of developments for indigenous Māori in Aotearoa/New Zealand, including Māori language education, is updated. Chapter 9 summarizes the arguments of the book, while also addressing ongoing challenges in securing minority language rights. Two in particular are foregrounded for further discussion: tolerability, or the need to gain the support of majority language speakers for minority language initiatives, and the balancing of national minority rights with rights attributable to other minority groups. I discuss the former by returning to the context of Wales and the attitudes of monolingual English speakers to Welsh language developments therein. I discuss the latter, by way of example, in relation to Pasifika peoples in Aotearoa/New Zealand.

Given all this, I am hopeful that those who have read the first edition will find enough new material here to re-engage with the book and its arguments. And, of course, I hope that those for whom this book is a new experience may find in it much of interest and provocation as well. As I said at the start, I believe many of the arguments, contentious though they may be to some, still hold, and I welcome the engagement and critique of new scholars with the material.

The cover of the first edition featured 'Light falling through a dark landscape (A)' (1972) by the New Zealand painter, Colin McCahon (1917–87). Another McCahon painting, 'Throw out the lifeline' (1976), graces the cover of this second edition – not least, because the metaphor seems so apt. For permission to reproduce both paintings, I am grateful to the Colin McCahon Trust. Other thanks are also due. To my redoubtable editor at Routledge, Naomi Silverman, whose unlimited forbearance and equally limitless resolve in the face of my many prevarications, got me there in the end, to the surprise of us both. To Graeme Aitken, my Dean at the Faculty of Education, University of Auckland, for granting me the necessary leave to finish this book. But also, more importantly, for being what a Dean should be (but seldom is): open, ethical and facilitative. To my wonderful children, Ella, Grace, Tomas and Luke, I promise that you will have more of my time again from hereon in. And, most of all, to Katie Fitzpatrick, who makes my world turn on its proper axis, and without whom I could not bear contemplation.

Stephen May
University of Auckland, New Zealand
April 2011

PREFACE TO THE
FIRST EDITION

This book is about language but it is not a 'language' book, or at least not in a narrow disciplinary sense. Rather, it is avowedly interdisciplinary. It encompasses debates in the sociology of language, ethnicity and nationalism, sociolinguistics, social and political theory, education, law and history. The principal advantage of interdisciplinary work is the opportunity it provides to draw together a wide range of disciplinary debates (often at variance with each other) on a particular topic – in this case, the contentious question of language and minority rights. In so doing, different disciplinary verities can be critically assessed and, where necessary, challenged and reformulated. The challenges of interdisciplinary work are, at least in my experience, twofold. The first is that it simply takes much longer to get to grips with all the material in question than it might otherwise. Thus, this particular project began life in 1994 and, apart from an eighteen-month hiatus in 1998–9, has preoccupied much of my time and energy since. But it also simply could not have been written at all had it not been for my own (almost wholly fortuitous) interdisciplinary background in sociolinguistics, education and sociology. The second challenge is actually to present something informed and worthwhile at the end of it all, rather than something superficial or, at worst, simply misinformed. I leave the reader to judge how well I have done here, but do take full responsibility for any oversimplification and/or misrepresentation that may occur in the following pages.

And while I am offering caveats, here are a few more. First, it will soon become apparent to the reader, if it is not so already, that I am personally committed both to the extension of minority language rights and, relatedly, to a greater recognition of cultural and linguistic plurality within modern nation-states. This in turn is a consequence of my long and active involvement in issues of multicultural and bilingual education over the years, beginning as a teacher and then teacher educator in Aotearoa/New Zealand. On this basis, some critics might suggest that my argument is a 'moralistic' one rather than a form of 'disinterested' academic enquiry (see, for example, J. Edwards, 1985: 144). I do not accept this critique or the distinction on which it is based. *All* positions that are taken on language and minority rights – academic or otherwise – involve a moral dimension, reflecting the particular values and ideologies of their exponents (cf. Woolard, 1998; Blommaert, 1999b). Ideology is not the sole preserve of minority language proponents, although it is often painted as such. Seen in this light, the equation of academic disinterestedness with skepticism toward, and/or criticism of minority languages may be seen for what it is – an ideological move in the wider politics of language, nothing more. Indeed, as I will argue, such a move may simply act to reinforce the hegemony of dominant ethnic groups, and the languages they speak, within modern nation-states.

Second, and more broadly, this position is consonant with debates in critical theory on the *situatedness* of any academic inquiry. As I have argued elsewhere (May, 1994, 1997a), all research is value-laden and, as such, a researcher *must* begin from a theoretical position of some description, whether this is articulated or not in the ensuing study. Accordingly, it is better to state one's position at the start than to cloak it in the guise of apparent neutrality. Not only that, critical social research, of which the following forms a part, is not content with the interpretive concern of 'describing' a social setting 'as it really is', since this assumes an objective, 'commonsense' reality where none exists. Rather, this 'reality' should be viewed as a social and cultural *construction*, linked to wider power relations, which privileges some and disadvantages other participants. As we shall see, the discourses of language and minority rights are prime sites where such power relations are articulated and outworked.

On a more technical note, since much of what follows is also concerned with the particular roles and functions of minority languages within modern nation-states, and the questions of their status, use and value, I have deliberately chosen not to follow the still usual publishing procedure of italicizing non-English words and phrases. This is not to imply their subsumption within English. Rather, it aims to act as a visual metaphor for a central tenet of my account – that the *normalization* of minority languages within the public domain is a legitimate and defensible sociological, political and linguistic activity.

INTRODUCTION

The contest between 'majority' and 'minority' languages[1] is, by definition, an uneven one – a mismatch. Much like a lightweight boxer taking on a heavyweight, we're almost certain what the outcome will be. Often the contest is quick as well as brutal. We see this clearly in the current plight of many of the world's approximately 6,900 languages (Lewis, 2009), with up to 90 percent of them predicted not to survive this century (Krauss, 1992; see also Crystal, 2000; Nettle and Romaine, 2000; Harrison, 2007).[2]

Of course, one cannot talk about languages without talking about their speakers. Languages don't just 'die' in the abstract. Language death occurs when the last speaker of that language dies. But, in effect, once a language ceases to be spoken by a *community* of speakers, it has effectively already perished. And more and more minority language communities, it seems, are choosing to express themselves instead through a majority language – that is, a language of greater power, prestige, influence and/or communicative reach. Thus, language decline and language death always occur in bilingual or multilingual contexts, in which a majority language comes to replace the range and functions of a minority language.

The process of language shift described here usually involves three broad stages. The first stage sees increasing pressure on minority language speakers to speak the majority language, particularly in formal language domains; a state of affairs described in sociolinguistics as 'diglossia'. This stage is often precipitated and facilitated by the introduction of education in the majority language. It leads to the eventual decrease in the functions of the minority language, with the public or official functions of that language being the first to be replaced by the majority language. The second stage sees a period of bilingualism, in which both languages continue to be spoken concurrently. However, this stage is usually characterized by a decreasing number of minority language speakers, especially among the younger generation, along with a decrease in the fluency of speakers as the minority language is spoken less, and employed in fewer and fewer language domains. The third and final stage – which may occur over the course of two or three generations, and sometimes less – sees the replacement of the minority language with the majority language. The minority language may be 'remembered' by a residual group of language speakers, but it is no longer spoken as a wider language of communication (Baker and Prys Jones, 1998).[3]

Of course, such language loss and language shift have always occurred – languages have risen and fallen, become obsolete, died or adapted to changing circumstances in order to survive, throughout the course of human history. But what is qualitatively and quantitatively different in the twenty-first century is the unprecedented scale of this process of decline and loss – some commentators have even described it as a form of 'linguistic genocide' (Skutnabb-Kangas, 2000). Such claims may seem overwrought and/or alarmist but there is plenty of evidence in support of them. For example, a survey by the US Summer Institute of Linguistics, published in 1999, found that there were 51 languages with only one speaker left, 500 languages with fewer than 100 speakers, 1,500 languages with fewer than 1,000 speakers, and more than 3,000 languages with fewer than 10,000 speakers. The survey went on to reveal that as many as 5,000 languages had fewer than 100,000 speakers each. It concluded, even more starkly, that 96 percent of the world's languages were spoken by only 4 percent of its people (Crystal, 2000). Given the processes of language shift and decline outlined above, and the current parlous state of many minority languages, it is not hard to see why. Even majority languages are no longer immune to such processes, not least because of the rise of English as a global language (Crystal, 2003; Graddol, 2007; see Chapter 6). Thus, if these predictions are to be believed, as few as 600 languages (less than 10 percent) will survive in the longer term – perhaps even as few as 300.

In response to these worrying trends, we have seen over the last thirty years the emergence of the broad paradigm of language rights. The discussion of language rights can be seen increasingly in the disciplines of sociolinguistics, the sociology of language, applied linguistics and language policy. However, the language rights paradigm also draws on related disciplinary areas, including sociology, political theory and international law. The key concern of the language rights paradigm is how to ensure that minority language speakers are able to continue to speak their language(s) for the foreseeable future. Given the increasing pressures on minority language speakers to shift to majority languages, this is clearly no easy task. It also raises some key questions. If speakers are choosing to willingly dispense with their languages, what right do we have to intervene? Surely, this is just misplaced social engineering (Edwards, 1994, 2010)? Or are we simply valuing the notion of languages in the abstract over the decisions of individual speakers to 'get ahead' socially and economically via another (invariably, majority) language (Mufwene, 2001, 2004; Wee, 2010)?

These questions need to be answered if proponents of language rights are ever to win the day. Let me attempt to do just that by outlining briefly the key academic concerns of the language rights paradigm. These are drawn from three distinct, albeit interconnected, constituent strands: language ecology; linguistic human rights (LHR); and a broader sociological and political defense of minority language rights. I place myself in the last of these strands. This is because, while I acknowledge the importance of both the language ecology and LHR movements, I also believe they demonstrate some key weaknesses that can only be addressed by a more interdisciplinary account of minority language rights.

Language ecology

A key strand of the language rights paradigm is language ecology. Language ecologists such as Peter Mühlhäusler and Luisa Maffi[4] argue that the current parlous state of many of the world's languages is analogous to processes of biological/ecological endangerment and extinction; indeed, it is far greater than the threat of extinction facing animal and plant species. Unless this process of language loss is seriously and urgently addressed, they argue, the world's linguistic 'gene pool', along with the cultural knowledge associated with these languages, will be irremediably diminished. The parallels that are drawn by language ecologists between linguistic and biodiversity have their merits, particularly in the clear resonances between the two processes. Thus, Steven Pinker observes that 'the wide-scale extinction of languages [currently underway] is reminiscent of the current (though less severe) wide-scale extinction of plant or animal species' (1995: 259). Likewise, James Crawford argues that each 'fall[s] victim to predators, changing environments, or more successful competitors', each is encroached upon by 'modern cultures abetted by new technologies' and each is threatened by 'destruction of lands and livelihoods; the spread of consumerism and other Western values' (1994: 5). Conversely, some commentators have observed that when biodiversity is high, so too are cultural and linguistic diversity (see Maffi, 2000, 2001).

But despite the usefulness of these parallels, there are significant limitations to language ecology arguments as well. One is an obvious tendency to present a 'preservationist' and 'romanticist' account of minority languages and their loss – amounting, in effect, to an overly utopian view of language and language change.[5] Another is that the language ecology paradigm actually reinforces, albeit unwittingly, the inevitability of the evolutionary change that it is protesting about. This is because while the biological/ecological metaphors drawn upon by language ecologists are useful in highlighting the scale and seriousness of the potential loss of languages to the world, they also contribute, ironically, to the equanimity with which potential language loss on such a scale is usually greeted. In effect, such metaphors reinforce, by implication, a widely held view that language loss is an inevitable part of the cycle of social and linguistic *evolution*. Thus, one could view the loss or death of a language as simply a failure on its part, or its speakers, to compete adequately in the world of languages where, of course, only the fittest can, and should, survive (see, for example, Ladefoged, 1992). Indeed, this kind of linguistic social Darwinism remains a prominent feature of many arguments against the retention of minority languages. They've had their day in the sun; time to move on.

The politics of language

What language ecology proponents fail to highlight sufficiently then are the wider political power relations that underlie language loss – or linguistic genocide, as Skutnabb-Kangas (2000) would have it.[6] Language loss is not only, perhaps not even primarily, a linguistic issue – it has much more to do with power, prejudice, (unequal) competition and, in many cases, overt discrimination and subordination. As Noam Chomsky asserts: 'Questions of language are basically questions of power' (1979: 191). Acknowledging the centrality of power relations also shifts the emphasis from examining the merits of languages in the abstract – as repositories of cultural knowledge, for example – to the actual predicaments of their speakers. When this occurs, we see immediately that the vast majority of today's threatened languages are spoken by socially and politically marginalized and/or subordinated groups. These groups have been variously estimated at between 5,000 and 8,000 in number and include within them the 370 million members of the world's indigenous peoples (United Nations, 2009; see Chapter 8), perhaps the most marginalized of all people groups. As Crawford (1994) notes, language death seldom occurs in communities of wealth and privilege, but rather to the dispossessed and disempowered. Moreover, linguistic dislocation for a particular community of speakers seldom, if ever, occurs in isolation from sociocultural and socioeconomic dislocation (Fishman, 1995a). The loss of a minority language almost always forms part of a wider process of social, cultural and political displacement.

Situating languages, and language loss, within the wider context of social and political power leads to a further recognition: that biological metaphors understate, or simply ignore the historical, social and political *constructedness* of languages (Hamel, 1997; Pennycook, 2004). If languages, and the status attached to them, are the product of wider historical, social and political forces, we can discount the process of 'natural selection' that a biological account would seem to imply. There is nothing 'natural' about the status and prestige attributed to particular majority languages and, conversely, the stigma that is often attached to minority languages, or to dialects.[7] Indeed, this is clearly illustrated by the fact that the same language may be regarded as both a majority *and* a minority language, depending on the context. Thus Spanish is a majority language in Spain and many Latin American states, but a minority language in the USA (cf. Chapters 6 and 7). Even the term 'language' itself indicates this process of construction since what actually constitutes a language, as opposed to a dialect for example, remains controversial (see Mühlhäusler, 1996; Romaine, 2000). Certainly, we cannot always distinguish easily between a language and a dialect on *linguistic* grounds, since some languages are mutually intelligible, while some dialects of the same language are not. The example often employed here is that of Norwegian, since it was regarded as a dialect of Danish until the end of Danish rule in 1814. It was only with the advent of Norwegian independence from Sweden in 1905 that Norwegian actually acquired the status of a separate language, albeit one that has since remained mutually intelligible with both Danish and Swedish. A more recent example can be seen in the former Yugoslavia, where we are currently seeing the (re) development of separate Serbian, Croatian and Bosnian language varieties in place of Serbo-Croat, itself a construct of the previous Tito-led Communist regime (see Chapter 4).

What these latter examples clearly demonstrate is that languages are 'created' out of the politics of state-making, not – as we often assume – the other way around (Billig, 1995). Independence for Norway and the break-up of the former Yugoslavia have precipitated linguistic change, creating separate 'languages' where previously none existed. These examples highlight, in turn, the centrality of the nation-state to the processes of language formation and validation, the significance of which I will examine more fully in the next section. The pivotal role of the nation-state here in determining what is and what is not a language might also help to explain the scale of the projected language loss discussed earlier. One only has to compare the 200 odd nation-states in the world today, with the 300 or so languages that are projected to survive long term, to make the connection. That many of these languages are already recognized as either national or regional languages, or are currently spoken by groups who wish them to become so, serves only to strengthen this connection further (see Gellner, 1983: 43–50). Such is the narrow concentration of 'officially recognized' languages that around 120 nation-states have actually adopted either English, French, Spanish or Arabic as their official language, while another fifty have a local language as the language of the state. In addition, there are another fifty or so languages that are accorded regional status (Colin Williams, 1996). In short, currently less than 1.5 percent of the world's languages are recognized officially by nation-states.

The nation-state model

Why then are nation-states, and the ideology of nationalism that underpins them, so central to the question of minority language loss? The first and obvious response to this question is that we continue to live in the era of the nation-state.[8] The nation-state remains the bedrock of the political world order, exercising internal political and legal jurisdiction over its citizens, and claiming external rights to sovereignty and self-government in the present interstate system. There are obvious advantages to the nation-state that help to explain its ongoing ascendancy. It liberates individuals from the tyranny of narrow communities, guarantees their personal autonomy, equality and common citizenship, and provides the basis for a collectively shared way of life (Parekh, 1995). Or at least it does so in theory. As such, it is often viewed as the apogee of modernity and progress – representing in clear political terms the triumph of universalism over particularism.

The 'triumph' of universalism with respect to language is evidenced by the replacement over time of a wide variety of language varieties spoken within a nation-state's borders with one 'common' national language (sometimes, albeit rarely, a number of national languages). This process usually involves the *legitimation* and *institutionalization* of the chosen national language (Nelde et al., 1996). Legitimation is understood to mean here the formal recognition accorded to the language by the nation-state – usually, via 'official' language status. Institutionalization, perhaps the more important dimension, refers to the process by which the language comes to be accepted, or 'taken for granted' in a wide range of social, cultural and linguistic domains or contexts, both formal and informal. Both elements, in combination, achieve the central requirement of nation-states: cultural and linguistic homogeneity in the civic realm or public domain. In the process, the chosen 'national' language comes to be associated with modernity and progress, while the remaining minority languages become associated with tradition and obsolescence.

The requirement to speak a common language is unique to nation-states, and a relatively recent historical phenomenon. It is unique because previous forms of political organization did not require this degree of linguistic uniformity. For example, empires were quite happy for the most part to leave unmolested the plethora of cultures and languages subsumed within them. The Greek and Roman Empires are obvious examples here, while 'New World' examples include the Aztec and Inca Empires of Central and South America respectively. More recent historical examples include the Austro-Hungarian Empire's overtly multilingual policy. But perhaps the clearest example is that of the Ottoman Empire which actually established a formal system of 'millets' (nations) in order to accommodate the cultural and linguistic diversity of peoples within its borders (Dorian, 1998).

It is historically recent because nation-states are themselves the product of the nationalisms of the last few centuries, beginning most notably with the French Revolution (see Chapter 2). Specifically, the emphasis on cultural and linguistic homogeneity associated with the rise of political nationalism is predicated on the notion of 'nation-state congruence'. Nation-state congruence holds that the boundaries of political and national identity should coincide. The view here is that people who are citizens of a particular state should also, ideally, be members of the same national collectivity. Ernest Gellner's definition of nationalism as a 'theory of political legitimacy which requires that ethnic boundaries should not cut across political ones' (1983: 1) clearly illustrates this standpoint.

The inevitable consequence of this political imperative is the establishment of an ethnically exclusive and culturally and linguistically homogeneous nation-state – a realm from which minority languages and cultures are effectively banished. Indeed, this is the 'ideal' model to which most nation-states, and nationalist movements, still aspire – albeit, as we shall see, in the face of a far more complex and contested multiethnic and multilingual reality. As Nancy Dorian summarizes it: 'it is the concept of the nation-state coupled with its official standard language ... that has in modern times posed the keenest threat to both the identities and the languages of small [minority] communities' (1998: 18). Florian Coulmas observes, even more succinctly, that 'the nation-state as it has evolved since the French Revolution is the natural enemy of minorities' (1998: 67).

And this brings me to the second response to the question of the interrelationship between the nation-state and language loss. The emphasis on cultural and linguistic homogeneity within nation-states and the attendant hierarchizing of languages are neither inevitable nor inviolate – particularly, in light of the historical recency of nation-states, and the related, often arbitrary and contrived, processes by which particular languages have been accorded 'national' or 'minority' status respectively. In short, the fundamental principles upon which the nation-state model has evolved are increasingly open to question. We see this process occurring from both above and below. From above, the inexorable rise of globalization, along with the burgeoning influence of multinational corporations and supranational political organizations, have required modern nation-states to re-evaluate the limits of their own political and economic sovereignty. The ascendancy of English as the current world language has also clearly impacted on the reach and influence of national languages other than English, while at the same time reconfiguring key language domains within and across nation-states such as the academy, business, technology and media (see Chapter 6).

From below, minority groups are increasingly exerting the right either to form their own nation-states – as seen in various secessionist and irredentist movements around the world – or for greater representation within *existing* nation-state structures. It is this last development, and its implications for the social, cultural and political organization of nation-states, which is most pertinent to the issue of minority language loss and displacement. In effect, minority groups are increasingly beginning to question and contest the principles and effects of nation-state congruence, not least because of the long historical proscription of minority languages and cultures that has usually attended it. In the process, national identity, its parameters and its constituent elements have been opened up for debate – particularly, with respect to questions of public bilingualism and multiculturalism (see Chapter 3).

Linguistic human rights

These questions are of central importance to another strand of language rights' commentary – linguistic human rights (LHR) – spearheaded by the work of Tove Skutnabb-Kangas and Robert Phillipson.[9] The LHR literature stresses the importance of first language retention and clearly highlights the wider political and social processes that have led increasingly to language loss. In response, LHR proponents argue that minority languages, and their speakers, should be accorded at least some of the protections and institutional support that majority languages already enjoy. These arguments are also echoed in much of the academic legal discourse that has developed in recent years with respect to minority group rights more generally (see Thornberry, 1991a, b; de Varennes, 1996a; Henrard, 2000). However, both these sets of literature seldom engage directly with the problematic questions, much discussed in social and political theory, of what actually constitutes a 'group' and, given the complexities involved in defining groups (see below), whether any rights (linguistic or otherwise) can actually be attributed to them.

The principal problem here is that LHR advocates tend to assume the identity of linguistic minority groups as given, the collective aims of linguistic minority groups as uniform and the notion of collective rights as unproblematic. Thus Skutnabb-Kangas and Phillipson (1995) argue that the notion of linguistic human rights is reflected at the level of linguistic communities by the *collective* rights of peoples to maintain their ethnolinguistic identity and difference from the dominant society and its language. I agree with this in principle, but the way the argument is formulated assumes that the linguistic community in question is easily definable in the first place – or, rather that all members of this group are (or will want to be) principally identified and identifiable by their language. And yet, this simply cannot be assumed, not least because of the processes of language shift and loss, discussed earlier, which may already have led many group members to abandon the minority language in question and/or any identification they may have had with it. This, in turn, highlights the essentially contested nature of 'collective' aims. Even if some level of collective consensus is reached about language, or indeed any other aspect of group life – and this in itself is no easy task – there will always be individuals who will choose to dissent from these conclusions (J. Edwards, 1994, 2001; Wee, 2010). This common disjuncture between 'individual' and 'collective' aims immediately problematizes the legitimacy of *any* claim to a group-based minority language right, whatever its social and political merits.

This key weakness in LHR theorizing has to be addressed directly via a more *contingent* understanding of linguistic identity – an acknowledgment that the languages we speak are not ineluctably linked to our (ethnic) identity. Accepting the contingency of the language and identity link addresses a key concern of some sociolinguistic commentators. John Edwards (1994, 2010) and Janina Brutt-Griffler (2002) argue, for example, that language does not define us, and may not be an important feature, or indeed even a necessary one, in the construction of our identities, whether at the individual or collective levels (see Chapter 4). This position on the detachability of language from ethnicity also closely accords with wider constructionist conceptions of ethnicity, which highlight the hybridity, fluidity and malleability of identity construction, as we will see shortly in Chapter 1.

Accordingly, I accept unreservedly a contingent understanding of language and ethnicity. However, there is a key caveat here. To suggest that language is not an inevitable feature of identity is *not* the same as saying it is unimportant. Yet many constructionist commentators in (rightly) assuming the former position have also (wrongly) assumed the latter. In other words, they assume that because language is merely a contingent factor of identity it cannot therefore (ever) be a *significant* or *constitutive* factor of identity. This additional presumption, as I will show, is neither necessary nor warranted.

Indeed, this position is extremely problematic, not least because it cannot explain the ongoing conundrum that, while language may not be a *determining* feature of ethnic identity, it remains nonetheless a *significant* one in many instances. Or to put it another way, it simply does not reflect adequately, let alone explain, the heightened saliency of language issues in many historical and contemporary political conflicts. In these conflicts, particular languages clearly *are* for many people an important and constitutive factor of their individual and, at times, collective identities. This is so, *even* when holding onto such languages has specific negative social and political consequences for their speakers, most often via active discrimination and/or oppression, as we shall see in the numerous contexts examined in this book.

Critical sociolinguistics

The tension between the individual and group is also reflected in important work within critical sociolinguistics over the last decade, most notably that of

Jan Blommaert, Alastair Pennycook and Lionel Wee, that has direct implications for language rights.[10] This work highlights the complex, fluid multilingual repertoires of individuals in their local context and how these differ significantly from more narrow conceptions of 'languages' (read: standardized language varieties) in the public domain or civic realm. The argument here is that narrow, reified conceptions of language will always fail to match the actual complexities and fluidity of individual multilingualism. On this basis, even if language rights are extended to minority language speakers, this does not necessarily lead to their greater social and political participation, or the diminishing of inequalities, because of the ongoing mismatch between formal language recognition and individual language use.

These critical sociolinguistic accounts acknowledge that such language use has been inevitably shaped by wider sociohistorical/sociopolitical factors, including discrimination and exclusion. However, language rights are still rejected in these accounts as a viable alternative for one of two related reasons, sometimes both. First, given the internalization over time of negative attitudes to a minority language, many of its speakers may no longer view a historically associated language as being particularly useful and may thus actively prefer to shift to a majority language. The second reason is that the transfer of a minority language from the private to the public domain inevitably raises questions about what constitutes the agreed norms and form of the language in question. If, as is likely, the language has been used in widely differing ways by individuals, there may be little initial agreement within a given language community about this.

This critical sociolinguistic critique highlights another of the key weaknesses of the broad language rights paradigm to date – its preference for a macro analysis that fails to account sufficiently for the micro sociolinguistic complexity 'on the ground'. Again, this is a point I have elsewhere conceded (May, 2005a). But the analysis also misses a key point. Put simply, it fails to recognize the *recursive* influence of the public recognition of minority languages on individual language use. As a result, these critical sociolinguistic accounts end up providing, in effect, a post-hoc validation of the *current* diglossic situation, the related language use(s) of speakers and their associated domain limitations.

My argument is a different one. It is not enough to continue simply to accept a current diglossic situation, where minority languages are used only in low-status domains and/or with delimited function and reach. Rather, we need to adopt a notion of linguistic complementarity that extends to the civic realm as well. By this, minority languages can (*re-*)*enter* key domains from which they have been historically excluded – education and governance being two key examples (see Chapters 7 and 8). When this happens, how minority languages are perceived and *used* can also change over time. This is because minority language speakers are then able to make *different* language choices that are not necessarily unidirectional – from a minority to a majority language – as in the past.[11]

If we acknowledge this possibility, we can also then address directly the pivotal question of exactly what we can accomplish in and through a minority language. Or whether, more bluntly, there is any point in maintaining a minority language if it stops us 'getting ahead' in the world today. For many, minority languages are viewed as doing precisely this – entrenching the social, political and economic marginalization of their speakers. Only through majority languages, and particularly English as the current world language, can upward mobility be assured. Or so the story goes (see Chapter 6).

But if minority languages can be reinstantiated successfully in the civic realm, then there is no reason why one can't get ahead in the world by maintaining one's (minority) language. Of course, this will almost certainly be in conjunction with existing majority languages, including English as a world language. But this notion of public linguistic complementarity, in itself, directly undercuts the language replacement ideology underpinning the nationalist valorization of majority languages – that one must choose a majority language *at the expense* of a minority language. Minority languages then can be seen as not only important as a means of identity, as language ecology and LHR proponents argue, but also as *instrumentally* useful.

Overview

It is with all these various questions in mind that I attempt in this book a theoretical and practical defense of minority languages in the (post)modern world. In **Chapter 1**, I highlight the pejorative perception of ethnicity – and, by extension, ethnic minority groups, and the languages they speak – apparent in much academic and political discourse. This is primarily a result of the unfavorable juxtaposition of ethnicity with the nation-state – the one associated with primitivism and particularism, the other associated with modernity and universalism. From this, I explore in detail the various academic debates on ethnicity and, in particular, the broad polarization between 'primordial' and 'situational' perspectives that marks the field. The former ascribes to ethnicity an enduring, intrinsic character that is associated with, and determined by, particular objective cultural characteristics – the 'cultural stuff' of ethnicity such as language, ancestry and history. The latter rejects this position as essentialist[12] and argues instead for the social and political constructedness of ethnicity, its fluidity and malleability, and its instrumental mobilization to particular political ends. A situational account of ethnicity also specifically rejects any significant or even any particular link between ethnicity and language.

I tend largely to concur with a situational view of ethnicity. On this basis, I argue that language *is* a contingent marker of ethnic identity and that adopting any other position involves, inevitably, an essentialized view of the language-identity link. However, I believe that constructionist accounts of ethnicity have, at the same time, understated the collective purchase of ethnicity, and its often-close links to particular, historically associated languages. Thus, as I have already suggested, a situational view of ethnicity cannot account adequately for the often-prominent role that historically associated languages play in the identity claims and the political mobilization of many minority movements in the world today. In theory, language may well be just one of many markers of identity. In practice, it is often much more than that.

In order to explain these apparent contradictions, I argue that the primordial/situational dichotomy of ethnicity is in the end unhelpful and unnecessary and that one can, and should, combine elements of the two. Thus, ethnicity needs to be viewed *both* as constructed and contingent, *and* as a social, political and cultural form of life. In this sense, ethnic identities are not simply representations of some inner psychological state, nor even particular ideologies about the world. Rather, they are social, cultural and political *forms of life* – material ways of being in the modern world. To this end, I employ Bourdieu's (1977, 1990a, b) notions of 'habitus' and 'field', and Anthony Smith's (1995a, 2009) notion of 'ethnie' as useful means to theorize this position. In so doing, I also draw on related debates on the significance (and limits) of postmodernist conceptions of hybridity, syncretism and 'new ethnicities'.

I take much the same stance in **Chapter 2**, where I examine parallel debates on nationalism and the construction and constructedness of nation-states. Debates on nationalism, like those on ethnicity, have tended to polarize around primordial and modernist accounts. The former position, which is most often articulated by nationalists themselves, views nations as 'perennial', as if they have always existed in one form or other. In its most extreme form, it also equates nations directly with ethnocultural communities that are, in turn, defined by fixed cultural characteristics – particularly, but not exclusively, a common language. The modernist position, which most academic commentators on nationalism have adopted, points to the formation of nation-states as a specific product of eighteenth/nineteenth-century nationalisms and the related processes of industrialization and modernization (see especially, Gellner, 1983; Hobsbawm, 1990; Anderson, 1991). This modernist view thus attempts to debunk the central claim of many nationalist movements in the modern world – that the right to nationhood is based principally on *pre-existing* ties of ethnicity. Rather, it stresses the contingent nature of national identities. National identities, like any other, are created out of particular sociohistorical conditions, are variable in salience depending on context, are subject to change and are always worked out in a complex interrelationship with other forms of social relations and identity.

Again, I tend to concur broadly with modernist accounts of nationalism. Be that as it may, the key problem with such accounts is their inability to explain away the *ongoing* influence of ethnicity and nationalism in the world today. After all, if modernism has now largely been achieved, and the nation-state is its apogee, so too surely should ethnic and national movements have atrophied. And yet this is clearly not the case. Thus, I suggest that a middle position may again be a more helpful way forward here – one that acknowledges not only the 'legal-political' dimensions of nationalism but also the 'cultural-historical' (Anthony Smith, 1995a, 2009). This avoids the modernist mistake of privileging the legal-political over the cultural-historical – that is, perceiving the end product of nationalism, the nation-state, as principally a political rather than an ethnocultural/ethnolinguistic community (when in fact it is both). This in turn arises from the modernist concern to disavow *any* link between ethnicity and nationalism (see, for example, Hobsbawm, 1990). As we shall see, however, such a position conflates the nation and the state (Guibernau, 1996, 1999). In so doing, it fails to explore adequately the differential power relations that underlie the representation of the language and culture of the dominant ethnie, or majority ethnic group, *as that* of the *civic* culture of the nation-state (cf. Billig, 1995; Kymlicka, 1989, 1995a, 2001). The result is the marginalization of a range of sociological minorities within modern nation-states whose languages and cultures are consigned to the private sphere.

In **Chapter 3**, I explore further the claims of minorities for greater representation within existing nation-states – particularly with respect to their languages and cultures – in relation to political theory. Here, I examine the prominent debate between liberal and multiculturalist commentators on the respective merits of individual and group-differentiated rights. Much of the debate favors the liberal preference for individual over group rights. Liberal commentators valorize individual rights, which are associated with citizenship and the apparent neutrality of the civic realm, for their universalism, their protection of fundamental liberal freedoms and their strict impartiality. Liberal commentators view group-differentiated rights, associated with multiculturalism, far more skeptically, often hostilely. In these accounts, multiculturalism is often linked with ethnic particularism and the potential illiberality that may result – some would argue, *always* results – when one apportions rights differently between groups. I examine here the arguments of John Porter, Albert Schlesinger Jr. and Brian Barry as broadly representative of this anti-multiculturalist position.

My own position, following the work of Will Kymlicka and Iris Marion Young, is that group-differentiated rights and the associated politics of multiculturalism are defensible as long as they retain within them the protection of individual liberties. Of course, combining the two is not always easy. Nonetheless, I argue that such an alternative is necessary because the present articulation of individual rights within political liberalism implicitly, and at times explicitly, supports the hegemony[13] of the dominant ethnie within nation-states, along with the languages they speak.

The literature on multiculturalism is also useful in helping to distinguish between differing levels of group-based rights available to particular minority groups. Following Will Kymlicka (1995a, 2001), such groups can be described variously as national, ethnic and other social/cultural minorities. National minorities, including indigenous peoples, comprise those groups who retain a historical association with a particular territory but who have been subject to conquest, colonization and/or confederation in that territory. Ethnic minorities comprise those individuals and groups who have migrated to another country, and have subsequently settled there. Other social and cultural minorities include 'new social movements' such as gay, lesbian and queer communities, women, and the disabled. To each of these groupings, Kymlicka accords particular group-based rights: 'self government', 'polyethnic' and 'special representation' rights, respectively (although groups may well have access to more than one set of rights, depending on their circumstances).

Self-government rights acknowledge that the nation-state is not the sole preserve of the majority (national) group and that legitimate national minorities have the right to equivalent inclusion and representation in the civic realm. Polyethnic rights are intended to help ethnic (and/or religious) minority groups to continue to express their cultural, linguistic and religious heritage, principally in the private domain, without it hampering their success within the economic and political institutions of the dominant national society. Finally, special representation rights are a response to some systemic disadvantage in the political process that limits a particular group's view from being effectively represented. In line with Kymlicka's general argument, I will suggest that, with respect to language, national minorities have access to qualitatively greater rights than other minority groups. However, this does *not* presuppose that the latter have no basis for greater linguistic rights, a key point that I argue in Chapters 4 and 5 and to which I return in the final chapter.

The arguments outlined thus far help to unravel the complex dynamics that link nationalism, language and identity, and their equally complex and contested political articulation in the form of individual and group-based rights. Having thus addressed these questions and controversies, I turn again directly in **Chapter 4** to questions of language loss and language shift, and the social, political and linguistic processes underlying them. Drawing principally upon sociolinguistic and sociology of language literature, I explore the link between *particular* languages and *particular* ethnic and/or national identities. In line with my previous discussions on ethnicity and nationalism, I argue here that a historically associated language is not a necessary marker of such identities, not least because of the growing prevalence of 'minority language shift' (Fishman, 1991). The loss of Irish and its replacement by English in Ireland provides an apposite example that I discuss at length. However, I also critique the view held by some sociolinguists, notably John Edwards and Janina Brutt-Griffler, that particular languages are peripheral to one's identity, and the related implication that minority language shift is an inevitable, voluntary and beneficial process for minority groups. Rather than being about 'modernization', as it is often constructed in these accounts, this process is more often about differential power relations than anything else. Bourdieu's (1982, 1991) notions of 'linguistic markets', 'symbolic violence' and 'misrecognition' provide an explanatory framework for this discussion – particularly with regard to the differential status and value accorded to majority and minority languages. The ascendancy of the former is principally achieved by their legitimation and institutionalization within nation-states and the subsequent marginalization of a wide range of other language varieties, as discussed earlier. I illustrate this process by examining the historical development of French as the national language of France.

Chapter 5 explores the specific links between education and minority language policy. Since education has often played a key role historically in facilitating, and at times enforcing, the transition to a majority 'national' language, one can assume that it might also be used effectively to promote a minority language. That said, it is also acknowledged that education cannot by itself effect language change, or reverse language shift (Fishman, 1991). Following Stacy Churchill (1986), various approaches to minority language policy are examined here, ranging from the complete disavowal of minority languages to their formal inclusion within all significant institutional and language domains of the nation-state.

In examining the variety of educational approaches adopted toward minorities in modern nation-states, this chapter also develops further the idea, first introduced in Chapter 3, that differing language rights can be accorded to minority groups. I draw here on Heinz Kloss's (1971, 1977) important distinction between 'tolerance-oriented' and 'promotion-oriented' language rights. Tolerance-oriented rights ensure the right to preserve one's language in the private, non-governmental sphere of national life. Promotion-oriented rights regulate the extent to which minority language rights are recognized within the *public* domain or civic realm of the nation-state. I argue that all groups must have, as a minimum, tolerance-oriented language rights. However, only national minority groups can claim the *automatic* right to promotion-oriented language rights – for example, via formal representation of their language in the public domain and/or through state-supported minority language education. Ethnic minority groups cannot claim promotion-oriented language rights as of right. Nonetheless, I argue that they can still lay claim to them, most notably in the realm of education, on the basis of the principle in international law 'where numbers warrant'.[14] The chapter concludes by discussing developments in international law that support the granting of such rights – notably, Article 27 of the (1966) International Covenant on Civil and Political Rights and the (1992) European Charter for Regional or Minority Languages.

In **Chapter 6**, I explore the impact of globalization on debates about language rights and, in particular, the increasingly pervasive influence of English as the current world language. This raises questions, in turn, about the relationship between language choice and social and economic mobility. Can we get by in the world today without English? Should English replace other languages? How does English contribute to what I term the 'monolingual norm'? I examine and critique the work of cosmopolitan theorists Daniele Archibugi and Abram de Swaan with respect to these questions. I also critically examine debates within political theory that argue for English monolingualism and against bilingual education, notably in the work of Thomas Pogge, and David Laitin and Rob Reich. I then turn to an examination of the 'English Only Movement' in the USA. This movement advocates that English should be made the official language of the US. But more significantly, it argues against *any* public support for languages other than English. The movement's principal target here is, once again, the provision of bilingual education, particularly for Latino communities in the US.

In the next two chapters, I continue to explore particular contexts in which language rights are highly salient. In **Chapter 7**, I look at the rise of regionalism and the opportunities it has afforded for the re-establishment of national minority languages as *civic* languages in particular regions. The three cases that I discuss at length are French in Quebec, Catalan in Catalonia and Welsh in Wales. Each of these contexts is widely regarded as having been largely 'successful' in reinstantiating their national minority language in the public domain, despite the ongoing dominance of an overarching national language (English in Canada and Britain; Spanish in Spain). The large degree of general support that now obtains toward such minority language policies is in itself a remarkable achievement, given the long historical derogation and proscription of these minority languages within their respective nation-states. However, as I will show, each example also demonstrates clearly the ongoing contested, and contentious, nature of minority language policy development. This is particularly evident in the negative, sometimes hostile, attitudes of majority language speakers in these contexts. The oppositional discourses of majority language speakers include the following, sometimes uneasy, combination of claims. The first is a societal discourse that equates minority language developments with ethnic/linguistic particularism and/or minority nationalism. The second employs a more personalized defense against having to learn a minority language – arguing that it amounts to an illiberal imposition and asserting the associated 'right' to remain monolingual in the majority language. The last deploys ostensibly 'multiculturalist' claims as a means of countering the obvious 'preferences' accorded to the national minority language. I examine the legitimacy of these various claims in each context and generally find them wanting.

Chapter 8 examines these same issues with respect to the claims of indigenous peoples for greater cultural and linguistic rights and recognition.

Indigenous peoples present us with easily the starkest example of the cultural and linguistic genocide that I referred to at the beginning of this Introduction. In the process of colonization, indigenous peoples have been consistently, often violently, dispossessed of their cultures, languages and lands, not to mention their very lives. The chapter focuses first on recent developments in national and international law that aim to gain a measure of justice and restitution for indigenous peoples from those who colonized them. Particularly in the last thirty or so years, indigenous peoples, and the political movements associated with them, have mounted a sustained assault on the established nation-state system by arguing for greater self-determination or autonomy within that system. In so doing, they have highlighted the limits of democracy and the colonial underpinnings of nation-state formation. They have also consistently brought to our attention the ongoing processes of imperialism and disadvantage to which they have been subjected in the name of both.

The central claim of indigenous movements – represented most clearly in the (2007) United Nations Declaration on the Rights of Indigenous Peoples (UNDRIP) – is that they are 'peoples'. This, in turn, entails associated rights of self-determination in international law, including the active protection and promotion of indigenous languages and cultures within nation-states. This view has gained considerable credence in recent times, not least because of the effective advocacy of indigenous peoples themselves. However, like the national language policies described in Chapter 7, such a 'differentialist' view of group-based rights continues to be controversial and contested. I explore the developments, setbacks and related controversies over indigenous self-determination in relation to international law and various national contexts. I then turn to examine in detail the case of the indigenous Māori of Aotearoa/ New Zealand.

By way of conclusion, **Chapter 9** reiterates my position that minority language rights are both sociologically and politically defensible in the world today. This necessarily entails major social and political – not to mention, theoretical – consequences. The most significant of these is the need to radically rethink, or *reimagine* the traditional organization of nation-states. After all, it is this, more than anything else, which has marginalized minority languages in the first place, and perpetuated the linguistic (and wider) inequalities experienced by their speakers. The first step in such a process is to deconstruct the orthodoxy that ascribes 'majority' or 'minority' status to particular languages, valorizing the former and stigmatizing the latter. This must be recognized for what it is – a social and political process, deeply imbued with power relations, and arising out of the political nationalism of the last few centuries. As such, it is neither inevitable, nor inviolate. Similarly, the apparently inexorable association of majority (national) languages with modernity and progress – and, conversely, of minority languages with tradition and obsolescence – is a product of the same historical, social and political forces, and needs to be interrogated accordingly.

Second, the process of rethinking the nation-state in relation to minority languages must involve, to my mind, the legitimation and institutionalization of the languages of national minority groups in the civic realm of the nation-state. If national minority languages are legitimated and institutionalized in this way, most often via a proactive minority language policy, they have the opportunity to assume at least some of the status and range of majority 'national' languages. In so doing, national minority languages can break out of the private familial domain and 'invade' the public or civic realm (while bearing in mind Fishman's (1991) caveat that the latter cannot act as a substitute for the former). This is crucial to the long-term survival of any minority language, since languages that are not accorded at least some degree of formal status or role in the public realm are the ones most likely to become marginalized and/or endangered in the longer (and sometimes shorter) term. History, if nothing else, teaches us this all too clearly. This also helps to explain my ongoing skepticism toward more recent critical sociolinguistic accounts that dismiss language rights as an option in multilingual contexts.

But this is not all. A third key requirement for rethinking the linguistic orthodoxy of the nation-state is the *active* protection of all other minority languages – at the very least in the private domain, and where numbers warrant, in the public domain as well. This additional 'move' equates broadly with more radical forms of multiculturalism. It is crucial to establishing a genuinely pluralist conception of the nation-state, not least because it guards against the propensity of many nation-states to 'play' the claims of different minority groups off against one another. I return to Aotearoa/New Zealand here, and the position of Pasifika peoples therein, to explore this issue in more detail.

Prospects for change

So where does this leave us? While continuing to uphold the importance of citizenship and individual rights, it is my contention that a greater accommodation of minority languages and cultures within the nation-state provides a more just representation of the (at times differing) interests of all its citizens. Such a position inevitably entails an acceptance of the legitimacy of some form of group-differentiated rights in modern liberal democracies. Establishing group-differentiated rights with respect to language – as with differentiated group-based rights more generally – remains a fraught, contested and contentious process. If one is to avoid a return to the reified and essentialized group rights models of the past, it requires a continuing acknowledgment of the ongoing interspersion of groups, the complex interconnections between ethnic and national identities and other forms of identity, and their varied (and variable) cultural and linguistic expression. However, group-differentiated minority language rights also recognize a central point too often overlooked in modern liberal democracies – that these language and identity processes can continue to be negotiated from *within* rather than determined from *without*. Or, to put it another way, the complex processes of language and identity can be negotiated on one's own terms (both individually and collectively), rather than the terms set by others, as has so often been the case historically for minority groups.

More pragmatically, the accommodation of minority language rights may become a political necessity, given the growing discontent with existing nation-state structures evident among minorities today. And this highlights a more general point. If the increasing demands of minority groups for greater cultural and linguistic representation are not met, they may lead, in turn, to secessionist pressures and the potential fragmentation of nation-states. Given the likely consequences of such fragmentation, and the hardening of ethnic and national boundaries that normally ensues, we should avoid this wherever we can. The still relatively recent spectres of Rwanda and the former Yugoslavia are sufficient reasons alone for doing so.

However, there is also a positive dimension to this. If nation-states are reimagined in more plural and inclusive ways, there is potential for the recognition of not only greater political democracy but greater *ethnocultural* and *ethnolinguistic* democracy as well. Thus, far from undermining democratic principles – a common assumption among opponents of minority rights – the accommodation of cultural and linguistic group-based rights may well *extend* them. Indeed, my argument throughout this book is that ethnic and national conflicts are most often precipitated when nation-states *ignore* demands for greater cultural and linguistic democracy, not – as is commonly assumed – when they accommodate them (see also Parekh, 2000; Kymlicka, 2001, 2007). Given the increasingly parlous state of the world's minority languages, the related ongoing disadvantages facing minority language speakers and the increasing fractiousness of modern social and political life, these questions, and their potential resolution, take on an even greater urgency.

1

THE DENUNCIATION OF ETHNICITY

In order to begin to understand why minority languages are held in such low esteem in the world today, we need first to examine related debates on ethnicity. This is a crucial first step because the 'ideology of contempt' (Grillo, 1989) exhibited so consistently toward minority languages has more to do with the (minority) ethnicities with which they are historically associated than with the languages themselves. Indeed, criticisms of minority languages almost always occur within a wider critique and/or dismissal of the particular ethnic affiliations of their speakers. If, as Grillo suggests, 'subordinated languages are despised languages' (1989: 174), then inevitably so too are those who speak them. Indeed, languages, in the end, only reflect the status of their speakers (Dorian, 1998). I will thus begin this chapter by charting briefly the long-held pejorative perception of ethnicity in much academic and popular commentary.

The predominantly negative view of ethnicity in academic and popular discourses arises from its consistently unfavorable juxtaposition historically with national identity and, more recently, as the longevity of the nation-state has itself come into question, with globalization and new forms of global identity. For example, it is almost de rigueur now in academic discourse to view ethnicity as socially and politically constructed; an essentially anti-modern and regressive phenomenon that is mobilized instrumentally by particular groups to achieve certain (self-interested) political ends. As a result, the 'cultural stuff' of ethnicity – that is, the ancestry, culture, religion and/or language to which such groups regularly lay claim – is regarded as largely fictive or fabricated. Indeed, many academic commentators view ethnicity as simply a convenient construction of an ethnic group's *supposed* distinctiveness that is employed *retrospectively* to engender 'ethnic solidarity' as a basis for social and political action.

Certainly, this is the view of ethnicity that has dominated in social anthropology over the last forty years, particularly since Frederik Barth's (1969b) seminal essay on ethnic group boundaries, a perspective viscerally encapsulated by Roger Sandall's (2001) notions of 'culture cult' and 'designer tribalism'. It is evident in a parallel sociological consensus on the arbitrary constructedness of ethnic groups – a process Rogers Brubaker (2002) has dismissively described as 'groupism' – and a related rejection of the apparent fixity of such identities. The latter has in turn been heavily influenced by postmodernist understandings of multiple, fluid identity formation – that individuals are never limited to just one form of identity – as championed by, among others, Homi Bhabha (1994) and Paul Gilroy (2000). This acceptance of multiple identities, and related notions of (unfettered) identity choice, is also clearly reflected from within political theory in the increasing promotion of (heterogeneous) cosmopolitan identities as the 'new' form of global citizenship, replacing ethnic, racial and even national identities. Jeremy Waldron (1993, 1995, 2000), Martha Nussbaum (1997, 2001) and Seyla Benhabib (2002, 2004) are broadly representative of this cosmopolitan position.

I will revisit each of these academic traditions in more detail in due course. Meanwhile, popular commentary reflects a similarly skeptical bias toward ethnicity, albeit of a somewhat different kind. Fueled by lurid media reports of the immolation attending yet another 'ethnic conflict', the wider public locate in ethnicity the principal cause of many of today's social and political problems. Places such as Rwanda, Sri Lanka, Northern Ireland and the former Yugoslavia – to name just a few examples – suggest starkly the destructive and unproductive nature of ethnicity and ethnic mobilization. Indeed, since the end of the Cold War, the most common sources of political violence in the world have been ascribed to these so-called 'ethnic conflicts' (Gurr, 1993, 2000).[1]

Such developments are closely related, in turn, to the proliferation of a variety of 'ethnonational movements' – movements based on ethnic affiliation which aim to establish a national state of their own and which often, but do not always, resort to violence to achieve their ends (Fenton and May, 2002). The separatist ETA movement (Euzkadi 'ta Askatasuna) in the Basque Country, and the erstwhile Tamil Tigers in Sri Lanka and the IRA Republican movement in Northern Ireland are obvious examples. In addition, there are minority groups who, while not necessarily wanting to establish a state of their own, want greater recognition, representation and autonomy within existing nation-states. Most notable here, perhaps, are indigenous peoples groups such as the Māori of Aotearoa/New Zealand, the Aboriginal peoples of Australia, Sámi (Lapps), Inuit (Eskimos) and Native Americans.

Suffice it to say that, while these various developments present us with qualitatively different examples of ethnic minority affiliation and mobilization, they are widely held to be *negative* phenomena. This is so *even when* such groups may be seen to have legitimate and supportable claims. How (and why) has this negative perception of ethnicity come to hold such sway? I will attempt to answer this question in what follows by focusing in particular on the historical development of academic discourse in this area.

Academic denunciations of ethnicity

Over the last few centuries, the widespread dismissal of the legitimacy and value of ethnicity as a form of social and political identification has been juxtaposed historically against the valorization of *national* identity and the modern nation-state from which it springs. Itself a direct product of the era of nationalism (see Chapter 2), the nation-state in this view is something to which we can legitimately give our allegiance but ethnic groups are not. Nation-states are embracing and cohesive whereas ethnic groups are exclusive and divisive. Nation-states represent modernity while ethnic groups simply represent a harping, misinformed and misguided nostalgia. Or so the story goes. But it is a story long told and with an impressive academic pedigree. In the nineteenth century, the British liberal John Stuart Mill argued in *Representative Government*: 'Free institutions are next to impossible in a country made up of different nationalities. Among a people without fellow-feeling, *especially if they read and speak different languages*, the united public opinion, necessary to the working of representative government, cannot exist' ([1861] 1972: 361; my emphasis). Mill proceeds to elaborate on why he deems alternative ethnic affiliations (and their languages) to be so counter-productive to the political organization of the nation-state. In so doing, he invokes a clear cultural hierarchy between different groups, arguing that smaller nationalities – the equivalent of 'ethnic minorities' in modern political parlance – should be assimilated into the nation-state via its 'national' culture and language; that is, the culture and language of the dominant (national) group:

> Experience proves it is possible for one nationality to merge and be absorbed in another: and when it was originally an inferior and more backward portion of the human race the absorption is greatly to its advantage. Nobody can suppose that it is not beneficial to a Breton, or a Basque of French Navarre, to be brought into the current of the ideas and feelings of a highly civilised and cultivated people – to be a member of the French nationality, admitted on equal terms to all the privileges of French citizenship ... *than to sulk on his own rocks, the half-savage relic of past times*, revolving in his own mental orbit, without participation or interest in the general movement of the world. The same remark applies to the Welshman or the Scottish Highlander as members of the British nation [sic].[2] (1972: 395; my emphasis)

Likewise, the French nationalist and historian, Michelet – a near-contemporary of Mill – was to conclude of the French Revolution that: 'this sacrifice of the diverse interior nationalities to the great nationality which comprises them undoubtedly strengthened the latter ... It was at the moment when France *suppressed* within herself the divergent French countries that she proclaimed her high and original revelations' ([1846] 1946: 286; my emphasis). In this view then, a homogeneous national identity – reflected in the culture and language of the dominant 'national' group – should supersede and subsume alternative ethnic and/or national identities and their associated cultures and languages.

As we shall see in Chapter 3, many modern liberals continue to hold to this position. However, the merits of the dominant group's culture and language tend to be emphasized less overtly in contemporary commentary (although the cultural and linguistic hierarchies underpinning such assumptions remain). Rather, the argument is usually couched in terms of a defence of two ostensibly key liberal democratic principles – universal political citizenship, and the recognition of individual, as opposed to collective rights (see, for example, Barry, 2001). These two principles are seen as sufficient in themselves to repudiate the claims of other ethnic groups for greater social recognition in the public or civic realm of the nation-state – the private realm is seen as less problematic – and for associated cultural and linguistic recognition/representation. But more on this later.[3]

As for Marxist commentary on the legitimacy of ethnicity as a basis for social and political mobilization, Marx and Engels were themselves to adopt a remarkably similar position to that of their contemporary liberal commentators. In discussing the position of ethnic minorities, Marx and Engels drew on Hegel's distinction between nation and state – equating the 'nation' directly with the modern nation-state and 'nationality' with ethnic groups, or ethnocultural communities, which lacked a state of their own (Nimni, 1995). On this basis, Engels could observe (in 1849):

There is no country in Europe which does not have in some corner or other one or several fragments of peoples, the remnants of a former population that was suppressed and held in bondage by the nation [nation-state] which later became the main vehicle for historical development. These relics of nations [ethnic groups], mercilessly trampled down by the passage of history, as Hegel expressed it, *this ethnic trash* always become fanatical standard bearers of counter-revolution and remain so until their complete extirpation or loss of their national character, just as their whole existence in general is itself a protest against a great historical revolution. Such in Scotland are the Gaels ... Such in France are the Bretons ... Such in Spain are the Basques ... (Marx and Engels, 1976a: 234–5; my emphasis)

The position of Marx and Engels vis-à-vis ethnic minorities arises from their somewhat contradictory views on nationalism. On the one hand, Marx and Engels argued, as one might expect, that the working classes were the motor of history. In *The Communist Manifesto* (1848), Marx observes: 'The working men have no country ... National differences and antagonisms between peoples are daily more and more vanishing' (Marx and Engels, 1976b: 65). On the other hand, Marx and Engels also endorsed the nationalist causes of 'historic' nations where these were seen to facilitate and expedite the proletarian revolution. Thus Marx observes, again in *The Communist Manifesto*, that the struggle of the proletariat with the bourgeoisie is 'at first a national struggle' and that 'the proletariat of each country must, of course, first of all settle matters with its own bourgeoisie' (1976b: 60). In neither instance, however, were the claims of 'non-historic' nations or 'historyless peoples' (geschichtslosen völker) recognized – that is, ethnic and/or national groups which lacked the 'historical vitality' to consolidate a national state of their own. As Nimni concludes, in his lucid discussion of this question, 'Marx and Engels were, to put it mildly, impatient with and intolerant of ethnic minorities' (1995: 68; see also Guibernau, 1996: 13–21). In this regard, they were, like their liberal contemporaries, Mill and Michelet, very much a product of their times. Indeed, the pre-eminent Marxist historian Eric Hobsbawm (1990) argues that it is 'sheer anachronism' to criticize them for holding such views since they were shared by nearly all nineteenth-century political theorists on both the right and the left.

And yet, having said this, Hobsbawm's views are not too dissimilar to those of his nineteenth-century counterparts. For example, Hobsbawm (1990, 1995, 2008) contrasts a positive unifying nineteenth-century nationalism – modeled on the French Revolution and located in the political formation of nation-states – with a negative and divisive twentieth-century variant, largely centered on ethnocultural and linguistic differences (ethnonationalisms, in effect). This is clearly comparable with the distinction drawn by Marx and Engels between 'historic' and 'non-historic' nations, and the transitory and regressive nature attributed to the latter. Other Marxist commentators have been less skeptical about the legitimacy of ethnicity and ethnic mobilization,[4] although such commentators continue to vary widely in the degree to which they regard capitalism as *determining* the construction of ethnic relations. Strongly class determinist theories of ethnicity seek to reduce ethnic categories to the exigencies of more encompassing (class-based) experiences. Weaker versions attempt a more open-ended examination of the interconnections between ethnic and class mobilization(s). However, in both cases, Marxist analyses of ethnicity continue to be predicated principally on the pre-eminent influence of capitalism and on the subsequent subsumption of ethnic and national relations within class relations. Thus, Marxist perspectives on ethnicity have considerable difficulty in accounting for the *specificity* of ethnic form and meaning in the circumstances of their mobilization (Smaje, 1997; Fenton, 1999, 2003; see below). More problematically still, they cannot account for the fact that it is often ethnic identity, rather than class, that is the principal catalyst of such mobilization in the first place.

Resituating ethnicity in the era of globalization

The advent of globalization,[5] and related understandings of identity formation in a postmodern age, has seen the development of a potential counter-argument to this broadly articulated modernist position on ethnicity. Postmodernists argue that the rise of globalization – the next stage of the modernization process – has significantly undermined previous forms of identification and political mobilization. In this view, modern nation-states are finding it more difficult to impose a uniform national identity, given the rapid expansion of transnational flows of people, money, information and ideas (Appadurai, 1990). Consequently, a new decentered and 'hybridized' politics of identities is emerging.[6] In the place of the previous certainties of nationhood and national identity, local, ethnic and gender identities have emerged as alternative identity choices and bases for mobilization. As Stuart Hall observes, the result is the simultaneous rise of new 'global' *and* new 'local' identities and the consequent proliferation of supra- and subnational identities:

> Increasingly, the political landscapes of the modern world are fractured ... by competing and dislocating identifications ... National identities remain strong, especially with respect to such things as legal and citizenship rights, but local, regional, and community identities have become more significant. Above the level of the national culture, 'global' identifications begin to displace, and sometimes override, national ones. (1992a: 280, 302; see also James, 2006)

Postmodernist analyses thus provide a possible space for the re-emergence of ethnicity as a valid social and political form of identification and mobilization. However, ethnicity in this context faces some stiff competition. The fragmented, dispersed and decentered individual of the postmodern world is supposedly able to choose from a bewildering range of identity styles and forms of political mobilization, and ethnicity, it seems, is just one of them. Moreover, while advocating freedom of identity choice, there is still a lingering preference for the (new) global over the (old) local identities in these analyses.[7] As I will argue in this chapter, this position significantly understates, and sometimes simply ignores, the key ongoing role that ethnicity often assumes in the processes of identity formation and social and political mobilization. Relatedly, postmodernists may also have underestimated the salience and resilience of 'national cultures' in which liberal and Marxist commentators have historically placed such store. Michael Billig cogently argues, for example, that national allegiances cannot simply be exchanged like 'last year's clothes'. As he asserts:

> There is a sense of 'as if' in some versions of the postmodern thesis. It is as if the nation-state has already withered away; as if people's national commitments have been flattened to the level of consumer choice; as if millions of children in the world's most powerful nation [the USA] do not daily salute one, and only one, style of flag; as if, at this moment around the globe, vast armies are not practising their battle manoeuvres beneath national colours. (1995: 139)

And so we come to a point where – despite both consistent negative attribution, and confident predictions of its imminent demise, for well over two centuries now – ethnicity continues to persist and prosper in the (post)modern world. Many contemporary liberals are confounded and dismayed by the resilience of ethnic ties, and the increasing advocacy of ethnic minority rights, within contemporary nation-states. Marxist commentators are similarly bemused by the emergent and ongoing claims of ethnonational movements in post-industrialist societies; a feature which the achievements of modernization (and class-based politics) should have rendered obsolete. Likewise, postmodernists, while they rightly highlight the contingent and multiple aspects of identity formation, cannot explain adequately why ethnicity (and nationality) should so often 'trump' the competition. The salience of ethnicity may well vary from context to context and, as we shall see, its interrelationship with nationalism and national identity, and with other forms of social relations and social identity, may be complex, overlapping and at times contradictory. Nonetheless, ethnicity cannot be as easily discounted as we have been led to believe.

Moreover, the rejection of ethnicity as a valid form of social and political action is in itself problematic. If ethnicity has survived and prospered – despite, it seems, insuperable odds – this suggests that it has at least *some* basis in social reality. This accords with Steve Fenton's succinct conclusion that ethnic groups 'are both actual and constructed' (2003: 6; see also Cornell and Hartmann, 2007; R. Jenkins, 2007). Ethnicity cannot *simply* be a convenient and largely fictive construction, although such elements are clearly apparent within it. The 'cultural stuff' of ethnicity – ancestry, culture and (for our purposes) language – *does matter* to a significant number of people. Likewise, ethnicity has meaning not only at the level of social and political *mobilization* but also as a principal form of individual and collective social *identity*. Whether we like it or not, ethnicity continues to have a special claim on the individual and collective allegiances of many people in the world today and we need to understand why this should still be so.

Ethnicity and modernity

So what exactly is ethnicity and what are the key sociological questions that surround it? Before examining these questions in detail, I want to flag a central theme which should already be apparent from my discussion thus far and which pervades much of what will follow – that is, ethnicity's complex and ambiguous relationship to modernity (Fenton, 2003). There is a dualistic tension in much of the academic debate about ethnicity that posits 'ethnic groups', ironically, as at once both a modernist creation – defined socially and politically by their *partial* incorporation into the modern nation-state – and as essentially *anti-modern*. The former is signaled by the usual collocation of 'ethnic' and 'minority'. Indeed, most of the discourse concerning ethnicity still tends to concern itself primarily with subnational units, or minorities of some kind or another (Kaufmann 2004).[8] The latter is suggested by the unflattering comparison of ethnic (minority) groups as atavistic and regressive, in contrast to the modernity of the nation-state; a position that is particularly evident in nineteenth-century academic commentary, as we have seen, but is by no means exclusive to it. Thus, while these ethnic minority groups may argue that their apparently distinct ethnicity pre-dates their (incomplete) incorporation within the modern nation-state, ethnicity is generally viewed here as a *construction* of modernity – a byproduct, in effect, of the political, cultural and ideational processes of nation-state formation – rather than an antecedent to it. Yet, at the same time, ethnic claims for social and political recognition are rejected on the basis that they fail to reach or reflect appropriate standards of modernity!

As I will argue in Chapter 2, both these assertions are problematic and have much to do with the primacy ascribed to political nationalism(s), and to its institutional embodiment in the modern 'nation-state', over the last three centuries. At this stage, however, it is enough to point out that this central dualism can be traced through much of the academic (as well as social and political) commentary on ethnicity.

Terminology

This dualism is also evident in the very terminology used, and the various attempts over the years to define both 'ethnicity' and 'ethnic group'. Glazer and Moynihan (1975) attributed the first use of the term 'ethnicity' to the American sociologist David Riesman in 1953, although other commentators suggest an earlier genesis in the 1940s (Sollors, 1989; Fishman, 1989a, 1997). Here we are talking specifically about ethnicity as a noun, 'signifying, like social class, either a sub-field of the study of stratification, or a type of status group, or both' (Anthony Smith, 2004a: 17–18). Its adjectival origins, however, are far older, since ethnicity actually derives from the Greek word 'ethnos', first used by Homer, meaning people or tribe. The equivalent term for ethnos in English – 'ethnic' – was used from the mid-fourteen century to the mid-nineteenth century to describe someone as heathen or pagan (R. Williams, 1976).[9] This etymological association was subsequently to fit well with the pejorative construction of ethnic groups in relation to the nation-state. The related collocation of 'ethnic' and 'minority' is also reflective of this positioning since it assumes that majority groups are somehow not 'ethnic'; that they simply represent modernity, or the modern (civilized) way of life. However, as I will argue, *all* groups – both minority and majority ones – incorporate an ethnic dimension and the failure of the latter to recognize or acknowledge this has more to do with differential power relations between groups than with anything else.

Subsequent discussions of the term ethnicity in the social sciences continue to reflect these ambiguities and tensions. Isajiw (1980), for example, found in a review of sixty-five studies of ethnicity, that fifty-two gave *no* explicit definition of the concept. If a particular view of ethnicity was assumed in these studies, it tended to accord de facto with the 'cultural stuff' of ethnicity – ancestry, culture and language. This position is reflected in its broadest terms by Glazer and Moynihan's much cited assertion that ethnicity is 'the character or quality of an ethnic group' (1975: 1). More recently, however, a contrasting view of ethnicity as *subjective* and *situational* has come to the fore; a position which has much to do with Barth's (1969a) elaboration of ethnic *boundaries* and which is characterized by Eriksen's counter-description of ethnicity as essentially 'an aspect of social relationship' (2010: 16), rather than a property of a group.

These seemingly contradictory aspects of ethnicity are encapsulated within Max Weber's early definition of the associated term 'ethnic group'. Weber argued, in his posthumously published masterpiece, *Economy and Society*, that ethnic groups are 'those human groups that entertain a subjective belief in their common descent because of similarities of physical type or of customs or of both, or because of memories of colonization and migration' ([1922] 1968: 389). This definition highlights how ancestral, cultural, and at times racialized traits are commonly associated with particular ethnic groups, both by members of the groups themselves and by others. However, along with these traits, Weber also specifically emphasizes the subjective nature of ethnic group membership – the *belief* in 'their' common descent. For Weber, objective characteristics such as language and particular cultural practices do not in themselves constitute an ethnic group; they simply facilitate that group's formation. Rather, he stresses that it is the political community that engenders such sentiments of likeness, although ethnic bonds, once created, contribute in an ongoing way to the solidarity of the group (Guibernau, 1996; Fenton, 2003). In other words, Weber seems to be suggesting that belief in ancestry and shared culture and language is a *consequence* rather than a *cause* of collective political action, acting in turn as a means of defining group membership, eligibility and access (R. Jenkins, 2007).

As Richard Jenkins concludes of Weber's formulation, ethnic groups are, in the end what people (both within and beyond the group) believe or think them to be.

Polarities and their like

Max Weber's formulation is an early attempt to highlight, and where possible reconcile, the countervailing tensions between the objective and subjective aspects of ethnicity. Like most contemporary commentators (see below), it is clear that Weber tends to favor the latter over the former, adopting in the end a more constructionist approach to ethnic identity formation. Nonetheless, Weber is able to hold the two in tension in a way that many who have come after him have not. Thus, much subsequent debate within sociology and anthropology has tended to a more dichotomous approach, where ethnic identity has been viewed as *either* the product of objective cultural (and linguistic) characteristics *or* (much more commonly) the result of a malleable, fluid and at times fictive process of identity construction. Accordingly, such analyses have largely been framed within and by the following kinds of polarities. Is ethnicity a premodern or a modern phenomenon? Is it an intrinsic attribute of human identity or a social construction that is mobilized to achieve certain political ends? Can it be defined by particular objective cultural attributes or is it subjectively maintained by shifting relational boundaries that allow groups to distinguish themselves one from another? Does it only apply to minority groups or does it encompass dominant/majority groups as well? Is ethnicity primarily material or symbolic, political or cultural, voluntary or involuntary, individual or collective? These dichotomies around ethnicity overlap in many instances and may be summarized as follows:

* premodern or modern
* primordial or situational
* intrinsic or instrumental
* content or boundaries
* objective or subjective
* category or group
* involuntary or voluntary
* individual or collective
* material or symbolic
* minority or majority.

In the remainder of this chapter, I will critically evaluate these debates on ethnicity and the various oppositions to which they give rise. In so doing, I will frame my analysis within the bifurcated approach that has been largely characteristic of these discussions until now – working, in particular, within the broad distinction commonly drawn between *primordial* and *constructionist* accounts of ethnicity. However, this should *not* be seen as an endorsement of this practice. I adopt it here simply as a useful heuristic device in order to compare and contrast the various positions adopted in these debates.

My own argument is that such an approach is unhelpful. Adopting an oppositional stance, though a favorite pastime of social scientists, inevitably results in a partial view of the phenomena analyzed. Self-evident as it may seem, the only sensible way forward is to endorse a middle ground – combining, where appropriate, salient elements of traditionally bifurcated positions. Thus, after presenting an overview of the relevant debates on ethnicity, including postmodernist conceptions, I will conclude the chapter by arguing that Bourdieu's concepts of 'habitus' and field, along with Anthony Smith's notion of 'ethnie', in combination, provide us with the means of developing a more integrative – and, in the end, more adequate – account of ethnicity. Such an account will also help to explain not only the continuing influence of ethnicity in the (post)modern world but also its complex interconnections with nationalism and national identity, the subject of the next chapter.

Ethnicity as primordial

One of the key reasons proffered for the enduring nature of ethnicity in the modern world is that it constitutes a primary aspect of human nature and human relations. This stance, which is broadly termed 'primordialism', is actually represented by a range of positions (Anthony Smith, 1995a). The extreme version, elaborated in the linguistic nationalism of the eighteenth-century 'German Romantics', Herder, Humboldt and Fichte, posits ethnic – and, by extension, national – identity as natural and immutable. Human beings are viewed, by nature, as belonging to fixed ethnic communities, which are, in turn, defined by the constitutive elements of 'language, blood and soil' (see also Chapter 2). This particular ideology of primordialism naturalizes ethnic groups and justifies ethnic chauvinism (R. Jenkins, 2007). A second stream of primordialism is represented by the sociobiology of Pierre van den Berghe (1979, 1995) who argues that ethnic groups are 'natural' because they are extensions of biological kin groups, selected on the grounds of genetic evolution (see Anthony Smith, 1998: 147–51 for a useful summary). The third, and most plausible stream, is associated most prominently with Geertz (1963, 1973), Isaacs (1975) and Shils (1957, 1980). Clifford Geertz, for example, in a much-cited passage, develops Shils's (1957) argument that the political actions of ethnic groups are often attributable, in the first instance, to primordial attachments. These primordial ties are regarded as a fundamental basis for collective action because they are rooted in our earliest socialization, in kinship and in the wider ties and solidarities built on and around kinship. As Geertz outlines:

> By a primordial attachment is meant one that stems from the 'givens' of existence, or more precisely ... the *assumed* givens of social existence: immediate contiguity and live connection mainly, but beyond them the givenness that stems from being born into a particular ... community, speaking a particular language ... and following particular social practices. These congruities of blood, speech, custom and so on, are seen to have an ineffable, and at times overpowering, coerciveness in and of themselves. One is bound to one's kinsman, one's neighbour ... as the result not merely of personal affection, tactical necessity, common interest or incurred moral obligation, but at least in great part by virtue of some unaccountable absolute import attributed to the very tie itself. (1973: 259; my emphasis)

Geertz argues that these perceived 'primordial' attachments toward other co-ethnics are categorically defined (most often by notions of common descent and via designated cultural practices) rather than being the result of social interaction. That is, patterns of interaction arise out of prior categorical distinctions, not the other way around (Gil-White, 1999). This helps to explain why such attachments often trump what Geertz describes as 'civil sentiments' – those sentiments and allegiances that arise from civic participation in the modern nation-state. Geertz is not arguing here that ethnic ties or affiliations *are* primordial in any real sense – hence, his deliberate qualification in the above quote regarding 'the assumed givens of social existence'. Rather, he is arguing that people *perceive* these ties as primordial and thus as pre-eminent over other affiliative ties. Such a position then does not necessarily entail the view that ethnic groups are fixed and static, as with the other primordialist strains, although ethnic groups are still equated in this conception with certain historical/cultural characteristics – the 'congruities of blood, speech, custom and so on'.

Be that as it may, much subsequent criticism of primordialism within anthropology and sociology has consistently misrepresented, even caricatured, Geertz's arguments as doing precisely that. The most common complaint is that Geertz is endorsing unproblematically a view of ethnic ties as presocial, unreasoning and, by extension, fixed or immutable (Eller and Coughlan's 1993 contribution is perhaps the nadir in this respect).[10] Critics have achieved this by a twofold process: first, by conveniently eliding the psychological significance of ethnic belonging to its members with the objective reasons why such groups may form; second, by then charging Geertz, along with all other 'primordialist' commentators, with maintaining that ethnic groups are *objectively* primordial, with impermeable boundaries (Gil-White, 1999). The result is to dismiss all so-called primordialists for apparently justifying, rather than simply attempting to explain, the influence of notions of common descent and culture in relation to ethnic identification (Horowitz, 2002; Bayar, 2009). The intellectual solecism of this position arises, as Steve Fenton (2003) argues, from asking the wrong question in the first place: 'Is ethnicity a primordial construction?' The question that Geertz is actually exploring is quite different: 'What does the term primordial mean and what assistance, if any, can it provide in explaining ethnic ties and identities?' As Fenton succinctly concludes: 'The first is not a sensible question, the second is' (2003: 76).

This is not to say, of course, that primordialist explanations are unproblematic. A number of valid key objections clearly remain. First, constructionist critics argue that while cultural attributes, as identified by Geertz and others, are often associated with ethnic distinctiveness, they do not constitute a *sufficient* explanation for ethnicity. To attempt to equate the two does, in fact, amount to cultural determinism. Nor does an emphasis on cultural characteristics explain adequately why some cultural attributes – language, for example – may be salient markers of ethnic identity in some instances but not in others. In effect, cultural differences do not always correspond to ethnic ones (see also my ensuing discussion of situational ethnicity). As Robert Thornton argues, an understanding of culture must thus involve more than 'simply a knowledge of differences, but rather an understanding of *how* and *why* differences in language, thought ... and behaviours have come about' (1988: 25; my emphases). Second, and relatedly, cultural forms thus require a historical examination; as indeed do all aspects of ethnic group formation (Anthony Smith, 1998, 2009). This is not something which a primordialist account can adequately provide. By situating the search for ethnicity within 'the assumed givens of social existence', which is, even in Geertz's account, usually stated rather than examined, the primordialist position conveniently explains both everything and nothing. It lacks, in effect, explanatory power and predictive value and is, at best, an ex post facto argument (Rothschild, 1981; Stack, 1986; Horowitz, 2000, 2002). As John Stack elaborates, the primordial approach 'fails to explain why ethnicity disappears [as an organizing social category] during one historical period and reintensifies in another' (1986: 2). Third, and most tellingly perhaps, primordial accounts also underplay the multiplicity of social groups to which individuals may belong and the role of individual choice in selecting among and within them.

Ethnicity as constructed

The emphasis on individual choice is reflected in the alternative endorsement of social constructionist accounts, which highlight the *situational* or *circumstantial* characteristics of ethnicity. This view of ethnicity, which now predominates in sociology and anthropology, is outlined most clearly in Frederik Barth's influential (1969b) *Ethnic Groups and Boundaries* (see also Moerman, 1965, 1974).

Building on Weber's earlier formulation of ethnic groups (see above), Barth, in his introduction, argues that ethnicity is *not* some bundle of unchanging cultural traits which can simply be examined and enumerated in order to determine differences between ethnic groups. Indeed, the 'cultural stuff' of the group – language, culture, ancestry – is not even a key consideration for Barth. Rather, ethnic groups are situationally defined in relationship to their social interactions with other groups, and the boundaries established and maintained between them as a result of these interactions. As Barth asserts:

> ethnic categories provide an organisational vessel that may be given varying amounts and forms of content in different sociocultural systems ... The critical focus of investigation from this point of view becomes the ethnic boundary that defines the group, not the cultural stuff that it encloses. (1969a: 14–15)

For Barth, ethnicity is about social relationships rather than specific cultural properties since 'we can assume no simple one-to-one relationship between ethnic units and cultural similarities or differences' (1969a: 14). Cultural attributes are not significant in themselves since any one of a range of cultural properties could be used to fill the 'organizational vessel' of a particular ethnicity. This may help to explain the diversity of cultural diacritica employed by ethnic groups in the world today to distinguish themselves from others. Instead, it is the *perceived* usefulness of these cultural attributes in maintaining ethnic boundaries which is central. Cultural attributes only become significant as markers of ethnic identity when a group deems them to be *necessary*, or socially effective, for such purposes. Thus, particular cultural attributes (such as a group's language) may vary in salience, may be constructed or reconstructed, and may even be discarded by an ethnic group, depending on the particular sociohistorical circumstances of their interactions with other groups, and the need to maintain effectively the boundaries between them. It is these ethnic boundaries which determine in the end who is and who is not a member of a particular ethnic group, as well as designating which ethnic categories are available for individual identification at any given time and place (Nagel, 1994). Shared culture in this model is thus best understood as generated in and by the processes of ethnic boundary maintenance rather than the other way around (R. Jenkins, 2007).

Barth's emphasis on the relational, processual and negotiated aspects of ethnicity (Eriksen, 2010) also presupposes that the formation of ethnic identity is largely shaped by the group itself – that ethnic identity formation is largely an *internal* process of ascription. This process will be in response to those on the other side of the ethnic boundary, and to changing circumstances, certainly. Likewise, the success of ethnic ascription will depend to a large extent on the reciprocity of other parties in recognizing and accepting the distinctions involved. Nonetheless, Barth sees ethnicity as a product of *intra*group processes of negotiation rather than the direct result of outside forces. In short, an ethnic group is ultimately defined by its own members. As Barth clearly states, it 'makes no difference how dissimilar members may be in their overt behaviour – if they say they are A, in contrast to another category B ... they declare their allegiance to the shared culture of A's' (1969a: 15).

Ethnicity as subjective

In adopting this position, Barth's account can be said to be a subjectivist one. It emphasizes the role of individual agents, rather than social structure, as the primary force in the construction of ethnic identities. As such, it has been criticized for underplaying (or even ignoring) the social and cultural constraints facing actors in their ethnic choices (Worsley, 1984; Wallman, 1986; Gil-White, 1999). As these critics argue, ethnogenesis, or the creation of new ethnicities, does not just happen. Identities are not – indeed, *cannot* – be freely chosen and to suggest otherwise is to adopt an ahistorical approach which reduces life to the level of 'a market, or cafeteria' (Worsley, 1984: 246).

While this criticism is a valid one, the answer probably lies somewhere in between both positions. As Eriksen astutely observes, 'ethnic identities are neither ascribed nor achieved: they are both. They are wedged between situational selection and imperatives imposed from without' (2010: 66). Joane Nagel likewise suggests that ethnic identity:

> is the result of a dialectical process involving internal and external opinions and processes, as well as the individual's self-identification and outsiders' ethnic designations – i.e., what you think your ethnicity is, versus what they think your ethnicity is ... Ethnic boundaries, and thus identities, are constructed by both the individual and the group as well as by outside agents and organisations. (1994: 154–5)

In other words, ethnic groups are both internally and externally defined; distinguishing 'us' from 'them' is always a two-way process. Where the balance might lie between internal and external definitions of ethnicity, however, remains an open question. In any given instance it is a question of degree. The continuum that is possible here is perhaps best illustrated by the commonly drawn distinction between ethnic *categories* and ethnic *communities*. Anthony Smith (1991) argues that the former are identified by others as constituting separate cultural and historical groupings. However, they may have little self-awareness at the time that they form such separate collectivities. Ethnic categories, in short, are named, characterized and delineated principally by others (R. Jenkins, 1996, 2007). Ethnic communities, in contrast, define themselves, their name(s), their nature(s) and their boundaries, and are thus more akin to Barth's notion of an ethnic group. As Paul Brass describes it, an ethnic community 'has adopted one or more of its marks of cultural distinctness and [has] used them as symbols both to create internal cohesion and to differentiate itself from other ethnic groups' (1985: 17). Such communities are thus characterized by a sense of ethnic *solidarity* which, in turn, is usually mobilized via an insistence on certain social and political rights. These rights are said to derive from the specific 'group character' (Glazer and Moynihan, 1975) and often involve an association with a particular territory or homeland. I will return to the notion of ethnic community in my later discussions of Anthony Smith's (1986, 1991, 1995a, 2004a, b, 2009) use of the comparable French term 'ethnie'.

Ethnicity and 'race'

Discussion of the balance between internal and external ascription also allows us to explore the crucial distinction between ethnicity and 'race'. Michael Banton, for example, argues that this distinction can be made on the basis that 'membership in an ethnic group is usually voluntary; membership in a racial group is not' (1983: 10). In other words, ethnicity is internally defined, 'race' is externally ascribed. There are serious weaknesses with Banton's argument here – not least, the implicit assumption that racial groups are somehow real[11] – to which I will return. However, the distinction he draws is useful in highlighting the processes of ascription which have led to the stigmatizing of certain groups on supposedly racial grounds and, from that, the establishment of social (and, in some cases, political) hierarchies between various groups.

Historically, the process of racialization has occurred in two principal ways. One has been via the imputation of biologically determined characteristics as a means of distinguishing between various groups. This process has been most prominently associated with the scientific racism of the nineteenth century (see Gould, 1981), although it continues to be represented in current academic discourse (see M. Kohn, 1995) and is still widely held at a popular 'commonsense' level (Omi and Winant, 1986; Miles, 1993; Miles and Brown, 2003).

A second, comparable process of ascribing essentialized cultural differences to groups has also become increasingly widespread, particularly post-9/11. This has led to the rise of 'new racisms' which describe group differences principally in cultural and/or historical terms – ethnic terms, in effect – without specifically mentioning 'race' or overtly racial criteria (Barker, 1981; van Dijk, 1993; Small, 1994; Schmidt, 2002). New racisms, in this sense, can be described as a form of *ethnicism* which, as Avtar Brah describes it, 'defines the experience of racialised groups primarily in "culturalist" terms' (1992: 129). By this, she argues, 'ethnicist discourses seek to impose stereotypic notions of common cultural need upon heterogeneous groups with diverse social aspirations and interests' (ibid.).

An obvious example, post-9/11, is the construction of Muslims and Islam as a homogeneous collective threat to Western nation-states and, individually, as representing and/or practicing an antediluvian, illiberal, religious identity. This reductionist construction of Muslims may simply talk of cultural or religious differences (and not mention race at all), but it is clearly racialized nonetheless (Modood, 2007).

Before proceeding further, however, a number of additional caveats need to be raised in relation to Banton's initial distinction between 'race' and ethnicity. First, the distinction considerably understates the reciprocal nature of group identification and categorization discussed in the preceding sections. As Richard Jenkins (1994) argues, the definition of 'them' in terms of 'race' is likely to be an important aspect of our definition of 'us' (which may, in turn, incorporate a 'racial' dimension). Second, while many examples of ethnic categorization do involve the imputation of essentialized notions of racial and/or cultural difference – and, from that, the positing of a hierarchy of group difference[12] – many also do not. In this sense, racism in its various forms can be viewed as a particular subset – or, more accurately perhaps, specific subsets – of ethnic categorization. However, they are not reducible one to the other. Ethnic categories may be essentialized in the same way as 'race' categories have been historically but they need not be. Nor are ethnic relations necessarily hierarchical, exploitative and conflictual in the same way that 'race relations' invariably are (Rex, 1973; R. Jenkins, 2007). Indeed, it has often been the case that the global impact of racism has overridden previously non-hierarchized ethnic categories (Balibar, 1991; Fenton, 1999). As such, it is simply wrong to conflate 'race' with ethnicity as some commentators are in the habit of doing (see, for example, Wallman, 1986; Anthias and Yuval-Davis, 1992; Gunaratnam, 2003). Third, groups as well as being identified negatively by others may actually seek to identify themselves in positive 'racial' terms; a feature which is notable in many forms of black nationalism and also within some indigenous peoples' movements. Finally, 'racial' and ethnic ascriptions both remain, in the end, comparable processes of social and cultural *construction*. As the development of 'new racisms' indicates, and as Richard Jenkins argues, 'it is emphatically not the case that the difference between ethnicity and "race" is a simple difference between the physical and the cultural, although it may be a difference between *purported* physical and cultural characteristics' (1994: 208; my emphasis; see also Goldberg, 1993). Paul Gilroy, in his discussion of 'race' and racism, similarly asserts:

> Races are not ... simple expressions of either biological or cultural sameness. They are imagined – socially and politically constructed ... Dealing with these issues in their specificity and in their articulation with other [social] relations and practices constitutes a profound and urgent

theoretical challenge. It requires a theory of racisms that does not depend on an essentialist theory of races themselves. (1990: 264; see also 2000)

Much the same could be said for the broader concept of ethnicity. Acknowledging that ethnicity is a social and cultural construction allows us to explore its articulation with other social forces and the various, or multiple, manifestations which may result (including various racisms). In so doing, the way in which ethnicity is deliberately employed – or mobilized – in specific contexts becomes central, as do the particular ends pursued in the process of mobilization. The mobilization of ethnicity here can be summarized as 'the process by which a group organises along ethnic lines in pursuit of collective political ends' (Stack, 1986: 5). In order to examine this process more closely, we need to turn to discussions on the *instrumental* utility of ethnicity.

Ethnicity as intentional

Accepting a situational or circumstantial view of ethnicity invites an obvious corollary, at least to its advocates: if ethnicity is primarily an aspect of social relationships, then it can best be analyzed through the various uses to which individuals and/or groups put it. This is where ethnic mobilization comes in. It follows that ethnicity can be regarded principally as a social and political *resource* and ethnic groups as specific *interest groups*, comparable to other groups that might mobilize on the basis of social class, or trade unionism, for example. This appears to be the consensus of most commentators on ethnicity over the last four decades.[13] However, the accepted instrumentalist position also regularly posits such ethnic mobilization as no more than self-interested, even cynical, attempts at social and political aggrandizement, most often promoted and led by an elite substrata within the minority ethnic group. Peter Worsley summarizes this view in its most trenchant form: 'Cultural traits are not absolutes or simply intellectual categories, but are invoked to provide identities which legitimise claims to rights. They are strategies or weapons in competitions over scarce social goods' (1984: 249; see also below).

Such a view also presupposes the *fluidity* or *malleability* of ethnicity. In effect, the origin, content and form of ethnicity are all open to negotiation, reflecting the creative choices of individuals and groups as they define themselves and others in ethnic ways (Nagel, 1994). Such choices involve a wide range of possibilities. At one level, ethnic choices may be limited to what Gans (1979) has termed 'symbolic ethnicity'. This is common among many immigrant minority groups and, as Gans suggests, is 'characterised by a nostalgic allegiance to the culture of the immigrant generation, or that of the old country; a love for and pride in a tradition that can be felt without having to be incorporated in everyday behaviour' (1979: 9). In this regard, many hyphenated white identities in the United States (Italian-Americans, Jewish-Americans, etc.) continue to exhibit a 'symbolic ethnicity', even when previously demarcated ethnic boundaries within the white population (such as language, religion and endogamy) have atrophied over time (see Alba, 1990; Waters, 1990; Kivisto, 2002).

At the other end of the spectrum, ethnicity may be constituted as a (or the) principal form of social identity and political organization – a context which is literally *saturated* by ethnicity (Fenton, 1999). As Fenton argues, ethnicity becomes here a more or less dominant element of the framing of political power, its legitimation and exercise, as seen historically in Nazi Germany and apartheid South Africa. Similar circumstances are evident in contemporary times in such places as Rwanda (Hintjens, 2001, 2008) and the former Yugoslavia (Glenny, 1996; Wilmer, 2002; Rogel, 2004). In addition, the immolation in the former Yugoslavia throughout the 1990s usefully demonstrates the varying *salience* of ethnicity over time with regard to social and political organization. For example, from the time of the Second World War to the beginning of the major ethnic conflicts of the late 1980s, ethnicity had *not* been mobilized as a principal form of social and political delineation in the relations between Serbian, Muslim and Croatian groups in the area.

When viewed in this (instrumental) light, ethnic histories and ascriptions can be *adopted* and *adapted* by individuals and/or groups according to the particular social and political aims being pursued at the time. Eugeen Roosens (1989) provides one of the most pointed examples of this process at group level in his depiction of the Huron Indians of Quebec. Roosens argues that the Huron developed – or rather reconstituted – their history as a Native American tribe in order to claim access to the political rights and rewards associated with 'indigenousness'. This 'invention of tradition' (Hobsbawm and Ranger, 1983) involved the establishment of a pan-Indian identity where before there was none. It also saw the development of a reified 'ethnic counterculture' (Roosens, 1989) in which the uniformly positive characteristics of Huron 'culture' were juxtaposed against the largely negative depictions of the colonial cultures which supplanted it. Of course, such reconstructions are not limited to indigenous peoples and, indeed, are a common characteristic of national as well as ethnic histories – a point which I will elaborate upon in the following chapter on nationalism and national identity. However, Roosens's principal argument – that the construction of ethnicity may comprise a largely fictive element in some instances – is a hard one to ignore (see also Sollors, 1989).

A comparable degree of skepticism is directed at individuals who decide to adopt or change a particular ethnic affiliation. As Roosens again observes, 'many people change their ethnic identity only if they can profit from doing so' (1989: 13; see also Steinberg, 1981). In his ensuing discussion of ethnic minority group members in the USA, Roosens elaborates on the particular utility of choosing to mobilize on the basis of an ethnic identity rather than, for example, on the basis of social class:

> It becomes more interesting to appear socially as a member of an ethnic group than as a specimen of a lower socioeconomic category. In a world where a reevaluation of 'oppressed' cultures is in vogue in many circles, this is a way of self-valorisation that cannot be achieved by considering oneself, for example, a member of the working class or the lower middle class. (1989: 13–14)

Similarly skeptical views have been expressed about the authenticity of other indigenous people group identities (see, for example, Sandall, 2001; Waldron, 1995, 2000, 2002). Suffice it to say at this point that a pejorative view of any notion of individual choice with regard to such (minority) ethnicities predominates, particularly among majority group members in any given society. This rejection of an apparent 'designer ethnicity' among minority groups occurs despite the fact that majority group members may exhibit considerable latitude in their own ethnic choices and social identifications (Alba, 1990; Waters, 1990; Kivisto, 2002). Conversely, the latter may mobilize a composite 'white' identity to similar instrumental ends (McLaren, 1995; Dyer, 1997: Roediger, 1999; McLaren and Torres, 1999).

Mobilizing particular identities will also depend, to a large extent, on the audience(s) being addressed. This may produce a pattern of 'ethnic layering' for different ethnic groups (Nagel, 1994). For example, Cornell (1990) discusses the various levels of ethnic identity available to Native Americans, including subtribal, tribal, regional and pan-Indian identities. A similar pattern is found for Māori in Aotearoa/New Zealand – ranging from whānau (extended family), through hapū (subtribe) and iwi (tribe), to a pan-Māori identity (May, 2002; R. Walker, 2004; see Chapter 8). A variety of situational levels of ethnic identification can also be found among African Americans (Waters, 1990; Song, 2001), Hispanic Americans (F. Padilla, 1985; Jiménez, 2004), white Americans (Waters, 1990, Kivisto, 2002), Asian Americans (Song, 2001, 2003; Hunt et al., 2010), British Asians (Modood, 1992, 1997; Raj, 2003; Song, 2003), and African Caribbean/Black British (Goulbourne, 1991a; Gilroy, 1987, 1993a, 2000; Twine, 2010).

Of course, the variety of ethnic identifications available to these – and, by implication, all other – ethnic groups should not surprise us. A social constructionist view of ethnicity requires it. As Joane Nagel observes, a 'chosen ethnic identity is determined by the individual's perception of its meaning to different audiences, its salience in different social contexts, and its utility in different settings' (1994: 155). Relatedly, these various identities may overlap with, or crosscut other social identities. For example, one may be a woman, a

Muslim, a Bangladeshi, a Bengali speaker, an Asian, working class, a Londoner, English, an English speaker and British, all at the same time. However, which of these identities predominate in any given circumstance, and how they interact with each other, will depend on the context, the audience, and the ongoing balance between the internal definition and external ascription of social identities, discussed earlier. This complex dialectic also suggests that there will be significant *intra*ethnic differences evident within any given ethnic group. The varying confluence of ethnicity, language, class, religion and gender will result in a full repertoire of social identifications and trajectories among individual members of a particular ethnic group. In this light, it also needs to be constantly borne in mind that ethnic, linguistic, class, religious and gender groups are themselves not solidary groups but have their own broad-based internal divisions. Paul Brass is thus surely right when he argues in relation to ethnicity and class (and one can add linguistic and other forms of identity here also):

> that the processes of ethnic – and class – identity formation and of intergroup relations always have a dual dimension, of interaction/ competition with external groups and of an internal struggle for control of the group ... It [thus] becomes critical to have analytical categories that can be used to analyze both the internal conflicts and the external relations of the group and the points of intersection between the two. (1985: 33)

I will outline such analytical categories in my ensuing discussions of habitus, field and ethnie. However, before doing so, it is important to explore briefly where this complex, crosscutting conception of ethnic (and other) identities might eventually take us. For this, we need to turn to postmodernist conceptions of identity, and particularly the notion of 'hybridity'.

Hybridity: the postmodernist politics of identity

The articulation of cultural hybridity – and related concepts such as mestisaje and creolization – is a prominent feature of the work of British theorists Stuart Hall, Homi Bhabha and Paul Gilroy, among others. Hall's (1992a) discussion of 'new ethnicities', Bhabha's (1994) celebration of creolization and subaltern voices from the margin, and Gilroy's (1993b, 2000) discussion of a Black Atlantic – a hybridized, diasporic black counter-culture – all foreground the transgressive potential of cultural hybridity. Hybridity is viewed as being able to subvert categorical oppositions and essentialist ideological movements – particularly, ethnicity and nationalism – and to provide, in so doing, a basis for cultural reflexivity and change (Werbner, 1997a; Hutnyk, 2005). Out with the old singular, in with the new plurality – a plurality of cultures, knowledges, languages and their continuous interspersion, where 'ethnic absolutism' has no place and 'where "race" will no longer be a meaningful device for the categorisation of human beings' (Gilroy, 1993b: 218). Within the discourses of hybridity, and of postmodernism more broadly, the new social agents are plural – multiple agents forged and engaged in a variety of struggles and social movements (Giroux, 1997). Conversely, hybridity theory is entirely opposed to universalism, traditionalism and any idea of ethnic or cultural (or linguistic) rootedness. In line with postmodernism's rejection of totalizing metanarratives, exponents of hybridity emphasize the contingent, the complex and the contested aspects of identity formation. Multiple, shifting and, at times, nonsynchronous identities are the norm for individuals. Like constructionist accounts of ethnicity, this position highlights the social and historical contingency of culture and its associated fluidity and malleability. It also posits contingent, local narratives – what Lyotard (1984) has described as 'petits récits' – in opposition to the totalizing narratives of ethnicity and nationalism.

In short, postmodernist commentators reject any forms of 'rooted' identity based on ethnicity, nationality and (one must also assume) language. Rooted identities such as these are branded with the negative characteristics of essentialism, closure and conflict. Instead, postmodernist commentators such as Homi Bhabha (1994) argue that it is the 'inter' and 'in-between', the liminal 'third space' of translation, which carries the burden of the meaning(s) of culture in this postmodern, postcolonial world. Others have described this process as one of 'border crossing' (see Anzaldúa, 1987; Rosaldo, 1989; Giroux, 1992). In the postmodern world we thus have access to a wide range of identities and an even wider range of their various permutations. Suffice it to say that in this brave new world any notion of historical continuity – ethnic, cultural or linguistic – is regarded as entirely unnecessary, if not irremediably passé.

Limits to the social construction of ethnicity

If this is the case, the argument for maintaining particular ethnic affiliations – and by extension, linguistic ones – comes into serious question. But before we dismiss such affiliations out of hand, we need first to examine critically the limitations of these various constructionist accounts of ethnicity. Can we be satisfied that ethnicity is a modern construction (an invention even), only incidentally related to culture, as 'situational' commentators would have it? Is it completely fluid and malleable – able to be mobilized at will, in virtually any form, by individuals and groups in their pursuit of social and political gain as 'instrumentalists' argue? And is the locus of identity now irretrievably in the 'gaps' rather than the substance as hybridity theorists now surmise? The answer to each of these questions is: not entirely.

For all its persuasiveness, there is an obvious degree of overstatement in social constructionist accounts of ethnicity. For a start, accepting that culture is contingent to identity – the situational aspect of ethnic identity – does not necessarily entail the assumed corollary that ethnic groups are thus merely self-interested, rational, actors, often controlled by minority elites for political ends – the instrumental dimension. And yet, most constructionist commentators on ethnicity over the years have simply elided these two positions, in the process collapsing important distinctions between ethnic identity formation and ethnic mobilization. As Francisco Gil-White argues, such commentators 'often confuse explaining ethnic groups as such with the related problem of explaining ethnic mobilization, arguing as though ethnic groups regularly sprang suddenly into being, where none existed, in order to address the political interests of their members' (1999: 804; see also Bayar, 2009).

An additional problem lies with the constructionist and postmodern emphases on the voluntaristic nature of identity choices, which, if taken to its extreme, mean that all ethnic choices become possible, a position represented by the methodological individualism of rational choice theory (see Hechter, 1986, 1987; Banton, 1987). Methodological individualism assumes that groups are constituted from individual behavior and are subject to continuous change as individuals respond to changing circumstances. In this view, social relations become a form of market relations with individuals making rational choices about their ethnic alignment(s) solely on the basis of the social and material gain it will bring them. As Michael Banton observes of this process, an individual will join in ethnic group mobilization 'only when he expects the benefits of his participation to exceed the costs' (1987: 136). On this basis, it is argued that the ethnic options of individual actors can be predicted. However, serious limitations can be attributed to this analysis. The central premise that rationality equals self-interest is too narrow; one may also act rationally in someone else's – or a collective group's – interest. Likewise, such a position fails to address adequately the external constraints facing actors in their ethnic choices (see below). Given this, rational choice theory presents us with a socially and economically reductive account of ethnicity (for a useful critique, see Figueroa, 1991).

Ethnicity may well be a social construction but it is clear that not everything will function equally well in the social legitimation of ethnic identities. Even avowed social constructionists, such as Eugeen Roosens, concede this point. As Roosens observes, 'Ethnic groups and their cultures are not merely a completely arbitrary construct: there is always a minimum of incontestable and noninterpretable facts necessary to win something from the opponent ... The reality [of ethnicity] is very elastic but not totally arbitrary' (1989: 156; see also below). Thomas Eriksen puts it even more directly:

> If the agents themselves hold that a certain description of their culture is obviously false, it cannot provide them with a powerful ethnic identity. If a group's version of its cultural history is seriously contested by other

groups ... it may also be problematic to maintain the identity postulated by that account of history. So we cannot conclude that anything goes and that everything about ethnicity is deception and make-believe ... rather, [ethnic] identities are ambiguous, and ... this ambiguity is connected with a negotiable history and a negotiable cultural content. (2010: 88–9)

Negotiation is a key element here to the ongoing construction of ethnicity, but there are also limits to it. Individual and collective choices are circumscribed by the ethnic categories available at any given time and place. These categories are, in turn, socially and politically defined and have varying degrees of advantage or stigma attached to them (Nagel, 1994). Moreover, the range of choices available to particular individuals and groups varies widely. A white American may have a wide range of ethnic options from which to choose on the basis of their ancestry. An African American, in contrast, is confronted with essentially one ethnic choice – black; irrespective of any preferred ethnic (or, for that matter, other) alternatives they might wish to employ.[14] As Nagel observes 'the extent to which ethnicity can be freely constructed by individuals or groups is quite narrow when compulsory ethnic categories are imposed by others ... [such] ethnic boundaries can be powerful determinants of both the content and meaning of particular ethnicities' (1994: 156).

The above example also suggests that the different ethnic choices available to majority and minority group members are a product of *unequal* power relations in the wider society. In particular, it is the differing location(s) of particular ethnic groups within the nation-state that shapes and constrains the ethnic options available to them, a theme I will pursue more fully in the following chapters. Suffice it to say at this point, that when ethnicity is viewed solely as an instrumental resource these differences in power are not adequately addressed. Similarly, the power differentials *within* a particular ethnic group, and the broad-based divisions that may result, are also ignored (Brass, 1985; Song, 2003).

Second, there are serious limits to the central instrumentalist notion that ethnic groups are simply one of many interest groups seeking resources in and from the nation-state. Such a view is problematic because it fails to answer the question of *why* ethnicity is so often chosen as a means of mobilization over other possibilities – often dashing class-based interests along the way.[15] In attempting to answer this question we can leave aside the somewhat limited suggestion that ethnicity is simply more effective in attaining social and political goals. In some cases it may well be (see, for example, Roosens's earlier observations on the Huron). In other instances, it clearly is not. It is difficult, if not impossible to explain, for example, why ethnically based claims should still hold sway in the face of direct political persecution. One only has to think of the various ethnolinguistic minorities in Franco's Spain (see Chapter 7), Kosovans in the former Yugoslavia, Kurds in Saddam Hussein's Iraq, or, still currently, Tibetans in China and Roma across Europe. These examples demonstrate that ethnic groups will continue to reproduce their ethnicity *even when* it reduces their chances of attaining prosperity and political power (Eriksen, 2010).

Why is this? The reasons lie principally in the 'ineffable' cultural and symbolic attributes of ethnicity largely dismissed in instrumental accounts. Ethnic groups differ from other interest groups precisely in their particular concern with cultural attributes and symbols, language, kinship and historical memory. These features are predicated principally on 'belonging' rather than 'accomplishment' (Kymlicka, 1995a; Margalit and Raz, 1995; Calhoun, 2003, 2007) and provide the basis not only for political action but also, crucially, for identity and meaning (Melucci, 1989; Guibernau, 1996; see also Chapters 3 and 4). They may well be socially constructed (or reconstructed) but their enduring influence cannot be explained on the basis of functionality alone. Ignoring the cultural matters that are important to ethnic groups is thus an analytical error since these are central to their distinction from other interest groups. Paul Brass argues to this end:

> Ethnic groups, by definition ... are concerned not only with material interests but with symbolic interests. Moreover, no matter how old or new, 'genuine' or 'artificial', rich or superficial, the culture of a particular ethnic group may be, its culture and the definition of its boundaries are crucial matters that do not arise in the same way for other interest groups. (1985: 31)

The ongoing influence of culture and cultural affiliations are also not adequately resolved by hybridity theory. For example, the heterogeneous, hybrid and plural identities so enamored of hybridity theorists are assumed by them to be somehow unique to the (post)modern world, replacing the homogeneous, bounded identities of the past (particularly, ethnicity and nationalism). But this is simply wrong, or at the very least lousy history. Cultural mixture and adaptation have been features of all societies, in all historical periods, as Lévi Strauss (1994) has rightly argued. Thus, the historicist model adopted by hybridity theorists – of closed to open, absolutist to relativist, static to dynamic – is simply implausible (R. Jenkins, 2007). It is also highly modernist in its teleological view of 'progress'. And perhaps most ironically, in assuming that heterogeneous identities have now replaced previously bounded and homogeneous ones, hybridity theory ends up treating cultures as complex wholes. This perpetuates an essentialist conception of culture rather than subverting it (Friedman, 1997; Wicker, 1997; Bader, 2001). The juxtaposition of purity/hybridity, authenticity/mixture – so central to hybridity theory – is thus fundamentally misconceived (Caglar, 1997; Modood, 1998a; Hutnyk, 2005).

And if this were not enough, it is also abundantly clear that there is considerable disparity between the intellectual celebration of hybridity (whatever its merits) and the reality of the (post)modern world. There are two key points at issue here. The first relates to my earlier discussion on the limits of social constructionist accounts of ethnicity. Namely, the comparable failure of hybridity theorists to distinguish between the far greater possibilities of identity choices afforded to the privileged (including themselves) and the far more constrained identity choices, and 'emancipatory' possibilities, of the poor, minoritized and/or marginalized. This 'flattening of difference', as Peter McLaren (1997) argues, ignores how, in the real world, class, ethnic and gender stratification, objective constraints and historical determinations inevitably structure identity choices (see also Chow, 1998). A similar critique has been made against the advocacy of cosmopolitanism within political theory in recent years, which, like hybridity theory, champions new (multiple) forms of global citizenship, at the perceived expense of local or ethnic identities (I discuss cosmopolitanism further in Chapter 3).

Second, there is a confirmed reluctance among many hybridity theorists to engage with the world as it is, rather than as they imagine or wish it to be. This world *is* increasingly one of fractured and fracturing identities. But these identities are generally *not* hybrid; just the opposite, in fact. As we shall see in the next two chapters, nation-states are facing a plethora of ethnic, regional and other social and cultural minority demands, many of which are couched in singular, collectivist terms. The tendency to rootedness and to boundary maintenance (often expressed via ethnicity) thus militates against ecumenism, and these tendencies are generated and reinforced by the real fragmentation occurring within and between nation-states in a global era (Friedman, 1997). Given this, as Jonathan Friedman asserts, the valorization of hybridization is largely self-referential and self-congratulatory:

hybrids, and hybridisation theorists, are products of a group that self-identifies and/or identifies the world in such terms, not as a result of ethnographic understanding, but as an act of self-definition – indeed, of self-essentialising – which becomes definition for others via the forces of socialisation inherent in the structures of power that such groups occupy: intellectuals close to the media; the media intelligentsia itself; in a sense, all those [and, one might add, only those] who can afford a cosmopolitan identity. (1997: 81)

Ahmad (1995), in a similarly scathing critique, argues that articulations of hybridity fail to address adequately the social and political continuities and transformations that underpin individual and collective action in the real world. In that world, he argues, political agency is 'constituted not in flux or displacement but in given historical locations'. Moreover, it is sustained by a coherent 'sense of place, of belonging, of some stable commitment to one's class or gender or nation' (1995: 16, 14). In short, hybridity theory might sound like a good idea, but it is not in the end consonant with many people's individual and collective experiences. This disjuncture also holds true with social constructionist accounts of ethnicity more generally. After all, there is surely something strange going on when theorists proclaim that ethnicity is 'invented' and set out to 'decenter' it, while at the same time the news is full of ethnic cleansing and genocide (Levine, 1999). As Anthony Smith acidly observes, '[p]eople do not lay down their lives for a discursive construction' (2009: 14). Consequently, we need to explain more adequately why ethnicity does seem to continue to mean something to so many people. Perhaps more importantly, we also need to be able to explain why, when ethnicity matters, it can *really* matter (R. Jenkins, 2007).

Finding common ground – ethnicity, habitus and field

A useful first step to this end is to dispense with the dichotomous approach adopted to date in much of the primordialist/constructionist debate on ethnicity. Like so many dichotomies posited in the social sciences, it seems to have led us to a theoretical and practical impasse. Indeed, as Richard Jenkins has observed, 'the debate about whether or not ethnicity is "situational" or "primordial" seems futile; it confuses the *ubiquity* of a social phenomenon such as ethnicity with "naturalness", implying fixity, determinism and some kind of presocial power of causation' (1994: 220).

Given this, I want to suggest that primordial and constructionist views do not form mutually exclusive conceptualizations of ethnicity but that each formulation represents a *partial* representation of the underlying social and cultural movements that they seek to describe. Following Jenkins, ethnicity can thus be viewed as both a cultural creation *and* a primary or first-order dimension of human experience: 'on the one hand, ubiquitous and, on the other, possessing a particular immediacy and compelling urgency in many social situations' (R. Jenkins, 1996: 72). As Jenkins argues, despite its limitations, the 'primordialist' position outlined by Geertz, Isaacs and Shils rightly highlights that ethnicity is something in which we actively participate, an integral aspect of ourselves, rooted in our earliest socialization (see also Gil-White, 1999; Fenton, 1999, 2003). John Rex muses along similar lines that this may well explain 'why it is that, despite the very strong pressure in complex societies for groups to be formed on the basis of congruence of interest, many individuals do in fact stubbornly continue to unite with those with whom they have ties of ethnic sameness, even though such alliances might run contrary to patterns of group formation determined by shared interests' (1991: 11).

However, to take ethnicity seriously as a primary social sentiment in this way does not necessarily entail its reification as a set of fixed cultural properties. Stack (1986) asserts, for example, that the arguments of Geertz, Shils and Isaacs in relation to primordialism have never denied the significant role of socioeconomic and political factors as intervening variables in the crystallization of ethnicity. Nor, as I suggested earlier, has it conceptualized ethnicity as immutable and static (see, for example, Geertz, 1973: 258). We do not need to abandon the social constructionist consensus on ethnicity. Nor do we need to naturalize ethnicity as a sociobiological phenomenon as, for example, do van den Berghe (1979, 1995) and Kellas (1998). Ethnicity can still be viewed as socially constructed and fluid, *within certain limits*. Likewise, its mobilization by individuals and groups in the social and political domain, and within specific temporal and historical contexts, can be fully acknowledged and explored – albeit, as I will argue below, in broader, more useful, ways than most constructionists have hitherto managed.

Similarly, acknowledging the constructedness of ethnicity does not necessarily foreclose the possibility that the 'cultural stuff' of ethnicity – including, for example, a historically associated language – may still have ongoing and significant influence and importance. Indeed, even Barth (1994), some thirty years after his initial seminal intervention, has admitted as much. As Richard Jenkins argues, a constructionist recognition of ethnicity as transactional and changeable does not mean that ethnicity is *always*, or *has* to be so, only that it *may* be. As he concludes, 'the recognition that ethnicity is neither static nor monolithic should not be taken to mean that it is definitively and perpetually in a state of flux. It isn't' (2007: 52). A sense of continuity does *not* preclude cultural and linguistic change and adaptation, *and vice versa*.

A way in which these apparent dualisms can be effectively incorporated and expressed is through Bourdieu's related concepts of habitus and field. Both help us to overcome the primordialist/constructionist divide: the first in relation to ethnic identity formation, the second, in relation to ethnic mobilization. Bourdieu's analysis of habitus is principally concerned with social class (see Bourdieu, 1984, 1990a, 1990b; Bourdieu and Passeron, 1990; Bourdieu and Wacquant, 1992). However, since Bourdieu describes habitus as 'a system of dispositions common to all products of the same conditionings' (1990b: 59), habitus is equally applicable to ethnicity and ethnic identity formation.[16] For Bourdieu, habitus comprises all the social and cultural experiences that shape us as a person; his use of the term 'dispositions' is an attempt to capture fully this meaning. Specifically, there are four key aspects of habitus highlighted in Bourdieu's work which are useful to our discussion here: embodiment; agency; the interplay between past and present; and the interrelationship between collective and individual trajectories (Reay, 1995a, b). I will look at each of these elements in turn.

First, habitus is not simply about ideology, attitude or perception, it is a *material* form of life, which is 'embodied and turned into second nature' (Bourdieu, 1990a: 63). It is, in effect, an orientation to social action (Bourdieu, 1990b). Thus, via the concept of habitus, Bourdieu explores how members of a social group come to acquire, as a result of their socialization, a set of *embodied* dispositions – or ways of viewing, and living in the world. This set of dispositions – what Bourdieu would call 'bodily hexis' – operates most often at the level of the unconscious and the mundane and might comprise in the case of ethnicity such things as language use, dress, diet and customary practices (Smaje, 1997). The key point for Bourdieu is that habitus is both shaped by *and also shapes* the objective social and cultural conditions which surround it. As Roy Nash observes, the habitus is 'a system of durable dispositions inculcated by objective structural conditions, but since it is embodied the habitus gains a history and generates its [own] practices [over] time even when the objective conditions which give rise to it have disappeared' (1990: 433–4). Ethnic attitudes and practices, including language use, may thus be lived out implicitly as a result of historical and customary practice. As such, they may provide the parameters of social action for many. However, in the course of those very actions they may also begin to take on a life of their own (see below).[17]

Second, Bourdieu's notion of habitus foregrounds the interrelationship between agency and structure. While many have dismissed Bourdieu's position as structurally determinist (for a critique of this position, see Harker and May, 1993; Swartz, 1997), his specific aim is actually to overcome the agency/structure dichotomy in sociological thought – 'to escape from structuralist objectivism without relapsing into subjectivism' (Bourdieu, 1990a: 61). Thus, Bourdieu argues that habitus does not *determine* individual behavior. A range of choices, or strategic practices, is presented to individuals within the internalized framework of the habitus. Moreover, these practices, based on the intuitions of the practical sense, *orient* rather than strictly determine action. Choice is thus at the heart of habitus. However, not all choices are possible. As Bourdieu observes, 'habitus, like every "art of inventing" ... makes it possible to produce an infinite number of practices that are relatively unpredictable (like the corresponding situations) but [which are] also limited in their diversity' (1990b: 55). These limits are set by the historically and socially situated conditions of the habitus's production; what Bourdieu terms both 'a conditioned and conditional freedom' (1990b: 55). As he elaborates,

> being the product of a particular class of objective regularities, the habitus tends to generate all the 'reasonable' and 'commonsense' behaviours (and only those) which are possible within the limits of these regularities, and which are likely to be positively sanctioned because they are objectively adjusted to the logic characteristic of the field, whose objective future they anticipate. At the same time ... it tends to exclude all 'extravagances' ('not for the likes of us'), that is, all the behaviours that would be negatively sanctioned because they are incompatible with the objective conditions. (1990b: 55–6)

In short, improbable practices, or practices viewed as antithetical to the mores of a particular group, are rejected as unthinkable. This process of 'constrained change' (Chandra, 2006) or 'path dependency' (Wimmer, 2008) means that only a particular range of possible practices is usually considered, although this range of possibilities may evolve and change over time in relation to changing circumstances. Thus, Bourdieu posits that individuals and groups operate strategically *within the constraints* of a particular habitus – for our purposes, in order to establish and/or maintain ethnic boundaries – but also that they react to changing external conditions, economic, technological and political (Harker, 1984, 1990; Harker and May, 1993; May, 1999a).

This recursive position allows Bourdieu to argue that the habitus is both a product of our early socialization, yet is also continually modified by individuals' experience of the outside world (Di Maggio, 1979). Within this complex interplay of past and present experience – the third key dimension highlighted here – habitus can be said to reflect the social and cultural position in which it was constructed, while also allowing for its transformation in current circumstances. However, the possibilities of action in most instances will tend to *reproduce* rather than *transform* the limits of possibility delineated by the social group. This is because habitus, as a product of history, ensures the active presence of past experiences, which tend also to normalize particular cultural and linguistic practices, and their constancy over time (Harker and May, 1993). Nonetheless, this tendency toward reproduction of group mores and practices does not detract from the *potential* for transformation and change.

The fourth element of habitus – the interrelationship between individual action and group mores – also reflects this tension. In many instances, individual practices will conform to those of the group since, as Bourdieu argues, 'the practices of the members of the same group ... are always more and better harmonised than the agents know or wish' (1990b: 59). Yet Bourdieu also recognizes the potential for divergence between individual and collective trajectories. In effect, habitus within, as well as between, social groups, including ethnic groups, differs to the extent that the details of individuals' social trajectories diverge from one another: 'Each individual system of dispositions is a structural variant of the others, expressing the singularity of its position within the [group] and its trajectory' (Bourdieu, 1990b: 60).

There is, in all of this, a certain sense of vagueness and indeterminacy in Bourdieu's rendition of habitus, and debates about its efficacy in bridging the structure/agency divide remain ongoing.[18] However, if the concept is employed as social *method* rather than as social *theory* – that is, as a way of thinking and a manner of asking questions, which is actually Bourdieu's preference (see Harker et al., 1990) – it can be usefully applied to a discussion of ethnicity. As Gilbert summarizes it, Bourdieu's approach 'suggests an explanation of the regularities of social practice [in this case, ethnicity] as structured by the relations between, on the one hand, an objective set of historically produced material conditions, and on the other, historically produced definitions of those conditions and predispositions to act in certain ways in any historical conjuncture' (1987: 40–1). In other words, ethnicity as socially constructed *and* as a material form of life is addressed by the concept of habitus. This avoids the 'primordialist' mistake of assuming a realist definition of ethnicity, without diminishing the *significance* of ethnicity and the processes of cultural and linguistic identification that may be associated with it, which is the key constructionist error (see also Bentley, 1987; Smaje, 1997). As Bourdieu observes of social class, for example – and one can clearly add ethnicity here:

> My work consists in saying that people are located in a social space, that they aren't just anywhere, in other words, interchangeable, as those people claim who deny the existence of 'social classes' [or ethnic groups], and that according to the position they occupy in this highly complex space, you can understand the logic of their practices and determine, inter alia, how they will classify themselves and others and, should the case arise, think of themselves as members of a 'class' [or ethnic group]. (1990a: 50)

The dichotomy between the 'ineffable' nature and the 'calculated' or 'instrumental' use of ethnicity is also rendered negotiable by the concept of habitus, in conjunction with Bourdieu's notion of field. As Gilbert again observes: 'The notion of habitus, while recognising conscious intention, need not inflate it in explaining action, nor relegate the dynamic of social action to an ineffable consciousness' (1987: 41). Instead, it

> offers an explanation of human understanding and action which goes beyond individualism, but does not resort to abstract social forces, functionalist mechanisms or reified institutions as agents of social practice. ... it allows us to see how ideologies through their symbols and representations [including, one assumes, language] are part of the objective presentation of the contexts of practice, the means for defining a situation, and the medium in which past and present practices are installed in the interpretive and generative operations of the habitus. (Ibid.)

The notion of 'contexts of practice' highlighted by Gilbert is equivalent to Bourdieu's notion of field, which Bourdieu defines as a specific site of economic, cultural and/or intellectual reproduction, with its own 'logic of practice' (Bourdieu and Wacquant, 1992: 97). Central to the logic of practice in any given field are the types of capital (economic, cultural, linguistic, etc.) that are valued, recognized and/or rewarded within it. Fields are thus structured (and structuring) spaces that shape/influence individual and collective choices and options and which are 'characterised by their own distinctive properties, by distinctive forms of capital' (Thompson, 1991: 15). In this sense, fields are essentially relational – any individual or collective action undertaken in the field will have implications (positive and/or negative) for all others within that field. They are also intrinsically competitive spaces, or arenas of struggle. Fields, as such, continuously reflect (changing) positions of relative dominance and/ or subordination in determining what counts as capital in the field, including categorical divisions or distinctions. As Swartz (1997) argues:

> Fields are 'tightly coupled' … relational configurations where change in one position shifts the boundaries among all other positions. Field struggle pits those in dominant positions against those in subordinate positions. The struggle for position in fields opposes those who are able to exercise some degree of monopoly power *over the definition and distribution of capital* and others who attempt to usurp the advantages. (p. 124; my emphasis)

In conjunction with habitus, Bourdieu's notion of field helps to explain more adequately the resulting practices of ethnic identity formation and maintenance, and allied processes of ethnic mobilization. In contrast to the intrinsically limited instrumentalist notions of calculated self- and/or collective interest, these practices are rather a combination of the *interrelationship* between the structure of the relevant field – the nation-state, as we will see in Chapter 2 – and the (ethnic) habitus of the agents involved (Bourdieu, 1984).[19]

This combined understanding also highlights just how much is at stake for ethnic groups – the very 'definition and distribution of capital' – and related power differentials, particularly between dominant and subordinate groups. As Bourdieu argues, the individual and collective habitus of the former are invariably constituted as *cultural capital* – that is, recognized as socially valuable – whereas the habitus of the latter are not. This has obvious parallels with the negative, and commonly expressed views of ethnic minority cultures and practices (including the speaking of a minority language) as regressive and 'premodern'. It is members of ethnic majorities, or 'dominant ethnies' (Kaufmann, 2004; Kaufmann and Haklai, 2008; Anthony Smith, 2009; see below), who most often express these views – a process that Lukes (1996) has aptly described as the product of 'ascriptive humiliation'. However, minority group members also often express these views themselves, usually as the end result of a process of negative internalization. Bourdieu (1991) terms the process by which the latter is achieved as 'méconnaissance' or 'misrecognition' and its inevitably deleterious consequences as 'symbolic violence'.

While I have already briefly addressed the historical antecedents of this pattern of negative ascription in the early part of the chapter, I will explore its social and political implications for ethnic minority groups more fully in

Chapters 3–5. At this point, it is sufficient to observe that the habitus of ethnic minority individuals and groups, including their language use, tend to be specifically marginalized and devalued, both as a legitimate means of identity, and for their apparent lack of 'relevance' to the modern world.

Ethnies

If Bourdieu's concepts of habitus and field provide us with a useful methodological framework for exploring ethnicity, Anthony Smith's notion of ethnie provides a consonant explanation of how the actual *particularities* of ethnicity and ethnic identity are *enacted* by individuals and groups. Smith's central argument – as in this account – is that the competing primordialist/ constructionist accounts of ethnicity lead us into a theoretical cul-de-sac:

> By fixing attention mainly on the great dimensions and 'fault lines' of religion, customs, language and institutions, we run the risk of treating ethnicity as something primordial and fixed. By concentrating solely on the attitudes and sentiments and political movements of specific ethnie or ethnic fragments, we risk [seeing] ethnic phenomena ... as wholly dependent 'tools' or 'boundary markers' of other social and economic forces. (1986: 211)

In order to avoid this dichotomy, Smith argues that any realistic account of ethnicity and ethnogenesis must 'reconstitute the notion of collective cultural identity itself in historical, subjective and symbolic terms' (1991: 25). As Smith elaborates, a conception of ethnic identity along these lines:

> refers not to a *uniformity of elements* over generations but to a *sense of continuity* on the part of successive generations of a given cultural unit of population, to shared memories ... and to notions entertained by each generation about the collective destiny of that unit and its culture. (1991: 25; my emphases)

The parallels with habitus and field are obvious here. Particular sets of social networks are formed on the basis of believed or actual (ethnic) connectedness and are sustained, crucially, by a collective sense of continuity. This continuity is rooted in cultural elements of symbol, myth, memory, value, ritual and tradition. Meanwhile, these cultural elements in turn are reinforced by a distinctive symbolic repertoire that includes language, religion, customs, institutions, etc. (Anthony Smith, 2009). Thus, ethnic groups in Smith's conception change more slowly than is often assumed by constructionist commentators of ethnicity and may express deeply held group values and meanings (Anthony Smith, 2004b;

see also Hutchinson, 1994, 2000, 2008). Nonetheless, an ethnic group may still rise or fall, subject to the vicissitudes of history. In this sense, Smith argues, such collectivities are doubly 'historical' since 'not only are historical memories essential to their continuance but each ... is the product of specific historical forces and is therefore subject to historical change and dissolution' (1991: 20).

For Smith, the concept of ethnie, or ethnic community, best expresses the historical and symbolic processes highlighted here. Specifically, ethnies comprise:

- a collective proper name
- a myth of common ancestry
- shared historical memories
- one or more differentiating elements of common culture
- an association with a specific homeland
- a sense of solidarity (see Anthony Smith, 2009: 27).

As can be seen, most of these characteristics reflect a significant cultural and historical content and, except for aspects of a common culture, a strongly subjective component also. Given this, ethnies are not incompatible with a social constructionist view of ethnicity (see Anthony Smith, 1998: 192). For example, in relation to the characteristic of common ancestry, Smith argues that it is 'myths of common ancestry, not any fact of ancestry (which is usually difficult to ascertain), that are crucial. It is fictive descent and putative ancestry that matters for the sense of ethnic identification' (1991: 22). Likewise, attachments to a specific territory or homeland may be most significant to ethnic identity for their mythical and subjective qualities; the 'sense of place' that they evoke. Even in relation to the more objective aspects of a common culture – language, religion and kinship, for example – it is the *diacritical significance* attached to these elements which makes them salient to ethnic identity, not the actual elements themselves (cf. Barth, 1969a). Finally, while Smith argues that these attributes are clearly characteristic of ethnies, they are also malleable and fluid. They may vary in their salience; singly and in relation to each other, within and between historical periods, and among individual group members and thus the group itself. As we shall see, the languages associated over time with particular ethnies are clearly one such example.

Smith's notion of ethnie allows us then to see ethnic identification as a *dynamic* quality of group relations. More importantly perhaps, it provides us with an operational concept that encapsulates 'the central paradox of ethnicity: the coexistence of flux and durability, of an ever-changing individual and cultural expression within distinct social and cultural parameters' (Anthony Smith, 1991: 38). Interestingly, this position ends up actually being quite close to Barth's later (1989) formulation of 'streams of tradition' or 'universes of discourse' in which individual actors differentially participate but which possess a degree of stability over time (see also R. Jenkins, 1995). An additional benefit of the concept of ethnie is that it allows us to explore effectively the close interrelationship between ethnic and national identities, the subject of the next chapter.

2
NATIONALISM AND ITS DISCONTENTS

Many of the academic arguments surrounding ethnicity have also been rehearsed at length in relation to national identity and nationalism. Indeed, the field of nationalism studies reveals a very similar constructionist/essentialist dichotomy, with modernist commentators on nationalism adopting the former position, and 'perennialists' adopting the latter (see below). Given this, it is perhaps surprising that discussions of ethnicity and nationalism have until recently been conducted largely in isolation from one another. As Eriksen (2010) observes, the remarkable congruence between theories of nationalism and national identity and anthropological theories of ethnicity seems to have gone unrecognized, or at least unremarked, by many theorists of nationalism (see, for example, Gellner, 1983; Hobsbawm, 1990; Anderson, 1991). This lack of cross-referral may well be attributable to the well-known solidity of academic boundaries (May et al., 2004b). However, it may also be due to the prevailing modernist view among theorists of nationalism that ethnicity and nationalism are separate phenomena. Hobsbawm argues, for example, that nationalism and ethnicity are 'different, and indeed non-comparable, concepts' (1992: 4). Consequently, any connection between the two is seen as more or less coincidental. By this, modernist commentators on nationalism have attempted to debunk the central claim of many nationalist movements in the modern world: that the right to nationhood is based principally on *pre-existing* ties of ethnicity. In its most extreme form, this latter position equates nations directly with ethnocultural communities which are, in turn, defined by fixed cultural characteristics – particularly, but not exclusively, a common language. While this view is now largely limited to nationalist proponents themselves, it also has some early currency in the academic writings of the late eighteenth-century 'German Romantics', Herder,

Humboldt and Fichte. However, like the debates on ethnicity in the previous chapter, the common orthodoxy nowadays among theorists of nationalism is to reject this position as essentialist and to argue for a more subjective, situational and socially constructed account of nationalism and nationhood.

I will explore these debates more fully in due course. However, before doing so, I want to foreshadow my own position. As in the previous chapter, my argument will be that the polarization of primordial/perennial and modernist accounts of nationalism has been unhelpful – resulting in limited and partial accounts of the phenomena of nationalism and nationhood which they seek to explain. Thus, after outlining the key countervailing tenets of these debates, I will once again advocate an alternative position – one that combines salient elements of both extremes and, in so doing, returns ethnicity to the study of nationalism. This alternative can broadly be described as 'ethno-symbolic', a position most prominently associated with Anthony Smith's long-standing work on nationalism.[1] An ethno-symbolic perspective avoids the trap of essentialism associated with primordial/perennial accounts while still being able to explain the crucial interrelationship of ethnicity with nationalism and national identity, via its cultural antecedents, something modernist accounts have seen fit to ignore. As such, it provides an appropriate basis for the ensuing arguments in Chapters 3–5 in support of minority rights – both generally, and in particular relation to language and education. It is my view here that the historical denigration of ethnic minority language(s) and culture(s) within modern nation-states, and their related exclusion from the public or civic realm, are fundamentally misguided. Moreover, for those groups that can claim to be national minorities (ethnies) in their own historic territory, such an approach can actually be said to be illegitimate (Guibernau, 1996, 1999; Kymlicka, 1995a, 2001).

The processes of denigration and exclusion to which minority groups have been subject stem from the long-standing pejorative views of ethnicity in both political and social science commentary, discussed in Chapter 1. As I will argue in this and the next chapter, these views can be traced historically to an overemphasis on *political* nationalism and its institutional embodiment in the modern nation-state, and to the associated valorization of civic over ethnic ties; the latter usually being invoked in support of liberal democracy (Barry, 2001). Such a position suits well the interests of majority ethnic groups, or dominant ethnies, in nation-states (see Kaufmann, 2004; Brown, 2008; Kaufmann and Haklai, 2008), since it ends up representing their ethnic affiliations, particularly their language and cultural traditions, *as those of* the nation-state. In effect, the *ethnic* interests of the majority group are legitimated and naturalized as *civic* ones, which, in turn, are equated directly with modernity. By this, the legitimate claims of minorities for similar recognition and inclusion in the public or civic realm are ignored, discounted and/or suppressed on the basis that they are merely 'ethnic'. At best, minority group members may be able to continue to maintain their ethnic habitus in private, although the pressure to assimilate to the civic language and culture may remain intense. At worst, minority language(s) and culture(s) may be actively suppressed – a practice which remains an all too common feature of modern nation-state policy. The wide-ranging suppression of Kurdish in Turkey up until the early 1990s is one recent prominent example of the state-sanctioned linguistic suppression of minority languages (see Chapter 5). Another was the exclusion of Albanian from Kosovan schools, under the Serbian-controlled regime of the 1990s, which was also a key catalyst in the subsequent bid for Kosovan independence from Serbia. A still current example is the exclusion of Tibetan from schools in Chinese-controlled Tibet.

Terminology

Before proceeding further, however, it is necessary once again to clarify our terms. Indeed, if it is not already apparent, one of the principal difficulties in discussions of both ethnicity and nationalism has been the indeterminacy and confusion that have surrounded the meaning and use of key terms. As such, it is crucial at the start to define and distinguish between the following four central concepts: the 'nation', 'nationalism', the 'state' and the 'nation-state'. In due course, I will also examine the distinctions that can be drawn between 'political nationalism', 'cultural nationalism', the 'multinational state' and the 'polyethnic state', and will specify in detail how a variety of ethnic and national minority groups are positioned in relation to all of the above.

Following Guibernau (1996), a 'nation' refers to a group of people who are conscious of forming a distinct community and who may be said to share:

- a historic territory, or homeland,
- common historical memories,
- a common culture,
- a common (political) destiny and, relatedly,
- a desire for at least some degree of social and/or political self-determination.

Thus, the 'nation' includes five key dimensions – psychological (consciousness of forming a group), territorial, historical, cultural and political. This has distinct echoes of the notion of ethnie, discussed in Chapter 1, although the two are not one and the same, not least because not all ethnies become nations (Anthony Smith, 2009). However, for my purposes here, the two terms may be regarded as broadly comparable, or at least complementary.[2]

Following John Breuilly (1993) and Anthony Smith (1994), the ideology of nationalism can be broadly summarized as follows:

- The world is divided into nations, each with its own identity and destiny.
- The nation is the sole source of political power, and the interests and values of the nation take priority over all other interests and values – loyalty to the nation is pre-eminent.
- Everyone must belong to a nation, if everyone is to be truly free.
- To realize themselves, nations must be as politically independent as possible – political autonomy, or at least some degree of self-determination, is a central tenet of nationalism.
- To maintain peace and justice in the world, nations must be both sufficiently free and sufficiently secure to pursue their own (national) interests. (See Breuilly, 1993: 2; Anthony Smith, 1994: 379.)

Admittedly, it needs to be stressed here that the history of nationalism(s) is replete with numerous and wide variations. Accordingly, some commentators have despaired of finding, or even attempting a universal definition of nationalism (Tishkov, 2000). John Hall, for example, makes the blunt assertion that 'no single, universal theory of nationalism is possible. As the historical record is diverse, so too must be our concepts' (1993: 1). Other commentators, while not endorsing this degree of relativism, argue that explanations of nationalism must at least take due account of the temporal and societal context (see, for example, Gellner, 1983; Anthony Smith, 1995a, 2004a, b; R. Jenkins, 2007). However, these caveats notwithstanding, there is sufficient consistency among nationalist proponents to present the above as the 'core doctrine' of nationalism, particularly as it has been mobilized historically and politically in the establishment of 'nation-states'.

Which brings us to the 'state' and the 'nation-state'. The 'state', following Max Weber, has been defined in Western social science theory as an entity a) with political sovereignty over a clearly designated territorial area, b) with monopoly control of legitimate force and c) consisting of citizens with terminal loyalty to it (Giddens, 1984; Oommen, 1994). The 'nation-state' – the raison d'être of so many historical and current nationalisms – is the confluence of the nation and the state. As Gellner asserts in his hugely influential *Nations and Nationalism*, 'nationalism is *primarily* a political principle, which holds that the political and the national unit should be congruent' (1983: 1; my emphasis). In other words, the core tenet of what might be termed 'political nationalism' is the belief that 'the national state, identified with a national culture and committed to its protection, is the natural political unit' (Gellner, 1993: 409). It follows directly from this principle that all nations should aspire to be represented in and by a state of their own. Moreover, as Gellner's latter comment implies, once this coincidence of nation and state has occurred, the principal aim of the institutional nation-state is, recursively, to create (or *recreate*) and maintain a particular conception of nationhood and/or national identity. Thus, the Italian nationalist Massimo d'Azeglio could declare: 'We have made Italy, now we have to make Italians' (cited in Hobsbawm, 1990: 44). In so doing, the nation-state conflates the historical-cultural and the legal-political dimensions of nationhood in order to create a homogeneous national culture with which its members can identify and to which they will be committed. This is achieved principally through the establishment and promotion of a common language and civic culture, and via the agencies of the state – most notably, education.

The nation-state is thus a specifically modern phenomenon; the product, in effect, of the nationalism of the last two to three centuries. And yet, despite its historical recency, such is the pervasiveness of the nation-state in the modern world, and so unquestioned are the political principles upon which it is predicated, that it has come to be largely naturalized and taken for granted. So much so, in fact, that the 'nation-state' is often seen as synonymous with both 'society' and 'modernity'. The naturalization of the nation-state as the normative societal model in much social science commentary has been described as 'methodological nationalism' (Wimmer and Schiller, 2002). Zygmunt Bauman comments on its effects within Western social science generally, and sociology in particular:

> Sociology, as it came of age in the bosom of Western civilisation and as we know of it today, is endemically national-based. It does not recognise a totality broader than a politically organised [nation-state]: the term 'society' ... is, for all practical purposes, a name for an entity identical in size and composition with the nation-state. (1973: 42–3; see also Halle, 1962; Tilly, 1984)

Of the correspondence of modernity and the nation-state, Eric Hobsbawm asserts that 'the basic characteristic of the modern nation and everything associated with it is its modernity' (1990: 14). These two tenets combine when nation-states – or, more specifically, those 'nations' whose culture is currently represented within and by a 'state' – are compared with nations without a corresponding state. As David McCrone observes in this regard, of the early development of *British* sociology:

> British sociology simply accepted that 'society' was coterminous with the British state, unitary and highly centralised, driven by social change in the political and cultural heartland of southern Britain [i.e. England]. If there was a particular sociology of the 'periphery' – in Wales, Ireland and Scotland – it had to do with analysing a 'traditional', pre-capitalist way of life. It was judged to be the task of the sociologist of these parts merely to chart its decline and ultimate incorporation into 'modern' society, or so it seemed. (1992: 5)

And so, by implication, we return once again to the pejorative distinction between 'ethnicity' and the modern 'nation-state', first discussed in Chapter 1. However, we can also now specifically include within the former category the sublimation of 'national minorities', or nations not currently represented by a (corresponding) state. Hroch (1985, 1998) has described these as 'smaller nations'. Guibernau (1999) has termed them more accurately, albeit prosaically, as 'nations without states', while Keating (1996, 1997) refers to them as 'stateless nations'. In order to explore further the origins, nature and validity of the particular construction on which this distinction is based, I want now to turn to a closer examination of nationalism and the various debates and controversies which have surrounded it.

Linguistic nationalism

For many nationalists, nations are perennial; they have always existed in one form or another. In this view, modern nations can trace their antecedents to the Middle Ages and, in some cases, to 'nationes' in antiquity (Anthony Smith, 2004b). Relatedly, in a position that closely parallels the primordial conceptions of ethnicity, the enduring influence of nations, and nationhood, is explained by an ideology of pre-existing kinship or ethnic ties. From this, the nation is objectified via a range of 'national' characteristics – including language, history and a variety of specific cultural practices. Nationalists thus regularly invoke both primordial ties and the weight of history in their assertions of (and for) nationhood. Indeed, it is this 'deep-seated sense of kinship which infuses the nation' (Connor, 1993) that nationalist leaders have so effectively employed in mobilizing individual members of nations on behalf of nationalist causes.[3]

This view of nations as objective, pre-given and fixed social entities has been principally expounded by nationalists themselves, although it was also to gain some early currency in academic commentary on nationalism. Friedrich Schleiermacher (1768–1834), for example, viewed the nation as 'a natural division of the human race, endowed by God with its own character' (cited in Kedourie, 1960: 58). However, it was the late eighteenth-century triumvirate of Herder, Humboldt and Fichte – the 'German Romantics' as they have come to be known – who have been most closely associated with this essentialist position[4] in the social sciences. Thus, Johann Gottfried Herder (1744–1803) argued, along very much the same lines, for the divine inspiration of the nation as a natural form of human organization: 'a nation is as natural as a plant, as a family, only with more branches' (1969: 324; see Bauman and Briggs, 2003: Ch. 5, for further discussion). From this, Herder and Humboldt, and subsequently Fichte, were to advocate an 'organic' or 'linguistic' nationalism where culture – and particularly, language – was viewed as central to the essence or character (Volksgeist) of the nation. In this perspective, language came to be the *most* important distinguishing characteristic of nationhood – indeed, its very soul. The interrelationship between language and the soul or spirit of the nation is most clearly stated by Wilhelm von Humboldt (1767–1835): '[the nation's] language is its spirit and its spirit is its language' (see Cowan, 1963: 277). Or, as he observes elsewhere: 'From every language we can infer backwards to the national character' (Humboldt, 1988: 154). Indeed, Humboldt is credited as a result with the development of the twin theories of linguistic determinism and linguistic relativism – that language plays a significant role in determining culture, and that each language has a different way of 'looking at the world' (Clyne, 1997; Joseph, 2004; see Chapter 4). As Kedourie observes of the German Romantics, language was seen as 'an outward sign of a group's particular identity and a significant means of ensuring its continuation' (1960: 71). Or, put another way, the continuing existence of a nation was inconceivable without its own language. Without a language, Herder argued, a Volk is an absurdity (Unding), a contradiction in terms (see Barnard, 1965: 57).

The culturalist and linguistic emphases of the German Romantics – highlighting 'language, blood and soil' as constitutive elements of the Volk – were established in direct opposition to the political nationalism of the French Revolution and its associated notions of equality and popular sovereignty. Indeed, the anti-French feeling of Herder, Humboldt and Fichte, and their general ethnocentrism, are prominent features of their writings. Fichte (1762–1814) is the most extreme in this regard. In his *Addresses to the German Nation* (1807), he argued that of all the 'Teutonic' peoples only the Germans retained their original language: 'the German speaks a language which has been alive ever since it first issued from the force of nature, whereas the other Teutonic races speak a language which has movement on the surface but is dead at the root' (1968: 58–9). On the basis of this anthropomorphic view of language, Fichte asserted that if German was superior to all other languages, then on Herder's principle of the centrality of language to nationhood, the German nation was also, by definition, superior to all others. Consequently, Fichte has been attributed with extrapolating Herder's (and Humboldt's) ideas about language distinctiveness into the wider sociocultural and political arena (Kedourie, 1960).[5] Thus, for Fichte, 'it is beyond doubt that, wherever a separate language can be found, there a separate nation exists, which has the right to take charge of its independent affairs and govern itself' (1968: 184). Kedourie succinctly summarizes the logic of this process of extrapolation as follows: 'a group speaking the same language is known as a nation, and a nation ought to constitute a state' (1960: 68).

I will have much more to say about the interrelationship between language, ethnicity and nationalism in Chapter 4. There, I will outline why language *can* be regarded as a significant marker of ethnic and national identity, albeit, I hasten to add, definitively *not* a determining one, as the German Romantics would have it. Suffice it to say at this point that the arguments of linguistic nationalism lack any kind of purchase or credibility. The view of nations as both natural and linguistically determined – or, as Richard Handler describes it, as 'bounded cultural objects' (1988: 27) – is clearly essentialist and determinist. It is widely dismissed by most commentators on nationalism, many of whom have instead opted for an overtly *modernist* perspective. In this latter view, nations and nationalism are a recent historical phenomenon, grounded in modernity, and any sensible discussion of them must be underpinned by two key principles:

1   Attempts to adduce a clearly definable set of 'national' criteria (such as language, for example) simply cannot account for all contexts and variants. Consequently, more subjective criteria are necessary to describe effectively the formation of nations and national identities.
2   Modern nations can be distinguished quite clearly from their historical antecedents; the link between the two is not necessarily continuous.

I will deal with each of these key tenets in turn.

The will to nationhood

As I have argued in my discussion of ethnicity, objectivist definitions exclude as much as they include; there are always variants and exceptions that do not fit easily into an established schema of objective criteria. Hans Kohn, for example, argues that nationalities 'come into existence only when certain objective bonds delimit a social group' (1961: 3). However, he also quickly concedes that these 'bonds' are not sufficient in themselves to provide an adequate definition of the nation. This 'subjectivist' view was first articulated in the nineteenth century – generally, in direct response and opposition to the tenets of cultural and linguistic nationalism outlined earlier. One of the most notable early proponents of this more subjectivist account of nationhood was Ernest Renan (1823–92). In his lecture, 'Qu'est ce qu'une nation?', delivered at the Sorbonne on 11 March 1882, he argued that various objective criteria – language, religion, material interest, geography and 'race' – were all insufficient delimiters of the nation. In relation to language, for example, and in direct contravention to Fichte, he states: 'Language may invite us to unite but it does not compel us to do so' (1990: 16). This leads him to conclude that the nation is, in essence, 'a soul, a spiritual principle' (1990: 19) that is not directly linked to any particular objective marker(s).[6] Rather, two aspects constitute this principle for Renan, one of which lies in the past, one in the present:

One is the possession in common of a rich legacy of memories; the other is present-day consent, the desire to live together, the will to perpetuate the value of the heritage that one has received in an undivided form. A nation is therefore a large-scale solidarity ... It presupposes a past; it is summarised, however, in the present by a tangible fact, namely consent, the clearly expressed desire to continue a common life. A nation's existence is, if you will pardon the metaphor, a daily plebiscite ... (1990: 19)

The *will* to nationhood both unifies historical memory – that history 'received in an undivided form' – and secures present-day consent. The former requires some serious forgetting, or sublimating, of countervailing and contradictory histories. As Renan famously observes, 'forgetting, I would even go so far as to say historical error, is a crucial factor in the creation of a nation' (1990: 11). The latter implies a continual renegotiation of the boundaries of consent – the desire to live together: 'the wish of nations is, all in all, the sole legitimate criterion, the one to which one must always return' (1990: 20). Both dimensions suggest our active participation in the *construction* of nationhood; that is, the construction of a particular 'discourse on society that *performs* the problem of totalizing the people and unifying the national will' (Bhabha, 1994: 160–1).

Max Weber, in his essay on the structures of power, reaches some remarkably similar conclusions. Near the outset of his brief analysis of the nation, he states:

If the concept of 'nation' can in any way be defined unambiguously, it certainly cannot be stated in terms of empirical qualities common to those who count as members of the nation. In the sense of those using the term at a given time, the concept undoubtedly means, above all, that one may exact from certain groups of men [sic] a specific sentiment of solidarity in the face of other groups. *Thus, the concept belongs in the sphere of values.* Yet, there is no agreement on how these groups should be delimited or about what concerted action should result from such solidarity. (1961: 172; my emphasis)

Weber's analysis, like Renan's, suggests the constructed nature of nationhood; its place 'in the sphere of values'. As a result, Weber goes on to explore, and discount, a number of commonly invoked prerequisites of nationhood. With regard to a common language, for example, he suggests that 'national solidarity among men [sic] speaking the same language may be just as well rejected as accepted' (1961: 173). Likewise, he dismisses the notion of 'ethnic solidarity' as a *sufficient* condition of nationhood, although he does concede that 'the idea of the "nation" is apt to include the notions of common descent and of an essential, *though frequently indefinite,* homogeneity' (1961: 173; my emphasis), a point to which I will return.

The conclusions drawn by Renan and Weber clearly emphasize the subjective over the objective in the development of nationhood; a central characteristic of modernist accounts. The will to nationhood, in Renan's evocative terms, is both a conscious choice and a particular construction of history and therefore cannot be equated directly with pre-existing ethnic, cultural and/or linguistic communities. This position seems to be given credence by the many instances where the use of objective 'national' criteria is shown to be clearly inadequate as a predictor of nationhood and nationalism. With regard to ethnic affiliation, for example, Connor (1991) notes that modern Greeks are not descended from their alleged ancestors, the ancient Hellenes, but from Slavs who first migrated to mainland Greece in the sixth century AD. Language and religion are also problematic as national indicators. Language may or may not be a key focus of national identity, as seen in the nationalist movements of Wales and Scotland respectively. Even where it is, as in Wales, it may not be so across the population as a whole (see Chapter 7). Likewise, religion differs in significance from one national context to another. For example, the Catholic/Protestant religious divide is a principal factor in nationalist struggles in Northern Ireland but not in Scotland.[7] More complicated still, objective characteristics such as religion and language may vary in salience both internally within a national group and across different historical periods. When the Belgium state was established in 1830, for instance, religious differences were far more important than linguistic ones. However, since the early 1960s, there has been far greater emphasis in Belgium on the linguistic differentiation between French and Flemish speakers (Blommaert, 1996; Mnookin and Verbeke, 2009; see Chapter 5). A similar trend is observable in Quebec where nationalist claims since the Quiet Revolution, with its genesis also in the early 1960s, have focused increasingly on the French language at the expense of an earlier focus on Catholicism (Handler, 1988; Oakes and Warren, 2007; see Chapter 7).

In short, no single distinguishing feature fits all national contexts. As Anthony Smith observes, 'a national identity is fundamentally multidimensional; it can never be reduced to a single element' (1991: 14). The strident claims of linguistic nationalism can thus be safely dismissed since language, it seems, is only one of many characteristics, which may (or may not) be salient at any given time and place. Where national symbols do achieve significance in particular national contexts, and/or in particular historical periods, it is principally because of their role in differentiating 'us' from 'them'. As Armstrong (1982) observes, objectified national characteristics act in this way as symbolic 'border guards'. These border guards are closely linked to specific cultural codes and function to identify people as members or non-members of the specific national collectivity. This is not too dissimilar a position to a situational account of ethnicity with its emphasis on ethnic boundaries (cf. Barth, 1969a, b).

The modern (nation-)state

The second, and related, tenet of the modernist position on nationalism is the argument that modern nations are just that – modern – and thus fundamentally distinct from previous forms of collective organization. In short, modernists proclaim that nations – by which they actually invariably mean nation-*states* (see below) – are the product of the age of nationalism.[8] Moreover, it is argued that this age of nationalism arose out of the specific historical and social developments of modernization and its concomitants – industrialization, political democracy, and universal literacy – in eighteenth- and nineteenth-century Europe. Prior to this, the feudal, dynastic and largely agrarian societies of the day had little notion of national sentiment – those feelings of collective 'national' belonging – that characterizes the modern nation. In this view, to equate the modern nation with its ancient predecessors is to commit the sin of 'retrospective nationalism'. As Anthony Smith summarizes it: 'according to the modernist perspective, nations and nationalism are not logically contingent; they are sociologically necessary only in the modern world' (1994: 377).

The important distinctions between premodern and modern nations highlighted by modernists can be summarized as follows. First, modern nations tend to be equated directly with their political representation in the nation-state. In other words, modern nations are seen as 'mass' nations, based on the notion of universal enfranchisement, and with the specific goal of administrative and political representation in the form of the nation-state (Anthony Smith, 1995a). In this, they are a product of post-Enlightenment political rationalism and the ideology of nationalism, both of which emerged only in the eighteenth century. One only has to look to the nation-states that comprise the United Nations to confirm this since most did not exist, either in name or as an administrative unit, more than two centuries ago. Indeed, as Immanuel Wallerstein argues, there are actually very few nation-states that can trace a name and a continuous administrative entity in a particular geographical area to a period prior to 1450. Of some 200 contemporary nation-states, perhaps only France, Russia, Portugal, Denmark, Sweden, Switzerland, Morocco, Japan, China, Iran and Ethiopia can claim such a lineage. However, even these claims are somewhat problematic since it can still be argued that these states came into existence as modern sovereign nation-states only with the emergence of the present world system. A number of other modern nation-states such as Egypt, India and Greece have perhaps had a longer lineage but theirs has been discontinuous (see Wallerstein, 1991: 80–1).

Second, and relatedly, the term 'nation' in its modern sense embodies two interrelated meanings – the 'nation' as the people living *within* a nation-state and the 'nation' as *the* nation-state (Billig, 1995). Accordingly, the modern nation is viewed as both an 'historical culture-community' and a 'legal-political' one

(Anthony Smith, 1995a), with the latter invariably taking precedence over the former. These two dimensions, and their coalescence in the institutionalized nation-state, are again products of the ideology of political nationalism. Thus, on the one hand, nationalism legitimates the construction of a particular sense of national identity for those historical culture-communities that are said to inhabit their own nation-state. This involves the exercise of *internal* political and legal jurisdiction over its citizens and the construction (or attempted construction) of a homogeneous national culture in which political and ethnic boundaries are seen to coincide (Gellner, 1983). On the other hand, political nationalism also includes the general principle that nations should, if at all possible, possess their own state. For already established nation-states this latter principle involves the exercise of *external* rights to sovereignty and self-government in the present inter-state system, along with the defence of these rights – by war if necessary. For those historical culture-communities that do not currently possess their own state, this principle is expressed via the many secessionist and irredentist nationalist movements in the world today.

Third, the link between the modern nation, and its institutional embodiment in the nation-state, is further predicated on the rise of a bureaucratic state organization, a capitalist economy, and a 'high' literate and scientific culture; the latter based, usually, on a single and distinctive vernacular language. All of these are characteristic of modernization (see below). In contrast, previous cultural communities tended to be localized, largely illiterate, and culturally and linguistically heterogeneous (Birch, 1989; Hutchinson, 1994).

In the modernist view then, nations (as represented in and by the nation-state) are the product of very specific social, economic and political circumstances. Their emergence as the primary social community in the modern era is directly related to the advent of modernization and the concomitant rise of the state and the ideology of nationalism. This is an important qualification to Renan's and Weber's emphasis on the 'will to nationhood' discussed earlier. As Gellner (1964, 1983, 1997) argues, for example, the volitional aspect of nationhood is an important but insufficient identifier of the modern nation since other collectivities have also possessed this in various historical periods. In Gellner's view, the emergence of the modern nation is thus primarily associated with the structural changes brought about by modernization.

Following from this, some modernist commentators – Hobsbawm (1990) and Balibar (1991) to name just two – argue that any attempt to present the nation as a natural and/or ancient form of human organization must involve what we saw described in our discussion of ethnicity in Chapter 1 as 'the invention of tradition'. Like proponents of a situational view of ethnicity, such commentators view nations as, at best, socially constructed and, at worst, simply invented. That said, the degree to and fervor with which this constructionist position is held varies considerably among modernist commentators on nationalism, as does the related disavowal of any link between nationhood and a pre-existing ethnicity. With respect to the latter, some do acknowledge, albeit begrudgingly, a connection between ethnicity and nationhood (see, for example, Gellner, 1983, 1997; Anderson, 1991), while others, such as Hobsbawm (1990), argue that the two phenomena are entirely unrelated. But, these differences notwithstanding, modernists *are* all agreed that nationhood is the *result* of political modernization – expressed in nationalism and the construction of the nation-state – and *not* the result of pre-existing ethnicity.

The modernists

The preceding discussion suggests that what is broadly termed the modernist position on nationalism is by no means undifferentiated. In particular, modernists differ over the historical timing of nationalism and the nation-states to which it gave rise, and over the key influences which have surrounded the development of nationalism. In relation to the historicity of nationalism, a range of starting points is offered. Hans Kohn (1961) and Liah Greenfeld (1992) suggest the seventeenth-century British rebellion against the monarchy, Anderson (1991) the American Revolution, Best (1988) and Alter (1989) the French Revolution, and Kedourie (1960) and Breuilly (1993) the German response of the German Romantics (Herder et al.) to the political implications of the French Revolution.[9] All broadly agree, however, about the historical recency of nationalism[10] and its rapid and widespread development. As Best (1982) succinctly observes, by the beginning of the nineteenth century the world was full of it.

Modernist writers also attribute a range of key influences to the rise of nationalism. Gellner (1964, 1983, 1997) has argued, for example, that the emergence of nationalism is predicated on the impact of industrialization, Anderson (1991) on the role of print capitalism, and Giddens (1984), Brubaker (1996) and Breuilly (1993, 2005a, b) on the development of the modern state and its institutional mechanisms.

It is not my intention here to explore in any depth the full range of modernist theories; there are numerous books already devoted to such a task.[11] However, I do intend to examine in some detail two exemplars of this position – Ernest Gellner (1983) and Benedict Anderson (1991). These two theorists illustrate the modernist position writ large and their work on nationalism has been particularly prominent and influential. As we shall see, both theorists also highlight the interconnections between nationalism, language and education, a concern which is central to this account and which will be explored more fully in the following chapters.

Gellner's theory of industrialization

In his seminal book, *Nations and Nationalism* (1983), Gellner argues that the rise of nationalism cannot simply be explained ideologically – that is, as the result of a contest of ideas – but must be rooted in the material changes brought about in Europe at the end of the eighteenth century by industrialization. In this, his analysis is essentially functionalist, although it bears similarities to some Marxist perspectives on nationalism.[12] For Gellner, nationalism developed within the context of the transition from traditional agrarian societies to modern industrial societies. In the former, literacy performed a specialized function and, along with occupational mobility, was limited to a small elite. Mass public education was unheard of. Political control was also largely decentralized and populations spoke a variety of languages and dialects. Localism in both speech form and cultural identification was the norm and, consequently, there was little, if any, emphasis on achieving a uniform state culture. As Gellner observes, 'what is virtually inconceivable within such a system is a serious and sustained drive for linguistic and cultural homogeneity ... Both the will and the means [and, one might add, the *need*] for such an aspiration are conspicuously lacking' (1987: 15).

Thus, prior to industrialization, political forms of organization required neither the demarcation of clear territorial boundaries nor the fostering of internal integration and homogeneity. Feudal elites, for example, controlled wide territories but exercised little centralized control. Empires, larger in scale again, demanded political loyalty from their diverse people groups and acceptance of one's place in the social/political hierarchy, but made little, if any, demands for cultural and linguistic homogeneity (Grillo, 1998). As long as due honor was given to Caesar and taxes were paid, all was well.

In contrast, the modern industrialized society – with its literate, mobile and occupationally specialized division of labor – required cultural and linguistic continuity and, where possible, cultural and linguistic homogeneity in order to function effectively. While work in premodern society had been predominantly manual, work in modern industrial society was now predominantly semantic (Anthony Smith, 1998). The latter also required its workers to be 'substitutable'. In effect, workers had to be able to cope with and move between the increasingly complex and differentiated roles created by the division of labor. What made the individual substitutable in this way was a significant degree of cultural and linguistic *standardization*. Here the development of a standardized, context-free and unitary language becomes crucial, with this in turn facilitating and reflecting the development of a 'high' literate and, crucially, *common*, culture.

In his earlier 1964 account, *Thought and Change*, Gellner had placed greatest emphasis on the role of a unitary language as the cement of modern society – bringing together a wide range of people from different regions and backgrounds in developing urban centres. However, by the time of *Nations and Nationalism*, language, though still a factor, had come to be viewed as subsidiary to the role of mass education systems in establishing an effective common culture (see Laitin, 1998; O'Leary, 1998; Anthony Smith, 2004b) – a process he describes as 'exo-socialization'. For Gellner, mass education – established, maintained and monitored by the state – provided the literacy and 'technological competence' necessary for producing 'full' or 'effective' citizens in modern industrial societies.

The principle of 'one state, one culture' thus saw the state, via its education system, increasingly identified with a *specific* language and culture (Taylor, 1998). As Gellner asserts: 'whereas in the past the connection [between state and culture] was thin, fortuitous, varied, loose and often minimal ... now it [became] unavoidable. That is what nationalism is all about ...' (1983: 38). The result was the emergence of the nation-state in which cultural and political boundaries were seen to conveniently converge. In Gellner's view, the rise of nationalism is thus inextricably linked to the *prior* development of a strong state culture *from which* a homogeneous nation could be shaped. As he observes:

It is not the case that the 'age of nationalism' is a mere summation of the awakening and political self-assertion of this, that, or the other nation. Rather when general social conditions make for standardised, homogeneous, centrally sustained high cultures, pervading ethnic populations and not just elite minorities, a situation arises in which *well-defined educationally sanctioned and unified cultures* constitute very nearly the only kind of unity with which men willingly and often ardently identify. The cultures now seem to be the natural repositories of political legitimacy. Only *then* does it come to appear that any defiance of their boundaries by political units constitutes a scandal. (1983: 55; my emphasis in the first instance)

Gellner's analysis situates nationalism in the social, economic and political changes attendant upon modernism, while also linking nationalism specifically to the development of a literate, national 'high' culture. Nationalism has flourished, he suggests, because 'well-defined, educationally sanctioned and unified cultures', as he puts it, offer a path to modernity, a basis of political legitimacy, and a means of shared cultural and linguistic identity.

Anderson's 'imagined communities'

Benedict Anderson's likening of the modern nation to an 'imagined political community' evokes a similar conception. In his equally influential analysis of nationalism, Anderson argues that all national communities are '*imagined* because the members of even the smallest nation will never know most of their fellow-members, meet them, or even hear of them, yet in the minds of each lives the image of their communion' (1991: 6). This is not to say that a sense of national consciousness or identity is *imaginary*. It is merely to suggest that the idea of a collective 'national' community, like all large-scale collectivities, has to be *specifically* and *consciously* cultivated, since it involves conceiving of something that is beyond one's immediate day-to-day experience. As he outlines, 'my point of departure is that nationality, or, as one might prefer to put it in view of that word's multiple significations, nation-ness, as well as nationalism, are cultural artefacts of a particular kind' (1991: 4).

Anderson argues that the development of the modern nation 'conceived as a solid community moving steadily down (or up) history' (1991: 26) arose from the congruence of industrial capitalism and print technology in fifteenth- and sixteenth-century Europe. The convergence of capitalism and print technology at this time saw the rapid spread in print of previously localized vernacular languages, aided in part also by the Protestant drive to vernacularize scripture. These developments gave a new fixity to language and created unified fields of exchange and communication below Latin (the dominant administrative language of the day in Europe) and above the spoken vernaculars. They were also aided by the concurrent, albeit haphazard, elevation of vernaculars as languages of political administration. As a result, vernacular languages came to assume many of the administrative functions previously enjoyed only by Latin and rose to be 'languages-of-power'. As speakers of languages with widely different dialects became capable of comprehending one another, via print, they also came to recognize themselves as belonging to one particular language (and cultural) group among many. With the advent of modernization and the increasing centralization of state control, this was to lead, in turn, to an emerging sense of national consciousness. Via this process a *shared* sense of a particular nation's history – along with its associated language(s) and cultural symbols – began to be cultivated.

Anderson argues that this emerging national consciousness 'could arise historically only when substantial groups of people were in a position to think of themselves as living lives *parallel* to those of other substantial groups of people – if never meeting, yet certainly proceeding along the same trajectory' (1991: 188). In this way, a new kind of indirect relationship was formed in which the biographies of individuals, and the nation as a whole, could be joined in a common historical narrative (Calhoun, 1993a). We may all have our own personal histories but the claim to nationhood provides us with a *collective* sense of history:

- by linking us to past and future generations,
- by situating us in the global context as a member of one nation among many,
- by providing formal equivalence for us as one member among many of a specific nation.

As I have already discussed, other modernist commentators (see, for example, Hobsbawm and Ranger, 1983; Hobsbawm, 1990; Balibar, 1991) would suggest at this point that the construction of such collective histories is largely, even entirely, fictive, recalling Renan's earlier observation about the primacy of 'historical error' (1990: 11) in many national histories. If we take British history as just one example, we can see this demonstrated in the invented traditions of Scottish tartans and Highland culture (Trevor-Roper, 1983) and the druidic inventions of the Welsh eisteddfodau (see Chapter 7), both developed only in the nineteenth century. A similar process of historical (re)creation can be seen in the supposed centrality of the monarchy to conceptions of British identity (Cannadine, 1983; Kumar, 2003; Colley, 2009).

This 'inventionist' position, most trenchantly outlined by Hobsbawm (1990), has clear parallels with Roosens's (1989) account of the construction of Huron ethnicity discussed in Chapter 1. Anderson, however, is less concerned here with outlining a moral(ist) position on nationalism (a feature of much political and social science commentary, dating from Lord Acton's critical account in 1862). He argues simply that *all* modern nations are imagined in this way. It is not so much the falsity/genuineness of nations which is thus in question but the *style* in which they are imagined. In this sense, Anderson adopts a position that is closer to earlier modernists such as Kedourie (1960), Deutsch (1966), Seton-Watson (1977) and Tilly (1975). These earlier commentators highlighted the fictive elements of nation-formation. However, they also assumed that nations, once formed, were real communities of culture and power; a Durkheimian 'social fact', in effect (Anthony Smith, 1995b, 2004b).

Like Gellner then, Anderson asserts that the rise of nationalism has *effected* the construction of the modern nation as we know it in its nation-state form – an anonymous, socially differentiated and large-scale collectivity with its basis in the categorical relationships of equivalent individuals (see also Calhoun, 1993a, b, 1997). The sense of commonality that results has seen 'the "imagined community" ... spread out to every conceivable contemporary society' (1991: 157). Nonetheless, the nation and nationality are, for all that, still cultural artifacts. Nationalism has produced nations (as nation-states) and national identity, not the other way around.

Limits of the modernist account

Modernist accounts of nationalism appear, at first brush, to be particularly compelling. They certainly effectively repudiate the claims of many nationalists that 'their' nations are perennial; highlighting, instead, their very specific emergence in the modern, post-Enlightenment era, via the nation-state model. Along with most commentators on nationalism, I broadly concur with these analyses, at least with respect to the issue of historical recency (although see

Anthony Smith, 2008). However, modernist conceptions of nationalism and national identity, in rightly situating nation-states within the modern era, may have overstated the supposed radical disjuncture between pre-existing ethnicity and nation-state formation. This is because the more trenchant modernists also regularly argue that nationalism creates nations/nation-states ex nihilo (Anthony Smith, 2004b). In so doing, they ignore the often-crucial role that cultural (and linguistic) antecedents play in the formation of national identities. This is a similar weakness to constructionist accounts of ethnicity, discussed in Chapter 1, which disavowed any meaningful role for language and culture in relation to ethnic identity formation.

Modernists have thus been rightly skeptical of primordial/perennial accounts that attempt to 'naturalize' nationhood via a pre-existing ethnicity and/or language, and have also highlighted the apparent disjunctures between modern nation-states and earlier collectivities. However, on this basis, modernists cannot account for the ongoing *persistence* of nationalism in the modern world – particularly in situations where political modernization has already been achieved. After all, the logic of the modernist argument is that as nationalism supersedes ethnicity, so should internationalism replace nationalism as the next stage of the modernization process. Instead, neither has really occurred. The rise today of an increasing internationalization appears *in conjunction with* nationalism rather than as a replacement for it (Robertson, 1992; Held et al., 1999; James, 2006; see Chapter 1). Likewise, ethnicity continues to feature prominently in relationship to nationalism, as the increasing proliferation of 'ethnonationalisms' in the modern world highlights (Conversi, 2002; Fenton and May, 2002).

Part of this inability to predict the ongoing salience of ethnicity and nationalism, and their interconnections, can be explained by Anthony Smith's observation that, in rejecting primordial accounts entirely, modernist commentators on nationalism have confused individual and collective levels of ethnicity. As I argued in Chapter 1, we may, as individuals, demonstrate a considerable degree of latitude in our attachment to and choice of particular social and political identities. As such, ethnic choices and identifications may vary in their salience – both in themselves, and in relation to other social identities – at any given time and place. However, this view needs to be balanced by the recognition that 'at the collective as opposed to the individual level, ethnicity remains a powerful, explosive and durable force' (Anthony Smith, 1995a: 34).

Some modernists have countered here with an economic 'core–periphery' explanation, that ethnonationalism persists because modernization proceeded unequally, leading to the uneven economic development of certain historical, cultural and linguistic groups within particular nation-states and, thus, to the growth of ethnonationalist movements (see, for example, Deutsch, 1966; Wallerstein, 1979). An obvious example here is the 'internal colonialist' thesis advanced by Hechter (1975; see also Nairn, 1981). Hechter argued that uneven economic development in Britain led to a stratified 'cultural division of labor' in the 'Celtic fringe' of Wales, Ireland and Scotland that, in turn, could account for their respective nationalisms:

> To the extent that social stratification in the periphery is based on observable cultural differences, there exists the probability that the disadvantaged group will, in time, reactively assert its own culture as equal or superior to that of the relatively advantaged core. This may help it conceive of itself as a separate 'nation' and seek independence. (1975: 10)

However, the model of internal colonialism has since been widely contested. McCrone (1992, 1998), for example, points out that while the Scottish Highlands, or Gaeltachd, could be seen as a suitably appropriate example of the model, the 'culturally anglicized' and 'overdeveloped' Lowlands of Scotland certainly are not. Likewise, in relation to Wales, internal colonialism considerably understates the centrality of south Wales to the rapid development and expansion of *British* industrialization (Gwyn Williams, 1982, 1985). In Williams's view, the industrialized south of Wales was no mere satellite of an imperial economic core based in London, as Hechter would have it. Rather, the imperial core came to Wales. This can be demonstrated by the huge influx of migrants to the area in the late nineteenth century, and by the consequent reconstruction of local Welsh issues and concerns as British ones (Colin Williams, 1994; see Chapter 7).

If one looks more widely, the relatively prosperous Catalan, Basque and Québécois nationalist movements also illustrate the limits of the core–periphery approach. The Catalan national minority, for example, was politically and culturally oppressed under Franco's fascist regime until his death in 1975. However, the Catalan region itself has been historically one of the strongest economic regions in Spain. Thus, in 1980, Catalans comprised 16 percent of the Spanish population but 20 percent of GDP, while per capita income was 30 percent above the Spanish average. Moreover, this longstanding economic and demographic power had, in the nineteenth century, formed the basis of the cosmopolitan and high culture Catalan language movements Renaixença and Modernista (Miller and Miller, 1996; see Chapter 7).

In short, while adverse economic factors may play a significant part in some ethnonationalist movements, they are not a *sufficient* explanation for the ongoing prominence of such movements in the modern world. Moreover, economic considerations aside, a modernist conception still cannot answer the question of *why* ethnicity – as opposed to religion, regionalism or class, for example – is so often chosen as the principal focus of nationalist mobilization. Nor can it explain why ethnonational claims persist, even when such claims may entrench, rather than ameliorate socioeconomic and/or political disadvantage – that is, when there appears to be no immediate (or even long-term) 'pay off' (see Anthony Smith, 1998: 63–9; cf. Chapter 1).

Ethno-symbolic accounts of nationalism

For a more adequate explanation, we need to consider an approach that returns ethnicity and ethnic identity to the study of nationalism.[13] As Richard Jenkins argues, if the concept of nationalism 'is to retain its analytical value, the varieties of what we persist in calling "nationalism" must also have something in common' (1995: 369). On this basis, he concludes: 'Although not the only common thread – political membership conceived as citizenship might be another – ethnicity, personal and collective identity which draws upon a repertoire of perceived cultural differences, is the most ubiquitous and plausible' (ibid.).

Ethno-symbolic analyses of nationalism, championed most prominently by Anthony Smith and John Hutchinson (see n. 1), provide us with the strongest, most effective, means of explicating the links between ethnicity and nationalism. Ethno-symbolic approaches accept many of the tenets of the modernist thesis – particularly the recency of nationalism, and the, at times, constructed nature of national identity. However, they also directly address three of its key weaknesses: its historicity, its conflation of the 'nation' and the 'nation-state' and its separation of political and ethnic nationalism(s) (see also Castells, 1997). I will deal with each of these key issues in turn.

Historical continuity

First, while ethno-symbolic commentators acknowledge the distinctive characteristics of the modern nation, they also argue that the processes of nation formation need to be examined within and through a longer, more cyclical account of history than modernist accounts usually allow (Hutchinson, 2005; Anthony Smith, 2008). To this end, ethno-symbolic analyses have attempted to distinguish national sentiment – understood here as those feelings of collective belonging to a nation – from the ideology and movement of nationalism itself. This is important because, as Anthony Smith (1994, 1998, 2008) argues, one can have nationalist movements and ideologies among a given population without any corresponding diffusion of national sentiment in that population. The reverse can also be found, and it is from this latter scenario that historians such as Seton-Watson (1977), Armstrong (1982), Hroch (1985), Greenfeld (1992), and Colley (2009) have convincingly argued that the emergence of national sentiment was evident some centuries before the development of nationalism itself.

This more diachronic approach – examining nation formation over the longue durée – does not necessarily entail a perennial view of nations (see

Anthony Smith, 1998: 159–76). Rather, it attempts to situate nationalism within a wider theory of ethnic formation, emphasizing *commonalities* as well as *differences* between the premodern and modern eras. As Anthony Smith argues, while ethno-symbolic accounts share the modernist view of the historical embeddedness of nations and nationalism, they reject their 'relatively restrictive definition or periodisation' (2009: 29), which ruptures nation-state formation from any connection with pre-existing ethnies. The rise of nationalism and the nation-state *has* been shaped by premodern ethnic identities (ethnies), whatever modernists might say, and thus can be situated within a larger cycle of ethnic resurgence and decline in history.[14] Smith's position specifically links 'the consequences of modernity with an understanding of the continuing role played by cultural ties and ethnic identities which originated in premodern epochs' (1995a: 47). Richard Jenkins reiterates this view in his observation that 'nationalism is an aspect of the growth of ... complex political units, based, to some degree, on notions of ethnic and cultural commonality (however much, *pace* Anderson, imagined)' (1995: 370).

Following this argument, the formation of modern nations is seen to involve the appropriation of some of the key attributes of pre-existing ethnies. In the process, many extant memories, myths and symbols are assimilated, while additional ones are invented where necessary. These cultural elements, in combination, play a key role in establishing a common (national) consciousness and a related symbolic repertoire, including language, religion, customs and institutions. This process, in turn, provides a sense of historical continuity for particular national groups (Anthony Smith, 2009). Elites have a key role, to be sure, in propagating such national(ist) histories, as modernists have been quick to point out. However, as with comparable debates in ethnicity (see Chapter 1), modern national cultures are not wholly inventions, even if they do clearly contain within them some fictive elements. Rather, 'they are connected to, and often continuous with, much older cultures which the modernizing nationalists adapt and standardize' (Anthony Smith, 2004b: 72) to their own ends. Cultural continuity – and for our purposes, linguistic continuity also – is not the same as cultural fixity.

Crucially, this view also allows us to extend the principle of nation formation beyond established nation-states to include those nations which are currently not represented by a corresponding state (see below), something not countenanced in modernist accounts. Thus, for example, the modern Breton nationalist movement draws heavily on the persistence of Breton traditions, myths, memories and symbols (including language) which have survived, in various forms, throughout the period of French domination since 1532. Likewise, Catalan nationalism – first instigated in 1880, revived in the 1930s, and again in the 1980s – draws on Catalonia's long maritime history and the attraction and prestige of the Catalan language and culture (Castells, 1997; see

Chapter 7). Accordingly, the difference between modern nations and ethnies becomes a question of degree rather than kind. As Richard Jenkins observes, 'the boundary between "ethnicism" and "nationalism" ... becomes indeterminate, lying somewhere along a continuum of change within historically evolving traditions or universes of discourses' (1995: 372).

In adopting a more evolutionary position, however, ethno-symbolic commentators do not make the mistake of assuming a *causal* relationship between prior ethnies and the subsequent formation of modern nations. As Hutchinson observes, 'to do so without empirical examination is to make uncritical assumptions about continuities between premodern ethnic and modern national identities and to fall into the post hoc ergo propter hoc fallacy' (1994: 26: see also Fishman, 1989b, c). Nonetheless, they hold that modernists have drawn the distinction between modern nations and premodern ethnic communities too starkly. Thus, a modernist account such as Gellner's can be criticized for its teleological overtones in emphasizing a single and revolutionary transition from preindustrial to industrial society as an explanation for nationalism.[15] Gellner's difficulty here is that in many contexts nationalism predates industrialization. In Serbia, Ireland, Mexico and Japan, to name just a few examples, there was no industrial development at the time that nationalism emerged in these contexts. One could even argue that nationalism was already a significant force before the onset of industrialization in France and Germany (Anthony Smith, 1998, 2008). The role of mass education as an agent of nationalism may be similarly overstated, since nationalist movements again often predated the former (Hroch, 1985, 1993). Relatedly, the advent of industrialization also at times significantly predated formal education, most notably Britain where mass education was not established formally until 1870, some one hundred years after the advent of industrialization there.

In ethno-symbolic accounts then, nationalism is viewed not only as a means to achieve modernity but also, crucially, as a means of (re)creating a sense of distinctive collective identity and autonomy (Hutchinson, 1994, 2005). The nation is not seen just as a *political* community represented by the nation-state, as in modernist accounts of nationalism. It is viewed also as an *ethnocultural* community that may or may not be so represented and yet which is still shaped by shared myths of origins, and a sense of common history and ways of life. Moreover, it is principally this latter dimension, the 'inner world' of ethnicity and nationalism (Anthony Smith, 2009: 23), which endows its members with identity and purpose. The motive force of nationalism here, its emotional reach and pull among the wider population (and not just elites), is something modernist accounts are not able adequately to explain. In this sense, nationalism and national identity can be understood in relation to the notion of habitus and field, and to the related limits concerning the constructedness of ethnic identities, discussed in Chapter 1. Bhikhu Parekh argues, for example, that national identity is a process of self-creation that does not occur in a historical vacuum. Rather,

> A [national] community *inherits* a specific way of life ... which sets limits to how and how much it can change itself. The change is lasting and deep if it is grafted on the community's suitably reinterpreted deepest tendencies and does not go against the grain. A community's political [and cultural] identity then is neither unalterable and fixed, nor a voluntarist project to be executed as it pleases, but a matter of *slow* self-recreation within the limits set by its past. (1995: 264; my emphases[16])

Such a position shifts the focus away from the increasingly arid debates surrounding the historical and political legitimacy of nationalism. As Joshua Fishman has argued, in an essay first published in 1972, 'we must not ask if [nationalism] is "good", if it is "justified", if it is based on "valid arguments". Rather, we must ask "why does it occur, and when, and how can its obvious power be most productively channelled"?' (1989b: 104). These questions are crucial to unraveling the ongoing salience and alliance of ethnicity and nationalism in the modern world. By attending to the popular base and cultural framework of nationalism – an area which modernists have seen fit to ignore – ethno-symbolic accounts provide us with a plausible explanation to these questions. After all, it is not chronological or factual history that is the key to the nation but *sentient* or *felt* history (Connor, 1993).[17] As Craig Calhoun observes, 'ethnicity or cultural traditions are bases for nationalism when they effectively constitute historical memory, when they inculcate it as habitus ... not when (or because) the historical origins they claim are accurate' (1993a: 222).

Uncoupling the nation-state

In so doing, an ethno-symbolic approach also allows us to untangle the confluence of the historical-cultural and legal-political dimensions of nationhood as they have come to be represented in the institutionalized form of the nation-state. As I have already suggested, this has arisen from the central principle of political nationalism – nation-state congruence – which holds that the boundaries of political and national identity should coincide. The view here is that people who are citizens of a particular state should also, ideally, be members of the same national collectivity. Gellner's definition of nationalism as a 'theory of political legitimacy which requires that ethnic boundaries should not cut across political ones' (1983: 1) clearly illustrates this standpoint. The end result of nationalism, in this view, is the establishment of the ethnically exclusive and culturally homogeneous nation-state.

This attempt to make both state and national culture coextensive entities has resulted in the nation-state system as we know it today and continues to form the basis of many of the current nationalist claims for self-determination. And yet, interestingly, the earliest uses of the term 'nationalism' did not actually conflate the nation and the state in this way (Connor, 1978). However, by the nineteenth century nationalist doctrine had come to hold that nation and state were coterminous; that every nation deserved a state. Not only this, an important corollary had also by then emerged – that each state should represent one nation. As Gellner describes it, nationalism holds that the nation and state 'were destined for each other; that either without the other is incomplete, and constitutes a tragedy' (1983: 6). Max Weber would appear to concur in his observation that 'a nation is a community which normally tends to produce a state of its own' (1961: 176). This crucial interlinking of the idea of nation and its political representation in the state is perhaps not too surprising. As Immanuel Wallerstein observes:

> Why should the establishment of any particular sovereign state within the interstate system create a corresponding 'nation', a 'people'? This is not really difficult to understand. The evidence is all around us. States in this system have problems of cohesion. Once recognised as sovereign, the states frequently find themselves subsequently threatened by both internal disintegration and external aggression. To the extent that 'national' sentiment develops, these threats are lessened. The governments in power have an interest in promoting this sentiment, as do all sorts of subgroups within the state ... States furthermore have an interest in administrative uniformity that increases the efficacy of their policies. Nationalism is the expression, the promoter and the consequence of such state-level uniformities. (1991: 81–2)

Wallerstein argues, along with other modernist commentators, that nationalism arose *out of* the emergence of the modern state system: 'in almost every case statehood precede[s] nationhood' (1991: 81). Political expression in the form of the nation-state thus *legitimates* and *institutionalizes* nationhood. However, a sense of national sentiment is also at the same time promoted by the agencies of the state – particularly education and the media – and this acts recursively to maintain the nation-state's internal cohesion. This, in turn, provides a basis on which to counter possible outside threats to its autonomy. The state's role is thus crucial in accomplishing the three recurrent goals of nationalism that I outlined at the beginning of this chapter – national identity, national unity and national autonomy (see Anthony Smith, 1994, 1998, 2008). The process of imbuing citizenship with 'national' sentiment also helps to explain for modernists why 'national' identities commonly 'trump' other personal or group identities (Calhoun, 1993a).

The principal difficulty with the formulation of nation-state congruence, however, is *its inability to accommodate and/or recognize the legitimate claims of nations without states, or national minorities*. This limitation has both a theoretical and a practical dimension. Theoretically, the conflation of the nation and the state assumes that the two concepts are reducible to each other when they clearly are not. Nations are often but *not always* represented in and by a (nation-)state. Or, to put it another way, *citizenship* does not always equate directly with *nationality*. Practically, and following from this, the 'nation-state' is actually a misnomer since its construction as ethnically exclusive and culturally homogeneous is directly contradicted by demographic and political realities.

In relation to nations without states, or national minorities, it is worth noting that Weber's earlier comment on the link between nation and state contains an important qualification: 'a nation ... *normally tends* to produce a state of its own' (1961: 176; my emphasis). The qualification suggests a distinction between nation and state and Weber reiterates this distinction even more clearly elsewhere in his observation that a '"nation" is ... not identical with the "people of the state", that is, with the membership of a given polity' (1961: 172). In short, nation and state are not one and the same thing. As such, the 'nation' should be seen as a separate ideological and political construct from that of the 'nation-state' (Anthias and Yuval-Davis, 1992).

In relation to the decoupling of nation and state, even the most cursory examination of the world's nation-states should make clear that the happy coincidence of national and state loyalties, while the central aim of political nationalism, seldom actually occurs. There are invariably considerably more nations than existing states – even in Europe, where, arguably, the ideal of the nation-state is strongest (Anthony Smith, 1983). Likewise, several nations can coexist within the boundaries of a particular state – Britain and India are obvious examples here. The Welsh nationalist Dafydd Elis Thomas is at pains to point out this distinction between nation and state in the British context:

> Britain is a state rather than a nation. The British state, imposed upon the English, Scottish, Welsh and part of the Irish peoples and then imposed worldwide, is an inherently imperial and colonial concept at home and abroad. The British state cannot and should not be an object of affection, save for those who want to live in a form of authoritarian dependency. (Cited in Gilroy, 1990: 263)

A comparison of the terms 'nationalism' and 'patriotism' may help to illustrate this distinction further. As Walker Connor argues, 'Nationalism, in correct usage, refers to an emotional attachment to one's people – one's ethnocultural group. It is therefore proper to speak of an English, Scottish, or Welsh nationalism, but not of "British" nationalism, the latter being a manifestation of PATRIOTISM' (1993: 374; emphasis in original). On this argument, nationalism and patriotism will only coincide in 'true' nation-states; that is, in states where the population is ethnically homogeneous. However, Connor proceeds to point out that this is extremely rare since most states, by this definition, are not actually nation-states at all. For example, in 40 percent of all states there are at least five or more statistically and/or politically significant ethnic groups, while in nearly one-third of all states (31 percent) the largest national group is not even the majority (Connor, 1993; see also Nielsson, 1985). These groups comprise national and indigenous minorities such as Irish, Scots and Welsh in Britain, Hawaiians and Native Americans in the USA, Québécois and Aboriginal peoples/Native Canadians in Canada, Sámi in 'Sápmi' (which includes areas of Russia, Finland, Norway and Sweden), and Māori in Aotearoa/New Zealand. They also include a wide variety of immigrant groups. The result is that most states are *multinational* (comprising a number of national minorities) and/or *polyethnic* (comprising a range of immigrant groups). Indeed, most countries in the world have been historically, and remain today, a combination of the two (Kymlicka, 1995a, 2001, 2007). I will explore the distinctions between multinational and polyethnic states, and between national, indigenous, and immigrant minorities, more fully in the final section of this chapter. But for now, we can surely agree with Anthias and Yuval-Davis that: 'Today there is virtually nowhere in the world in which ... a pure nation-state exists, if it ever did, and therefore there are always settled residents (and usually citizens as well) who are not members of the dominant national collectivity in the society' (1992: 21). As they conclude, the fact that the notion of nation-state congruence remains so powerful is an 'expression of the naturalising effect of the hegemony of one collectivity and its access to ideological apparatuses of both state and civil society. This constructs minorities into assumed deviants from the "normal", and excludes them from important power resources' (1992: 21–2).

If, as these commentators suggest, the ethnically exclusive and culturally homogeneous 'nation-state' is a misnomer, how has it come to so dominate conceptions of nationalism and nationhood? This, in turn, leads us to another question. Even if we acknowledge the primacy of multinational and polyethnic states – and it is hard not to – why does the majority ethnic group, or dominant ethnie, in these states so often continue to perceive the state as the political expression of *their* particular ethnic group (and, usually, theirs alone)? I will explore these questions more fully in the final section of this chapter. Before doing so, however, I want to turn to the third key limitation of modernist conceptions of nationalism – which is closely related to much of the preceding discussion – that is, the dominance of statist (or political) nationalisms over what might be termed 'cultural nationalisms'.

Statist and cultural nationalisms

An inevitable corollary of the modernist rejection of ethnicity as a central variable in nation formation is, as we have seen, an over-emphasis on the political and civic elements of nationalism at the expense of its cultural dimensions. In effect, this has involved the legitimation of the 'Staatsnation' over the 'Kulturnation'. The latter, accordingly, has often been relegated to an 'ethnic' rather than a 'national' concern, a move illustrated by the commonly invoked distinction between ethnicity and nationalism in the academic literature. Anthias and Yuval-Davis provide us with a representative example of this distinction: 'there is no inherent difference (although sometimes there is a difference in scale) between ethnic and national collectivities' (1992: 25), they argue. Rather, '[what is specific to the nationalist project and discourse is the claim for a separate political representation for the collectivity. This often – but not always – takes the form of a claim for a separate state' (ibid.).

However, in reality, the distinction drawn here between ethnicity and nationalism is not nearly so straightforward. As Craig Calhoun observes, in a more nuanced analysis:

> The relationship between nationalism and ethnicity is complex ... Nationalism, in particular, remains the preeminent rhetoric for attempts to demarcate political communities, claim rights of self-determination and legitimate rule by reference to 'the people' of the country. Ethnic solidarities and identities are claimed most often when groups do not seek 'national' autonomy but rather a recognition internal to or cross-cutting national or state boundaries. The possibility of a closer link to nationalism is seldom altogether absent from such ethnic claims, however, and the two sorts of categorical identities are often invoked in similar ways. (1993a: 235)

Even this analysis though does not go far enough, since it continues to assume, unproblematically, nationalism's principal preoccupation with *political* and *civic* legitimation – externally via the principle of self-determination in the inter-state system, and internally via the establishment of national citizenship. In this regard, the aspiration of nations for statehood may be overdrawn. While attaining statehood is often the central aim of nationalist movements, it may not always be, and nationalist movements may be content to pursue more limited political aims in relation to greater autonomy and/or self-determination within existing nation-state structures (see Chapters 7 and 8). Nationalist sentiments need not therefore be limited to the questions of state formation or secession; indeed, statehood need not even be the central issue at stake. The long-held emphasis on statist definitions of nationalism has thus tended to preclude the recognition of a much wider range of *cultural* nationalisms (Fishman, 1989b; Hutchinson, 1987, 1994, 2005). These cultural nationalisms are a recurring force in the modern world and, ironically perhaps, seem currently to affect most those Western nations whose state power and boundaries have long been settled. Such nationalisms are concerned principally with what constitutes national *identity*, and with the moral regeneration of the national *community*, or 'way of life', rather than with state secession as such. Via this communitarian emphasis, cultural nationalisms attempt to reconstruct tradition (be it historical, cultural or linguistic) in order to meet more adequately the demands of modernity (Hutchinson, 1994, 2005). Indeed, this central emphasis of cultural nationalism on 'modernization from within' counters the often-invoked criticism that such movements are merely traditionalist and reactionary (see, for example, H. Kohn, 1961; Gellner, 1964, 1983; Schlesinger, 1992). They may well be, but they need not always be. I will explore these criticisms, and their inherent weaknesses, more fully in the following chapters.

Cultural nationalisms can thus be seen as contrapuntal to political nationalisms. They are often present when the aims of political secessionist nationalisms have been exhausted, or are simply no longer feasible or relevant – hence the prominence of cultural nationalisms in established Western nation-states. Cultural nationalisms accordingly differ from political nationalisms in the nature and extent of their political organization, comprising largely small-scale 'grass roots' movements which have as their principal foci specific historical, linguistic and educational concerns (Hutchinson, 1994, 2005).[18] That said, cultural nationalisms will always incorporate some political aims and, as such, may themselves develop into political nationalisms with their attendant claims to independent statehood – as seen, for example, in Belgium and Quebec in recent times (see Chapter 7). In effect, as Calhoun's previous comment suggests, both political and cultural emphases are likely to be present at any given time in nationalist movements, even if different weightings are ascribed to them. These weightings may also vary in salience over time. Nonetheless, cultural and political nationalisms can be seen as distinct variants, with differing emphases and concerns.

Wales provides us with a clear example of cultural nationalism here. As Richard Jenkins (1991, 1995) argues, Wales has had a long history of political and economic incorporation into the British state; much more so than Scotland, for example, which has managed throughout to retain its own church, law and education system. Despite the establishment of devolved models of governance in Britain in the late 1990s, which have seen the establishment of a Welsh Assembly and a Scottish Parliament (D. Smith and S. Wright, 1999; Deacon and Sandry, 2007), the degree of Welsh political incorporation into the British state remains considerable. Given this, Welsh nationalism has sought its legitimacy historically largely in 'cultural continuity' and collective memory (Colin Williams, 1994). This can be seen particularly in the promotion of Welsh culture, and its associated traditions, and in the particular importance placed on the Welsh language. As Richard Jenkins argues: 'In Wales, the defence and promotion of Welsh culture – symbolized most sharply by the Welsh language – [has been] the dominant item on the nationalist agenda, with some form of devolved self-government coming a poor second' (1991: 32). Indeed, given this historical tendency, the actual referendum for the approval of Welsh devolution, conducted in September 1997, was only just passed, again in contrast to Scotland where the comparable referendum was strongly supported (May, 1999d). The history of Welsh nationalism thus clearly demonstrates that there are means other than state recognition by which national distinctiveness can be attained and maintained. Moreover, the move to greater regional autonomy in Britain, and elsewhere, does not necessarily fuel the fires of political nationalism at the expense of former culturalist emphases. In the European Union, for example, the increasing move toward regional autonomy, particularly via the notion of 'Europeanization', has strengthened rather than weakened the tenets of some cultural nationalist movements there (D. Smith and S. Wright, 1999; Keating, 2009; Fitjar, 2010). Certainly, this is the case in both Wales and Catalonia, as will be evident in Chapter 7.

It is also the case, in a different political arena, for indigenous peoples' movements. In recent years, Sámi (Lapps) in Norway, Inuit (Eskimos) and Native Canadians in Canada, Māori in Aotearoa/New Zealand and, to a lesser extent, Aboriginal peoples and Torres Strait Islanders in Australia, have all been granted varying degrees of cultural, linguistic, educational and administrative autonomy, albeit in the face of at times considerable opposition. As I will discuss further in due course, these developments have been the direct result of indigenous advocacy, in national and international arenas, for greater autonomy *within* the nation-states that colonized them, rather than for secession as such (May, 1999c, d, 2002; see also Chapter 8).

The modernist mistake then has been to assume that cultural and political nationalisms are entirely separate phenomena – the former related only to 'ethnic' groups, the latter only to 'national' ones – rather than distinct variants of the same phenomenon. This dominance of statist or political forms of nationalism, and the consigning of cultural nationalism to the realms of 'mere ethnicity', can be traced back to the principle of nation-state congruence discussed in the preceding section. Nationalism is only nationalism (and therefore justifiable), it seems, when it is tied to the modernizing state (Calhoun, 1993a). This is to miss an essential element of the power of nationalism, its protean or chameleon-like quality (Anthony Smith, 1995a; Brubaker, 1998). However, as Anthony Smith argues:

It is also crucially to misunderstand the relationship between culture and politics in nationalism. Nationalism cannot be reduced to the uniform principle that the cultural unit must be made congruent with the political unit. Not only does this omit a number of other vital nationalist tenets, it fails to grasp the fact that the development of any nationalism depends on bringing the cultural and moral regeneration of the community into a close relationship, if not harmony, with the political mobilisation and self-determination of its members. (1995a: 13)

In short, the principal consequence of this approach has been to legitimate the 'legal-political' dimensions of nationhood over the 'cultural-historical'. For majority ethnic groups, or dominant ethnies, the result has been relatively unproblematic since the latter dimension (their ethnic habitus, in effect) is seen to correspond directly with the former. In the process, their 'ethnic' ties are elided with, and normalized and legitimated as, 'civic' ones within the field of the nation-state. For minority groups, however, their ethnic habitus is seen to be distinct from and oppositional to the legal-political interests of the nation-state. Accordingly, any claims which are made for some degree of ethnic autonomy vis-à-vis the nation-state, and/or greater civic representation within it, are viewed as inherently parochial and destabilizing (see Chapter 3).

Dominant ethnies

The fundamentally different treatment of majority and minority ethnic groups within the nation-state is indicative of what Michael Billig (1995) describes as the 'projection' of nationalism onto 'others' and the 'naturalization' of one's own. Billig describes the latter process as *banal* nationalism and he equates this, as I have, with contemporary 'civic' loyalties to nation-states. The naturalization of such ties means that banal nationalism – that is, the nationalism of the dominant ethnie – 'not only ceases to be nationalism ... it ceases to be a problem for investigation' (1995: 17). By this, the *hegemonic* construction of the nation-state is overlooked, or at the very least is viewed as unproblematic. And yet, as Billig again observes:

> The battle for nationhood is [specifically] a battle for hegemony, by which a part claims to speak for the whole nation and to represent the national essence ... The triumph of a particular nationalism is seldom achieved without the defeat of alternative nationalisms and other ways of imagining peoplehood. (1995: 27, 28)

Walker Connor (1993) uses the term 'Staatsvolk' to illustrate the process by which the dominant ethnic group comes to determine the 'national essence' of the nation-state. Staatsvolk describes a people who are culturally and politically pre-eminent in a state, even though (as we have seen) other groups may well be present in significant numbers. Connor suggests that, by their pre-eminence, the dominant group's culture and language come to be represented as the core or *national* culture and language. Minority groups, and their languages and cultures, consequently tend to be excluded from 'national' recognition. At the same time, minority groups are also variously encouraged and/or coerced by the dominant ethnie to assimilate to 'national' (i.e. dominant ethnie) norms. These countervailing pressures place minority groups in a double bind. If they resist, their attempts at maintaining a distinct identity are often labeled as a parochial and anti-national form of communalism. This is despite the fact that the dominant ethnie's advocacy of a 'universalistic' national consensus is simply a majoritarian version of the same process (Dench, 1986; Brown, 2008). If they acquiesce, and assimilate, minority groups may still face exclusion from the full benefits of a 'national' identity determined and delimited by the dominant ethnie. This latter trend is increasingly evident in the widespread retrenchment of multiculturalism, and related citizenship rights, in many nation-states over the last decade, particularly with respect to immigrant minorities.[19]

The ethnic hegemony that results sees a situation in which members of the Staatsvolk control knowledge/power, and thus the creation of sociocultural reality, through both their socioeconomic dominance and their control over the major institutions of the state (Bullivant, 1981). At the same time, many members of the Staatsvolk, or dominant ethnie, are often largely unaware of this process of ethnic hegemony. In the British context, for example, England, and particularly its southeast region, has long held dominance over the affairs of the British state (see, for example, Hechter, 1975; Nairn, 1981; Kumar, 2003). A consequence of this dominance is that many English people use the terms 'English' and 'British' interchangeably – assuming implicitly that one amounts to the other, when in fact one describes a national affiliation and the other a state affiliation. This, of course, simply reminds the Welsh, Scots and other non-English peoples living in Britain that they live in a multinational state dominated by the English (Connor, 1993; Crick, 1989, 1995; Miles, 1996).

Most modernist accounts of nationalism accept this process of ethnic hegemony uncritically, assuming it to be the necessary price of modernization. Gellner, for example, has argued that the requirements of a modern industrialized society led to the perceived need for a homogeneous national culture in the first place, particularly in the form of a common language and culture. This was reflected in the 'one state, one culture' principle discussed earlier. As he states:

> the culture needs the state and the state *probably* needs the homogeneous cultural branding of its flock, in a situation in which it cannot rely on largely eroded sub-groups either to police its citizens, or to inspire them

with that minimum of moral zeal and social identification without which social life becomes very difficult ... (1983: 140; my emphasis)

The need for a 'minimum of moral zeal and social identification' is the basis on which a homogeneous national culture is advanced. Accordingly, any alternative form of ethnic and cultural identification is seen as *oppositional* to this overarching conception of national culture and, thus, undermining of social cohesion (see Chapter 3 for further discussion). Moreover, since the nation-state represents in the modernist view the end point of the transition from tradition to modernity, alternative ethnic and cultural identifications are also, by definition, seen as regressive and premodern. As such, the nation-state appears as a new form of group life *at odds* with that of separate ethnic groups; these being, no doubt, the 'largely eroded sub-groups' to which Gellner refers (Rex, 1991). This position is not too dissimilar to the nineteenth-century views of Mill, Michelet and Engels on minority groups, outlined in Chapter 1. For Gellner, the best such groups can hope for – aside from assimilation or the (unlikely) prospect of secession – is to be represented in the modern nation-state 'in a token and cellophane-packaged form' (1983: 121; see also 1994: 108).

The construction of sociological minorities

To recapitulate, it has been my argument that modernist accounts of nationalism fail adequately to explain the ongoing link between ethnicity and nationalism in the modern world. This inadequacy is demonstrated in both the historical and cultural realms. In relation to the former, explaining the rise of nationalism via the transition to modernity in the eighteenth and nineteenth centuries leads to a teleological account of history that over-emphasizes the role of modernism and underplays, or ignores, the influence of pre-existing ethnies. In relation to the latter, nation-state congruence leaves little or no room for minority ethnies to have their historical, cultural and linguistic concerns recognized by and expressed within appropriate state hierarchies. As Richard Jenkins concludes, both these dimensions are interconnected:

> Historically, the [modernist] argument tends towards tautology: nationalism is what supersedes ethnicity, which is what precedes nationalism. Culturally, we are left with no authentic place within modern nation-states for ethnicity, other than an axiomatic homogeneity on the one hand, or an immigrant or peripheral presence on the other. (1995: 372)

The result has seen the juxtaposition in today's nation-states of (modern) 'national' and (premodern) 'ethnic' identities and, relatedly, of *dominant ethnies* and a wide range of *sociological minorities*. The distinction drawn here between dominant ethnies and sociological minorities highlights two often overlooked features of national life. The first relates to its *heterogeneity* – a characteristic which, at the individual level, we may take for granted but at the level of the polity we tend to ignore. As I noted earlier, for example, Max Weber highlights this disjuncture in his observation that the idea of the nation includes 'an essential, *though frequently indefinite*, homogeneity' (1961: 173; my emphasis). As he observes:

> If one believes that it is at all expedient to distinguish national sentiment as something homogeneous and specifically set apart ... one must be clearly aware of the fact that sentiments of solidarity, very heterogeneous in both their nature and origin, are comprised within national sentiments. (1961: 179)

The second, and related, aspect is that if some 'sentiments of solidarity' take precedence over and/or subsume others in the construction of the nation-state, they must do so on the basis of a differential apportionment of status and value. As Billig succinctly comments, 'the aura of nationhood always operates within contexts of power' (1995: 4; see also Hall, 1992a). Given this, sociological minorities can be defined as groups which are a numerical minority in a given state *and* which are also politically non-dominant (Minority Rights Group, 1997). Indeed, in this context, while the term 'minorities' tends to draw attention to numerical size, its more important reference is to groups with few(er) rights and privileges (see Chapter 5). This is not to suggest that majority/minority relationships are fixed since, by definition, they are relative and relational and may differ from one context to the next (Young, 1993; Eriksen, 2010). Nonetheless, sociological minorities are usually characterized by a history of social, economic and political marginalization and/or exploitation by dominant ethnies within given 'nation-states' (Hechter, 1975; Dench, 1986; Tully, 1995; Carens, 2000).[20]

In this final section, I want to outline briefly the key distinctions that can be drawn between various sociological minorities. In so doing, I will employ Eriksen's (2010) useful attempts at a typology along these lines. Given the inevitable limitations of typologies, I will also draw on a number of complementary categorizations where appropriate.[21] However, this attempt at a more nuanced categorization notwithstanding, the following distinctions should be seen primarily as useful heuristic devices rather than as definitive and/or exhaustive categories. It should also be borne in mind that these minority ethnies are no more homogeneous than any other grouping and will, accordingly, reflect significant *intra*group as well as *inter*group differences, along with a considerable degree of overlap (see Chapter 1).

Indigenous peoples

Indigenous peoples are aboriginal groups who are politically non-dominant and who are not, or are only partially, integrated into the nation-state. They include such groups as Māori, Sámi, Australian Aboriginal peoples and Torres Strait Islanders, Native Americans, Hawaiians and Inuit. These groups are associated historically with a non-industrial mode of production and a stateless political system (Minority Rights Group, 1997; Paine, 2000). The extreme disadvantages faced currently by many indigenous groups in modern nation-states are the result of colonization and subsequent marginalization within their own historic territories. Such historic processes have usually seen the expropriation of land, and the destruction, or near-destruction of their language(s) and traditional social, economic and political practices – not to mention the very groups themselves (see Chapter 8). In Australia, for example, British colonizers in the nineteenth century declared sovereignty on the basis that the land was terra nullius. In effect, Australian Aboriginal peoples were deemed to be so uncivilized as to be safely ignored. Indeed, as late as 1953, the Australian delegate to the United Nations Sub-Commission on the Prevention of Discrimination and the Protection of Minorities could state that 'there were no minority problems in Australia ... There were, of course, the aborigines [sic], but they had no separate competing culture of their own' (cited in Kingsbury, 1989: 145).

Accordingly, the predominant concerns of indigenous peoples are for separate political and cultural recognition *within* the nation-state and, where possible, for political and economic redress for past injustices. In this regard, political pressure from indigenous peoples has led to a limited range of reparative legislation within nation-states in recent times. Examples here include Canada, Aotearoa/ New Zealand, Australia, Brazil, Norway and, most recently (2009), Bolivia. These developments at the national level have also been influenced by the growing articulation of indigenous rights and reparations within international law, and via supranational organizations such as the United Nations (UN). The nearly three-decade negotiations in the UN on a United Nations Declaration on the Rights of Indigenous Peoples (UNDRIP) included key participation and advocacy from the World Council of Indigenous Peoples (WCIP) and the United Nations Working Group on Indigenous Populations (WGIP). It led, in the first instance, to a (1993) Draft Declaration, which, after much subsequent prevarication and/or obstruction by UN member states, was finally recognized as a full UN Declaration in 2007.[22]

As Eriksen (2010) observes, however, the concept of 'indigenous peoples' is not an accurate analytical one since it excludes groups such as the Welsh, Catalans and Basques who could also claim to be 'indigenous' but who do not share all the attributes ascribed to these groups as they have come to be defined in international law. In this regard, Stacy Churchill's (1986) distinction between 'indigenous' and 'established' minorities is a useful addendum here. Churchill argues that 'established' and 'indigenous' minorities are both minority groups that have been long established in their native countries. However, where indigenous peoples are characterized by a 'traditional' culture that is often regarded as being at odds with that of the majority group, established minorities are characterized by a lifestyle similar to the remainder of the national society, although sometimes falling behind in rate of evolution. As such, established minorities are more likely to be able to lay claim to a right to conserve their identity and to back it with political might. This distinction is not entirely unproblematic. However, it does point to the overlap of established minorities with the next group in Eriksen's typology, 'proto-nations'.

Proto-nations

Proto-nations are most commonly associated with the growing number of secessionist and irredentist nationalisms in the world today that have come to be termed 'ethnonational movements' (see Fenton and May, 2002). As discussed previously, these comprise historical culture-communities which are territorially based and which do not currently possess their own nation-state – 'nations without states' in Guibernau's (1999) terms. Such groups are usually no more or less modern than other national groups and are fully differentiated along class and educational lines. Their numbers may be said currently to include Kurds, Palestinians, Southern Tamils, Tibetans, Basques, and the Québécois, among others. The most commonly associated aim of ethnonational movements is to (re)claim statehood and to be recognized subsequently in the world inter-state system. As such, their concerns more closely reflect political nationalisms (see above). However, there is also often a considerable degree of overlap within such movements between an overtly separatist political approach and one that favors more culturalist (and non-secessionist) emphases. The distinctions between the Basque separatist ETA organization and moderate Basque politicians, and the separatist Parti Québécois and other Francophone nationalist organizations in Québec, illustrate these differences.

Modern (urban) migrants

Unlike the preceding groups, which can be broadly classified as national minority ethnies – that is, as previously self-governing and with a historic claim to a particular territory – modern migrants comprise those who have emigrated and settled subsequently in a new country. Usually such groups have come to be concentrated in urban areas, although this may not have been the case historically. Thus, Indian and Chinese minorities in Malaysia, Fiji and Aotearoa/ New Zealand were initially employed as predominantly agricultural migrant labor in the nineteenth century, before subsequently settling in cities in the twentieth century. African Caribbeans in Britain provide a more recent example of direct migration to urban areas in the 1950s as part of a postwar British employment policy to fill low-skill, low-wage positions in the depleted labor market of the time.

Often described as 'ethnic minorities', these groups may retain elements of their culture, language and traditions – sometimes over the course of a number of generations – in the new host society. However, their general aim is to integrate into the host society and to be(come) accepted as full members of it. As such, ethnic minorities can be distinguished from national minority ethnies since their ethnic and cultural distinctiveness is manifested primarily in the private domain and is not inconsistent with their institutional integration into the nation-state (Kymlicka, 1995a). This is not to suggest that ethnic minorities do not face racism, discrimination and exclusion within the host nation-state, or that they may resist assimilation to the norms of the dominant ethnie. Quite the reverse in fact, since the so-called 'ethnic revival' that emerged in the 1960s has seen such groups increasingly assert the right to express their ethnic particularities (see Chapter 3). However, ethnic minorities do not usually seek separate and self-governing status within the nation-state, as is typically demanded by national minorities. Rather, they argue for a more *plural* and *inclusive* conception of national identity and culture, which recognizes their contribution to and influence on the historical and contemporary development of the host nation-state. In the process, the boundaries of nationhood – what it is that constitutes the national community – is opened up for debate. Of central concern in this debate are the questions of who is (and who is not) to be included in the national collectivity, and on what (and whose) terms are the criteria for inclusion to be based.

That said, there are a number of caveats that need to be made before proceeding further. First, ethnic minorities may become national minorities over time if they settle together and acquire self-governing power in the interim (Kymlicka, 1995a). This is particularly evident in ex-colonial societies such as the USA, Canada, Australia and Aotearoa/New Zealand where white settler groups have subsequently come to constitute the dominant ethnie(s) in the modern nation-state. Likewise, the one possible exception to the broad distinctions so far outlined is the example of African Americans in the USA. African Americans clearly do not fit either the national or immigrant category. They have no historic territorial claim to the Americas (unlike Native Americans) and their historical subjection through slavery clearly precludes voluntary immigration.

The apparently anomalous position of African Americans led Steve Fenton (1999), who used an earlier version of Eriksen's typology as a useful starting point, to add the category of 'post-slavery minorities', a category Eriksen has since incorporated into his own schema (see 2010: 18–19). Another useful means of analysis is via John Ogbu's (1987) distinction between 'voluntary' (immigrant) and 'involuntary' (caste-like) minorities (see also Gibson and Ogbu, 1991). Adopting a predominantly culturalist approach, Ogbu argues that all minority groups are subject to racism and discrimination to some degree, as well as facing cultural and language discontinuities in relation to their (uneven) integration in the nation-state. However, for voluntary minorities these discontinuities are seen as *primary cultural/linguistic differences* – that is, they existed prior to their immigration to the host country and are thus viewed as barriers to be overcome. As such, voluntary minorities are more likely to accommodate to the 'cultural model' of the majority group or dominant ethnie. In contrast, involuntary minorities – including in Ogbu's view, African Americans and indigenous people groups – are characterized by a history of exploitation and/or subjugation *within* a particular nation-state. Accordingly, involuntary minorities tend to develop a *secondary cultural system* in which cultural differences are viewed in light of that history, and in opposition to the majority group.

Cultural and language differences thus come to serve a boundary-maintenance function (see Chapter 4). They are seen as symbols of identity to be maintained rather than barriers to be overcome and may consequently develop into oppositional cultural (and political) nationalist movements. Such political nationalism has been represented among African Americans principally through the call for a separate black state. This was first supported in the 1930s, resurfaced again briefly in the 1960s in association with the 'Nation of Islam' movement, and again gained prominence in the 1990s under the leader of the Nation of Islam, Louis Farrakhan. These developments notwithstanding, much of the political effort among African Americans – including the principal concerns of the civil rights movement – has centered on gaining full and equal rights and benefits for African Americans *as US citizens*. As such, the concerns of African Americans approximate more closely immigrant minorities than national ones (Kymlicka, 1995a).

Ethnies in plural societies

Eriksen (2010) makes one final distinction based on ethnic groups within so-called 'plural societies'. Plural societies are most prominently associated with the work of Furnivall (1948) on Burma and M. G. Smith (1965) on the British West Indies. They have come to refer to ex-colonial societies, primarily Asian and Caribbean, with self-consciously culturally heterogeneous populations. The groups that make up these societies are divided internally by class and rank but are also clearly identifiable through ethnic and cultural differences. They are compelled to participate in uniform political and ethnic systems, although one particular group will usually dominate. Ethnic relations are characterized consequently by intergroup competition. Secessionism is usually not an option, since the groups involved have no external nation-state to which they realistically relate.

Having said this, the utility of the term 'plural society' has more recently been brought into question (see R. Jenkins, 1986, 1997; Eriksen, 1998). This is because plural societies are not the exception, as the above formulation suggests, but are actually the norm. As I have already discussed, most contemporary states can be regarded as plural or *polyethnic* in this way. In short, contemporary 'nation-states' increasingly comprise a variety of ethnic groups which are in competition for the resources of the state – a process I outlined more fully in my discussion of situational ethnicity in Chapter 1. The USA is perhaps the clearest example of a plural or polyethnic state in this regard. To complicate matters further, polyethnic states are often *multinational* ones as well. In other words, indigenous and national minority groups are also present in many of the same states (the USA being no exception; see Chapter 3). However, what has tended to happen up until now is that both these types of minority group have been treated *in the same way* by the dominant ethnie. As a result, indigenous peoples and other national minorities have been denied their historical rights as ethnies and have been treated as merely one of a number of competing 'ethnic minorities' laying claim to the nation-state's (invariably) limited social, economic and political resources.

As I have argued, this elision has been the inevitable result of the exclusion of ethnicity from the realms of nationalism, which has, in turn, been predicated on the principle of nation-state congruence and the related separation of political and cultural nationalisms. It may also help to explain the continued spread of ethnonationalism(s) in the modern world. The voices of dissenting national minorities are increasingly questioning the pejorative distinction drawn between the (modern) 'national' identity of the dominant ethnie and their own supposedly (premodern) 'ethnic' identities. Not only this, they are also increasingly dissatisfied with the concomitant rejection by the former of their claims for greater civic recognition and inclusion within the nation-state. As Homi Bhabha argues, we are confronted with the nation-state 'split within itself, articulating the heterogeneity of its population ... a liminal signifying space that is *internally* marked by the discourses of minorities, the heterogeneous histories of contending peoples, antagonistic authorities and tense locations of cultural difference' (1994: 148).

Of course, such minority disenchantment is by no means a new phenomenon, nor is the state–minority relationship from which it springs. However, what I have argued here is that these developments include a growing number of indigenous and established national minorities who are less concerned with independent statehood – although it may inevitably spill over into this – than with challenging and changing the hegemonic construction of 'national' culture upon which nation-states have traditionally been based. As Colin Williams observes, 'it is clear that as many societies become increasingly multiethnic in composition the question of national congruence will have to be redefined and more appropriate answers given than those which are currently practised in many states' (1994: 12). What might be involved exactly in redefining or *rethinking* the nation-state to this end, particularly with respect to questions of language and education, is the focus of the next three chapters.

3

LIBERALISM AND MULTICULTURALISM

It has been my argument thus far that the construction of national and ethnic minorities and their pejorative and marginalized status are the result of what Stacy Churchill (1996) has termed the *philosophical matrix of the nation-state*. A philosophical matrix denotes 'a combination of ideas, not easy to separate or define, that embodies the expectations of society as to how it should function' (MacLachlan, 1988: pp. x–xi). The philosophical matrix of the nation-state, rooted in the political nationalism of the eighteenth and nineteenth centuries, has also been usefully described by Will Kymlicka (2001) as the 'nation-building' model of modern state formation. It is predicated on the confluence of nation and state and on the establishment (often retrospectively) of a common civic or 'national' language and culture.

Interestingly, it was Fichte who first advocated this linking of nation, state and language into an indissoluble whole. Fichte, as we have seen, incorporated Herder's views on language and culture within a statist account of nationalism (Hutchinson, 1994). This led to the development of the linear 'one language, one nation, one state' principle of linguistic or organic nationalism, a principle which has since rightly been widely discredited as essentialist and which has also been associated (pejoratively) with many contemporary ethnonationalisms (Fenton and May, 2002). In contrast, political nationalism argued that it was the state that preceded and precipitated the rise of the nation, not the other way around. The key principle that followed from this can be summarized as 'one state, one nation, one language' and it has since come to represent the common modernist orthodoxy in discussions of nationalism, not to mention the development of modern nation-states themselves. Indeed, as early as 1862, Lord Acton argued unequivocally on this basis for the superiority of political nationalism over linguistic nationalism:

The State may in course of time produce a nationality ... but that a nationality should constitute a State is contrary to the nature of modern civilisation ... [Such a position is] in defiance of the modifying action of external causes, *of tradition and of existing rights*. It overrules the rights and wishes of the inhabitants, absorbing their divergent interests in a fictitious unity, sacrifices their several inclinations and duties to the higher claim of nationality and crushes all natural rights and established liberties for the purpose of vindicating itself. (1907: 288; my emphasis)

And yet political nationalism, and the modern nation-state with which it is associated, can be accused of the very same proclivities. The nation-state, as it has come to be constructed, *creates* sociological minorities by establishing a civic language and culture that is largely limited to, and representative of, the dominant ethnie or Staatsvolk. Minorities are, in turn, denied legitimate rights to their *existing* language and cultural traditions where these differ from those of the dominant ethnie. Political nationalism may thus have prided itself on the reversal of the linguistic nationalists' language–nation–state connection but it has left the *linearity* of the principle untouched. As such, what results is still ethnic and linguistic hegemony, albeit from the opposite direction. Moreover, the hegemonic construction of the nation-state is far less readily apparent than more 'overt' ethnonationalisms. Cloaked as it is in the apparently neutral representation of a modern 'national' language and culture, the legitimation and valorization of the dominant ethnie's habitus often escapes notice or critical comment. As Michael Billig observes, this 'banal nationalism' is simply 'overlooked, forgotten, even theoretically denied' (1995: 17) which perhaps helps to explain why dominant groups so seldom come to define themselves (or their language(s)) as 'ethnic'.

A further explanation of the uncritical acceptance of this elision of civic and ethnic ties rests with the key liberal democratic principles of universal political citizenship, and the related primacy of individual over collective rights. These principles have been regularly invoked over the last two centuries by liberal commentators in their dismissal of ethnicity as a valid form of collective social and political organization and identity (cf. Chapter 1). They have also been consistently employed in support of the present political organization of the nation-state. In this chapter, I will examine the cogency of this orthodox liberal defence of the nation-state, and the key tenets on which it is based, and will argue that these accounts are invariably framed within, and thus constrained by, the notion of nation-state congruence arising from political nationalism. If this assumption is dropped, the recognition of a more plural conception of the nation-state – based, at least to some degree, on group-differentiated rights – becomes a possibility. In this regard, it is my view that national minorities (including indigenous and established minorities) have rights to greater inclusion within the civic realm of the nation-state – that is, 'civil society' in Gramsci's (1971) sense[1] – than many currently enjoy. Moreover, these rights of inclusion are *distinct* from those of other ethnic minorities (see Chapter 2). Accordingly, I will concentrate in much of what follows on the particular rights of national minorities. However, I will return to the question of other ethnic minority groups, and the wider implications of my own position with regard to them, in Chapters 5 and 9.

The pluralist dilemma

A central concern in current debates surrounding the organization and legitimacy of modern nation-states has to do with what Brian Bullivant (1981) has termed 'the pluralist dilemma'. The pluralist dilemma, for Bullivant, is 'the problem of reconciling the diverse political claims of constituent groups and individuals in a pluralist society *with the claims of the nation-state as a whole*' (1981: p. x; my emphasis), what he elsewhere describes as the competing aims of 'civism' and 'pluralism'. Other commentators have suggested similar distinctions: 'roots' and 'options' (Rokkan and Urwin, 1983); 'state' and 'community' (Anthony Smith, 1981); and, drawing on de Saussure, 'parochialism' and 'intercourse' (J. Edwards, 1994, 2010). All these distinctions emphasize, like Bullivant's, the apparent polarities involved in the task of national integration; the difficulties of reconciling social cohesion on the one hand with, on the other, a recognition and incorporation of ethnic, linguistic and cultural diversity within the nation-state. In an earlier analysis, Schermerhorn has described these countervailing social and cultural forces as *centripetal* and *centrifugal* tendencies. As he observes:

> Centripetal tendencies refer both to cultural trends such as acceptance of common values, styles of life etc., as well as structural features like increased participation in a common set of groups, associations, and institutions ... Conversely, centrifugal tendencies among subordinate groups are those that foster separation from the dominant group or from societal bonds in one way or another. Culturally this most frequently means retention and presentation of the group's distinctive tradition in spheres like language, religion, recreation etc. (1970: 81)

How then can the tensions arising from the pluralist dilemma best be resolved in the social and political arena? Drawing on political theory, two contrasting approaches have been adopted in response to this central question, which Gordon (1978, 1981) has described as 'liberal pluralism' and 'corporate pluralism'. Liberal pluralism, exemplified in the seminal contribution of John Rawls (1971), is characterized by the absence, even prohibition, of any ethnic, religious or national minority group possessing separate standing before the law or government. Its central tenets can be traced back to the French Revolution and Rousseau's conception of the modern polity as comprising three inseparable features: freedom (non-domination), the absence of differentiated roles and a very tight common purpose. On this view, the margin for recognizing difference within the modern nation-state is very small (Taylor, 1994). In contrast, corporate pluralism – now more commonly known by the term 'multiculturalism' (see May, 2001; Kymlicka, 2007; Modood, 2007) – involves the recognition of minority groups as legally constituted entities, on the basis of which, and depending on their size and influence, economic, social and political awards are allocated.[2] Glazer (1975) and Walzer (1992, 1994) draw similar distinctions between an approach based on 'non discrimination' – which involves, in Glazer's memorable phrase, the 'salutary neglect' of the state toward ethnic minorities – and a 'corporatist' (Walzer) or 'group rights' (Glazer) model.

It is clear, however, that for most liberal commentators the merits of liberal pluralism significantly outweigh those of a group-rights or multiculturalist approach. In effect, the answer to the pluralist dilemma has been consistently to favor civism over pluralism.[3] On this basis, the 'claims of the nation-state as a whole' – emphasizing the apparently inextricable interconnections between social cohesion and national homogeneity – have invariably won the day over more pluralist conceptions of the nation-state where ethnic, linguistic and cultural differences *between different groups* are accorded some degree of formal recognition. This should perhaps not surprise us, since the former is situated squarely within the 'philosophical matrix of the nation-state' to which I referred earlier. Relatedly, liberal pluralism also accords closely with the longstanding pejorative distinction between *citizenship* and *ethnicity* – a distinction first illustrated in Chapter 1 by the likes of the nineteenth-century liberals, Mill and Michelet, and the socialists, Marx and Engels. In this light, it is perhaps worth observing that the consensus between liberal and Marxist commentators on the position of ethnic and national minorities within the nation-state has also been reflected in the subsequent construction of liberal-democratic and socialist states. As such, while I will concentrate in what follows on the political organization of liberal democracies, it should be pointed out that socialist and other non-democratic states have also tended to adopt a very similar position vis-à-vis national and ethnic minorities. In this latter regard, Will Kymlicka (1995a: 69–74) and Valery Tishkov (1997, 2000) provide useful discussions of the history of the former Soviet Union with respect to its treatment of minorities.

The result of this broad consensus has been the construction in contemporary orthodox liberal accounts of a range of interrelated, and at times overlapping, polarities, which are outlined below. In each, the former feature is associated (positively) with liberal pluralism while the latter is associated (negatively) with a multiculturalist approach:

- universal or particularist
- individual or collective
- autonomy or identity
- private or public
- informal or formal
- fluid or bounded
- dialogic or ghettoized
- changing or static
- modernity or tradition
- commonality or difference
- cohesion or fragmentation.

In orthodox liberal accounts, individual and universal 'citizenship' rights are invariably constructed in opposition to collective and particularist 'ethnic' rights, the latter associated exclusively with multiculturalism (Barry, 2001). As such, formal differentiation within the nation-state on the grounds of (ethnic) group association is rejected as inimical to the individualistic and meritocratic tenets of liberal democracy. Where countenanced at all, alternative ethnic affiliations should be restricted solely to the private domain since the formal recognition of collective (ethnic) identity is viewed as undermining personal and political autonomy, and fostering social and political fragmentation. As Will Kymlicka observes, 'the near-universal response by liberals has been one of active hostility to minority rights ... schemes which single out minority cultures for special measures ... appear irremediably unjust, a disguise for creating or maintaining ... ethnic privilege' (1989: 4). Any deviation from the strict principles of universal political citizenship and individual rights is seen as the first step down the road to apartheid. Or so it seems.

In a similar vein to postmodernist commentators (see Chapter 1), many liberal critics of multiculturalism also argue that any acknowledgment and accommodation of group-related differences must significantly understate the fluid and dialogic nature of inter- and intragroup relations.[4] The resulting liberal consensus is well illustrated by Brian Bullivant:

> Certain common institutions essential for the well-being and smooth functioning of the nation-state as *a whole* must be maintained: common language, common political system, common economic market system and so on. Cultural pluralism can operate at the level of the *private*, rather than public, concerns such as use of ethnic [sic] language[5] in the home ... But, the idea that maintaining these aspects of ethnic life and encouraging the maintenance of ethnic groups almost in the sense of ethnic enclaves will assist their ability to cope with the political realities of the nation-state is manifestly absurd. (1981: 232; emphases in original)

Defending liberal democracy

This 'de-ethnicized' view of liberal democracy, and the various polarities which characterize it, are clearly evident in the work of three prominent liberal commentators – John Porter, Arthur Schlesinger Jr. and Brian Barry. In what follows, I want to explore briefly their respective arguments. Before doing so, however, I should point out that Porter and Schlesinger tend toward the politically conservative end of the liberal continuum while Barry's position originates from a political position somewhat further to the left. This raises an important point. The orthodox defence of liberal democracy, in the form of liberal pluralism, is advocated by commentators on both the left and right of the political spectrum – albeit for somewhat different reasons, as we shall see (cf. May, 1999a; Bonnett, 2000; Chapter 5). Nonetheless, the wide support that liberal pluralism garners reinforces the degree to which the political tenets of nation-state congruence underlying it have come to be taken as given.

Porter's 'vertical mosaic'

John Porter wrote extensively (1965, 1972, 1975) on pluralism in Canada, particularly in relation to the 'ethnic revival' of the 1960s and 1970s. In this regard, he was a strong advocate of liberal pluralism and a sharp critic of the multicultural model. As he observes, 'the organisation of society on the basis of rights or claims that derive from group membership is sharply opposed to the concept of a society based on citizenship, which has been such an important aspect in the development of modern societies' (1975: 297). From this, Porter argued that the maintenance of collective ethnicity in modern societies was regressive and historically naive. Moreover, it resulted in a form of ethnic stratification which, in combination with social class, reduced the social and economic mobility of individuals. Thus, in his influential study *The Vertical Mosaic* (1965), Porter argued that ethnicity was a principal factor in the formation and persistence of the social stratification system in Canada. In his view, this stratification process, or vertical mosaic, was initiated by the colonial contest between the British and French. When the French settlers lost this contest, they were accorded secondary status to their British counterparts. Subsequent immigrant groups were assigned an 'entrance status' which located them at various positions lower down the social hierarchy, while Native Canadian and Inuit occupied the lowest levels (see also Chapter 7).

Consequently, the stark choice facing Canadians, he asserted, was 'between ethnic stratification that results from ethnic diversity and the greater possibilities for equality that result from a reduction of ethnicity as a salient feature of modern society' (1972: 205; see also 1975: 288–304). Like many other liberals, Porter directly equated 'modern society' here with the homogeneous civic culture of the nation-state. On this basis, he advocated the *assimilation* of ethnic minorities into Canadian national life and rejected any form of multiculturalism that would perpetuate ethnic and/or cultural distinctiveness. This was clearly in the best interests of ethnic minority groups, he believed, since in modern society: 'the emphasis was on *individual* achievement and in the context of a new nation with *universalistic* standards of judgment it meant forgetting ancestry and attempting to establish a society of equality where ethnic origin did not matter' (1975: 293; my emphases).

In advocating this position, Porter does allow for some recognition of minority languages. As he concedes, 'identification with and the use of their own language, particularly in school, may be important in providing opportunity for very low status groups' (1975: 302). However, he quickly proceeds to argue that 'such use of language is quite different from the goal of having ethnic communities become a permanent compensation for low status, or as psychic shelters in the urban-industrial world' (1975: 303). For Porter, it was only *citizenship* that could provide minority ethnic group members with the individual social mobility and achievement necessary to make their way in the modern world. This, in turn, implied 'a commitment to the values of modernism and a movement away from the [minority] ethnic community with each succeeding generation' (1975: 302). The reason for this was obvious enough. Minority cultures were 'tradition bound' and 'less and less relevant for the post-industrial society' (1975: 303). As Porter concludes, ethnicity in the modern world is simply an anachronism: 'Many of the historic cultures are irrelevant to our futures. Opportunity will go to those individuals who are future oriented in an increasingly universalistic culture. Those oriented to the past are likely to lose out' (1975: 304).

Schlesinger's 'cult of ethnicity'

These themes were echoed during the 1990s in the United States in the often-vituperative debates surrounding multiculturalism, bilingualism and 'Afrocentrism'. Much of the populist commentary in the US over that period was increasingly opposed to multiculturalism and heralded the subsequent retrenchment, post-9/11, of many of its most significant policy accomplishments, particularly within education (May, 2009; May and Sleeter, 2010). Since then, for example, decades of affirmative action and related civil rights advances for African Americans have been dismantled, most notably in relation to access to higher education (Crosby, 2004; Kellough, 2006). The comparable retrenchment of bilingual education for Latino students is another example of the retreat from multiculturalism in the US (Crawford, 2000; Dicker, 2003; May, 2008a), a point to which I will return in Chapter 6.

An exemplar of this populist, conservative critique of multiculturalism can be found in Arthur Schlesinger Jr.'s *The Disuniting of America* (1992).[6] As his title suggests, Schlesinger, a noted liberal historian, has argued to much public acclaim against the 'disuniting' of America by the 'cult of ethnicity':

> A cult of ethnicity has arisen both among non-Anglo whites and among non-white minorities to denounce the idea of the melting pot, to challenge the concept of 'one people', and to protect, promote, and perpetuate separate [ethnic] communities ... The new ethnic gospel rejects the unifying vision of individuals from all nations melted into a new race [sic]. Its underlying philosophy is that America is not a nation of individuals at all but a nation of groups, that ethnicity is the defining experience for most Americans, that ethnic ties are permanent and indelible .... The ethnic interpretation, moreover, reverses the historic theory of America as one people – the theory that has thus far managed to keep American society whole. (1992: 15–16)

For Schlesinger, this 'ethnic cheerleading' is preservationist rather than transformative and results in a view of America which, instead of being 'composed of individuals making their own unhampered choices', is increasingly 'composed of groups more or less ineradicable in their ethnic character'. The result is a 'multiethnic dogma [which] abandons historic purposes, replacing assimilation by fragmentation, integration by separatism' (1992: 16–17). In the face of this assault, Schlesinger gloomily wonders: 'The national ideal had once been *e pluribus unum* [out of many, one]. Are we now to belittle *unum* and glorify *pluribus*? Will the center hold? Or will the melting pot give way to the Tower of Babel?' (1991: 14; see also 1992: 18).

Schlesinger directs particular opprobrium here at the emergence among African Americans of an 'Afrocentric' view of American (and world) history, along with its formal promotion in schools under the rubric of multiculturalism.[7] For Schlesinger, these developments are simply nationalist myth-making, along the lines of Hobsbawm's (1990) 'invention of tradition', and lead inevitably to cultural reification and essentialism. The rise of Afrocentrism may be understandable, he argues – given the consistent exclusion of black voices in previous historical accounts of the USA – but it is still *bad* history, albeit of a manifestly different kind from that which preceded it. Moreover, the whole notion of using history as therapy, whose principal function is to raise minority self-esteem, is misguided. After all, as Schlesinger points out, 'the absence of historical role models seems [not] to have handicapped two other groups in American society – Jewish Americans and Asian Americans' (1992: 89).

In saying this, Schlesinger does acknowledge the effects of racism – both historically and currently – on the African American community, albeit within an implicitly pathological frame of reference. As he observes, 'black Americans, after generations of psychological and cultural evisceration, have every right to seek affirmative action for their past. ... For blacks the American dream has been pretty much a nightmare and, far more than white ethnics, *they are driven by a desperate need to vindicate their own identity*' (1992: 60; my emphasis). However, in his view, Afrocentrism is not the answer to the problem since it simply replaces one form of ethnic and/or cultural exclusiveness (and exclusion) with another. Indeed, Schlesinger argues that the end game of this 'filiopietistic commemoration' (1992: 99) – or, more prosaically, the worship of ancestors – will actually confirm rather than reduce self-pity and self-ghettoization among African Americans. Rather, he asserts, a more appropriate approach would surely be to encourage ethnic minority students 'to understand the American culture in which they are growing up and to prepare [them] for an active role in shaping that culture' (1992: 90). 'As for self-esteem', he opines, 'is this really the product of ethnic role models and fantasies of a glorious past? Or does it not result from a belief in oneself that springs from achievement, from personal rather than [ethnic] pride?' (1992: 92).

Finally, Schlesinger extends his apocalyptic critique to include an attack on bilingualism and the bilingual movement in the USA, along with its strong links to various Latino communities there.[8] Unlike Porter, who was at least prepared to countenance a limited role for minority languages, Schlesinger rejects out of hand the official recognition of minority languages – a position presaged by his previous allusion to the Tower of Babel:

> The separatist movement is by no means confined to the black community. Another salient expression is the bilingualism movement ... In recent years the combination of the ethnicity cult with a *flood* of immigration from Spanish-speaking countries has given bilingualism new emphasis. The presumed purpose is transitional ... Alas, bilingualism has not worked out as planned: rather the contrary ... indications are that bilingual education retards rather than expedites the movement of Hispanic children *into the English-speaking world* and that it promotes segregation more than it does integration. Bilingualism shuts doors. It nourishes self-ghettoization, and ghettoization nourishes racial antagonism ... using some language other than English *dooms* people to second class citizenship in American society. (1992: 107–8; my emphases)

I will return to the contentious issue of bilingual education in the US when discussing Brian Barry in the next section. I will also explore more fully the wider arguments about bilingualism, the role of English and the particular preoccupation with Latino communities in Chapter 6, where I examine the key tenets of the US 'English Only' movement. Suffice it to say at this point, that in attributing to bilingualism the same fractious and regressive characteristics as Afrocentrism, Schlesinger invokes, once again, the rhetoric of national cohesion. 'A common language is a *necessary* bond of national cohesion in so heterogeneous a nation as America ... *institutionalized* bilingualism remains another source of the fragmentation of America, another threat to the dream of "one people"' (1992: 109–10; my emphases). His parting comments echo this conclusion when he returns directly to the question of the pluralist dilemma: 'The question America confronts as a pluralistic society is how to vindicate cherished cultures and traditions without breaking the bonds of cohesion – common ideals, common political institutions, common language, common fate – that hold the republic together?' (1992: 138). His answer, by now, should come as no surprise: 'the bonds of social cohesion in our society are sufficiently fragile, or so it seems to me, that it makes no sense to strain them by encouraging and exalting cultural and linguistic apartheid. The American identity will never be fixed and final; it will always be in the making' (1992: 138). QED, or so it seems.

Brian Barry and the egalitarian liberal 'answer'

The final example of liberal pluralism, broadly defined, that I want to discuss is the provocative and trenchant rejection of multiculturalism by the political philosopher, Brian Barry, in his 2001 book, *Culture and Equality*. Barry's contribution here is important for a number of reasons. The first relates to his personal politics. Over the course of his life, Barry was closely associated with the politics of the left. As a result, much of his work was motivated by a concern for redressing social and economic inequalities and a related advocacy of a politics of redistribution.[9] Indeed, one of the principal motivations for his critique of multiculturalism was that it undermined broader egalitarian aims via its (unnecessary) preoccupation with the politics of identity. As he observes toward the end of *Culture and Equality*, multiculturalism makes the achievement of egalitarian policies more difficult in two ways: 'At the minimum, it diverts political effort away from universalistic goals [of equality]'. More seriously, he concludes, 'it may very well destroy the conditions for putting together a coalition in favour of across-the board equalization of opportunities and resources' (2001: 325). Barry is not the only commentator from the left to advocate this broad position (see also Goulbourne, 1991a, b; Michaels, 2006; Phillips, 1997, 2009), but he is certainly the most prominent.

And that brings me to the second reason for the importance of *Culture and Equality* – its ongoing, widespread influence, particularly within political theory. Barry's intervention is regarded as the most comprehensive challenge to the theoretical tenets of multiculturalism and its policy implications in modern nation-states. Its polemical and dismissive tone – lambasting 'the latest piece of foolishness' defended 'in the name of multiculturalism' (2001: p. viii) – adds further to its visibility and purchase.[10]

Barry's principal premise is that the institutionalization of cultural diversity, via the politics of multiculturalism, overstates the importance of cultural identity at the specific expense of the principles of equality and freedom. The latter principles, he argues, are both fundamentally necessarily for the achievement of the egalitarian principle of universal justice – hence, his advocacy of egalitarian liberalism – and can only be achieved by a 'difference blind' approach, grounded in individual autonomy and disembedded from any cultural referents. In contrast, the politics of cultural identity leads inevitably in his view to ethnic particularism, promoted most often by ethnic minority elites for their own political ends. As he dismissively observes, multiculturalism

> rewards the groups that can most effectively mobilize to make claims on the polity, or at any rate it rewards ethnocultural political entrepreneurs who can exploit its potential for their own ends by mobilizing a constituency around a set of sectional demands. (2001: 21)[11]

Such sectional politics promotes cultural relativism, the misplaced assumption that all cultures and cultural practices have equal value. This position is untenable, Barry argues, because it does not allow for any critique of the patently illiberal cultural practices of certain ethnic and/or religious minorities, such as forced marriage or genital mutilation. In so doing, it entrenches cultural essentialism, 'the endemic tendency to assume that distinctive cultural attributes are the defining feature of all groups' (2001: 305), identified with the ethnic primordialists and romantic nationalists discussed in Chapters 1 and 2, respectively. The consequence of this 'culturalization' of groups is also the 'systematic neglect of alternative causes of group disadvantage' (ibid.), returning to his wider concern with the politics of redistribution.

For Barry, minority groups, of whatever hue, must realize that maintenance of particular cultural and linguistic practices is a *luxury* that can only ever be afforded in the private domain, and then only voluntarily, allowing individuals the right of exit at any time. Barry also argues that this right of exit should extend to children, particularly with respect to education. The decision of Latino parents in the US to school their children via bilingual education programs, he avers, is demonstrably not in the latter's best interests. As with Schlesinger, Barry contends these bilingual education programs privilege Spanish language maintenance – a cultural imperative – at the specific expense of wider social and economic mobility, gained (only) via English in the wider US society (2001: 215–20, 226–8).[12]

Barry argues that such educational choices also result, in practice if not always in actual intent, in de facto segregation, which fatally undermines common understandings of the good life – what he terms 'the politics of solidarity'

(2001: 300). Commonality can only be achieved then by the active, concerted, participation of minorities in a shared and purposeful *national* identity, or 'civic nationality' (2001: 80). This is a comparable position to Bullivant's advocacy of civism as the answer to the pluralist dilemma. On this view, it is simply naive to think that different groups can live together peacefully without having anything in common; a position that echoes Furnivall's (1948) and M. G. Smith's (1965) discussions of ethnies in plural societies (see Chapter 2). Rather, the core of a common national identity must be 'a common commitment to the welfare of the larger society made up of the majority and the minority (or minorities), and mutual trust in others to abide by that commitment even when it entails sacrifices' (2001: 88).

However, for Barry, it is also clear that it is minority group members who must disproportionately bear the responsibility for making these sacrifices. As Barry asserts: 'I think that it is an appropriate objective of public policy in a liberal democratic state [that] all immigrants – or at least their descendants – become assimilated to the national identity of the country in which they are settled' (2001: 72). He proceeds to qualify this position, by acknowledging that assimilation has often been a forced choice for many minority group members, given that the retention of the culture or language of group may result in stigmatization and discrimination. But, so be it. As he concludes:

> Linguists and anthropologists may well have professional regrets if as a result a certain language ceases to be spoken or a certain cultural trait disappears. But preferences of these kinds are surely not an adequate basis on which to force people to perpetuate the language or cultural traits against their own judgment as to where the advantage lies. (2001: 75[13])

In sum, Barry's position is that 'the choice of solidarity with one's cultural group should not give rise to any sort of relative disadvantage, compared with participation in the mainstream [national] society' (2001: 95). Adapting one's ethnic or linguistic habitus is thus the necessary price for minority group members if they are to make their way successfully in the modern nation-state. Only by this, can they acquire a good education (preferably, it seems, one conducted solely in English), enhance their employability and, via both, achieve greater social and economic mobility. These are all central concerns of Barry's egalitarian liberalism and are, he argues, solely afforded by its difference blind approach rather than the segmented politics of multiculturalism. The price of not doing so should also by now be clearly evident: minority group members who continue to privilege the maintenance of their cultural distinctiveness over cultural adaptation and/or transformation 'will tend to cluster in occupations at the lower end of the hierarchy of money, status and power' (2001: 91). If so, they only have themselves to blame for it.

Critiquing liberal democracy

Such is the current orthodoxy among liberals to the question of the pluralist dilemma. When in doubt, the historical and political imperatives of nation-state congruence should prevail. So too should the related prerogative of the dominant ethnie to determine civic culture and minorities to accede and adapt to it, so defined. But how satisfactory is this broadly articulated position and what viable alternatives are there, if any? We can begin to unravel these questions by first highlighting some of the key inconsistencies that are evident in each of the preceding accounts.

John Porter's strong advocacy of assimilation, for example, was based on his long-held and principled commitment to egalitarianism. His arguments did not stem principally from a sense of nativism, racism or exclusion toward ethnic minorities. Rather, his advocacy of assimilation was promoted specifically on behalf and for the benefit of ethnic minority groups. In this sense, Porter represents the 'old' liberal position of the likes of Mill and Michelet. 'Ethnic' practices were seen as antediluvian and, it was assumed, would thus atrophy and eventually die in the face of modern (and modernist) civic culture. Consequently, the sooner ethnic groups were disabused of such 'traditional' practices, including the speaking of a minority language, the sooner they could contribute in and to the forward march of progress and civilization. This march of progress was also, by implication, most clearly evident in the dominant ethnie. However, its actual representation was couched almost exclusively in terms of the more 'objective' notions of 'individual achievement' and 'universalistic standards of judgement', with the state assuming the role of neutral arbiter. From this, all individuals were to be treated as 'equal' members of the civic polity – irrespective of their personal, social, religious and ethnic backgrounds – in order to 'establish a society of equality where ethnic origin did not matter' (1975: 293).

Porter's position is consistent here with an orthodox view of liberalism that addresses the person *only* as a political being with rights and duties attached to their status as *citizens*. Such a position does not countenance private identity, including a person's communal membership, as something warranting similar recognition. These latter dimensions are excluded from the public realm because their inevitable diversity would lead to the complicated business of the state mediating between different conceptions of 'the good life' (Rawls, 1971, 1985; Dworkin, 1978). On this basis, personal *autonomy* – based on the political rights attributable to citizenship – always takes precedence over personal (and collective) *identity* and the widely differing ways of life that constitute the latter. In effect, personal and political participation in liberal democracies, as it has come to be constructed, ends up denying group difference and posits all persons as interchangeable from a moral and political point of view (Young, 1993, 2000).

However, this strict separation of citizenship and identity in the modern polity understates, and at times disavows, the significance of wider communal affiliations, including ethnicity, to the construction of individual identity. As Michael Sandel (1982) observes, in a communitarian critique of liberalism, there is no such thing as the 'unencumbered self' – we are all, to some extent, *situated* within wider communities which shape and influence who we are.[14] Likewise, Charles Taylor argues that identity 'is who we are, "where we're coming from". As such, it is the background against which our tastes and desires and opinions and aspirations make sense' (1994: 33–4). These arguments have clear parallels with my discussion of habitus and field in Chapter 1. They also highlight the obvious point that certain goods such as language, culture and sovereignty cannot be experienced alone; they are, by definition, *communally* shared goods. A failure to account for these communal goods, however, has led to a view of rights within liberal democracy which is inherently individualistic and which cannot appreciate the pursuit of such goods other than derivatively (Van Dyke, 1977; Taylor, 1994; Coulombe, 1995).[15]

In short, individualistic conceptions of the good life may preclude shared community values that are central to one's identity (Kymlicka, 1995a, 2001). Conversely, as Habermas has put it, 'a correctly understood theory of [citizenship] rights requires a politics of recognition that protects the individual in the life contexts in which his or her identity is formed' (1994: 113). Following from this,

A 'liberal' version of the system of rights that fails to take this connection into account will necessarily misunderstand the universalism of basic rights as an abstract levelling of distinctions, a levelling of both cultural and social differences. To the contrary, these differences must be seen in increasingly context-sensitive ways if the system of rights is to be actualised democratically. (1994: 116)

Criticism of the inherent individualism of orthodox liberalism is not limited to communitarian critiques, however. This is an important point since communitarian critiques have themselves been widely criticized for essentializing group identities.[16] Thus, Will Kymlicka (1989) argues from a liberal perspective that the attempts of theorists like Rawls (1971) and Dworkin (1978) to separate citizenship from communal identity actually still retain an implicit recognition of cultural membership as a primary good. The only reason they do not explicitly give it status as a grounds for differential rights claims, Kymlicka suggests, is because they accept uncritically the notion of the nation-state as politically and culturally coterminous (see Chapter 2). If this assumption is dropped, cultural membership has to be explicitly recognized as a possible source of injustice and/ or inequality – a point which earlier theorists of liberalism, such as Hobhouse and Dewey, actually recognized. I discuss this latter point, and the significance of Kymlicka's wider contribution, more fully later in the chapter.

The dissociation of citizenship from individual identity, and the social and cultural context in which the latter is inevitably formed, highlights a related problem with orthodox liberal accounts such as Porter's – their inherent belief in the ethnic neutrality of the state. In other words, for orthodox liberals, the civic realm of the nation-state is a forum in which ethnicity does not (and *should* not) feature. However, as I have argued in the preceding chapters, ethnicity is *never* absent from the civic realm. Rather, the civic realm represents the particular (although not necessarily exclusive) *communal* interests and values of the dominant ethnie *as if* these values were held by all. In Charles Taylor's analysis, the 'supposedly neutral set of difference-blind principles [that constitute the liberal] politics of equal dignity is in fact a reflection of one hegemonic culture ... [it is] a particularism masquerading as the universal' (1994: 43–4). In a similar vein, Iris Marion Young argues that if particular groups 'have greater economic, political or social power, their group related experiences, points of view, or cultural assumptions will tend to become the norm, biasing the standards or procedures of achievement and inclusion that govern social, political and economic institutions' (1993: 133).

This hegemonic process is clearly illustrated in Porter's direct equation of citizenship with modernity and the associated valorization of homogeneity as simply the proper application of Reason (Goldberg, 1994). It is even more starkly apparent in Schlesinger's advocacy of a common American culture. In Schlesinger's account, the possibilities of heterogeneity are at least acknowledged by him, albeit somewhat grudgingly. However, his overall argument is unequivocal about homogeneity as the historically prevalent condition of social life and, as such, an ideal to be pursued and recaptured at all cost. This conclusion is encapsulated in his bald assertion of American history as 'the dream of one people' (1992: 110); a far from unproblematic assertion, as it turns out, since it can be accused of the very same features of 'bad history' and 'history as therapy' which he has leveled at Afrocentrism. As Robert Hughes, another liberal commentator, more candidly concedes, America 'has always been a heterogeneous country and its cohesion, whatever cohesion it has, can only be based on mutual respect. There never was a core America in which everyone looked the same, spoke the same language, worshipped the same gods and believed the same things' (1993: 12; see also Chapter 6).

The idea of a homogeneous common culture is thus simply another variant of nationalist myth-making. After all, as we saw in Chapter 2, *all* nationalist histories are therapeutic to some extent and contain inevitable elisions and absences. The key question then becomes not so much the teaching of bad or therapeutic history but *whose* history one wants to teach. National histories have tended, inevitably, to be the history, writ large, of the dominant (victorious) ethnie, as the growing number of revisionist histories in many ex-colonial contexts make clear. And this returns us once again to the central issue of hegemonic power relations. As Peter McLaren asserts, these 'conservative attacks on multiculturalism as separatist and ethnocentric carry with them the erroneous assumption by White Anglo constituencies that North American society fundamentally constitutes social relations of uninterrupted accord' (1995: 126–7). By this,

> [t]he liberal view is seen to underscore the idea that North American society is largely a forum of consensus with different minority viewpoints accretively added on. We are faced here with the politics of pluralism which largely ignores the workings of power and privilege. (1995: 127)

McLaren's analysis allows us to question the very notion of a commonly shared (American) culture and the supposedly unified and consensual history underpinning it. Common to whom, one might ask, and on whose terms? Who determines its central values and/or sets its parameters? Who is subsequently included and/or excluded from full participation in its 'benefits' and, crucially, *at what cost*? After all, those whose cultural and linguistic habitus are not reflected in the public realm are more likely to pay a far higher price for their subsequent participation in that realm. In contrast, those whose habitus are consonant with the civic culture and language – and, as such, are regarded as cultural and linguistic capital – have no such difficulties, as I will discuss further in the next chapter.

Brian Barry's account does not include the same degree of animus toward minority groups, the result of his broad-based left politics. However, his trenchant dismissal of multiculturalism for a difference-blind egalitarian liberalism ends up sharing many of the same misplaced premises as that of Porter and Schlesinger. Crucially, it is almost indistinguishable from their accounts in relation to the political *consequences* for minority groups. How so? First, by endorsing, through his advocacy of 'civic nationality', the same presentist, ahistorical conception of the supposedly homogeneous nation-state. As Oliver Schmidtke observes of this, '[b]y implicitly reifying the nation-state as the superior – if not exclusive – container for a universalistic liberal democracy, Barry misses the opportunity to reinvigorate political communities and democratic practices beyond the territorial confines of the nation-state' (2002: 274). This 'ahistoric, quasi-ontological quality ... attributed to the nation-state' (2002: 277) is then used in much the same way as Porter and Schlesinger to assert that the values of the 'nation-state as a whole' are universalistic, to be subscribed to by all. At no point is the historical recency of nation-states, and the principle of cultural and linguistic homogeneity, critically evaluated (cf. Norman, 1999). Nor, as a result, is the historical impact of exclusion and/or disadvantage faced by minority groups. Following from this, the claims of minority groups are dismissed as particularist and self-interested, rather than situated within, and arising from, the historical inequalities attendant upon nation-state congruence.

There is a convenient elision accomplished here, exemplified most clearly in Barry's account. On the one hand, the politics of recognition is repeatedly parodied for its excesses, while the politics of interests, of a more just and equitable engagement for minority groups within the wider national culture, is ignored. So too is the intrinsic link between the two that almost always underpins minority group rights claims. In other words, demands for recognition by minority groups are invariably linked to wider issues of exclusion and related social and/or political disadvantage, the latter often (but not always) including economic disadvantage as well (Squires, 2002; Kymlicka, 2007).[17]

Second, and relatedly, Barry, along with Schlesinger, makes no meaningful distinctions between the historical locatedness of particular minority groups and their associated rights claims. Rather, he treats all minority groups as equal supplicants upon the existing social, cultural and linguistic hierarchies of the (pre-existing) nation-state. As McLaren again comments, this approach wants to assimilate such minorities 'to an unjust social order by arguing that every member of every ethnic group can reap the benefits of neocolonialist ideologies and corresponding social and economic practices. But a prerequisite of "joining the club" is to become denuded, [de-ethnicized] and culturally stripped' (1995: 122). Indeed, even those minority members who advocate this position – and who are often much trumpeted as a result as 'good' or 'successful' minorities – generally do so from a position of personal ethnic and/or cultural dislocation (see Rodriguez, 1983, 1993). The result leaves little or no room for negotiation; little or no opportunity for changing 'the rules of the game'. And why is this? Because 'our' common bonds are too fragile, too easily dismembered or dismantled by the demands of particularism. One wonders what should be so fragile about Western civilization and, conversely, what is so radical about multiculturalism that this should be the case (Hughes, 1993)? But this, commentators such as Barry and Schlesinger insist, is what is centrally at stake.

There is a third parallel discourse going on here as well. Unlike Porter and Schlesinger, Barry does acknowledge that the liberal state is not culturally neutral. But he still holds that it is fair. His argument is that neutrality is not achievable, since a particular cultural worldview, and associated cultural practices, will inevitably be privileged in the construction of national identities. Neutrality comes, rather, from equal, or even-handed, treatment of extant cultural differences in the public or civic realm, via a common law for all. Any positive public accommodation of cultural differences, aka multiculturalism, is thus unnecessary. But what we see here, alongside the consistent downplaying of the links between culture and inequality discussed above, is the rejection of any meaningful contribution of minority groups to the wider debate about what actually constitutes equality and fairness. It is only liberals, it seems, who have anything meaningful and useful to contribute to such a discussion, and then, at least for Barry, only those who explicitly endorse an orthodox liberal view.[18] As Andrew Wright observes, '[t]he egalitarian [liberal] claim to tolerate difference is only skin deep; reducing the debate to the single value of equality ignores the equally important liberal values of empathy, respect and openness' (2004: 300–1). A more broad-based conversation between majority and minority group members about what constitutes national identity, and the associated toleration and limits of diversity, would encompass these latter values more effectively. Barry argues in relation to minority groups, for example, that 'we cannot expect the outcomes of democratic politics to be just in a society that contains large numbers of people who feel no sense of empathy with their fellow citizens and do not have any identification with their lot' (2001: 79). But this must surely work both ways. As Wright concludes, 'a society is unlikely to flourish if the liberal majority is unwilling or unable to engage sympathetically with minority groups on anything other than its own egalitarian terms' (2004: 310). Similarly, David Miller argues that what equal treatment entails 'is not self-evident in a culturally plural society, but has to be worked out through democratic dialogue in which the full range of different points of view are represented' (2002: 264).

A reconfigured national conversation along these lines would also entail a more differentiated understanding of identity than orthodox liberals allow, addressing a notable double standard apparent in their accounts. We see this double standard clearly in relation to the issue of cultural essentialism. On the one hand, liberal critics of multiculturalism rail against the supposed essentialism attendant upon all minority-group claims – the result of the 'culturalization' of groups, in Barry's overtly pejorative terms. The regular elision of multiculturalism with communitarianism in their accounts (particularly, Barry's) reinforces this view, since the latter is seen as necessarily reifying groups and essentializing their cultural, religious and/or linguistic practices.[19] This process of culturalization, it is argued, also invariably traps individual members of minority groups within the confines of their espoused collective identity, requiring them to conform to the supposed norms of the group. In similar vein to social constructionist critics of ethnicity, discussed in Chapter 1, this is seen to result from an overemphasis on *inter*ethnic differentiation at the expense of the inevitable traffic between cultures, the fluidity of individual ethnic identification(s), and the possibilities therein of significant *intra*ethnic differences, all of which may operate in combination with a variety of other social, cultural and political allegiances. Relatedly, the limiting of individual freedom in the face of supposedly fixed group norms is regarded as patently illiberal, as well as being linked directly to the entrenchment, rather than amelioration, of wider social disadvantage. We see this clearly illustrated, for example, in both Schlesinger and Barry's rejection of bilingual education as a form of self-imposed cultural and linguistic ghettoization and, in addition in

Barry's account, an illiberal imposition by minority parents on their children (see also Laitin and Reich, 2003; Pogge, 2003).[20]

All very convincing at one level, it seems, until one deconstructs the (only) alternative apparently on offer in such orthodox liberal accounts, the acceptance of a national identity at the specific expense of any alternative group identities that minority groups might wish to maintain. This zero-sum game requires minorities to accept a prior, inviolate, *majoritarian-determined* national identity that trumps all others (Calhoun, 1993a, 1997). This position specifically forecloses the possibility of a more dynamic and multifarious conception of nationhood, arising, in turn, from the more democratic, reciprocal discussion of what might constitute such national identities, discussed earlier. Requiring minorities to choose between various levels of identity is a consequence of the unquestioned acceptance of nation-state congruence, not a necessary condition of liberal democracy, as orthodox liberals aver. Such a position also fails to reflect adequately the possibilities of holding dual or multiple identities, except oppositionally. And yet it is clear that many of us can and do hold multiple and complementary identities – social, political and linguistic – at one and the same time, albeit not always easily (see Chapter 1). Certainly, one can hold both a regional and a national identity without these necessarily being conflictual. Why then should this not also be the case for ethnic and national identities (Stepan, 1998; Taylor, 1998)? Likewise, the juggling of different linguistic identities is an everyday activity for many minority language speakers, not least because they invariably have to operate in a majority language as well (see Chapter 4).

It is surely a delicious irony then that orthodox liberals end up endorsing a form of communitarianism not that dissimilar from the ethnic essentialism that apparently so invokes their ire. The only difference, it seems, is that theirs is a majoritarian form of 'ethnic cheerleading', reasserting the dominant ethnie's unbridled role in determining the scope (and limits) of national identity. Then again, all this might prove moot, if national identities are themselves increasingly passé in a globalized world where new cosmopolitan identities that transcend national boundaries are now the order of the day (Heller, 2011; cf. Chapter 1). Before turning in the final section of this chapter to a discussion of how we might rethink liberal democracies, and national identities, in ways that can and do accommodate minority group rights, let me first briefly address this important caveat.

The cosmopolitan alternative

Cosmopolitan theorists, much like those who advocate the merits of hybridity, celebrate loudly the multiplicity of identity choices available in the postmodern world. As Edward Said argues, 'no one today is purely one thing. Labels like Indian, or woman, or Muslim, or American are no more than starting points'

(1994: 407). Following from this, some cosmopolitan theorists, such as Martha Nussbaum (1997), have championed a new politics of belonging. Nussbaum advocates the notion of 'citizen of the world', a global form of citizenship that is no longer rooted in, or confined to, local, ethnic or national identities, but specifically transcends them. Again, the underlying principles are of individual transformation and the related movement away from the 'confines' of localized identities toward more broad-based identities (Calhoun, 2003, 2007). In effect, this amounts to a transnationalization of the national identity arguments endorsed by orthodox liberals.

One of the most trenchant advocates of cosmopolitanism is the political theorist Jeremy Waldron although, as a forerunner to the likes of Nussbaum, his focus of critique is still primarily on ethnic rather than national identity. Waldron objects to the idea that our choices and self-identity are defined by our ethnicity and asserts, instead, the need for a 'cosmopolitan alternative'. As he dismissively observes, 'though we may drape ourselves in the distinctive costumes of our ethnic heritage and immure ourselves in an environment designed to minimize our sense of relation with the outside world, no honest account of our being will be complete without an account of our dependence on larger social and political structures that goes far beyond the particular community with which we pretend to identify' (1995: 104). On this view, people can pick and choose 'cultural fragments' from various ethnocultural sources, without feeling an allegiance to any one in particular. Thus, Waldron argues, an Irish American who eats Chinese food, reads Grimm's Fairy Tales to their child, and listens to Italian opera actually lives in 'a kaleidoscope of cultures'. While Waldron concedes that we need cultural meanings of some kind, he argues that we do not need *specific* cultural frameworks: 'we need to understand our choices in the contexts in which they make sense, but we do not need any single context to structure our choices. To put it crudely, we need culture, but we do not need cultural integrity' (1995: 108; see also Hannerz, 1992).

The result is a purposefully freewheeling identity, with no deeply held affiliations, either publicly or privately, except, perhaps, as an acknowledged interdependent participant in the wider global community. All other, more situated, identities are dismissed out of hand. As Waldron provocatively concludes of these more situated, localized, identities:

From a cosmopolitan point of view, immersion in the traditions of a particular community in the modern world is like living in Disneyland and thinking that one's surroundings epitomize what it is for a culture really to exist. Worse still, it is demanding the funds to live in Disneyland and the protection of modern society for the boundaries of Disneyland, while still managing to convince oneself that what is happening inside Disneyland is all there is to an adequate and fulfilling life. … It is to

> imagine that one could belong to Disneyland while professing complete
> indifference towards, or even disdain for, Los Angeles. (1995: 101)

A not too dissimilar conclusion then to orthodox liberal commentators and
constructionist critics of ethnicity: ethnicity, apparently, is a fantasy world,
essentialist, isolationist, antediluvian and thus intrinsically delimited (and
delimiting), not to mention, irremediably passé. End of story. However, as
with the critique of hybridity theory, discussed in Chapter 1, this cosmopolitan
position has some key limitations of its own. It too largely ignores the class-
based, privileged, nature of so-called cosmopolitans – the 'frequent flyers' of
the contemporary world. As Craig Calhoun acerbically observes, advocacy of
cosmopolitan identities 'obscures the issues of inequality that make [such]
identities accessible mainly to elites and make being a comfortable citizen of
the world contingent on having the right passports, credit cards, and cultural
credentials' (2007: 286). In framing cosmopolitanism appeals to humanity in
individualistic terms, he continues, 'they are apt to privilege those with the most
capacity to get what they want by individual action' (2007: 295). More broadly,
cosmopolitanism ideas

> reflect the attractive illusion of escaping from social determinations into
> a realm of greater freedom, and from cultural particularity into greater
> universalism. But they are remarkably unrealistic, and so abstract as
> to provide little purchase on what the next steps of actual social action
> might be for real people who are necessarily situated in particular webs
> of belonging, with access to particular others but not humanity in
> general. Treating ethnicity as *essentially* (rather than partially) a choice of
> identifications, [cosmopolitan theorists] neglect the omnipresence of
> ascription and discrimination as determinations of social identities. (2007:
> 300–1; emphasis in original)

Problematic as well is the by now increasingly tiresome charge that any
recognition of group-based identities, and associated rights claims, necessarily
entails an essentialist construction of group identity. Not so: a group-based
approach *can* accommodate a view of ethnic and cultural groups as dynamic
and fluid while still retaining some sense of distinct cultural identity, as I will
elaborate on in the next section. In this regard, Margalit and Raz (1995) argue
that people today may well participate in a wide range of different social and
cultural activities but that this does not necessarily diminish their allegiance
to an 'encompassing group' with which they most closely identify. Nor does
an approach that acknowledges the importance of cultural membership to the
allocation of rights within a liberal democracy necessarily conflict with and/or
supersede the rights of individuals as citizens.

So where does this leave us? Critics of multiculturalism and minority rights consistently construct these as communitarian and thus entirely incompatible with liberalism and the primacy of individual rights, autonomy and mobility. But this need not be the case. As Pierre Coulombe observes: 'No one (I hope) wants to live in a society which only protects our personal autonomy. Nor does anyone (I'm sure) want to be treated as a heteronomous being. The challenge, therefore, is to rethink a political community that springs from our self-image as self-authored, yet situated, citizens' (1995: 21), while avoiding the pitfalls of reductionism or essentialism. This difficult balancing act can be found in the work of two key political theorists: Iris Marion Young and Will Kymlicka.

Rethinking liberal democracy

Those theorists who have become increasingly disenchanted with the orthodox liberal position on minority rights, and the philosophical matrix of the nation-state which underpins it, have begun to ask a number of key questions in their quest for a viable alternative approach. Following Mallea (1989), these questions may be summarized as follows:

- How can the values of individualism and pluralism be pursued simultaneously?
- Does the existence of ethnic and cultural diversity necessarily result in reduced levels of social cohesion?
- Can any society that embraces a monistic view of culture be considered democratic?
- What form might consensual theories of government take in plural societies?
- How much decentralization can political systems cope with in responding to the legitimate aspirations of national and ethnic minority groups?
- Does the concept of valid community lie in the extent to which it creates and maintains its own cultural norms?
- What levels of tolerance for contradiction and ambiguity can and should exist in plural societies?

Young and Kymlicka provide us with two of the most influential attempts at addressing these questions (see also Taylor, 1994) – attempts which, as we shall see, can usefully inform the issue of minority language rights as well. It is not my intention here to examine each of the questions outlined above in specific detail. However, it will soon become apparent that their various themes resonate throughout the work of both Young and Kymlicka. In what follows, I will discuss Young's postmodernist 'politics of difference' perspective,[21] which attempts to formulate an approach to rights within liberal democracies that is based on a recognition of group-related disadvantage and oppression, while at the same time recognizing and accommodating the relational and fluid nature of group identities. I examine Will Kymlicka's work for its development of the importance of cultural membership within a liberal (as opposed to communitarian) theory of rights. His central distinction between national and ethnic minorities, and the associated (and potentially differing) historical rights that underlie this distinction, also underpins my own position on minority language rights, as I will outline in subsequent chapters.

Differentiated citizenship

Iris Marion Young was a prominent critic of the conservatism and uniformity inherent in the notion of equal citizenship in liberal democracies. Her principal theoretical focus is on how this undifferentiated process impacts upon women as a disadvantaged social group. However, her work also has much broader application to a wide range of other disadvantaged groups including, for the purposes of this discussion, national and ethnic minority groups. Young argues, in effect, that the process of treating everyone as abstract individuals, undifferentiated by ethnicity, sex or class, actually reinforces the norms of the dominant group(s) within the nation-state at the expense of a wide variety of marginalized and/or oppressed groups. As she asserts:

> In a society where some groups are privileged while others are oppressed, insisting that as citizens persons should leave behind their particular affiliations and experiences to adopt a general point of view serves only to reinforce privilege; for the perspectives and interests of the privileged will tend to dominate this unified public, marginalizing or silencing those of other groups. (1989: 257)

Instead, she advocates a form of 'differentiated citizenship' where group representation rights are accorded to marginalized and oppressed groups within a single polity on the basis of their systemic disadvantage: 'the solution lies at least in part in providing institutionalized means for the explicit recognition and representation of oppressed groups' (1989: 258; see also 1990: 183–91). Her suggested list of those groups in the USA for which such recognition might be appropriate is extremely broad. It includes: 'women, blacks, Native Americans, Chicanos, Puerto Ricans and other Spanish-speaking Americans, Asian Americans, gay men, lesbians, working class people, poor people, old people and mentally and physically disabled people' (1989: 261). The inclusion of such diverse groupings is not without its problems, as I will discuss later in relation to Kymlicka's more focused position. However, Young's argument for a more heterogeneous conception of the nation-state is an important one. Various social, cultural and ethnic minority groups have the right in her view to a differentiated place in the civic realm. This right, in turn, is based on the *mutual* recognition and valuing of their specificity and worth in the public domain (Young, 1993). The notion of social justice is central here to Young's argument: 'Besides guaranteeing civil and political rights, and guaranteeing that the basic needs of individuals will be met so that they can freely pursue their own goals, *a vision of social justice provides for some group related rights and policies*' (1993: 135–6; my emphasis). From this, 'group institutions will adhere to a principle that social policy should attend to rather than be blind to group difference in awarding benefits or burdens, in order to remedy group based inequality or [to] meet group specific need' (ibid.).

Young is thus principally preoccupied with questions of justice and oppression, particularly as these affect a wide range of disadvantaged and/or oppressed groups within modern nation-states. In this respect, she is concerned both with the recognition of oppressed groups via political and institutional devices, and the recognition of cultural differences as a basic principle of equality and justice (see 1990: 174). However, in arguing for the recognition of group-based rights, she also meticulously tries to avoid the mistake of reifying groups. In fact, she specifically rejects the two common alternatives in addressing the pluralist dilemma – assimilation and separatism – for doing exactly this. Assimilation, she suggests, rightly champions individual freedom, equality and self-development. However, it wrongly assumes that *any* assertion of group identity and difference is, by definition, essentialist. Separatism may help establish cultural autonomy and political solidarity for oppressed groups and does challenge the hegemonic construction of the nation-state. However, it tends also to understate the historical *interrelations* between different groups – particularly, in modern mass, urban societies – and to simplify and freeze its own group identity in ways that fail to acknowledge intragroup differences. In this sense, Young can be seen to criticize both orthodox liberal and communitarian approaches to rights and identity. Her rejection of separatism – that is, the key tenet of political nationalism – is also broadly consonant with a more culturalist conception of nationalism, as discussed in Chapter 2. Indeed, in her later work she argues for a relational concept of self-determination that closely accords with the key tenets of cultural nationalism (Young, 2004, 2005; cf. Chapter 8).

For Young, both assimilation and separatism end up reinforcing the notion of difference as 'Otherness'. In this view, each group has its own nature and shares no attributes with those defined as Other. In effect, difference as Otherness 'conceives social groups as mutually exclusive, categorically opposed' (1993: 126). Moreover, in a similar vein to the discussion in Chapter 1 of 'ascriptive humiliation' (Lukes, 1996), and 'misrecognition' and 'symbolic violence' (Bourdieu, 1991), Young argues that when this process of social relations occurs between a privileged group on the one hand, and a disadvantaged group on the other, the attribution of Otherness invariably takes on a pathological characteristic for the latter. As she argues, the 'privileged group is defined as active human subject' while 'inferiorized social groups are objectified, substantialized, reduced to a nature or essence' (1993: 124–5). Similarly, '[whereas the privileged groups are neutral, exhibit free, spontaneous and weighty subjectivity, the dominated groups are marked with an essence, imprisoned in a given set of possibilities' (1993: 125). She concludes: 'Using its own values, experience, and culture as [universal] standards, the dominant group measures the Others and finds them essentially lacking' (ibid.).

More broadly, Young argues that this particular logic of identity essentializes and substantializes group natures, generates dichotomy at the expense of unity (even when it is couched in terms of the latter) and runs counter to the relational and fluid nature of inter- and intragroup relations. In a position which echoes Eriksen's observation that ethnicity is essentially 'an aspect of social relationship' (2010: 16; see Chapter 1), Young observes:

> Defining groups as Other actually denies or represses the heterogeneity of social difference, understood as variation and contextually experienced relations. It denies the difference among those who understand themselves as belonging to the same group; it reduces the members of the group to a set of common attributes ... The practical realities of social life, especially but not only in modern, mass, economically interdependent societies, defy the attempt to conceive and enforce group difference as exclusive opposition, there are always ambiguous persons who do not fit the categories ... partial identities [that cut] across more encompassing group identities. (1993: 127–8)

In contrast, Young argues that her conception of a differentiated approach to public policy is better able to recognize heterogeneity and the interspersion of groups. Such an approach does not posit a social group as having an essential nature composed of a set of attributes defining only that group, nor does it repress the interdependence of groups in order to construct a substantial conception of group identity. Rather,

> a social group exists and is defined as a specific group only in social and interactive relation to others. Social group identities emerge from the encounter and interaction among people who experience some differences in their way of life and forms of association, even if they regard themselves as belonging to the same society ... Group identity is not a set of objective facts, but the product of experienced meanings. (1993: 130)

This position is closely parallel to the conclusions drawn about situational ethnicity in Chapter 1. It is also akin to Charles Taylor's (1994) emphasis on the *dialogical* nature of identity formation in his comparable discussion on 'the politics of recognition' (see also Honneth, 1995). The result is a conception of difference which allows for specificity, variation and heterogeneity *within* the nation-state, as well as a central acknowledgment of the unequal power relations within which such difference is invariably framed. The expression of group differences is encouraged but within common institutions and a shared commitment to a larger political order. Moreover, groups are understood 'as overlapping, as constituted in relation to one another and thus as shifting their attributes and needs in accordance with what relations are salient' (1993: 123–4). As Young concludes, 'different groups always potentially share some attributes, experiences, or goals ... The characteristics that make one group specific and the borders that distinguish it from other groups are always *undecidable*' (1993: 130). Accordingly, a relational and contextualized conception of difference within the plurally conceived nation-state helps make more apparent 'the necessity and possibility of togetherness in difference' (1993: 124).

Inevitably, there are problems with Young's account (for a useful overview and critique, see Fletcher, 1998). For example, her concern to equalize political influence for marginalized and oppressed groups within the nation-state necessarily entails a wide-ranging remit – too wide-ranging perhaps, since the conglomeration of such groups is potentially unending. Her own description of the diverse range of groups who might be included in her formulations bears this out. Kymlicka observes, for example, that this 'list of "oppressed groups" in the United States would seem to include 80 percent of the population ... In short, everyone but relatively well-off, relatively young, able-bodied, heterosexual white males' (1995a: 145; see also Barry, 2001). There is also a problem with bringing such disparate groups together on the singular basis of disadvantage and/or oppression. One can argue, for example, that the rights of Native Americans as an indigenous people in North America, or of Māori in Aotearoa/New Zealand – both of whom she includes in her discussions of group-differentiated citizenship (see 1990: 175–83; 1993: 143–7) – are quite distinct from those of a broad social group such as poor people. Focusing on disadvantage as the principal criterion for their inclusion thus obscures the *particular* demands of these national minorities for greater self-determination within the nation-state. Native Americans and Māori can claim greater access to and representation within the state not simply because they are marginalized groups (although they *are* marginalized), but because of their legitimate historical and territorial rights as ethnies. Relatedly, an emphasis on disadvantage implies only *temporary* representation until such time as the disadvantage has been redressed (Loobuyck, 2005). This form of political affirmative action, in effect, is again clearly inadequate in addressing the long-term demands of national minorities for greater acknowledgment and representation in the civic realm (Kymlicka, 1995a, 2001; see below).

However, Young's failure to distinguish the rights of national minorities from other ethnic, cultural and social groups is not unusual in discussions of the pluralist dilemma. We have already seen this elision in the countervailing accounts of Porter, Schlesinger and Barry. It is clear, for example, that each of these more orthodox liberal accounts is characterized by an almost exclusive preoccupation with *ethnic* or *immigrant* minorities – that is, modern urban migrants and ethnic groups in plural societies, as defined in Chapter 2. Accordingly, the arguments employed in defence of the nation-state gain much of their moral suasion from the implicit underlying belief that immigrant groups should have less claim to official recognition by the state than the national 'majority' (cf. Kymlicka, 2007). Apart from a few desultory references to Canadian Aboriginal peoples, Native Americans in the US and the Welsh and Scottish in Britain, by Porter, Schlesinger and Barry, respectively, none addresses, or even acknowledges, the question of national minority rights. Thus, each fails to differentiate the claims of national minorities from those of other ethnic minority groups. Indeed, even within the latter category, both Schlesinger and Barry adopt an undifferentiated approach, as seen, for example, in their glib comparisons between the social and educational trajectories of African Americans and Jewish and Asian ethnic communities in the USA. Such a comparison is clearly both inadequate and inappropriate since it takes little, if any account of class as a significant factor, or the voluntary/involuntary status of these groups (Ogbu, 1987; see Chapter 2).

Multicultural citizenship

Will Kymlicka is one of the few theorists on either side of the pluralist dilemma debates to draw a clear distinction between the rights of national minorities (including indigenous peoples) and other minority ethnic, cultural and social groups (see also Walzer, 1982; Spinner, 1994; Taylor, 1994). As he observes in his seminal book, *Multicultural Citizenship* (1995a), most discussions of multiculturalism and/or minority rights 'focus on the case of immigrants, and the accommodation of their ethnic ... differences within the larger society. Less attention has been paid to the situation of indigenous peoples and other nonimmigrant "national minorities" whose homeland has been incorporated into the boundaries of a larger state, through conquest, colonisation, or federation' (1995a: p. vii). On this basis, Kymlicka defines national minorities 'as distinct and *potentially self-governing* societies incorporated into a larger state' and ethnic minority groups as 'immigrants who have left their national community to enter another society' (1995a: 19; my emphasis). The key distinction for Kymlicka is that national minorities, at the time of their incorporation, constituted an ongoing 'societal culture' – that is, 'a culture which provides its members with meaningful ways of life across the full range of human activities ... [and] encompassing both public and private spheres' (1995a: 76). Ethnic minorities, in contrast, may well wish to maintain aspects of their cultural and linguistic identities within the host nation-state but this is principally in order to contribute to, and modify the existing national culture rather than to recreate a separate societal culture of their own (see also Gurr, 1993, 2000).

Kymlicka's analysis here closely accords with my discussion in Chapter 2 of the key distinctions between ethnic and national minorities and the related significance of cultural and political nationalisms. As I argued there, political nationalism is not the only determining feature of nationalist movements since such a view, while received wisdom for many, relegates national minorities that are not (yet) politically active to the status of mere 'ethnic groups'. Kymlicka's emphasis on incorporation into the nation-state, rather than on political mobilization per se, provides a useful complement to my own argument. It allows for quiescent national minorities and highly mobilized immigrant groups without confusing the political status of the two.

In addition, both national and ethnic minorities in Kymlicka's formulation can be distinguished from 'new social movements' such as gay, lesbian and queer communities, women, and the disabled who have been marginalized within their own national society or ethnic group. Kymlicka thus provides us with a more nuanced analysis that allows for the possibility of attributing *differing* rights to various minority groups within the nation-state. In this regard, his position is a significant advance on much of the literature concerned with multiculturalism, which has largely failed historically to make these kinds of distinctions. This, in turn, has led to the valid charge of cultural relativism leveled against multiculturalism by its critics on both the right and the left, not to mention the attendant difficulties that such cultural relativism inevitably entails (May, 1999a, 2001; see also Chapter 4). In what follows, I will concentrate principally on the specific concerns of indigenous and other national minority groups, although I will also briefly address the specific rights attributable to ethnic minority groups and new social movements. I will return, however, to the wider implications of the latter, and specific ways of addressing the problems of cultural relativism, in Chapter 9.

Meanwhile, as we saw in Chapter 2, the distinction between the respective positions of national and ethnic minorities in modern nation-states can be illustrated by the terms 'multinational' and 'polyethnic'. As Kymlicka observes of this, most states are actually a combination of both: 'obviously, a single country may be both multinational (as a result of the colonizing, conquest, or confederation of national minorities) and polyethnic (as a result of individual and familial immigration)' (1995a: 17). However, most countries are also reluctant, more often than not, to acknowledge this combination in their public policy. Indeed, nation-states may well acknowledge neither, although this is rare, at least in liberal-democratic states. More usually, they may acknowledge one or the other. Thus, in the USA there is recognition of the country's polyethnicity – albeit, a grudging one among conservatives – but an unwillingness to distinguish and accept the rights of national minorities such as Native Americans, Hawaiians and Puerto Ricans. Likewise, Australia and Aotearoa/New Zealand have historically argued that they are settler colonies and hence have no national minorities; a position which ignores entirely the rights of Australian Aboriginal peoples and Māori who were subject to European colonization. In Belgium and Switzerland, however, the reverse applies. The rights of national minorities have long been recognized but an accommodation of immigrants and a more polyethnic society has been less forthcoming (for further discussion, see Kymlicka, 2007: 66–77).[22] Recognizing both dimensions then, and the respective rights attendant upon them, is the central challenge for developing a more plurally conceived approach to public policy in modern nation-states.

Following from this, Kymlicka argues that in addition to the civil rights available to all individuals, three forms of group-specific rights should be recognized in liberal democracies: 1) self-government rights; 2) polyethnic rights; and 3) special representation rights (see 1995a: 26–33). Self-government rights acknowledge that the nation-state is not the sole preserve of the majority (national) group and that legitimate national minority ethnies have the right to equivalent inclusion and representation in the civic realm. Accordingly, national minorities should be provided with rights to their autonomy and self-determination within the nation-state, which, if necessary, could be extended to incorporate the possibilities of secession. Ostensibly, this right of minority national groups to self-determination is not inconsistent with international law. The (1945) United Nations Charter, for example, clearly states that 'all peoples have the right to self-determination'. However, the UN did not define the term 'peoples' and the injunction has tended since to be interpreted only in relation to overseas colonies (the 'salt water thesis') rather than to national minorities, even though the latter may have been subjected to the same processes of colonization. Self-determination has thus been limited *in practice* to pre-existing (postcolonial) states. Meanwhile, attempts at broadening the principle to include the claims of national minorities, including indigenous peoples, have met with fierce resistance and, usually, limited success (Thornberry, 1991a, 1997; Young, 2004; San Juan, 2006; Robbins, 2010; although see Chapter 8).

Where national minorities have been recognized within existing nation-states, multinational and/or multilingual federalism has been the most common process of political accommodation that has been adopted. An obvious example here is the degree of autonomy given to French-speaking Quebec as part of a federal (and predominantly Anglophone) Canada. The establishment of seventeen regional "autonomías", including Catalonia and the Basque Country, in the post-Franco multinational Spanish state is another clear example (see Chapter 7). Self-government rights, then, typically involve the devolution of political power to members of a national minority who are usually, but not always, located in a particular historical territory. The key in providing for such rights is their *permanent* status. They are not seen as a temporary measure or remedy that may one day be revoked (cf. Loobuyck, 2005).

Polyethnic rights also challenge the hegemonic construction of the nation-state but for a different clientele and to different ends. Polyethnic rights are intended to help ethnic minority groups to continue to express their cultural, linguistic and/or religious heritage, principally in the private domain, without it hampering their success within the economic and political institutions of the dominant national society. One might add here that these rights are also available so that an undue burden of cultural and linguistic loss and/or change is not placed upon such groups (Kymlicka, 2001; see Chapter 4). Like self-government rights, polyethnic rights are thus also permanent, since they seek to protect rather than eliminate cultural and linguistic differences. However, their principal purpose is to promote integration *into* the larger society (and to contribute to and modify that society as a result) rather than to foster self-governing status among such groups. In this regard, integration comes to be seen as a *reciprocal* process rather than a simple accommodation of ethnic minority groups to the majoritarian national culture. It is a *revision* of integration rather than a *rejection* of it (see also Spinner, 1994; Spinner-Halev, 1999). Finally, special representation rights, along the lines outlined earlier by Young, are a response to some systemic disadvantage in the political process which limits a particular group's view from being effectively represented. Special representation rights aim to redress this disadvantage but do so principally on a temporary basis. Once the oppression and/or disadvantage has been eliminated the rights no longer apply.

Taken together, these three kinds of rights can be regarded as distinct but not necessarily mutually exclusive. Indigenous peoples, for example, may demand special representation rights on the basis of their disadvantage, and self-governing rights on the basis of their status as a national minority ethnie. However, the key point is that these claims need not go together. Thus, the disabled may claim special representation rights but would not be able to claim either polyethnic or self-government rights. Likewise, an economically successful ethnic minority group may seek polyethnic rights but would have no claim to special representation or self-governing rights, and so on. Assuming the validity of such group-differentiated rights in the first place, however, does return us to the central questions surrounding the legitimacy of minority rights in liberal democracies and the difficulties involved in ascribing and/or determining particular group identities for the apportionment of such rights. Kymlicka's response to both these concerns is to defend minority rights on the basis of liberal theory rather than from a communitarian stance (despite what Brian Barry might think; see n. 17). In so doing, he manages to uphold the importance of individual citizenship rights while, at the same time, developing an understanding of the importance of cultural membership to such rights.

Kymlicka brings a range of arguments to bear in support of his position. First, he rejects the assumption that group-differentiated rights are 'collective' rights which, ipso facto, stand in opposition to 'individual' rights. Group-differentiated rights are not necessarily 'collective' in the sense that they privilege the group over the individual – they can in fact be accorded to individual members of a group, or to the group as a whole, or to a federal state/province within which the group forms a majority. For example, the group-differentiated right of Francophones in Canada to use French in federal courts is an *individual* right that may be exercised at any time. The right of Francophones to have their children educated in French-medium schools, outside of Quebec, is an individual right also but one that is subject to the proviso 'where numbers warrant' (see Chapter 5). In contrast, indigenous land and fishing rights are usually exercised by the collective tribal group – as, for example, in the case of Native Americans in North America and Māori in Aotearoa/New Zealand. Finally, the right of the Québécois to preserve and promote their distinct culture in the province of Quebec highlights how a minority group in a federal system may exercise group-differentiated rights in a territory where they form the majority, an example I will discuss in more depth in Chapter 7.

In short, there is no simple relationship between group-differentiated rights accorded on the basis of cultural membership and their subsequent application. Thus, the common criticisms of 'collective rights' in the debates on the pluralist dilemma have little actual relevance to the question of group-differentiated rights. As Kymlicka concludes of the latter, 'most such rights are not about the primacy of communities over individuals. Rather, they are based on the idea that justice between groups requires that the members of different groups be accorded different rights' (1995a: 47).

Second, Kymlicka rejects the inevitable association of group-differentiated rights with illiberality – a key criticism of multiculturalism, particularly from those on the left. We have already seen the issue raised directly in Barry's work, for example. Feminist critics, concerned with the perpetuation of patriarchal practices within minority groups, have also consistently raised objections to group-based rights on this basis.[23] Kymlicka addresses this problem by drawing a key distinction between what he terms 'internal restrictions' and 'external protections' (1995a: 35–44; 2001: 22–3). Internal restrictions involve *intra*group relations where the ethnic or national minority group seeks to restrict the individual liberty of its members on the basis of maintaining group solidarity, creating in the process 'internal minorities' (Kymlicka, 2007). These rights are often associated with theocratic and patriarchal communities and, when excessive, may be regarded as illiberal. In contrast, external protections relate to *inter*group relations where an ethnic or national minority group seeks to protect its distinct identity by limiting the impact of the decisions of the larger society. External protections are thus intended to ensure that individual members are able to maintain a distinctive way of life *if they so choose* and are not prevented from doing so by the decisions of members outside of their community (see Kymlicka, 1995a: 204 n. 11). This too has its dangers, although not in relation to individual oppression in this case but rather the possible unfairness that might result between groups. The ex-apartheid system in South Africa provides a clear example of the latter scenario. However, as Kymlicka argues, external protections need not result in injustice: 'Granting special representation rights, land claims, *or language rights* to a minority need not, and often does not, put it in a position to dominate other groups. On the contrary ... such rights can be seen as putting the various groups on a more equal footing, by reducing the extent to which the smaller group is vulnerable to the larger' (1995a: 36–7; my emphasis).

Kymlicka argues that, on this basis, liberals can endorse certain external protections where they promote fairness between groups while still contesting internal restrictions which unduly limit the individual rights of members to question, revise or reject traditional authorities and practices (see also Kymlicka, 1999a, b). In relation to the various group-differentiated rights outlined earlier, Kymlicka concludes that 'most demands for group-specific rights made by ethnic and national groups in Western democracies are for external protections' (1995a: 42), a pattern that has been increasingly recognized by national and international law (McGoldrick, 2005; Kymlicka, 2007; see Chapter 5). Even where internal restrictions are also present, these are usually seen as unavoidable byproducts of external protections rather than as desirable ends in themselves. As we shall see in the ensuing chapters, this latter point has particular relevance to minority language rights. The likes of Barry and Schlesinger have already argued that the maintenance of a minority language, particularly via bilingual education, is a potentially illiberal imposition on children. However, as with Kymlicka, I will argue that such language rights are rather a form of external protection and neither intrinsically illiberal nor foreclosing of wider social and economic mobility (see Chapter 6).

Third, Kymlicka argues that a recognition of the importance of cultural membership to one's individual rights has historical precedent in both liberal theory and political practice. Indeed, the rigid separation of individual *autonomy* from individual and collective *identity* has only really occurred in liberal theory and practice since the Second World War. Prior to this, liberal commentators did not assume that the state should treat cultural membership as a purely private matter. On the contrary, 'liberals either endorsed the legal recognition of minority cultures, or rejected minority rights not because they rejected the idea of an official culture, but precisely because they believed there should only be *one* official culture' (1995a: 53–4). The latter position is clearly illustrated by the arguments of Mill discussed in Chapter 1. The former view is exemplified in the work of Hobhouse and Dewey in the early part of the twentieth century. They both argued, on the basis of the importance of cultural membership, that some accommodation should be made for the distinctive group-related rights of national minorities within the nation-state (Kymlicka, 1989). Hobhouse, for example, believed that if the claims of national minorities were satisfied by greater cultural equality, the distinctive problems of secession would not arise. In contrast, failure to address the legitimate rights of national minorities might actually hasten the break-up of the nation-state rather than the reverse. On this view, individual citizenship rights were *insufficient* to the continued maintenance of the nation-state:

> The smaller nationality does not merely want equal rights with others. *It stands out for a certain life of its own* ... [To] find the place for national rights within the unity of the state, to give scope to national differences without destroying the organisation of a life which has somehow to be lived in common, is therefore the problem which the modern state has to solve if it is to maintain itself. It has not only to generalise the common rights of citizenship as applied to individuals, but to make room for diversity and give some scope to common sentiments *which in a measure conflict with each other.* (1928: 146–7; my emphases)

Concern for the cultural protection of minorities was also reflected in political practices prior to the Second World War. In the nineteenth century, treaties were often employed for the protection of minority groups, initially on the basis of religion and later on the grounds of nationality (Thornberry, 1991a; Oestreich, 1999; Duchêne, 2008).[24] These practices culminated in the general organization of the League of Nations, established in the wake of the First World War. The League endorsed a range of bilateral treaties that were overseen by the League's Permanent Court of International Justice (PCIJ) and which subsequently became known collectively as the Minority Protection scheme. The principal focus of the scheme was the protection of 'displaced' minorities who had ended up on the wrong side of newly constituted borders as the result of the dissolution of the Russian, Ottoman and Habsburg Empires, and the reorganization of European state boundaries after the First World War (Wolfrum, 1993; Packer, 1999; Kymlicka, 2007).[25]

This approach was to change significantly, however, with the advent of the Second World War and the associated excesses and abuses of the said scheme by the Nazi regime, whereby Hitler used a supposed concern for the rights of German minorities elsewhere in Europe as a catalyst for the war. As a result, there was a postwar shift in emphasis to establishing generic human rights, irrespective of group membership, through the establishment and subsequent activities of the United Nations and other supranational agencies such as the

EU. In so doing, it was assumed that no additional rights need be attributed to the members of specific ethnic or national minorities (see also Chapter 5). As Claude has observed of these developments:

> The leading assumption has been that members of national minorities do not need, are not entitled to, or cannot be granted rights of special character. The doctrine of human rights has been put forward as a substitute for the concept of minority rights, with the strong implication that minorities whose members enjoy individual equality of treatment cannot legitimately demand facilities for the maintenance of their ethnic particularism. (1955: 211)

Consequently, all references to the rights of ethnic and national minorities were deleted from the (1948) United Nations Universal Declaration of Human Rights.[26] Relatedly, a widespread conviction began to emerge among liberals that minority group rights were somehow incompatible with national and international peace and stability. However, as Kymlicka asserts, these assumptions are fundamentally misplaced. As we have seen, individual autonomy is inevitably dependent, at least to some extent, on one's cultural membership. Moreover, the failure of modern liberal theory and practice to acknowledge the specific rights of minorities has left them subject to the majoritarian decision-making processes of the nation-state. The result has been to render minorities 'vulnerable to significant injustice at the hands of the majority, and to exacerbate ethnocultural conflict' (1995a: 5), trends which the UN and other supranational bodies have only more recently begun to address (see Kymlicka and Opalski, 2001; Kymlicka, 2007, for useful overviews of these international developments; see also Chapter 5).

Fourth, Kymlicka argues that Waldron's 'cosmopolitan alternative', which disavows the importance of one's *particular* cultural membership, is significantly overstated. On this basis, Waldron rejects the codification of minority rights as a misplaced and misguided anachronism since most people now move easily between cultures and thus do not *need*, it seems, to be attached to just one. We have already seen how social status affects the ability to 'move easily' between cultures, limiting the latter to social and cultural elites. What then of Waldron's related assertion that minority groups should simply dispense with their cultural and linguistic backgrounds and adopt those of the dominant ethnie?

Waldron's view here is reminiscent of the advocates of situational ethnicity, discussed in Chapter 1, who emphasize the fluid and multiple nature of ethnic (and other group) identities and the varied instrumental ends to which these are put. Not surprisingly, criticisms of Waldron's position are also similar to those directed at the more extreme instrumentalist positions adopted by some advocates of situational ethnicity. People do clearly move between cultures –

immigrants are an obvious example here – but cultural loss and/or subsumption is not nearly as easy and as unproblematic a process as Waldron suggests. Indeed, Margalit and Raz (1995) have argued that the transfer from one culture to another is often extremely difficult, even for voluntary migrants, not only because it is 'a very slow process indeed', but because of the importance of cultural membership to people's self-identity (see also Tamir, 1993; Taylor, 1994; Gutmann, 2003; Calhoun, 2007; Valadez, 2007). This is even more so for national minorities who are often forced, in effect, to renounce the language and culture of their own 'societal' or 'encompassing' group for another's (see Chapter 4). As Margalit and Raz observe, this ignores the fact that:

> membership of such groups is of great importance to individual well-being, for it greatly affects one's opportunities, one's ability to engage in the relationships and pursuits marked by culture. Secondly ... the prosperity of the culture is important to the well-being of its members ... people's sense of their own identity is bound up with their sense of belonging to encompassing groups and ... their self-respect is affected by the esteem in which these groups are held. (1995: 86–7; see also Taylor, 1994; Honneth, 1995)

In short, ethnic and national identities cannot simply be exchanged like last year's clothes, as we saw Michael Billig observe in Chapter 1. Moreover, if members of the dominant ethnie typically value their own cultural and linguistic membership, it is clearly unfair to prevent national minorities from continuing to value theirs. As Kymlicka concludes, 'leaving one's culture, while possible, is best seen as renouncing something to which one is reasonably entitled' (1995a: 90). Relatedly, he argues:

> The freedom which liberals demand for individuals is not primarily the freedom to go beyond one's language and history, but rather the freedom to move within one's societal culture, to distance oneself from particular cultural roles, to choose which features of the culture are most worth developing, and which are without value. (1995a: 90–1)

Kymlicka's (and Margalit and Raz's) position closely accords with my own view of ethnicity as habitus, outlined in Chapter 1.[27] In addition, Kymlicka's last observation provides us with a rejoinder to a related criticism of Waldron's, that a defence of minority rights inevitably reinforces a homogeneous conception of ethnic groups (see Waldron, 1995: 103–5). Waldron is particularly critical here of notions of cultural 'purity' and 'authenticity' which, he argues, are regularly employed by indigenous peoples and other national minorities in support of their claims to greater self-determination. These attempts at cultural delineation are manifestly artificial in his view and can only result in cultural stasis and isolationism. As such, liberals should regard them as anathema. However, as Kymlicka counters, the assertion of national minority rights does not preclude the possibilities of cultural adaptation, change and interchange:

> there is no inherent connection between the desire to maintain a distinct societal culture and the desire for cultural isolation. In many cases, the aim of self-government is to enable smaller nations to interact with larger nations on a more equitable basis. It should be up to each culture to decide when and how they adopt the achievements of the larger world. It is one thing to learn from the larger world; it is another to be swamped by it, and self-government rights may be needed for smaller nations to control the direction and rate of change. (1995a: 103–4)

Indeed, the desire of national minorities to survive as a culturally distinct society is most often *not* based on some simplistic desire for cultural 'purity'. Defenders of minority rights (including minority language rights) are rarely seeking to preserve their 'authentic' culture if that means returning to cultural practices long past. If it were, it would soon meet widespread opposition from individual members. Rather, it is the right 'to maintain one's membership in a distinct culture, and to continue developing that culture in the same (impure) way that the members of majority cultures are able to develop theirs' (1995a: 105). Cultural and linguistic change, adaptation and interaction are entirely consistent with such a position. As Kymlicka argues elsewhere (1995b: 8–9), minority cultures wish to be both cosmopolitan and to embrace the cultural interchange that Waldron emphasizes. However, this does not necessarily entail Waldron's own 'cosmopolitan alternative', which denies that people have any deep bond to their own historical cultural and linguistic communities. In similar vein, Kymlicka asserts that minority rights 'help to ensure that the members of minority cultures have access to a secure cultural structure *from which to make choices for themselves*, and thereby promote liberal equality' (1989: 192; my emphasis). On this view, national minorities continue to exercise their individual rights within their particular cultural and linguistic milieus and, of course, contextually, in relation to other cultural groups within a given nation-state (see Young, 1993). The crucial element, however, is that members of the national minority are themselves able to retain a significant degree of control over the process – something which until now has largely been the preserve of majority group members. The key issue thus becomes one of cultural and linguistic *autonomy* rather than one of retrenchment, isolationism or stasis. As Kymlicka concludes in his most recent book, 'this liberal view of multiculturalism is inevitably, intentionally, and unapologetically transformational of people's cultural traditions' (2007: 99).

Kymlicka's liberal defence of national minority rights is a cogent one. In reconceptualizing liberal theory – principally, by unshackling it from the 'philosophical matrix of the nation-state' within which it has come to be subsumed – he provides a powerful theoretical framework and intellectual justification for such rights. In so doing, he also comes closest to balancing what Hobhouse earlier highlighted as those 'common sentiments *which in a measure conflict with each other*' (1928: 146–7; my emphasis); namely, citizenship and (minority) ethnicity. This is not to say, however, that Kymlicka resolves the measure of conflict between such sentiments. Indeed, no account which deals with such issues could ever do so fully, nor indeed would it necessarily be helpful to do so, since the point in the end is that the various claims involved are *competing* ones (see also Chapter 9). As Homi Bhabha argues, 'the question of cultural difference faces us with a disposition of knowledges or a distribution of practices that exist beside each other, abseits designating a form of social contradiction and antagonism that has to be negotiated rather than sublated' (1994: 162). On this basis, what is required is a *negotiated* settlement that acknowledges difference, and accommodates it where it can, rather than a compromise that subsumes it and/or attempts to resolve all its contradictory aspects.

The inevitability of these ongoing tensions does mean though that Kymlicka has faced his own fair share of criticism. For example, communitarian critics such as Charles Taylor (1994) have argued that while Kymlicka's argument accounts for the cultural survival of existing groups who currently face pressure from majority cultural forces, it does not ensure their continued survival over generations, which, for such groups, is the central issue at stake. For the latter to occur, collective goals would in some circumstances have to be preferred to individual ones, a position that Kymlicka is reluctant to take. Indeed, for Kymlicka, the principal importance of cultural membership is that 'it allows for meaningful individual choices' (1989: 172). Thus, freedom of choice must be regarded as prior to the ties that bind us to community; in effect, community must remain commensurable with individual liberty (Coulombe, 1995). However, as Moore (1991) argues, there remains a certain contradiction in a position which claims that the value of autonomy is derived from its role in fostering community while also asserting that autonomy is the ultimate value on which that community is to be assessed (see also Tomasi, 1995). Relatedly, there is an ambiguity at times as to what actually constitutes a group for Kymlicka and, by extension, who might be eligible for the rights associated with such groups (Burtonwood, 1996). Kymlicka is rightly skeptical here of any notion of a group identity that is pre-given or fixed but articulates this less clearly than, say, Iris Marion Young. Accordingly, the problem of closure – the risk that institutionalized forms of group representation could block further development and change – is not completely obviated (Phillips, 1995), even if, as we have seen, cultural fluidity and change is clearly countenanced by Kymlicka.

Marrying a theory of rights to the complexities of political practice is a necessarily difficult and, at times, fraught process. Nonetheless, it remains my conviction that Kymlicka's arguments about rights, combined with Young's more nuanced conception of the fluidity and interfusion of groups, provide us with a powerful explanatory model for a legitimate defense of national minority rights within liberal theory. And yet, proponents of minority rights within political theory have seldom actually addressed, except by implication, how such rights might be applied specifically to minority languages and their speakers (De Schutter, 2007).[28] The most substantive attempt to date has been Kymlicka and Patten's (2003) important edited collection, *Language Rights and Political Theory*. Even here though, the majority of the contributors remain largely skeptical and/ or opposed to the recognition/implementation of such language rights.[29] The application of minority rights to language, and the links between language and identity that might underpin them, are the focus of the next chapter.

4

LANGUAGE, IDENTITY, RIGHTS AND REPRESENTATION

It should be abundantly clear by now that issues of language and education are central to the wider debates surrounding the pluralist dilemma (May, 2008b). Opponents of multiculturalism often direct particular opprobrium toward the maintenance of minority languages, such as Spanish in the USA, and the models of bilingual education that support such language maintenance. We saw this clearly in the previous chapter in the accounts of both Schlesinger and Barry. Likewise, advocates of cultural and linguistic pluralism often invest education with the capacity to transform public policy – and, by implication, public attitudes – to their more pluralist ends. This is particularly evident in the longstanding educational literature on multicultural education (see Modood and May, 2001; Banks, 2009; May, 2009, for useful overviews).

On the one hand, this preoccupation with language and education should not surprise us, given their centrality to the formation and maintenance of modern nation-states (see Chapter 2). In effect, the battle for nationhood is most often a battle for linguistic and cultural hegemony. Consequently, education – and, crucially, the language(s) legitimated in and through education – plays a key role in establishing and maintaining the subsequent cultural and linguistic shape of the nation-state. On the other hand, what should surprise us is how seldom relevant literature from within sociolinguistics[1] and educational research is meaningfully addressed in these broader discussions. Political theorists who oppose multiculturalism are particularly remiss in this regard. For example, a key premise underlying their often-stated antagonism toward bilingual education is that it precludes, or at least reduces, the effective learning of English (or other majority languages). The problem with this position is that any serious engagement with the educational research on bilingualism and bilingual education over the last forty years – or for that matter, any engagement at all – reveals it to be nonsense (May, 2003b). Bilingual education is not only effective in maintaining a minority language, but also in *enhancing* the learning of a second language, such as English, far more so than a monolingual educational approach.[2] I will return to this issue in more depth in Chapter 6.

Political theorists who support multiculturalism are often just as guilty of ignoring relevant research in language and education. Will Kymlicka is a case in point. He is one of the few political theorists to address language rights directly, and the role of education therein (De Schutter, 2007). Indeed, a key argument that he develops in his book *The Politics of the Vernacular* is one very similar to my own. He argues there (2001: 23–7, 242–53) for the importance of the link between language and culture as a basis for language rights claims. He also highlights the process by which nation-states invariably establish the language(s) of the dominant ethnie, or majority group, as an official language. The latter, in his view, actively disadvantages minority language speakers by ignoring and/ or stigmatizing their language varieties, as well as confining/consigning them to the private realm. Meanwhile, minority language speakers' access to, and opportunities to engage effectively within, the public or civic realm, where the official language dominates, is also necessarily limited. Both undermine, for him, the notion of liberal justice.

I agree with the conclusions Kymlicka draws, for reasons I will expand upon in this chapter. But the problem with Kymlicka's account is that he only engages briefly and tangentially with the sociolinguistic and educational research commentary that would further support his position. For example, he argues that there is 'strong evidence that languages cannot survive for long in the modern world unless they are used in public life, and so government decisions about official languages are, in effect, decisions about which languages will thrive, and which will die out' (2001: 78). However, as Clare Chambers (2003) observes, in her critique of Kymlicka's position, the only strong evidence he then cites is his own work. The extensive literature in sociolinguistics and the sociology of language on issues of language and identity, and their connection to cultural pluralism, goes unremarked. Chambers comments: 'until Kymlicka refers to more of that literature and makes clear what precisely his argument is for supposing that liberal justice is incompatible with the promotion of an official language, it is not really possible to assess his claims' (2003: 309). More broadly, she concludes, 'the idea that cultures are in some way dependent on language is a complex one that requires considerable discussion. … Kymlicka does not provide adequate answers, leaving his theory [of minority rights and its implications for language] vulnerable' (2003: 303).

I have singled out Kymlicka here simply because he is the most influential contemporary political theorist to support minority rights and one of the very few to discuss language rights directly. As I have already made clear, his wider arguments also provide me, crucially, with the basis for my own arguments about minority language rights. But as Chambers highlights, even his work is still largely constrained within disciplinary boundaries – much like the sociologists of ethnicity and nationalism discussed in Chapters 1 and 2, who, for many years, systematically failed to engage with each other's work. Thus, in this chapter, I want to explore directly the wider debates about language and identity in the sociolinguistic literature, particularly as these pertain to the pluralist dilemma, and associated notions of language rights and representation. I will then examine two specific national examples – Ireland and France – that illustrate the wider social and political issues at stake in these debates, especially for minority language speakers. In Chapter 5, I will explore more closely the central role of education in all of the above. However, in attempting to maintain some analytical distance between the two dimensions in what follows, I also acknowledge that it is often very difficult to separate them *in practice* when it comes to the pluralist dilemma.

Language and identity

In Chapter 1, we saw how language may be a salient marker of ethnic identity in one instance but not in another. While a specific language may well be identified as a significant cultural marker of a particular ethnic group, there is no inevitable correspondence between language and ethnicity. In effect, linguistic differences do not always correspond to ethnic ones – membership of an ethnic group does not necessarily entail association with a particular language, either for individual members or for the group itself. Likewise, more than one ethnic group can share the same language while continuing without difficulty to maintain their own distinct ethnic (and national) identities. Indeed, even where language *is* regarded as a central feature of ethnic identity, it is the *diacritical significance* attached to language which is considered crucial, not the actual language itself (cf. Barth, 1969a; see below). Moreover, languages, along with other cultural attributes, vary in their salience to ethnicity both within and between historical periods. Languages may come and languages may go, or so it seems. These themes were foregrounded in Chapter 2 when I examined the tenets of linguistic nationalism à la Herder, Humboldt and Fichte. There I concluded, along with most modernist commentators, that the view of nations as both natural and linguistically determined was little more than sociological (and linguistic) nonsense. As Ernest Renan has argued, language may well be a factor in national identity but it is certainly not the only one, nor is it even essential: 'language may invite us to unite but it does not compel us to do so' (1990: 16).

Given this, one might assume – as, indeed, do most modernist and postmodernist commentators on ethnicity and nationalism – that language has little actual significance to or bearing on questions of ethnic and national identity.

However, this would be to make a grave mistake, for a number of reasons. First, there is considerable evidence that while language may not be a *determining* feature of ethnic and national identity, it remains nonetheless a *significant* one in many instances. To say that language is not an inevitable feature of identity is not the same as saying it is unimportant. Yet many commentators in (rightly) assuming the former position have also (wrongly) assumed the latter. After all, as Adrian Blackledge observes: 'We can hardly argue theoretically that for students who died protesting the right to establish Bengali as the national language of East Pakistan in 1952, language was not a key feature of identity' (2008: 33). Thus, as I will argue, language may not be intrinsically valuable in itself – it is clearly not primordial – but it does still have strong and felt associations with ethnic and national identity. As such, language cannot simply be relegated to a mere secondary or surface characteristic of ethnicity.[3]

Second, and relatedly, the *cultural* significance of language to ethnic and national identity may help to explain, at least in part, its *political* prominence in many ethnic and ethnonationalist movements (see Blommaert and Verschueren, 1998; Blommaert, 1996, 1999c; S. Wright, 2000). In this regard, the interconnections between the cultural and political dimensions of language become central, most obviously in the official status accorded to particular languages within the nation-state (cf. Kymlicka, 2001). As Manning Nash observes:

> Language seems straightforwardly a piece of culture. But on reflection it is clear that language is often a political fact, at least as much as it is a cultural one. It has been said that 'language is a dialect with an army and a navy'. And what official or recognised languages are in any given instance is often the result of politics and power interplays. (1989: 6)

The official status of language(s) to which Nash refers is a key dimension in many of the debates on the pluralist dilemma and concerns majority group members as much as it does minorities. We have already seen the salience of language and language rights to the dominant ethnie from Schlesinger's comments in the preceding chapter, and we will encounter this preoccupation with language, from all sides, again and again in what follows. However, Nash's comment alludes to the fact that the official status ascribed to any one language is a somewhat arbitrary process – as much to do with political and social power relations as with anything else. This point is also presaged in Gellner (1983) and Anderson's (1991) accounts in Chapter 2 of the development of national languages, often retrospectively, within modern nation-states.

And it brings me to the third reason for not underestimating the significance of language to ethnic and national identity. Language construction and/or reconstruction may well be a somewhat arbitrary process at times. Nonetheless, a certain linguistic arbitrariness does not, ipso facto, diminish the affective and/ or political importance of the languages concerned for those who come to speak them. Indeed, if this were the case, it would be hard, if not impossible, to explain why particular national languages have such sociopolitical currency and meaning for their adherents, a currency which extends far beyond the reach of its solely 'linguistic' functions. In short, the legitimacy, or otherwise, of a language's provenance does not much matter. If a particular language comes to serve important cultural and/or political functions in the formation and maintenance of a particular ethnic or national identity, it *is* important. With this in mind, I want now to turn to a more detailed examination of each of the three key principles just outlined.

Identity in language

Toward the end of his influential account *Imagined Communities*, Benedict Anderson avers of language:

> What the eye is to the lover – that particular, ordinary eye he or she is born with – language – whatever language history has made his or her mother tongue – is to the patriot. Through that language, encountered at mother's knee and parted only at the grave, pasts are restored, fellowships are imagined, and futures dreamed. (1991: 154)

Some sociolinguistic commentators have read this subsequently as an endorsement of an essentialist view of language (see, for example, Silverstein, 2000; Joseph, 2004; Makoni and Pennycook, 2007). I think that this criticism is misplaced simply because what Anderson is actually trying to do here is to explain why national languages, which *are* clearly constructed, nonetheless can invoke such passion and commitment from their speakers. Anderson is the first to reject any suggestion of some kind of primordial status to language. It is always a mistake, he argues, to treat languages in the way that certain nationalist ideologues treat them – 'as *emblems* of nation-ness, like flags, costumes, folk dances and the rest'. Much the more important aspect of language is 'its capacity for generating imagined communities, building in effect *particular solidarities*' (1991: 133; emphases in original). The sociolinguist, Monica Heller, makes a similar point when she discusses the interrelationship between language and ethnic identity in a French immersion school in Toronto, Canada:

> Language use is ... involved in the formation of ethnic identity in two ways. First, it constrains access to participation in activities and to formation of social relationships. *Thus at a basic level language use is central to the formation of group boundaries.* Second, as children spend more and more time together

they share experience, and language is a central means of making sense out of that shared experience. (1987: 199; my emphasis)

Language, as a communally shared good, serves an important boundary-marking function (Tabouret-Keller, 1997; Bucholtz and Hall, 2004; Fought, 2006). In this sense, the boundary-marking function of language has clear parallels with Armstrong's (1982) notion of 'symbolic border guards', discussed in Chapter 2. After all, being unable to speak a particular language places immediate restrictions on one's ability to communicate – and, by extension, identify – with those who speak that language and any ethnic and/or national identities with which it is associated. This process of demarcation may be more salient for minority groups, since such groups are likely to be more conscious of the need for clear linguistic boundaries in relation to a surrounding dominant language and culture. The usefulness of linguistic demarcation may also thus help to explain why language often has a heightened sense of saliency in relation to identity when its role as only one of a number of cultural markers might suggest otherwise. Moreover, to the extent that language boundaries are employed as a demarcating feature of identity, then a decreasing emphasis on, or a blurring of, these boundaries would be regarded as a threat to a group's existence (Khleif, 1979).

Relatedly, where language is regarded as central to identity – or, as Smolicz (1979, 1993, 1995) terms it, where language is a 'core cultural value' – the *sharing* of that language may engender particular solidarities. Certainly, ethnic and nationalist movements have seen the potential this connection offers – often choosing language as a rallying point for the alternative histories, and associated cultural and political rights, that they wish to promote. In so doing, many such movements are simply reflecting long-held views of the language and identity link, which are reflected in the language itself. The Welsh word 'iaith', for example, originally meant both language and community; the word for foreigner, 'anghyfiaith', means 'not of the same language'; while the word for a compatriot, 'cyfiaith', means 'of the same language'. Likewise, the Basques define their territory 'Euskal Herria' on the basis of where 'Euskera', the Basque language, is spoken. Frequently invoked nationalist slogans also reflect the primacy given to the language and identity link: 'Sluagh gun chanain, sluagh gun anam' is Gaelic for 'A people without its language is a people without its soul', while 'Hep brezhoneg, breizh ebet' is Breton for 'without Breton there is no Brittany', and there are numerous other examples on which one could draw (see, for example, J. Edwards, 1994: 129; Fishman, 1997: 331–3).

From the above, it is clear that the link between language and identity encompasses both significant cultural and political dimensions. The cultural dimensions are demonstrated by the fact that one's individual and social identities, and their complex interconnections, are inevitably mediated in and through language. The political dimensions are significant to the extent that languages come to be formally (and informally) associated with particular ethnic and national identities. These interconnections help to explain why a 'detached' scientific view of the link between language and identity may fail to capture the degree to which language is *experienced* as vital by those who speak it. A supposedly detached, or 'disinterested' position on language may also significantly understate the role that language plays in social organization and mobilization (Fishman, 1997). In short, the 'shibboleth of language', as Toynbee (1953) coined it, still holds much sway. While the cultural and political dimensions of language and identity are inevitably closely intertwined, I want next to look briefly at each of these aspects in turn.

Language and culture

It does not take much to demonstrate that language is a communally shared good since language, almost by definition, requires dialogue. What is harder to determine is whether one's *own* language is a good. Is a particular language significantly related to one's cultural identity or would any language suffice? This is a crucial question since, if the latter is proved, the case for specific language rights – that is, rights relating to the protection and promotion of specific language varieties – is dealt a perhaps terminal blow. However, even if the former tenet is accepted, one must be able to account for the historical, social and political *construction* of the language and identity link and its clear *variability*, both at the inter- and intragroup level. This is not an easy task by any means but the work of the prominent sociolinguist Joshua Fishman provides us with a useful place to start.

Fishman (1991, see also 2001) argues that language and ethnocultural identity are crucially linked in three key ways: indexically, symbolically and in a part–whole fashion. First, a language associated with a particular culture 'is, at any time during which that linkage is still intact, best able to name the artifacts and to formulate or express the interests, values and world-views of that culture' (1991: 20). This is the indexical link between language and culture (cf. Silverstein, 1998). Such a link does not assume that a traditionally or historically associated language is a perfect isomorphic match with an attendant culture, or that other languages might not be able to replace this traditional link in the longer term. However, in the *short* term (that is, at any particular point in time), 'no language but the one that has been most historically and intimately associated with a given culture is as well able to express the particular artifacts and concerns of that culture' (1991: 21). In other words, the traditionally associated language reflects and conveys its culture more felicitously and succinctly than other languages, *while that language-in-culture link remains generally intact*.

Fishman's position here clearly echoes what is known in linguistics as the 'Sapir-Whorf hypothesis' – named after its proponents, Edward Sapir and

Benjamin Whorf – or, more accurately, the principle of linguistic relativity.[4] This theory of linguistic relativity was popular in the early part of the twentieth century and can be traced back, in turn, to Herder and Humboldt's views on language. Sapir's argument was that one's social and cultural experiences are organized by language and thus each language represents a particular worldview. As he observed, 'the "real world" is to a large extent unconsciously built up on the language habits of the group'. Thus, '[w]e see and hear and otherwise experience very largely as we do because the language habits of our community predispose certain choices of interpretation' (1929: 209). His pupil Whorf extended this by arguing that thought is not independent of the language used because language carves up experience according to its particular grammatical structure, categories and types. 'We dissect nature along lines laid down by our native languages. The categories and types that we isolate from the world', he argued, are not self evident but, rather, 'organized by our minds – and this means largely by the linguistic systems in our minds' (1956: 212). The key implication of linguistic relativity is that people who speak different languages are likely to have somewhat different cultural outlooks on the basis that the particular structure of each language results in a culturally specific structuring of reality. Indeed, a radical or strong version of the principle attests that languages are *causal* vis-à-vis culturally specific behaviors.

With the rise and subsequent dominance of constructionist accounts of language and identity over the last forty years, it should come as no surprise that this position quickly fell out of favor. In similar vein to discussions of primordialism or linguistic nationalism (cf. Chapters 1 and 2), subsequent sociolinguistic commentary and analysis was quick to dismiss the notion of linguistic relativity out of hand as linguistically determinist, à la Herder et al., based in turn on a preoccupation with its most radical or extreme versions. There are two problems with this. The first is that it has consistently both reduced and misrepresented the complexity of ideas underpinning Sapir and Whorf's work (Lee, 1996; Joseph, 2002; Glaser, 2007).[5] The second is that it has often resulted in the instant and fatuous dismissal of *any* meaningful interconnections between language, culture and thought. This latter position is problematic precisely because, as with Fishman's position, a weak version of the principle of linguistic relativity is clearly supportable – highlighting, as it does, the *influence* of language in shaping our *customary* ways of thinking. As such, it can be regarded as both reasonable and unsurprising (J. Edwards, 1994). 'Neo-Whorfian' research in cognitive science and the philosophy of language, particularly over the last decade, lends further weight to the validity of this position (Reines and Prinz, 2009).[6] Both suggest that if identity is understood in relation to habitus as 'the background against which our tastes and desires and opinions and aspirations make sense' (Taylor, 1994: 33–4), then a traditionally associated language would seem to have a significant part to play. Indeed, linguistic habitus, in Bourdieu's

(1991) terms, is a subset of the dispositions which comprise the habitus: it is that set of dispositions acquired in the course of learning to speak in particular social and cultural contexts.

If language and culture are linked indexically then they are also linked symbolically; that is, they come to stand for or symbolically represent the particular ethnic and/or national collectivities that speak them. Accordingly, the fortunes of languages are inexorably bound up with those of their speakers (Dorian, 1998; J. Edwards, 1994, 2001, 2010). Languages do not rise or fall simply on their own linguistic merits – indeed, it has long been accepted that all languages are potentially equivalent in linguistic terms. Rather, the social and political circumstances of those who speak a particular language will have a significant impact on the subsequent symbolic and communicative status attached to that language. This fact often escapes speakers of dominant national languages, and particularly speakers of English as the current world language, who take the 'natural' ascendency of these languages for granted. In contrast, the current international currency of a language like English has much more to do with the sociopolitical dominance of those nation-states, notably the USA, for which English is the accepted language of public discourse (Pennycook, 1994; Phillipson, 1992, 1998; Macedo et al., 2003; see Chapter 6). Likewise, national languages reflect the greater sociopolitical status of their speakers in relation to minority languages and cultures within the nation-state.

The final aspect – the part–whole link – reflects the partial identity between a particular language and culture. Since so much of any culture is verbally constituted (its songs and prayers, its laws and proverbs, its history, philosophy and teachings), there are parts of every culture that are expressed, implemented and realized via the language with which that culture is most closely associated. Fishman argues that it is within this part–whole relationship that

> child socialisation patterns come to be associated with a particular language, that cultural styles of interpersonal relations come to be associated with a particular language, that the ethical principles that undergird everyday life come to be associated with a particular language and that even material culture and aesthetic sensibilities come to be conventionally discussed and evaluated via figures of speech that are merely culturally (i.e. locally) rather than universally applicable. (1991: 24)

Fishman's analysis highlights the cultural significance of language to identity. This does not imply, however, the reification of the latter or the assumption that such identity can be 'preserved' in some pure, unaltered state. Nor does it link particular languages inexorably with particular identities. Rather, a traditionally associated language is viewed as a significant *resource* to one's ethnic identity, both at the level of societal integration and social identification (see also Ruiz,

1984). While such a resource may ultimately be discarded (see below), it remains important until such a time as this occurs. As Fishman concludes, 'a preferred, historically associated mother tongue has a role in [the] process of individual and aggregative self-definition and self-realisation, not merely as a myth (i.e. as a verity whose objective truth is less important than its subjective truth) but also as a genuine identificational and motivational desideratum in the ethnocultural realm' (1991: 7).

Given this, the constructionist tendency to repudiate language as a significant feature of identity may be considerably overstated. However, be that as it may, Fishman's argument still needs to account for the exceptions it implicitly acknowledges but does not necessarily explain. How do we accommodate those individuals and groups for whom a particular language is clearly not an important feature of their identity? How do we explain language shift, which suggests that these associations, while important, are by no means irreplaceable? And how do we counter the charge that the language and identity link is largely arbitrary – a social and political construction along the well-rehearsed lines of the 'invention of tradition' argument? To answer these questions we need to explore further the interconnections between the cultural and political dimensions of language and identity.

Language, culture and politics

The language and identity link cannot be understood in isolation from other factors of identity, nor from the specific political conditions in which it is situated. The relation between language and identity is thus *contingent* on both subjective factors and particular political circumstances (Coulombe, 1995). On this basis, it can be argued that the language we speak is crucial to our identity *to the degree to which we define ourselves by it.* This will obviously vary widely, both among individuals and within and between groups. As such, it may well be that some individuals and groups will regard a particular language as a largely superficial marker of their identities and have no great sense of loss in abandoning it. Immigrant ethnic minorities, for example, often adopt the language of the host country in which they reside, albeit usually over the course of two or three generations, on the basis of enhancing their integration and social mobility within that country. On this view, Carol Eastman has proffered the explanation that language use is merely a surface feature of ethnic identity and thus adopting another language would only affect the language use aspect of our ethnic identity, not the identity itself. As she asserts, 'there is no need to worry about preserving ethnic identity, so long as the only change being made is in what language we use' (1984: 275). Accordingly, immigrant ethnic groups may retain their original language as an 'associated' language – one that group members no longer use, or perhaps even know, but which continues to be a part of their heritage. Such an association is clearly comparable with Gans's (1979) notion of symbolic ethnicity, discussed in Chapter 1.

These arguments can be extrapolated to the relationship between language and national identity as well. Gellner, for example, has argued that 'changing one's language is not the heart-breaking or soul-destroying business which it is claimed to be in romantic nationalist literature' (1964: 165). Ireland is regularly invoked as an example here because, over the course of the last two centuries, English has come largely to supplant Irish as the ethnic (and national) language. A small minority may still speak Irish in the Gaeltacht (the Irish-speaking heartland),[7] and it still retains official status as the 'first official language' of Ireland.[8] However, the reality of Irish as a rapidly declining language has been clear for some considerable time now (Spolsky, 2004; S. Wright, 2004; Edwards, 2010). For example, an extensive sociolinguistic research study conducted in the 1970s, the Committee on Irish Language Attitudes Research (CILAR, 1975), found that less than 3 percent of the overall population used Irish in any regular way. There was also little interest in the restoration of Irish, hostility to the compulsory aspects associated with learning Irish (see below) and significant pessimism about the continued maintenance of the Irish still in use at the time. Nonetheless, a symbolic valuing of Irish was still evident and, as such, it was thought to continue to form part of Irish ethnic and national identity. As the CILAR observes: 'the average person would seem to place considerable value on the symbolic role of the Irish language in ethnic identification and as a cultural value in and of itself ... [but this] seems to be qualified by a generally pessimistic view of the language's future *and a feeling of its inappropriateness in modern life*' (1975: 29; my emphasis). This conclusion accords with Ussher's more succinct, and certainly more cynical observation: 'the Irish of course like their Irish, but they like it *dead*' (1949: 107; emphasis in original).

Two complementary explanations can be offered for this clear process of language shift in Ireland. One is that, while language is often a 'core cultural value' for many ethnic and national groups, it is not so in relation to Irish identity. Thus, Smolicz, who has promoted this notion of core cultural values, argues that the core values of the Irish ethnic group are 'unquestioningly centred on the Catholic religion' (1979: 63) rather than on the Irish language itself, a process that has been intensified by the fact that English was adopted as the language of Irish Catholicism from the late eighteenth century onwards. As Smolicz concludes of these developments: 'Bereft of their ancestral tongue, it was in Catholicism that the Irish found the refuge and shield behind which they could retain their identity and awareness of their distinction from the conquering British Protestants' (1979: 64). This might well explain the ongoing decline of the Irish language, despite the adoption from the nineteenth century onward of informal and subsequently formal language policies aimed at mitigating this language loss (Hindley, 1990; Ó Riagáin, 1997; Ó Catháin, 2007; see also below).

There is some merit in the 'core cultural value' explanation, although how the 'Irish ethnic group' is defined remains extremely problematic since intragroup differences are likely to be much more complex than such an analysis allows. In this regard, it is almost self-evident that different sections of the community, not to mention individuals, will have different relationships to their language(s) for a variety of political, social and/or religious reasons, thus significantly weakening the core value explanation (Clyne, 1997). In light of this criticism, Smolicz subsequently developed a more nuanced approach. While still holding that some cultures are more language-centered than others, Smolicz and Secombe (1988), for example, differentiate four broad approaches to minority languages that are evident among and within ethnic minority groups. These comprise: *negative evaluation* of the language; *indifference* – seeing no purpose in language maintenance and showing no interest in it; *general positive evaluation* – regarding the language as a vital element of ethnicity but not being prepared personally to learn it; *personal positive evaluation* – regarding the language as a core cultural value and putting this language commitment into practice (see also Clyne, 1990).

Even so, a more compelling explanation of language shift is likely to reside in the social and political processes that have seen the rise of English as the language of Ireland over the course of the last few centuries. These sociopolitical factors have linked English inextricably with modernization, thus providing the language with increasing symbolic and communicative currency in Ireland. Given this, the sociopolitical milieu of Ireland merits closer examination since it illustrates, writ large, the difficulties facing minority languages and cultures in the (post)modern world.

Language decline: the death of Irish?

Irish enjoyed its 'Golden Age' from the sixth to the ninth centuries when it was spoken as a common vernacular, alongside Latin, not only in what we now know as Ireland but also in the coastal areas of both southern and northern Britain. Indeed, Irish was so highly regarded at this time that by the eighth century it had supplanted Latin as the principal literary and religious medium, while the reach of the Irish-speaking community had extended over almost the whole area of present-day Scotland. The dominance of Irish first began to be undermined with the advent of the Norman invasions of the twelfth century. New towns were built by the Normans in Ireland, as elsewhere in Britain, and led to the introduction of a Norman French- and subsequently English-speaking bourgeoisie (Ó Murchú, 1988). Even so, this process, which continued until the sixteenth century, was a slow and limited one. Indeed, by the late fifteenth century most Normans living outside of the Dublin area had actually come to be assimilated into the wider Irish language and culture. Irish thus continued to have a strong societal and regional base and remained the dominant language among all classes in the countryside. It also remained the primary language of communication in urban areas (although English was used for public affairs) in what appears to have been some form of Irish–English diglossia.[9]

From the sixteenth century, however, English began to make its irrevocable advance. Henry VIII issued proclamations discouraging Irish (see Crowley, 1996, 2007) and, more significantly, plantation schemes were initiated to replace Irish with English settlers (Ó Riagáin, 1996). The latter proved to be crucial – resulting, as one writer has observed, in the 'Gaelic world [dying] from the top down' (de Paor, 1985; cited in Ó Riagáin, 1997: 4). By 1800, English – or, at least, an Irish variant of it – was spoken regularly by half the population; crucially, the most powerful half. Irish speakers were increasingly limited to the poor and underdeveloped Gaeltacht, while English speakers constituted the propertied rural and urban population. This language decline was compounded by the abandonment of Irish by the Catholic Church, its formal exclusion from the English-language National School system established in 1831 and the impact of rural depopulation (by both death and emigration) from the Famines of the 1840s. These trends, which can be regarded as largely external, were also hastened by the apparent willingness of Irish speakers themselves to abandon the language. As John Edwards observes, 'the mass of Irish people were more or less active contributors to the spread of English' (1984: 285). As a result, by the mid-nineteenth century, the percentage of the population who remained Irish-speaking had declined to just under 30 percent. Despite various attempts to revive Irish from the mid-nineteenth century on – exemplified most prominently in the activities of such nationalist-inspired language bodies as the Gaelic League (Conradh na Gaeilge), established in 1893 (see Tovey et al., 1989) – the decline of Irish continued into the twentieth century.

By the time the Irish Free State was established in 1922[10] the pattern of language decline appeared almost terminal. At most, only 10 percent of the population now used Irish as their daily language and this group was almost exclusively situated in the Gaeltacht (Ó Ciosáin, 1988; Ó Riagáin, 1996). Broader language trends were equally bleak. Census figures in 1926 indicated that only 18 percent could actually speak Irish and that very few of these were monoglot speakers (Ó Gadhra, 1988). Moreover, even this estimate would appear to have been overstated, since many of those returned as Irish speakers in the census were in older age groups and scattered across communities where Irish had ceased to be an everyday language (Ó Riagáin, 1997).

Given the parlous state of the language, a formal language policy was adopted by the Irish Free State with the specific aim of reversing this decline. Four main strategies were promoted, although the degree to which they were successfully implemented varied widely. In English-speaking areas, Irish would be compulsorily taught to all children in schools by immersion methods. This, it was hoped, would produce an adult population with functional competence in Irish within a generation. The second strategy was to strengthen and extend the use of Irish in the Gaeltacht, principally via economic regional development policies. The third element was a formal Irish language requirement in the public sector – most significantly in the Irish Civil Service. The final element focused on measures to standardize and modernize the language itself (Ó Riagáin, 1997; Ó Catháin, 2007).

It soon became apparent, however, that education was deemed to be the key element in this language policy. In this sense, the language policy reflected the previous emphases of Conradh na Gaeilge (the Gaelic League) at the end of the nineteenth century. At that time, the League had successfully lobbied for Irish to be used as a language of instruction in schools where it remained the first language of most of its pupils, and for its inclusion as an ordinary school subject elsewhere. It had also actively promoted teacher training in Irish via the establishment of its own teacher-training colleges. This almost transcendental belief in the power of education to effect language change arose in turn from the belief that, if the nineteenth-century education system had contributed to the demise of Irish via its advocacy of English, the reverse could also well apply. Indeed, such was the faith invested in schools that Timothy Corcoran, an educational adviser at the time of the establishment of the Irish language policy, could assert: 'the popular schools can give and can restore our native language. They can do it even without positive aid from home' (1925: 387; cited in J. Edwards, 1985: 56).

However, such optimism was to prove largely ill founded, at least in the Irish case. This is not to say that there haven't been important educational developments that have contributed positively to Irish language revitalization – most notably, Irish-medium education (see below). Nor is the role of education inconsequential to minority language revitalization policies, as I will argue in the next chapter. However, the example of Ireland does broadly demonstrate that the aim of restoring communicative competence in a language cannot be achieved on the backs of schools alone (Fishman, 1991, 2001; Colin Williams, 1994, 2008). This over-emphasis on education in the Irish context was further compounded by a lack of suitable teachers of Irish and by the ambivalence – and at times, outright opposition – of many teachers toward the language restoration project. Accordingly, by the 1960s/1970s the bulk of educational effort had been restricted to teaching Irish in the primary (elementary) sector. Even here though, teacher-training colleges were no longer instructing their students in Irish, with the result that teachers of Irish were themselves not particularly competent in the language. This has contributed to a subsequent decline in Irish language ability among primary students in 'ordinary' (mainstream) primary schools in Ireland since that time (Harris and Murtagh, 1999). The flow-on effects can also be seen in secondary (high) schools and universities, with Irish becoming more peripheral in both sectors (Williams, 2008).[11] Even schools in the remaining Gaeltacht areas have recently been found to be less effective than expected in maintaining high levels of fluency in Irish. This is the result in turn of resourcing and recruiting difficulties and the related challenges attendant upon meeting the needs of students with a wide range of Irish language abilities (Mac Donnacha et al., 2005).

That said, the growth in the Irish-medium education sector over the same period reflects a significant countertrend. This began with the development of Naíonraí – locally initiated Irish-immersion-speaking preschools, initially outside of the regular school system – which grew in number from one in 1968 to 260 in 2006. As a result, there has also been a subsequent re-emergence of Irish-medium schools to cater for Naíonraí graduates, most of which are situated outside of the Gaeltacht. In 2010, there were 169 such Irish-medium primary schools and thirty-eight post-primary schools, serving approximately 37,800 students, about 5 percent of all pupils (Walsh, 2011). Even here though, ongoing resourcing and recruitment issues, as well as the challenge of maintaining high levels of Irish, particularly written Irish, remain a concern.

Allied initiatives in the public sector between the 1970s and 1990s also met with variable success in Ireland. Bord na Gaeilge (Irish Language Board) was established in 1975 by the government to promote Irish in daily life and included within its remit the provision of language advice and information, language courses, and translation services. However, over the next twenty years, the activities of Bord na Gaeilge appeared to have little impact on the actual language use of ordinary Irish people themselves. Moreover, as the CILAR (1975) sociolinguistic study mentioned earlier found, and as more recent studies have confirmed (Ó Ciosáin, 1988; Ó Riagáin, 1988a), the compulsory dimensions associated with Irish – particularly, the Irish-language requirement for the Civil Service – engendered actual hostility toward the language. This hostility to the compulsory language requirement remained prominent until its eventual abandonment in 1974, and despite a generally favorable attitude to Irish and to bilingualism at the level of ethnic and cultural association.

Even economic measures aimed at preserving some measure of Irish in the Gaeltacht during this period backfired – largely because they did not link language maintenance effectively to wider development planning (Walsh, 2002, 2006). For example, efforts to discourage the emigration of Irish speakers from the Gaeltacht included industrialization projects aimed at improving employment prospects. However, rather than safeguarding and reinforcing the Irish-speaking community, such projects actually undermined them further by importing skilled and supervisory staff with no knowledge of Irish. Likewise, those Irish speakers who had been drawn back had, in the interim, acquired non-Irish-speaking partners, thus increasing the number of non-Irish-speaking households in the area (O'Cinnéide et al., 1985). Consequently, the Irish-speaking communities in the Gaeltacht have continued to decline. In 1991, for example, they accounted for 7.4 percent of all Irish speakers and 45 percent of all Irish-speaking families, but comprised only 2.3 percent of Ireland's total population. As Colin Williams concludes of this history, at least until the late 1990s:

> Despite communal and government efforts, the task of revitalising Irish has proved greater than the resources and commitment hitherto shown. The underlying fault is an over-optimistic assessment of the capacity of state intervention to restore Irish as a national language without a concomitant investment in socio-economic planning to bring about the necessary conditions to regulate the market forces which encouraged widespread Anglicisation [in the first place]. (2008: 220)

The result is that the 'Irish as a group seem not to have lost their national identity, but to have enshrined it in English' (J. Edwards, 1985: 62), a conclusion encapsulated in the title of Hindley's (1990) *The Death of the Irish Language*. Even those with a more optimistic view of Irish, such as Ó Riagáin, who argues that there has been 'some measure of revival', also concedes that it is 'of a scale that is continuously vulnerable to final submersion in the mainly English-speaking population' (1988b: 7; see also 2008). All of this would seem to indicate the futility – not to mention the naivety and misguidedness – of attempting to maintain minority languages in the face of modern social and political realities. But before consigning Irish – and, by extension, other minority languages – to what might seem to be their inevitable fate, let us examine more closely the constituent elements of the Irish case.

'Resigned language realism': is language revival just flogging a dead horse?

Ireland is an instructive example of a minority language policy that has met with variable success – indeed some go so far as to describe it as an archetypal failure. As such, skeptics and opponents of minority language rights regularly invoke it as a cause célèbre – an example of the apparent foolishness of attempting, as John Edwards argues, to revive languages 'in the face of historical realities' (1985: 64). Indeed, Edwards has tirelessly used the example of Ireland ever since (see 1994, 2001, 2010) to proclaim that language revival in these circumstances is inherently artificial and bound to fail. I have elsewhere (May, 2003a, 2005b) described this position as one of 'resigned language realism', and Edwards is its most consistent (and voluble) advocate. The apparent cogency of this position arises from the fact that one need not oppose the retention of minority languages, in principle – as do those commentators, such as Schlesinger and Barry, discussed in the previous chapter. Indeed,

Edwards often trumpets his general sympathy toward and support of minority languages, regularly reiterating his 'own personal preference for a world rich in all sorts of diversities' (2001: 239). However, as he immediately proceeds to observe: 'But preference alone, of course, is not the point' (ibid.). When faced with the 'Realpolitik' of the often-exponential shift and loss of their historically associated language(s), such as Irish, minority language groups must, it seems, simply acquiesce to the 'march of progress'. As Edwards asserts: 'Cutting across all perceptual and terminological matters ... are the powerful facts of social life, facts recognised by even the most sanguine supporters of linguistic diversity. Even the strongest will-to-revive may be dwarfed by societal pressures' (2001: 232). Or, as he has earlier observed:

> language shift reflects sociopolitical change and this, given the historical perspective, absolutely dwarfs efforts made on behalf of language alone. This is not to say ... that language cannot serve a vital rallying purpose in nationalistic political movements, but it only does so when it retains some realistic degree of communicative function. (1984: 288)

On this view, it is a profound error to think of language decline as anything other than a symptom of widespread social confrontation between unequal forces. If this is the case, the next question must surely be 'should we attempt to reverse language decline at all?' John Edwards and other like-minded commentators (see, for example, Coulmas, 1992; Bentahila and Davies, 1993; Brutt-Griffler, 2002) answer this question in the negative. Such a conclusion may seem to many simple commonsense. However, it betrays a number of inherent contradictions that I want to explore further, not only in relation to the Irish case but also with respect to some of its wider implications.

Edwards's view on Irish language policy highlights a number of key issues. The first is that *all* commentators on minority languages, and associated rights and representation, bring their own political agenda to the table. Thus, Edwards's attempts to paint his own position as one of mere 'Realpolitik', while at the same time dismissing proponents of minority language rights as 'idealists' and 'activists', must be seen for what is: a discursive, highly partial, *move* in the politics of language rights, not some impartial, disinterested stance.[12] Second, and relatedly, one's initial overarching perspective on minority languages, and associated rights and representation, will often presuppose (even predetermine) the conclusions drawn in relation to any given case study, such as Ireland. In this respect, those who dismiss Irish language policy as a definitive failure need themselves to be critiqued.

In saying this, let me again acknowledge, if it is not already sufficiently apparent, that Irish language policy clearly has met with variable – and, at times, limited – success. No one can deny this. But, given the historical circumstances of Irish, it can also be regarded as having achieved a number of significant, and often-overlooked, successes. For a start, Irish is still spoken in the wider society, and taught in schools, when, by now, it might not otherwise have been (Walsh, 2011). Given that, by the time serious language restoration attempts were promoted and implemented in the late nineteenth and early twentieth century, much of the language had already been lost to the majority of the population, this is a remarkable achievement in itself. That the proportion of Irish speakers continues to grow – in the 2006 Irish census Irish speakers comprised 41.9 percent of the population, compared with 32.5 percent in 1991 – is another key indicator of success. The highest number of Irish speakers in any of the decennial cohorts in this census were also in the 25–34 age group, highlighting the probable influence of Irish-medium education over the last thirty years, as well as the potential for its further expansion as the children of this group reach school age (Colin Williams, 2008).

Returning to a point I made earlier, this does not obviate the fact that education, on its own, is insufficient to carry or effect language revival. This is a key lesson that can be taken from the Irish case, but it is one that proponents of language rights, such as Joshua Fishman, also clearly make. Fishman (1991, 2001) consistently expresses caution over the influence/reach of education in language revival movements and emphasizes instead the centrality of intergenerational family transmission as the key to the continued survival of any minority language. While he argues that 'the family (and even the immediate community) *may not be enough* [to reverse language shift], particularly where outside pressures are both great and hostile ... without this stage safely under ... control the more advanced stages have nothing firm to build on' (1991: 94). In short, 'nothing can substitute for the rebuilding of a society at the level of ... everyday, informal life' (1991: 112).

Fishman develops this specific point further in the discussion of his well-known Graded Intergenerational Disruption Scale (GIDS) (Fishman, 1991: 81–121). GIDS highlights eight stages of support for minority languages, with the lower levels (6–8) focused on private language use and involving limited public support, while the higher levels (1–5) reflect more widespread public support and language use. Stage 6 of this scale involves intergenerational family transmission and is thus ostensibly at the scale's lower, more 'basic' end. However, Fishman argues that many language revitalization movements tend to overlook this crucial stage in their rush to establish ostensibly more 'advanced', public, stages such as minority language education (Stage 4). Invariably, he suggests, this proves counterproductive in the long term, as in the Irish case.[13] This conclusion is reiterated from within the Irish context itself by Ó Gadhra's observation that 'the failure to recognize, for a very long time, the extremely low [language] base from which we set out, has been one of the failures of the Irish revival effort' (1988: 254).

A related feature of the Irish case that merits discussion is the political context in which language restoration came to be situated. The well-known comment by the prominent Irish nationalist and politician, Eamon de Valera, clearly illustrates this context: 'If I had to make a choice between political freedom without the language [Irish], and the language without political freedom ... I would choose the latter' (cited in J. Edwards, 1994: 129). De Valera's assertion highlights the prominent political prerogative underpinning the motivation to restore Irish – namely, to employ the language as a distinguishing characteristic of the newly emergent nation-state of Ireland. However, this position was eventually to founder, both politically and linguistically.

In relation to the former, the attempt to promote the language as the unique heritage of *all* Irish people, including long-established English settlers and a much larger segment of 'native Irish' who had abandoned the Irish language in the nineteenth century, inevitably excluded more than it included (Ó Gadhra, 1988). From the start, the changed linguistic demography – coupled with long-standing forms of Irish identity not associated with the Irish language – militated against the successful adoption of the language as a unifying feature of modern Irish nationalism. In relation to the latter, the nationalists' advocacy of Irish did little, if anything, to reverse its linguistic decline. In fact, the formal language policy subsequently adopted by the nationalists may have further precipitated language loss by limiting itself largely to the promotion of the language's *symbolic* qualities. De Valera illustrates this process well since he himself made little effort to give the language much more than symbolic import (Dwyer, 1980).

This largely symbolic emphasis is thus likely to have been a contributing factor in the failure of the language to regain wider communicative currency. The public sector clearly highlights the limits of Irish language policy here. Despite the long-standing compulsory Irish language requirements for the civil service, the actual use of Irish in the delivery of services remained desultory and largely nominal. A similar pattern of ambivalence over the use(fulness) of Irish can be seen on the international stage when in 1973 Ireland failed to avail itself of the opportunity for Irish to be a full official and working language of the then European Economic Community. This made it the only constituent national language of a member state at that time to not be so represented, a situation only remedied by its belated inclusion as a working language of the now European Union (EU) on 1 January 2007.

And yet, alongside these clear limitations in Irish language policy, there have also been some significant policy successes, particularly over the last decade. For example, the advent of the British–Irish Agreement Act (1999), more widely known as the Good Friday Agreement, has resulted in the development of significant cross-border agencies between Ireland and Northern Ireland.[14] This has seen Bord na Gaeilge become Foras na Gaeilge, a modified language agency that is part of the North/South Language Body. In conjunction with the establishment in 2003 of an Irish Language Act, and the related appointment of a Language Commissioner, a much stronger regulatory system for promoting Irish is now in place (Nic Craith, 2007; Ó Catháin, 2007). This has been further strengthened by the publication in late 2010 of a new twenty-year strategy for the Irish language, the most significant language policy initiative in Ireland for decades (Walsh, 2011). These developments have occurred alongside the ongoing expansion of Irish-medium education, already discussed, and a similar expansion in Irish language media. The latter includes the growing reach of the Irish language television channel TG4, first established in 1996, and the emergence of Irish for an international audience via the worldwide web.[15]

More broadly, the Irish example demonstrates just how long it may actually take for the traditionally associated language of a particular ethnie to decline and be replaced – in this case, several centuries. This is not to suggest that language shift always occurs this slowly but it does demonstrate that the process of change is neither insignificant nor peripheral. Such a view is consistent with my previous discussions on the *slow* process of change associated with habitus and encompassing cultures and, relatedly, on the significance of language to ethnic identity. Language shift does clearly occur – it would be foolish to suggest otherwise. However, it is more problematic and traumatic than is often assumed, particularly for those ethnies for whom a certain language represented, at least at one time, an important feature of their collective identity (Taylor, 1994, 1998; Margalit and Raz, 1995; Valadez, 2007). Fishman reiterates this view when he asserts that 'language shift generally and basically involves cultural change as well indeed, initially, quite devastating and profound cultural change' (1991: 16).[16] This is not to say, using Fishman's terminology, that 'Xians'[17] cannot be Xians if they do not speak the language 'Xish'. Indeed, as we have already seen, the detachability of language from ethnic identity is clearly demonstrated by those Xians who have already come to speak 'Yish' – usually as a result of Yish being a language of greater power and opportunity, as in the Irish context. Nonetheless, we can assert on the basis of the link between language and identity, that it is a *different kind* of 'Xishness' that results. As Fishman concludes:

> The fact that the traditional symbolic relationship between Xish and Xishness can ultimately be replaced by a new symbolic relationship between Yish and Xishness merely indicates that in the fullness of time such transformations are possible and they have, indeed, occurred throughout human history. This does not mean that such symbolic redefinitions and self-redefinitions are either desirable or easily attained, or that Xishness is the same under both sets of linguistic circumstances. (1991: 34)

Fishman's argument raises another pertinent question, however. Adopting another language may result in a different kind of Xishness but if it is a more powerful and widely used language, if it results in a cultural shift toward greater modernity, surely this is a good thing (cf. Wee, 2010)? Again, this position is one adopted by most skeptics of minority language rights and it is one that bears remarkable similarities to the broadly pejorative views of ethnicity outlined in Chapter 1. On this view, minority languages are constructed as an impediment to modernization and social progress. Not only this, proponents of minority languages are peremptorily dismissed as self-interested and unrepresentative elites, intent on maintaining such languages solely for nostalgic and/or nationalistic reasons. This, their critics suggest, is invariably at the expense of the wider social mobility of those who speak the minority language and, concomitantly, largely against not only the latter's interests but also their wishes.

Schlesinger and Barry's views of bilingualism, discussed in the previous chapter, reflect well this dual attack on the twin 'perils' of linguistic self-ghettoization and the self-interested elites who perpetuate it. John Edwards (1985) is likewise dismissive of the apparent disparity between proponents of minority rights and their supposed constituents, and again uses the Irish case as an exemplar.[18] For the many who actually realize the 'benefits' of shifting to a more 'modern' language, Edwards argues that economic rationality plays a significant part. In effect, this amounts to a linguistic variant of rational choice theory, as discussed in Chapter 1 – loyalty to a particular language persists only as long as the economic and social circumstances are conducive to it (see also Dorian, 1981, 1982). As Edwards proceeds to observe, this contrasts with what he sees as the clearly regressive interests of minority language proponents:

> Note here how patronising and naive are attempts *to preserve people as they are*, on the grounds that they are really better off if only they knew it, that progress is not all it is made out to be ... Little wonder, then, that sensible populations themselves do not accept this line, and that the major proponents of the view are usually securely ensconced within that very segment of society they rail against ... looking backwards has been a favourite sport for disaffected intellectuals for a long time, but actually moving backwards has not been so popular. (1985: 95, 97; my emphasis)

Such views are also regularly advanced in relation to the developing world – as seen, for example, in Kay's (1993) arguments on the 'new African'. Kay's case study of Zambia demonstrates how the country is divided into seventy-two ethnic and seven regional languages but is united by one official language, English. From this, Kay argues for the displacement of African languages in favor of international languages such as English. African languages, with their reduced communicative power and symbolic purchase, reflect for Kay the old order, while the likes of English now represent the best means of escaping both poverty and the strictures of ethnic identity in Africa. More recently, the sociolinguist Janina Brutt-Griffler echoes both Edwards and Kay's views, when she also observes of the African context – in this case, in relation to Lesotho:

> If you make ethnicity, nationality, or minority status the unit of analysis, you can conclude that people would want to or have in their interest to maintain their mother tongue. If, on the contrary, you take class as the unit of analysis, their interest might dictate emphasis on access to 'dominant languages'… (2002: 225)

Suffice it to say, in all these examples, language loss is seen as a necessary aspect of modernization and development, even if, in the process, it risks the 'destruction' of cultures (see also Mazrui, 1975; Eastman, 1991; Makoni and Pennycook, 2007). Moreover as these aforementioned commentators repeatedly make clear, this process would also appear to be historically inevitable. We may not like the subsequent undermining of any 'utopian wishes [to maintain minority languages] in the face of harsh realities' (Brutt-Griffler, 2002: 222), but it is something we just simply can't (and shouldn't) fight. After all, as Edwards observes, 'history is the graveyard of cultures' (2001: 235). And even if one accepts the social justice arguments that underpin these attempts to 'preserve' minority languages and cultures, there are invariably more important battles to fight. As Brutt-Griffler concludes: 'It would seem, at the least, naïve to believe that a world that does not guarantee the majority of its inhabitants basic human rights will be able to assure them those of the specifically linguistic variety' (2002: 223).

How can one respond to this critique? For a start, it can be argued that the question of minority leadership is simply a red herring – merely a useful stick, in effect, with which to beat proponents of minority language rights. After all, the charges of self-interest and distinction from the 'rank and file' can be invoked against any leadership, including those advocating a majority language.[19] Likewise, it should be entirely unsurprising that a full range of opinion is expressed within minority groups about such central issues as language maintenance and shift. Internal differences are an inevitable characteristic of *all* groups. It is accordingly a reductio ad absurdum to imply that the presence of such differences negates the legitimacy of minority language claims. Indeed, critiques along these lines tend simply to obfuscate rather than clarify the competing goals, aims, values and opinions of the various protagonists involved in the minority language(s) debate (Fishman, 1991, 2001). Similarly, the charge of inherent *preservationism* – apparent in John Edwards's earlier comment – does not necessarily follow, as I will proceed to argue.

Nonetheless, the view presented here of minority languages as a brake on individual social mobility and collective modernization – as a *problem*, in effect – does seem convincing at first blush (although see Chapter 6). And such a view certainly has significant purchase among many actual minority language speakers themselves, as commentators such as Edwards and Brutt-Griffler are again all too ready to point out. Relatedly, those who advocate majority languages (however, disinterestedly they present themselves) generally pose as, and consider themselves to be, both humanitarians and realists, with nothing but the 'best interests' of minority language speakers at heart (Fishman, 1991). But this position, however benevolent it might seem, also harbors a number of significant problems of its own that are seldom acknowledged or addressed, and it is to these that I now want to turn.

Re-evaluating language shift

Language shift appears to be an increasing feature of the modern world. Certainly, there is a noticeably greater tendency for members of ethnolinguistic minorities to bring up their children in a majority language, rather than their first language(s), a process that often leads to the eventual displacement of the latter. This process of language displacement usually takes at least three generations, although it may occur more quickly. It involves: 1) initial language contact leading to minority status of the historically associated language; 2) bilingualism where the original language is retained but the new language is also acquired; 3) recessive use of the old language, limited largely to intraethnic communication; 4) increasingly unstable bilingualism, eventually leading to monolingualism in the new language (Brenzinger, 1997).

As I discussed in the Introduction, such trends have led to some dire predictions concerning the 'endangered' status of these former languages. J. Hill (1978: 69) estimates, for example, that in the last 500 years at least half of the languages in the world have disappeared, and Krauss (1992: 7), in a much cited article, argues that as few as 600, perhaps only 300, of the currently estimated 6,800 languages in the world will remain secure through the next century. Inevitably perhaps, there are disputes about the accuracy of such projections but the general trend is not in doubt (Grenoble and Whaley, 1996, 1998). To take just one example, when Australia was annexed to Britain in 1770 Australian Aboriginal peoples spoke more than 250 languages. Nearly 250 years on, only 145 of these languages remain in use. Of the latter, 110 are facing extinction, with a rapidly declining number of speakers and/or increasingly delimited use. Indeed, by the mid-1980s, only fifty Aboriginal languages had more than 100 speakers, twenty-eight of them more than 250 speakers, and only nine had more than 1,000 speakers (see Lo Bianco, 1987; Brenzinger, 1997; Lo Bianco and Rhydwen, 2001). In the 2006 Australian census, only 55,695 people, one in eight indigenous Australians, still spoke an Aboriginal language as the primary language of the home (Nathan, n.d.).

The reference to language 'extinction' here is a pertinent one since, again as noted in the Introduction, parallels are often drawn between endangered languages and endangered species. James Crawford draws such comparisons directly when he argues that endangered languages 'fall victim to predators, changing environments, or more successful competitors', are encroached on by 'modern cultures abetted by new technologies' and are threatened by 'destruction of lands and livelihoods; the spread of consumerism, individualism, and other Western values; pressures for assimilation into dominant cultures; and conscious policies of repression' (1994: 5; see also Hornberger, 1997, 1998; May, 1999c; May and Aikman, 2003). Lest the predatory allusion be taken too far, however, it should be stressed that most language shifts are not solely the result of coercion or 'language murder' (Calvet, 1974). However, neither are they solely the result of a 'voluntary' shift, or 'language suicide' (Denison, 1977), as critics of minority language rights are wont to suggest. Both internal pull and external push factors are invariably involved – although, as I will proceed to argue, it is usually the latter that direct the former. Likewise, it needs to be borne in mind that no two language contact situations are alike, nor do two language shifts resemble each other exactly (Brenzinger, 1997). Thus, while I will attempt to extrapolate general trends in what follows, it is regionally specific, or even community-specific, factors that dictate the ultimate patterns and effects of language shift in any given context (Grenoble and Whaley, 1996, 1998).

One further caveat needs to be made here. It is often thought that the *number* of actual speakers is the key variable in predicting the likelihood or otherwise of a particular language's survival. While numbers are clearly important – the fewer speakers, the less likely that a language will be maintained over time – this assumption is misplaced. It is not so much how many speak the language but *who* speaks it (and why) that is of most significance. For example, in a report on the situation of forty-eight minority language groups in the EU, Nelde et al. (1996) found that 'the demographic size of a language group is no guarantee of the group's [linguistic] vitality, with the existence of some of Europe's largest language groups being severely threatened' (Executive Summary). Two other variables were identified as far more influential in their analysis: the low status of many minority groups and their often related social, cultural and economic marginalization; and the degree to which minority languages were recognized by the state *and* supported within civil society – what Nelde et al. have termed the processes of 'legitimation' and 'institutionalization' (see below for further discussion). Both these variables highlight the importance of underlying *power relations* in situations of minority language shift, a key factor that is seldom acknowledged by its many apologists.

Acknowledging power relations

The significance of the often-unequal power relations that exist between minority and majority language communities tends to be ignored, or at least downplayed, by proponents of language shift. In this regard, it is interesting to note that language death seldom occurs in communities of wealth and privilege, but rather to the dispossessed and disempowered (Crawford, 1994). Even where unequal sociopolitical conditions are ostensibly recognized as a central factor, as in Edwards, Kay and Brutt Griffler's accounts discussed earlier, these are legitimized in the name of 'linguistic modernization'. However, this type of argument exhibits a curious schizophrenia. Edwards (1985), for example, is quite willing to acknowledge that language loss has little to do with linguistic merit and almost everything to do with the (unequal) exercise of social and political power. Yet, at the same time, he is prepared to endorse the arrogation of a majority language on the basis of its greater 'communicative currency'. In other words, the notions of 'communicative currency' or 'languages of wider communication' come to serve as linguistic proxies for the legitimation of the greater sociopolitical status of the majority language group.

Moreover, attempts to provide a minority language with a greater communicative currency of its own – via, most often, a sympathetic policy of status language planning[20] – are largely derided on the grounds that if another language already has such currency why bother?[21] The best that can be hoped for, it is argued, is the retention of some of the minority language's symbolic or totemic qualities but its continued communicative currency is ruled out of court (see J. Edwards, 1984: 289–91; 1985: 17–18). This is a specious, not to mention historically ill-founded argument though, since all the current major languages in the world today have at some time undergone a comparable process of communicative expansion. One wonders, for example, what the current status of English would be in Britain, let alone globally, had it not undergone its own significant social and lexical expansion in the sixteenth and seventeenth centuries. In the process, English was transformed within the British Isles from a language with a status lower than both Latin and French to effectively the 'national' language, or at least the accepted language of wider communication. This was a considerable achievement given that, prior to the fourteenth century, English was not even taught as a language. Latin was regarded as the language of record, or the literary language. Moreover, owing to the Norman invasion of 1066, French was the language associated with the nobility and thus social aspiration. Indeed, the first king of England since 1066 to speak English as a first language was Henry IV, who assumed the throne in 1399 (Graddol, Leith, and Swann, 2006; see also McCrum, Cran, and MacNeill, 2011).

Thus, while establishing a symbolic/communicative distinction to language may well help to explain the detachability of language from ethnic identity, the implicit assumption that the latter should atrophy and die is inherently a *political* not a *linguistic* judgment. Relatedly, if the loss of a particular language is the result largely of political processes, then apologists of such language shift demonstrate little credibility in their own decrial and/or dismissal of minority language promotion as 'politically motivated'. If we accept the assumption that the sociopolitical dominates the linguistic when it comes to questions of language shift, then we must also accept that arguments both for *and* against any language shift are inherently political. On this basis, Edwards's arguments, and their like, simply represent a particular *value judgment* – a judgment that equates minority language loss, and language shift to a majority language, with progress and modernity.

In effect, this position amounts to little more than linguistic social Darwinism – only the languages with the greatest communicative currency should and/ or will survive. Concomitantly, any efforts undertaken to protect minority languages from such 'inexorable' processes are viewed as antediluvian; as forlorn, Canute-like, attempts to maintain some kind of cultural and linguistic stasis. Edwards's earlier comments on the self-interested role of minority elites demonstrate this view clearly and he reiterates this position when he asserts: 'language in its communicative sense is ... an element of identity very susceptible to change. We may lament the fact, we may wish it were not so – but it is. To expect otherwise is tantamount to asking for change itself to cease' (1985: 97). Elsewhere he opines: 'Is the implication that stasis is the price of ethnolinguistic continuity? If so, history suggests it is a price higher than most have been willing to pay' (2001: 237). In this view, there is, it seems, very little room for agency – except of a prescribed kind, the *renunciation* of one's historically associated language(s). One must simply get with the (new) linguistic program, or be left behind.

Yet, as with the comparable criticism of minority rights more generally (see Chapter 3), this argument is simply wrong (and wrongheaded). There is no necessary correlation between the continued maintenance of one's minority language and cultural and linguistic stasis – cultural and linguistic continuity and change are always and inevitably intertwined (Fishman, 1991, 2001). Likewise, cultural nationalism, which often incorporates a defence of minority language rights, is principally concerned with the *reconstruction* of tradition – modifying it, where necessary – in order to meet more adequately the demands of modernity (Hutchinson, 1994, 2005; see Chapter 2). The key question in both these contexts is thus not one of stasis but rather one of greater *control* and *self-regulation* of the process of cultural and linguistic change. As Fishman argues:

> A call for RLS [reversing language shift] must ... be seen and explained [principally] as a call for cultural reconstruction and for greater self-regulation ... RLS is an indication of the dissatisfaction with ethnocultural (and, often, also with ethnopolitical and ethno-economic) life as it currently is, and of a resolve to undertake planned ethnocultural reconstruction. This change does not need to be backward looking in its thrust, regardless of the historical metaphors that it may utilise (because

of their recognised symbolic and emotional significance). Indeed, most RLS-efforts are actually syncretistic and modernistic with respect to their cultural implications and goals. (1991: 17)

This is not to say that all attempts to reverse language shift are shorn of their nostalgic elements. Nor does it preclude the unfortunate potential that still exists to reify language and culture. Nonetheless, the inevitable association of such movements with narrow provincialism is simply misjudged. As with the conclusions drawn in Chapter 3, maintaining one's minority language does not in any way preclude ongoing cultural and linguistic change, adaptation and interaction. Indeed, it can be argued that those who wish to maintain their historically associated language, usually alongside that of another more dominant language, actually exhibit a *greater* ability to manage multiple cultural and linguistic identities. Narrower identities do not necessarily need to be traded in for broader ones – one can clearly remain both Spanish-speaking and American, Catalan-speaking and Spanish, or Welsh-speaking and British – and to insist on doing so exhibits its own particular forms of reductionism and ethnocentrism.

But there is still a problem here. Arguments for the maintenance of minority languages are all very well, but if increasing numbers of people are *voluntarily* choosing to opt instead for a majority language, then the cause already appears to be lost, as critics suggest. This was certainly the basis of the case against Irish, for example. Likewise, Nathan Glazer argues, in the US context, that most immigrants want 'to become Americanized as fast as possible, and this [means appropriating] English language and culture ... while they often found, as time went on, that they regretted what they and their children had lost, this was *their* choice rather than an imposed choice' (1983: 149). However, it can equally be argued that the degree to which voluntary shift actually occurs is extremely problematic. After all, if minority languages are consistently viewed as low status, socially and culturally restrictive, and an obstacle to social mobility, is it little wonder that such patterns of language shift exist? In effect, these widely held views place minority language speakers in a seemingly intractable dilemma. This dilemma, as Fishman summarizes it, is 'either to remain loyal to their traditions and to remain socially disadvantaged (consigning their own children to such disadvantage as well), on the one hand; or, on the other hand, to abandon their distinctive practices and traditions, at least in large part, and, thereby, to improve their own and their children's lots in life via cultural suicide' (1991: 60). Thus, one can reasonably question here the legitimacy of this juxtaposition and the apparently forced choice it entails. To what extent is language shift *on these terms* actually necessary? Moreover, what are the *costs* involved in this process and to what extent can they be regarded as fair or warranted? And what, if anything, can be done to change 'the rules of the game' that constitute this dilemma in the first place? To explore these questions further, we need to examine the central issue of language status and the crucial role of the (nation-)state in its apportionment. In particular, the role of the state has a significant part to play with regard both to the official recognition of a language and its acknowledged and accepted domains of use within civil society.

A question of status

It is surprising the extent to which the relationship between language and politics has been overlooked in much sociological and political analysis. After all, language has been a contributing feature in many political conflicts, including those in the Baltics, the Balkans, Belgium, Canada, Spain, Sri Lanka, Algeria and Turkey, to name but a few (see Horowitz, 2000; Safran, 2004, 2010). Yet, as Weinstein (1983) observes, while commentators have had much to say about 'the language of politics', very few have had anything to say about 'the politics of language' (for similar observations, see also Grillo, 1989; Kymlicka, 1995a, b; Blommaert, 1996; Holborow, 1999).

What constitutes the politics of language then? Principally, it is a contest for linguistic control (and, by extension, social and cultural control) of the nation-state. In this regard, 'national' languages are so called because they have been *legitimated* by the state and *institutionalized* within civil society, usually to the exclusion of other languages (Nelde et al., 1996; Glyn Williams, 2005). Legitimation involves the formal recognition by the state of a particular language variety and this recognition is realized, usually, by the constitutional and/or legislative benediction of official status.[22] Accordingly, 'la langue officielle a partie liée avec l'État' (Bourdieu, 1982: 27) – the legitimate (or standard) language becomes an arm of the state – and other language varieties are consequently relegated to the lower status of 'dialects' or 'patois' (cf. Silverstein, 1996; Collins, 1999). This process of 'language standardization', as it is known in sociolinguistics, usually comprises four main aspects (see Leith and Graddol, 1996: 139; see also Bucholtz and Hall, 2004; Makoni and Pennycook, 2007):

1   *Selection*: of an existing language variety, usually that of the most powerful social or ethnic group;
2   *Codification*: reduction of internal variability in the selected variety, and the establishment of norms of grammatical usage and vocabulary;
3   *Elaboration*: ensuring the language can be used for a wide range of functions;
4   *Implementation*: promoting the language variety via print (cf. Anderson's account in Chapter 2), discouraging the use of other language varieties within official domains, and encouraging users to develop a loyalty to and pride in it.

Given this, it is important to stress that the often-invoked distinction between languages and dialects is not principally a linguistic one. Indeed, to attempt a linguistic distinction of the two is fraught with difficulty. One cannot distinguish, for example, a language and dialect on the basis of mutual intelligibility. There are some languages – such as Norwegian, Swedish and Danish – which are mutually intelligible and there are some languages which encompass dialects that are mutually incomprehensible. Rather, the distinction between language and dialect is primarily a political consequence of the language legitimation processes undertaken by nation-states (cf. Blommaert, 1999a, b). As Haugen (1966) observes, a 'dialect' is usually a language that did not succeed politically. Or, returning to an observation made at the beginning of this chapter, a language can be seen as a dialect with an army and navy! The boundaries between languages, and the classification of dialects, have invariably followed the politics of state making, rather than the other way around (Billig, 1995; see also Gramsci, 1971; Bakhtin, 1981; Harris, 1981). An inevitable corollary is that the status of languages and dialects may also change as the result of changes in nation-state formation. The dissolution in 1993 of the former Czechoslovakia, for example, saw the subsequent emergence of distinct Czech and Slovak language varieties, in the Czech Republic and Slovakia respectively, in place of a previously common state language. This, in turn, was built on a growing differentiation between the two language varieties in the former Czechoslovakia from the 1930s onwards (Tabouret-Keller, 1997). The former Yugoslavia provides an even more recent example. The (re)development of separate Serbian, Croatian and Bosnian language varieties in the newly constituted states of Serbia, Croatia, and Bosnia and Herzegovina respectively, have replaced Serbo-Croat, despite minimal linguistic differences among the varieties. Meanwhile, it should not be forgotten that Serbo-Croat was itself an artificial product of the communist Yugoslav federation under Tito which, despite attempts to make it the 'national' language of Yugoslavia, never reached much beyond the armed forces and diplomatic services (Jakšić, 1995: Grant, 1997; Rogel, 2004).

The legitimation of a language variety is thus an important first step in the political creation of a 'national' language. Moreover, it is a process bestowed upon only a privileged few since, as we saw in the Introduction, of the 6,800 or so living language varieties contained within approximately 200 nation-states, fewer than a hundred actually currently enjoy official status. Even so, legitimation of a language is not, in itself, enough to ensure a central role for that language variety within the nation-state, since it is possible to legitimize a language without this having much influence on its actual use. We saw this clearly demonstrated in the case of Irish, for example. Crucially, what is needed, in addition, is the institutionalization of the language variety within civil society. Indeed, this may be the more important aspect. By this, the language variety comes to be accepted, or 'taken for granted', in a wide range of social, cultural and linguistic domains or contexts, both formal and informal. The degree to which a language variety comes to be institutionalized in this way will also have a significant bearing on the subsequent status attached to the language in question and, by extension, its speakers. In effect, as Bourhis (1984) has convincingly argued, an ethnic group's cultural vitality, especially its linguistic vitality, is closely related to the degree of institutional support it enjoys. Likewise, Giles et al. (1977) have argued – in a broadly consonant, albeit more elaborate position – that ethnolinguistic vitality is based on a combination of the following components: economic status, self-perceived social status, sociohistorical factors and demographic factors (including institutional support). I will explore some of these other dimensions of ethnolinguistic vitality in my ensuing discussion of Bourdieu's notions of linguistic markets and symbolic violence.

The result of this joint process of legitimation and institutionalization is to *privilege* a particular language variety over others; imbuing it, in the process, with high status. Not only this, but the privileging of the language becomes *normalized* – it is simply accepted or taken for granted. Consequently, speakers of the dominant language variety are immediately placed at an advantage in both accessing and benefiting from the civic culture of the nation-state. A dominant language group usually controls the crucial authority in the areas of administration, politics, education and the economy, and gives preference to those with a command of that language. Meanwhile, other language groups are limited in their language use to specific domains, usually solely private and/or low status, and are thus left with the choice of renouncing their social ambitions, assimilating, or resisting in order to gain greater access to the public realm (Nelde, 1997).

If language conflict results, this is attributable, at least to some degree, to the differential social status and preferential treatment of the dominant language by the state and within civil society, and the related stigmatization of other varieties. Indeed, the dynamics of ethnic tension involving language, leading in some cases to political conflict, occur most often *not* when language compromises are made or language rights recognized, but where they have been historically avoided, suppressed or ignored (de Varennes, 1996a), a key point to which I will return in the final chapter. Such linguistic and political tensions are exacerbated by the continued assumption that the civic culture of the nation-state is somehow neutral and, relatedly, that the adoption of a national language depoliticizes that particular language variety. Yet, as I have argued, the establishment of a state-endowed or 'national' language must be regarded as an inherently deliberate (and deliberative) political act; an act, moreover, that advantages some individuals and groups at the expense of others. Fernand de Varennes summarizes the processes and its implications thus:

By imposing a language requirement, the state shows a definite preference towards some individuals on the basis of language ... In other words, the imposition of a single language for use in state activities and services is by no means a neutral act, since:

1) The state's chosen language becomes a condition for the full access to a number of services, resources and privileges, such as education or public employment. ...
2) Those for whom the chosen state speech is not the primary language are thus treated differently from those for whom it is: the latter have the advantage or benefit of receiving the state's largesse in their primary tongue, whereas the former do not and find themselves in a more or less disadvantaged position. ... Whether it is for employment in state institutions ... or the need to translate or obtain assistance ... a person faced with not being able to use his primary language *assumes a heavier burden.* (1996a: 86–7; my emphasis)

The public legitimation of a language, and its associated institutionalization in particular domains, thus become crucial to the ongoing maintenance of the dominant ethnie's cultural and linguistic hegemony within the nation-state. Relatedly, without these same processes being applied to minority languages, it is difficult to envisage a long-term future for them in a world that, while increasingly globalized, is still dominated by nation-states (Nelde et al., 1996; cf. Chapter 1). Given the spread of standardized education, the associated literacy demands of the labor force and the inevitable and widespread interaction required in dealing with state agencies, any language that is not widely used in the public realm becomes so marginalized as to be inconsequential. Using a particular language solely in the home domain, for example, limits its ultimate usefulness since speakers will be unable to deal adequately with the interpenetration of other domains such as talking about work or school at home (Clyne, 1997). The increasing marginalization of a language in turn limits the linguistic functions of the language itself while the latter, recursively, contributes further to the language's marginalization. As Florian Coulmas argues: 'Today the future of many languages is uncertain not only because their functional range is scaled down, but because they are never used for, and adapted to newly emerging functions which are associated with another language ... Lack of functional expansion is thus a correlate and counterpart of scaled-down use' (1992: 170). Such languages may persist among a small elite, as we have seen demonstrated in the case of Irish, or in a ritualized form, but not as a living and developing language of a flourishing culture (Kymlicka, 1995a).

Linguistic markets and symbolic violence

To explore further the implications of language legitimation and institutionalization for ethnolinguistic minorities, I want to turn again to the work of Pierre Bourdieu. Bourdieu has written widely, though disparately, on language, and his work in this regard includes the two seminal essays 'Le fétichisme de la langue' (Bourdieu and Boltanski, 1975) and 'The economy of linguistic exchanges' (1977). Where his thoughts on language (and linguistics) are perhaps most clearly articulated, however, are in *Ce que parler veut dire* (1982) and its English-language adaptation *Language and Symbolic Power* (1991). His principal concern in these various accounts is to situate language in its proper sociohistorical context. In this regard, he is particularly scathing of the preoccupation in modern linguistics with analyzing language in isolation from the social conditions in which it is used. As he comments ironically of this process: 'bracketing out the social ... allows language or any other symbolic object to be treated like an end in itself, [this] contributed considerably to the success of structural linguistics, for it endowed the "pure" exercises that characterise a purely internal and formal analysis with the charm of a game devoid of consequences' (1991: 34).

For Bourdieu, the inherent formalism of so much modern linguistics rests on a central distinction between the internal form of the language – a 'language system', in effect – and its outworking in speech. This distinction, in turn, arises from the conception of language as a 'universal treasure', freely available to all – a view that was first articulated by Auguste Comte and subsequently adopted by the founding fathers of modern linguistics, Ferdinand de Saussure and Noam Chomsky. De Saussure (1974) invokes the distinction via his celebrated comparison between 'langue' and 'parole', while Chomsky's (1972) notions of 'competence' and 'performance' reflect a similar conception. This is not to suggest that de Saussure's and Chomsky's conceptions are indistinguishable – Chomsky's model, for example, is more dynamic in its attempt to incorporate the generative capacities of competent speakers. However, both approaches rest on the notion that language can be constituted as an autonomous and homogeneous object, amenable to linguistic study (Thompson, 1991).

An allied critique of this preoccupation with linguistic formalism at the expense of a wider analysis of the social and political conditions in which language comes to be used can also be found in Vološinov (1973: 77–82) and Mey (1985). Vološinov argued cogently against the 'abstract objectivism' of structural linguistics, as represented by de Saussure, suggesting it created a radical disjuncture between the idea of a language system and actual language history. Mey observes 'that linguistic models, no matter how innocent and theoretical they may seem to be, not only have distinct economical, social and political presuppositions, but also consequences ... Linguistic (and other) inequalities don't cease to exist simply because their socioeconomic causes are swept under the linguistic rug' (1985: 26).

Bourdieu describes the resulting orthodoxy, which posits a particular set of linguistic practices as a normative model of 'correct' usage, as the 'illusion of linguistic communism that haunts all linguistic theory' (1991: 43). By this, Bourdieu argues, the linguist is able to produce the illusion of a common or standard language, while ignoring the sociohistorical conditions which have established this particular set of linguistic practices as dominant and legitimate in the first place – usually, as we have seen, as the result of nation-state formation. However, this dominant and legitimate language – this *victorious* language, in effect – is simply taken for granted by linguists (Thompson, 1991; see also Mühlhäusler, 1996). As Bourdieu asserts:

> To speak of *the* language, without further specification, as linguists do, is tacitly to accept the *official* definition of the *official* language of a political unit. This language is the one which, within the territorial limits of that unit, imposes itself on the whole population as the only legitimate language. ... The official language is bound up with the state, both in its genesis and its social uses ... this state language becomes the theoretical norm against which all linguistic practices are objectively measured. (1991: 45; emphases in original)

In addition to habitus and field (see Chapter 1), Bourdieu employs a number of key concepts that illuminate the processes that underpin language domination and legitimation. These include 'linguistic capital', 'linguistic markets', 'misrecognition' and 'symbolic violence'. Linguistic capital, in Bourdieu's terms, describes the 'value' given to one's linguistic habitus in particular linguistic markets. In a given linguistic market (such as the civic culture of the nation-state), some habitus are valued more highly than others. Accordingly, different speakers will have different amounts of linguistic capital depending on their ability to meet the requirements of the particular linguistic market concerned. Moreover, the distribution of linguistic capital is closely related to the distribution of other forms of capital (economic, cultural capital, etc.), which define the location of an individual within the social space (Thompson, 1991; cf. Ó Riagáin, 1997; Collins, 1999; Norton, 2000). Those whose habitus are consonant with the demands of the linguistic market are thereby able to secure an advantage, or 'profit of distinction', since the linguistic capital required is far from equally distributed. Meanwhile, those whose habitus are assigned a lesser value by the market come to *accept* this diminution as legitimate, a process which Bourdieu has described as 'symbolic violence'. Bourdieu argues here that symbolic violence occurs when a particular (linguistic) habitus, along with the hierarchical relations of power in which it is embedded, is 'misrecognized' (méconnaissance) as legitimate and tacitly accepted – *even by those who do not have access to it* – as a 'natural' rather than a socially and politically constructed phenomenon. To understand the nature of symbolic violence, Bourdieu argues, it is crucial to see that it presupposes a kind of active complicity, or implicit consent, on the part of those subjected to it; a process, in effect, which induces 'the holders of dominated linguistic competencies to collaborate in the destruction of their [own] instruments of expression' (1991: 49). While by no means limited to such a comparison, his conceptual analysis is clearly helpful here in explicating the unequal relationship that exists between 'majority' and 'minority' languages and the subsequent devaluation of the latter by both majority *and* minority speakers:

> In order for one mode of expression among others (a particular language in the case of bilingualism, a particular use of language in the case of a society divided into classes) to *impose* itself as the only legitimate one, the linguistic market has to be *unified* and the different dialects (of class, region or ethnic group) have to be measured practically against the legitimate language or usage. Integration into a single 'linguistic community', which is the product of the political domination that is endlessly reproduced by institutions capable of imposing universal recognition of the dominant language, is the condition for the establishment of relations of linguistic domination. (1991: 46–7; my emphases)

The single linguistic community, or the unified linguistic market, to which Bourdieu refers is most clearly represented in and by the homogeneous civic culture of the modern nation-state. Indeed, the triumph of official languages and the suppression of their potential rivals are prominent characteristics of the construction of statehood and the achievement of national hegemony, as we have seen. Bourdieu illustrates the particular processes of language domination involved here by tracing the emergence of his own language of French as the 'national' language of post-revolutionary France. It therefore seems appropriate to examine briefly the French example before drawing this chapter to a close.

Vive la France: the construction of la langue légitime

> I express my homage to the lay, Republican school system which often imposed the use of French against all the forces of social and even religious obscurantism. … It is time for us all to be French through that language. If it is necessary to teach another language to our children, let us not make them waste time with dialects they will only ever use in their villages. (Journal Officiel, 15 April 1994; cited in Ager, 1999: 20)

The above comment was made in the French National Assembly during discussion of the Toubon Act which, on being passed in 1994, made the use of French obligatory in five domains: education, employment, the media, commerce and public meetings (see also below). The sentiments of the speaker, and of the Act to which it refers, reflect, writ large, the modern French nation-state's historical and ongoing preoccupation with legitimating and institutionalizing French as the 'common' national language, and its related vitiation of minority languages. This dual process was most starkly demonstrated at the time of the French Revolution, and has subsequently been systematically reinforced, as the speaker suggests, via the French state education system, established during the early stages of the Third Republic (1870–1940). However, it was also present, at least in incipient form, well before the advent of the Revolution.

Prior to the French Revolution of 1789, three broad language groups were present in the territory we now know as France. The Langue d'Oïl, comprising a wide range of dialects, was spoken in the North. Of these, the Francien dialect, spoken in and around Paris, was the actual antecedent of modern French. The Langue d'Oc (Occitan), also comprising a wide range of dialects, was spoken in the South. And in central and eastern France, Franco-Provençal was spoken. But not only that, Basque was spoken in the southwest, as was Breton in Brittany, Flemish around Lille, German in Alsace-Lorraine, Catalan in Perpignan and Corsican (a dialect of Italian and Napoleon's first language) in Corsica (Ager, 1999). In addition, Latin was the administrative language, at least until the sixteenth century (see below), although it was as such largely confined to the church, the university and the royal administration (Johnson, 1993). Premodern 'France', like so many other administrations prior to the rise of political nationalism, was thus resolutely multilingual. As Peyre notes, citing the observations of the sixteenth-century chancellor Michel de l'Hôpital, linguistic divisions were not regarded as a danger to the kingdom. Rather, the key factors of unity were 'one faith, one law, one king': 'What the king demanded above all was loyalty … It mattered little then, *up to a certain point*, that custom and usage differed from one province to another' (1933: 10, 16; my emphasis).

The caveat 'up to a certain point' is an important one here because the sixteenth century was also to see the beginnings of a counter-movement against multilingualism that would reach its apogee soon after the French Revolution. The first sign of this can be found in the (1538) Ordonnance de Villers-Cotterêts, issued by King Louis XII. Article III of the Act made the 'maternal French tongue' (actually the Francien dialect of the Langue d'Oïl, spoken by the French court) the language of the law. The initial intent of the decree was not to make French the 'national' language – this, as we have seen, is peculiar to the political nationalism of subsequent centuries. It was simply to ensure that the language of the king's court would be used in the quarters significant to his power (E. Weber, 1976). In this sense, the Act's principal aim was the replacement of Latin as the language of administration. Nonetheless, the decree's admonition to transact and record all public acts in 'French' presaged the inexorable rise of modern French. In Benedict Anderson's terms, French came to be seen as the new 'language of power' (cf. Chapter 2). As a result, French began to replace Latin *and* other language varieties – both in court usage and in much state administration (Lodge, 1993; Schiffman, 1996) – although the various regional languages were still the normal means of communication for the wider population. From the sixteenth century to the time of the French Revolution most of France thus operated in diglossia, with French colonizing the higher status public language domains, while other languages were increasingly confined to the lower status private domains (Ager, 1999).

The establishment in 1635 of the Académie Française was to further reinforce the rise of French in the sixteenth century. Established by Cardinal Richelieu, the principal aim of the Académie was one of corpus planning – to systematically codify, standardize and 'purify' French. The Académie pursued these aims with zeal – as, indeed, it still does to this day. Its early work led to the publication of the *Grammaire Générale et Raisonnée* in 1660 and the first French-language dictionary in 1694. More significantly perhaps, the work of the Académie also reinforced a nascent, albeit growing belief at that time 'in the universality of standard French, in its innate clarity, precision, logic and elegance, and in its superiority over any other language and certainly over any … regional language' (Ager, 1999: 23; see also Moïse, 2007).

Both these developments in the sixteenth century foreshadowed the eventual proscription of other languages and dialects within France, most notably in the aftermath of the French Revolution. It is thus somewhat ironic that it was only during the early stages of the Revolution that the linguistic diversity of France was fully apprehended. A linguistic survey carried out by the abbé Henri Grégoire in 1790 revealed that over thirty 'patois' were spoken in France (for political reasons, he was reluctant to accord them the status of languages; see below). More pertinently perhaps, he concluded that as few as three million people – not more than a tenth of the actual population – could actually speak French with any degree of fluency (Johnson, 1993).

The initial response to this linguistic diversity was cautious magnanimity. For example, the new Assembly agreed on 14 January 1790 a policy of translating decrees into various 'idioms' and 'dialects' in order better to disseminate Republican ideas among the majority non-French-speaking population (Grillo, 1989). But this was soon to change. If we recall the French historian Michelet, and his comment in Chapter 1 advocating the 'sacrifice of the diverse interior nationalities to the great nationality', we can begin to understand why. In short, it soon became apparent to the Jacobins that the ideal of the Revolution lay in uniformity and the extinction of particularisms. For the revolutionaries, regional languages were increasingly regarded as parochial vestiges of the ancien régime, the sooner forgotten the better. This was reflected in their pejorative labeling as 'patois' rather than as languages. As Bourdieu observes of this process, 'measured de facto against the single standard of the "common" language, they are found wanting and cast into the outer darkness of *regionalisms*'. As a result, 'a system of *sociologically pertinent* linguistic oppositions tends to be constituted which has nothing in common with the system of *linguistically pertinent* linguistic oppositions' (1991: 54; emphases in original).

In contrast, French was seen as the embodiment of civilization and progress, a language fit for a new universalism. Consequently, the adoption of French as the single national language, representing and reflecting the interests of the new revolutionary order, was increasingly regarded as an essential foundation for the new Republic and its advocacy of liberté, égalité, fraternité. As the Jacobins came to insist: 'The unity of the Republic demands the unity of speech ... Speech must be one, like the Republic' (cited in E. Weber, 1976: 72). Bourdieu comments that this perceived imperative 'was not only a question of communication but of gaining recognition for a new *language of authority*, with its new political vocabulary, its terms of address and reference, its metaphors, its euphemisms and the representation of the social world which it conveys' (1991: 48; my emphasis).

The obvious corollary to this also came to be accepted and actively promoted – that the ongoing maintenance of other languages was specifically opposed to the aims of the Revolution. Indeed, Barère, in his Report of 1794, went so far as to assert:

> La fédéralisme et la superstition parlent bas-breton; l'émigration et la haine de la République parlent allemand; la contre-révolution parle l'italien, et le fanatisme parle le basque. Cassons ces instruments de dommage et d'erreur.

> Federalism and superstition speak Breton; emigration and hatred of the Republic speak German; counter-revolution speaks Italian, and fanaticism speaks Basque. Let us destroy these instruments of damage and error. (Quoted in de Certeau et al., 1975: 299)

These sentiments were also reflected, albeit somewhat less iconoclastically, in the final report of the abbé Grégoire on the linguistic state of the new republic. This report was eventually published in 1794, four years after the survey had been commissioned, and concerned itself principally with corpus issues – on 'perfecting' the French language (in a similar way to the Académie). However, its overall position on other languages in France is clearly indicated by its subtitle – 'Sur la nécessité et les moyens d'anéantir les patois et d'universaliser l'usage de la langue française' (On the need and ways to annihilate dialects and universalize the use of French). It should come as no surprise then that Grégoire went on to conclude that:

> Unity of language is an integral part of the Revolution. If we are ever to banish superstition and bring men closer to the truth, to develop talent and encourage virtue, to mould all citizens into a national whole, to simplify the mechanism of the political machine and make it function more smoothly, we must have a common language. (Cited in Grillo, 1989: 24)

The Grégoire Report proved a watershed. Earlier attempts at translation were quickly dispensed with in order to expedite this vision of a brave new world, represented in and through French. More importantly, the legitimation and institutionalization of French came to be inextricably intertwined in the minds of the Jacobins with the *active* destruction of all other languages. But there was still a problem. Such was the linguistic diversity highlighted by Grégoire that it could not be easily or quickly displaced. Even as late as 1863, official figures indicated that a quarter of the country's population, including half the children who would reach adulthood in the last quarter of the nineteenth century, still spoke no French (E. Weber, 1976). What to do? The answer lay in a combination of legal enforcement of the language, via a series of court decisions requiring the use of French in all legal documents (see Grau, 1992) and, more significantly, a central role for education.

The use of education as a key, perhaps *the* key agency of linguistic standardization began as early as 1793. At that time, French schools were established in the German-speaking Alsace region, while the ongoing use of German was banned (Grillo, 1989). This was to provide the template for the use of French education throughout the nineteenth (and twentieth) century. A central goal of the hussards noirs, the Republic's teachers, was to eradicate all regional languages, which were by then regarded as worthless, barbarous, corrupt and devoid of interest (Bourdieu, 1982). Given the ongoing linguistic diversity, this process took some time. It was not until the establishment of a fully secularized, compulsory and free primary system in the 1880s that education really began to have its full effect, principally through the formal proscription of all other languages from the school. But even prior to that time it had not been for want of trying. A poignant illustration of this is provided by a prefect in the Department of Finistère, the most western part of Brittany, who, in 1845, formally exhorted teachers: 'Above all remember, gentleman, that your sole function is to kill the Breton language' (cited in Quiniou-Tempereau, 1988: 31–2).

This state-led 'ideology of contempt' (Grillo, 1989) toward minority languages has resulted in their inexorable decline in France over the last two centuries to the point where less than 2 percent of the French population now speak these as a first language (see Nelde et al., 1996; Judge, 2007). It has also at the same time entrenched deep into the French national psyche a view that the promotion and even simply the maintenance of minority languages (and cultures) are fundamentally at odds with the supposedly universalistic principles and objectives of the French state, a form or ethnic particularism, in effect. As Bollmann observes of this, for France, '[une] logique ethniste … serait non seulement la negation de son histoire, mais le scenario politique le plus défavorable à l'intérêt national' (an 'ethnist' logic … would not only be the negation of its history, but [also] the political scenario which is most unfavorable to the national interest) (2002: 199).

Not surprisingly then, there have been remarkably few exceptions to this assimilationist imperative in French language and education policy. One such exception is the (1951) Deixonne Act, which gave formal status in education to four regional languages: Basque, Breton, Catalan and Occitan (see Schiffman, 1996). The Act was limited though in that it did not involve the *active* promotion of these languages, merely *permitting* the languages to be taught in a limited way within schools. (I discuss the distinction between active and permissive language and education rights more fully in Chapter 5.) Moreover, the Act itself was not actually implemented until 1969!

The advent of the Socialist government elected in 1997, however, did result in an apparent change in direction, or at least a discernible shift in emphasis, albeit briefly. Almost immediately on taking office, the government commissioned a report on France's regional languages – the first time that any French government had commissioned a report in this area. The Poignant Report, named after its author, was subsequently published in July 1998. While the report continued to uphold the primacy of French, it also advocated that 'the French Republic must acknowledge the existence on its territory of regional languages and cultures which are granted rights in accordance with the laws and regulations. The latter do not pose any threat to national identity' (cited in Louarn, 1998: 5). The report argued that the protection and promotion of France's regional languages was important because such languages constitute an important part of France's cultural and linguistic heritage. However, it also argued that some formal accommodation of regional languages might forestall the rise of potentially troublesome regionalisms at a later point, particularly in light of a growing emphasis on regionalism and devolution within the European Union (Ager, 1999: 38–9; see also Chapter 7). As Poignant concludes: 'The [twenty-first] century will have to deal with strong claims to regional identity. If this republic does not act in response, others will' (see Henley, 1999).

These developments suggested the nascent emergence of a more tolerant approach to minority languages within France in the late 1990s. But the last decade has proved that much of this potential has since been negated, or at least retrenched. Such is the legacy of French language and education policy that effecting even limited changes in this area remains a process fraught with difficulty. An obvious example of the significant obstacles that still remain in the way of adopting a more tolerant language policy in France is the (1994) Toubon Act. The Act was principally a response to a burgeoning fear of the impact of English as the current world language (see Chapter 6) on French speakers, both within France and beyond it. In particular, the growing fashion for English words, or what has come to be known as 'franglais', was deemed to be such a threat as to necessitate this specific legislative measure in addition to the general policing role performed by the Académie Française. Accordingly, the Toubon Act built upon a previous legislative measure, the (1975) Bas-Lauriol Bill, which was never fully implemented. Among a wide range of measures, it decreed that consumer goods must not be sold without a set of instructions in French, all-English advertisements must not be published either in the French press or in French cinemas, and bilingual signs must not give less prominence to the French part of their message.

It is not hard to see that the Act's aim 'to guarantee to French people the right to use their language and to ensure that it is used in certain circumstances of their everyday and professional life' (cited in Ager, 1999: 8) only serves to reinforce the ongoing legitimation and institutionalization of French. As such, it would seem to offer little, if anything, for France's minority language speakers. This is reinforced by the clear belief expressed in the Act that 'the mastery of French … is part of the fundamental aims of education' (cited in Ager, 1999: 65). Of course, this conclusion was even more baldly stated by the French Parliamentarian whose comments on the Act began this section. Plus ça change, or so it would seem.

Similar obstacles to any significant change can also be clearly seen in France's varied responses to the formal ratification of the European Charter for Regional or Minority Languages (see S. Wright, 2000; Judge, 2007; Moïse, 2007). The Charter, adopted in 1992 by the Council of Europe,[23] aims to promote the greater formal recognition of regional and minority languages within the Pan-European Community and, in so doing, to extend the provision of bilingual education (see also Chapter 5). By December 1998, eighteen of the then forty member states of the Council of Europe had signed the Charter, but not France. This was because the French Council of State (the Constitutional Court) had declared the Charter unconstitutional in 1996. The Council of State concluded that adoption of the Charter would result in the recognition of minorities as *groups* – an anathema to the Republican constitutional tradition, highlighted by Bollmann's quote above – and that it would contravene Article 2 of the Constitution that stipulates French as the 'language of the Republic'. However, as a result of a recommendation in the Poignant Report, a further legal opinion was obtained in 1998. This opinion adopted a more favorable stance, indicating that the minimum requirement necessary to sign up to the Charter – acceptance of thirty-five of its sixty-eight clauses – could be reached. The opinion also included the attendant observation that a minor change to Article 2 of the French Constitution would be all that would be required to ratify it.

The subsequent expectation at that time was that France would duly sign and ratify the Charter. This would give formal recognition for the first time not only to its historical regional languages of France but also to the languages spoken in its dependent territories, notably Creoles.[24] Even so, this recognition would be strictly limited. While bilingual provisions within education and the media would be facilitated and extended, French would remain the language of administration and the law. On this basis, France eventually signed the Charter in May 1999, the nineteenth member of the Council of Europe to do so. Nonetheless, the signing still created somewhat of a levée de bouclier (general outcry), with opponents of the Charter arguing that it undermined the '"neutralization" de l'espace public' (neutralization of public space) (Semprini, 1997: 209) central to French Republicanism, thus leading in their view to the inevitable 'balkanization' of France. Within a month of signing the Charter, the French Constitutional Court again ruled that the provisions of the Charter were contrary to the French Constitution 'en ce qu[ils confèrent] des droits spécifiques à des groupes de locuteurs de langues régionales ou minoritaires, à l'intérieur de territoires dans lesquels ces langues sont pratiquées' (in that they conferred specific rights to groups of regional or minority language speakers inside territories in which these languages are practiced) (cited in Moïse, 2007: 222). When the then Prime Minister, Lionel Jospin, moved as recommended to amend the constitution in light of this, Jacques Chirac, the then President, refused. Chirac's position played well among Republican purists who retain an almost visceral fear of minority languages. Subsequent conservative administrations in France have entrenched this position, particularly in light of increasingly incendiary debates about immigration and multiculturalism there and within Europe more broadly (Modood, 2007; Joppke, 2010). This period of retrenchment has included the publication of a report on domestic security by Alain Bénisti in 2004, which recommended that immigrant mothers be required to speak French to their children at home, rather than their first language(s). A further recommendation in light of lack of compliance reads as follows: 'si cette mère persiste à parler son patois l'institutrice devra alors passer le relais à un orthophoniste' (if the mother persists in speaking her patois, the school teacher will then have to refer the case to a speech therapist) (cited in Moïse, 2007: 232). Not surprisingly perhaps, these ongoing developments have meant that, at time of writing, France has yet to ratify the Charter. More broadly, the ongoing debates in France continue to highlight the tenuous, sublimated and still-often-reviled position of minority languages there.

Legitimating and institutionalizing minority languages

But the French example also offers us a useful means of critique. The rise of French provides us with one of the clearest examples of the centrality of power relations and associated language status in the construction of national languages. By implication, it also defuses the charge often leveled against many minority languages, and their related advocacy, concerning the arbitrary and/or artificial link between language and identity. After all, one cannot have it both ways. If there is a certain arbitrariness to the construction of national languages, one might expect a similar pattern to be evident among minority languages also. Moreover, in neither instance do questions surrounding a language's provenance necessarily diminish the affective ties associated with that language. For all their constructedness, evolution and change, both national *and* minority language varieties remain, for many of their speakers, important indicators of individual and collective identity. To accept this principle for one and not the other is clearly unjust.

Instead, we need to change the terms of the debate. If, as I have argued, the legitimation and institutionalization of a language are the key to its long-term survival in the modern world, there is a strong moral (and political) argument for providing national minority languages with these very same attributes. In so doing, national minority ethnies would be accorded the necessary cultural and linguistic capital to embark on their own process of linguistic modernization; a modernization initiated and shaped *from within* rather than from without as has largely been the case until now (cf. Kymlicka's notion of external protections, discussed in Chapter 3). Such a process does not preclude individuals from continuing to exercise their own language choices although, given the continuing balance in favor of dominant languages, and the questions this raises about so-called 'voluntary' language shift, the potential for conflict inevitably remains. Perhaps only when the new-found status of minority languages becomes firmly established might the tendency for individuals to shift to a majority language begin to change. Meanwhile, the association of modernity with one 'common' language and culture needs to be recognized as the nationalist myth-making that it is. Only if language change is separated from the current hegemonic imperatives of the nation-state can the prospect of more representational multinational and multilingual states be secured. The politics of language need not always remain subsumed by the language of politics. As Tollefson concludes:

> the struggle to adopt minority languages within dominant institutions such as education, the law, and government, as well as the struggle over language rights, constitute efforts to legitimise the minority group itself and to alter its relationship to the state. Thus while language planning reflects relationships of power, it can also be used to transform them. (1991: 202)

Changing the language preferences of the state and civil society, or at least broadening them, would better reflect the cultural and linguistic demographics of most of today's multinational (and polyethnic) states. Not only this, it could significantly improve the life chances of those national minority individuals and groups who are presently disadvantaged in their access to, and participation in public services, employment and education. As I have consistently argued, linguistic consequences cannot be separated from socioeconomic and sociopolitical consequences, and vice versa. This holds true too, of course, for other ethnic minority groups. Indeed, in concentrating once again here on national minority ethnies, I am not wishing to ignore or diminish the language rights attributable to these other groups. After all, the strong arguments in favor of the link between cultural and linguistic identities, which I have outlined in this chapter, clearly point to the right of *all* ethnic minorities to retain and maintain their traditionally associated language should they so wish (see also Chapter 5). Likewise, changing 'the rules of the game' that automatically presume an exclusive relationship between dominant languages and modernity should make the process of maintaining minority languages a little easier. However, as I have also consistently argued throughout this account, one can distinguish the rights of national minority ethnies from ethnic minority groups in relation to their *formal* inclusion in and representation within the civic culture of the nation-state. As such, the specific emphasis here on the legitimation and institutionalization of minority languages is necessarily limited to national minorities.

Even so, achieving a greater recognition and acceptance of the languages of national minority ethnies, let alone those of other ethnic minorities, remains a formidable task. As France illustrates all too starkly, the idea of national (and linguistic) congruence within the current nation-state system remains as deeply entrenched as ever. Crucially, it also continues to be rigorously defended by those who benefit most from it – majority language speakers. Indeed, in the long term, one must always concede the possibility of defeat – given the weight of the various forces that continue to arraign themselves against minority ethnies and the languages they speak. Nonetheless, I wish to argue in the next chapter that rethinking the nation-state along more plurilingual lines, and a reconceived role for education within this, also remain real – albeit, in many instances, still distant – possibilities.

5

LANGUAGE, EDUCATION AND MINORITY RIGHTS

Une langue qu'on n'enseigne pas est une langue qu'on tue.
You kill a language if you do not teach it.

(Camille Jullian)

In the preceding chapter, we encountered an apparent conundrum in relation to the role that education plays in language maintenance and shift. On the one hand, the example of Ireland demonstrates that, however much one might want it to, education is not sufficient in itself to stem societal change. Indeed, a consistent weakness of many minority language movements has been an overoptimistic view of what education can accomplish in halting, let alone reversing, language shift (see Fishman, 1991, 2001; Colin Williams, 2008). In short, the fate of a language cannot be borne on the back of education alone.

And yet to dismiss education as simply peripheral to the process of minority language maintenance, as do commentators such as John Edwards (1985, 1994), is also clearly wrong. After all, education is recognized as a key institution – perhaps *the* key institution – in the apparatus of the modern nation-state, a point that is acknowledged by a wide variety of sociological and educational commentators (see May, 1994: Ch. 2). To take just one prominent example, the nineteenth-century sociologist, Emile Durkheim, saw education as a pivotal agency in the inculcation of societal (i.e. nation-state) values, not least because of his own stated commitment to the French Republican tradition. As he argues: '[s]ociety can survive only if there exists among its members a sufficient degree of *homogeneity*; education perpetuates and reinforces this homogeneity by fixing in the child, from the beginning, *the essential similarities* that collective life demands' (1956: 70; my emphasis).

Durkheim's observation accords closely with the discussion in Chapter 2 of the key role education has played historically in establishing the homogeneous civic culture of the nation-state, a process which has led to the advent of much minority language shift in the first place. As Gellner (1983) has outlined, the nationalist principle of 'one state, one culture' saw the state, *via its education system*, increasingly identified with a specific language and culture – invariably, that of the majority ethnic group, or dominant ethnie. Indeed, a well-defined, educationally sanctioned and unified linguistic culture was seen as a prerequisite for modernity, a basis of political legitimacy and a means of shared cultural identity. The example of France, discussed in the previous chapter, clearly illustrates how education was employed to promote a state-sanctioned language, at the expense of other varieties, as a central part of a modernizing nationalist project.

If education is used so effectively to these assimilationist ends, its significance as an alternative vehicle for minority language aspirations should not therefore be underestimated. Those who dismiss the significance of education in this latter regard usually do so on the basis that education cannot be reasonably expected to cater for the language and identity needs of all pupils (see J. Edwards, 1985: 130–1). The Swann Report on multicultural education in Britain in the 1980s clearly outlines this position when it concludes: 'the role of education cannot be, and cannot be expected to be, to reinforce the values, beliefs, and cultural identity which each child brings to school' (DES, 1985: 321).

However, this begs a key question: given that education accomplishes this for majority group members – whose cultural and linguistic habitus are viewed as consonant with the school's – why can it not do so for minority group members as well? As I have argued consistently elsewhere (May, 1994, 1999a, 2001, 2009), there is a strong argument for schools extending and reconstituting what counts as 'accepted' and 'acceptable' cultural and linguistic knowledge. Moreover, the charge that such recognition would inevitably lead to a rampant cultural and linguistic relativism does not necessarily follow. As we shall see, the differing rights attributable to various minority groups, discussed in Chapters 2 and 3, can be applied directly to language and education. In short, greater ethnolinguistic *democracy* does not necessarily imply ethnolinguistic *equality* (Fishman, 1995b) – reasonable limits can still be drawn. Likewise, a recognition of minority habitus as cultural and linguistic capital in schools can coexist, albeit not always easily, with an ongoing valuing of a common or 'core' curriculum (see May, 1994, 1995).

These arguments have been most clearly articulated over recent years by a wide range of ethnic, cultural, linguistic and religious minority groups within education. The advocacy of such groups has focused on two key areas of concern. The first is that, despite their stated intentions to the contrary, previous educational policies have demonstrably failed to address and mitigate the comparative social and educational disadvantages faced by such groups (see Nieto and Bode, 2007; May, 1999b, 2009; May and Sleeter, 2010). While there are inevitably many intra- as well as intergroup differences here (Modood and May, 2001), a general pattern of differential status and achievement is clearly apparent among many minority groups. In short, minorities tend to be over-represented in unfavorable social and educational indices in comparison to majority group members. As Stacy Churchill observed of this a quarter of a century ago, an observation that still holds true today:

> Policy-making about the education of minorities must cope with an overriding fact: *almost every jurisdiction in the industrialized world is failing adequately to meet the educational needs of a significant number of members of linguistic and cultural minorities. ... Measured against the criterion of ensuring linguistic and/or cultural survival in the long term, the shortfall is much more serious* ... (1986: 8; emphasis in original[1])

Churchill's concluding comment introduces the second key area of concern – whether an education that requires minority students to dispense with their ethnic, linguistic and/or cultural identities is necessarily an educational opportunity *worth wanting* (K. Howe, 1992).[2] Thus, even if social and educational advancement were to be forthcoming – and, as the first concern suggests, it most often is not – the individual and collective costs of such cultural and linguistic evisceration are increasingly regarded by minority groups as too high a price to pay (see also Chapter 4). Secada and Lightfoot (1993) observe, for example, that the purported 'trade-off' between minority cultures and languages and access to opportunity is increasingly being seen (and rejected) as uneven by minority groups: give up your language and culture and you *might* have opportunity. When the latter is not forthcoming, communal anger has developed in response to prior generations being duped by this promise.

This increasing disenchantment among minority groups, and a related unwillingness to continue to accept the status quo, have contributed to a growing, albeit still tentative exploration of alternative educational approaches more accommodating of cultural and linguistic diversity. In what still stands as one of the most comprehensive and informed accounts of its kind, Stacy Churchill (1986) highlights these nascent developments by outlining the six principal policy responses to the educational and language needs of minority groups within the OECD. While he suggests that the differences between the various stages are not always clear-cut, he attempts the following ranking (in ascending order) by the degree to which such policies recognize and incorporate minority cultures and languages.

* *Stage 1 (Learning Deficit)*: where the educational disadvantages faced by minority groups are associated specifically and pejoratively with the use of the minority language. Accordingly, rapid transition to the majority

language is advocated, the minority language is actively discouraged and schooling occurs in and through 'submersion' in the majority language.[3]

- *Stage 2 (Socially Linked Learning Deficit)*: sometimes but not always arrived at concurrently with Stage 1, this stage associates a minority group's educational disadvantage with family status. Additional/supplementary programs are thus promoted which emphasize *adjustment* to the majority society.
- *Stage 3 (Learning Deficit from Social/Cultural Differences)*: most commonly associated with multicultural education, this stage assumes minority educational disadvantage arises from the inability of the majority society – particularly the education system – to recognize, accept and view positively the minority culture. However, a multicultural approach does not usually include a commensurate recognition of the minority language.
- *Stage 4 (Learning Deficit from Mother Tongue Deprivation)*: while still linked to the notion of deficit, the need for support of the minority language is accepted, at least as a transitional measure. Accordingly, transitional bilingual education programs, which use a minority language in the initial years of schooling to facilitate the eventual transition to a majority language, are emphasized.
- *Stage 5 (Private Use Language Maintenance)*: recognizes the right of national and ethnic minorities to maintain and develop their languages and cultures in private life to ensure these are not supplanted by the dominant culture and language. Maintenance bilingual education programs, which teach through a minority language over the course of schooling, are the most usual policy response here.
- *Stage 6 (Language Equality)*: the granting of full official status to a national minority language. This would include separate language provision in a range of public institutions, including schools, and widespread recognition and use in a range of social, institutional and language domains.

Educating for the majority

Stage 1 represents assimilation in its starkest form. For reasons already well rehearsed, it has historically been the predominant approach adopted by modern nation-states, and the mass education systems to which they gave rise. Such 'unitary language policies' (Grant, 1997) ignore or actively suppress minority languages, and view the latter as a threat both to the social mobility of the minority individual and to the majoritarian controlled institutions of the nation-state.

These policies, again for obvious reasons, had their heyday in the nineteenth century. The Irish and French state education systems are two examples already discussed in Chapter 4. Other examples abound. The Welsh language was formally proscribed from schools in Wales via the (1870) Education Act enacted by the British government in London. This legislation was in turn the culmination of a longstanding vitiation of the Welsh language within Britain, which dated back to the time of Henry VIII and the (1536) Act for the English Order, Habite and Language (see Chapter 7). In Aotearoa/New Zealand, a similar legislative pattern emerged in the nineteenth century with the (1847) Education Ordinance requiring that mission schools teach indigenous Māori children in English where previously they had taught in Māori. This was followed by the (1867) Native Schools Act, which established state educational provision for Māori and formalized an English-language-only policy (May, 1999c, 2004; Walker, 2004; see Chapter 8). Comparable educational legislation in Australia was enacted after the 1850s, leading to the 'linguistic genocide' (Skutnabb-Kangas, 2000) of most Australian aboriginal languages, the end results of which were briefly summarized in the previous chapter (see also Chapter 8).

These educational developments are not confined to the nineteenth century, however. Spain, under Franco's rule, proscribed the Catalan and Basque languages from all formal domains, including education, in favor of Castilian Spanish. These edicts, which were implemented just prior to the Second World War, were draconian to say the least and included the threat to exclude from the profession any teacher – even in private schools – who used a language other than Castilian. As stated in an order issued 18 May 1938: 'the Spain of Franco cannot tolerate aggressions against the unity of its language' (cited in de Varennes, 1996a: 22). With the death of Franco, and the return of democracy to Spain, these laws were revoked and a regional language structure implemented (see Chapter 7).

However, other comparable processes of language restriction and/or proscription remain in force to this day. One such example is Tibet where, in 1997, Chinese authorities proscribed the Tibetan language in Tibetan schools in favor of Mandarin Chinese. Ostensibly, this measure was aimed at 'improving' the educational attainment of Tibetan children. In reality, it was principally an attempt to curb Tibet's nationalist aspirations for independence from China, not least because language, along with religion, remains a central feature of a separate Tibetan identity (*Independent*, 5 June 1997). Despite regular protests over the last fifteen years, this situation remains unchanged.[4]

Another example is the longstanding repression of the Kurdish language within Turkey. Kurdish is an Indo-European language, specifically part of the northwestern Iranian language family. As such, it is linguistically far more closely related to Farsi/Persian than to Turkish, an Altaic language. It continues to be spoken predominantly in the territory of Kurdistan, an area with long historical associations for the Kurds that encompasses parts of present-day Turkey, Iran, Iraq and Syria. There are approximately 35 million Kurdish speakers in total and it is currently estimated that, of the 15 million Kurds within Turkey, 3.9 million speak Kurdish as a first language. However, the actual numbers of those who can speak Kurdish in Turkey is much greater than this, due to widespread bilingualism among Kurds and Turks. The ongoing repression of the Kurdish language – in Turkey and elsewhere – does make it difficult though to provide accurate estimates (see Baker and Prys Jones, 1998: 416–17; Skutnabb-Kangas, 2000: 61).

The active repression and proscription of Kurdish by the Turkish state form part of a wider denial/rejection of Kurdish nationalist claims to be a distinct people, with attendant rights to secession, or at least greater autonomy. This proscriptive language policy was first enshrined in Atatürk's Constitution of 1923, and reiterated in the Turkish Constitution of 1982 (see Skutnabb-Kangas and Bucak, 1995; Kirisci and Winrow, 1997). In the early 1990s there appeared to be a relaxation of these longstanding proscriptive laws but by the late 1990s they had once again been reinforced. This move was presaged in March 1997 when secret Turkish interior ministry documents were made public which stated that 'administrative and legal measures should be taken against those attempting to propagate the Kurdish language' (*Guardian*, 29 March 1997). Criminal proceedings were subsequently implemented in 1998 against the Foundation for Kurdish Culture and Research – the first non-governmental organization (NGO) in Turkey with an overtly Kurdish identity – for its promotion of Kurdish language courses. At the time, the Turkish National Security Council (NSC) summed up the key motivation behind this action. In its view, the ongoing use of the Kurdish language constituted a danger to 'the existence and independence of the state, the unity and indivisibility of the nation, and the well-being and security of the community' (Skutnabb-Kangas, personal communication).

Over the last decade, there has been some movement toward a more open approach to Kurdish in Turkey, although these developments remain both limited and uneven. In the media, Turkey allowed private television channels to air programs in the Kurdish language for the first time from March 2006. However, clear limits were also imposed: broadcasting in Kurdish could only be for a maximum of forty-five minutes a day or four hours a week and could not include any educational programs that taught the Kurdish language. These restrictions were only relaxed in 2009, with the advent of a new twenty-four-hour Kurdish television station, as part of the state-run Turkish Radio and Television Corporation (TRT).

Education for Kurds in Turkey, however, remains as circumscribed as ever. Kurdish education in private institutions is now allowed but the longstanding pejorative associations attendant upon it mean there is as yet little demand for these courses. Kurdish-medium schools remain actively proscribed by the Turkish state, and Kurdish children do not even have the right to study Kurdish as a subject in school (Skutnabb-Kangas and Fernandes, 2008). Suffice it to say, that the examples of both Tibet and Turkey serve to reinforce Eli Kedourie's well-worn observation concerning the central link between education and state nationalism: 'On nationalist theory ... the purpose of education is not to transmit knowledge, traditional wisdom, and the ways devised by a society for attending to the common concerns; its purpose rather is wholly political, to bend the will of the young to the will of the nation' (1960: 83–4). Relatedly, the quotation from the nineteenth-century French historian Camille Julian which began this chapter highlights the often-lethal consequences for a (minority) language when it is specifically excluded from schooling.

Of course, not all assimilationist policies are so overtly oppressive, and in recent years examples such as these have been limited for the most part to non-democratic, non-Western and/or newly formed states. But the same aims can be achieved as effectively, if not more so, by stealth – a process that Skutnabb-Kangas (2000) has described as 'covert linguicide'. These policies are much more apparent in contemporary Western democratic nation-states where 'submersion' or 'sink or swim' forms of language education – that is, requiring minority language speakers to be educated in the dominant language, come what may – continue to be widely promoted and practiced. Assimilation in this sense also retains considerable public support, as we shall see for example in Chapter 6 when discussing the US 'English Only' movement.

One reason for this ongoing support of assimilationist education, aside from the apparent imperative of maintaining a common language and culture, is the still-popular conception that the 'family background' of ethnic minority students may be an obstacle to their educational and wider social mobility. This approach equates with Stage 2 of Churchill's typology and need not detain us long here since it is, in effect, no more than a modified form of assimilation. Language education policies that fall within this category may best be described as *compensatory*; that is, they aim to compensate for the supposed inadequacies of the minority student's 'family background' in order to address, and mitigate, the ongoing relative 'underachievement' of many ethnic minority students within schools.

The variables regarded as most salient with respect to family background vary but may include the immediate family environment, child-rearing practices and/or the cultural and linguistic repertoires employed within the family (see Shields et al., 2005; Valencia, 1997, 2010, for useful critical reviews). Whatever variables are focused upon, however, the starting premise is invariably one of cultural and linguistic 'deficit' in relation to majority group cultural and linguistic 'norms'. It follows from this view that the principal function of educational programs is to facilitate and/or expedite the minority student's *adjustment* to 'mainstream' schooling and the cultural and linguistic mores of the dominant group, which such schooling invariably reflects. One of the most prominent examples of such programs, launched in 1965 and still in use today, is the Head Start preschool program in the USA, aimed primarily at poor, black and Latino inner-city children. The more recent Sure Start program (launched in 1998) is its British equivalent.

Stage 3 includes within it those policies and programs that come under the rubric of 'multicultural education', broadly defined. I have written at length elsewhere about multicultural education (see especially 1999b, 2001, 2009) but for the purposes of this present discussion, the following brief analysis will suffice. Multicultural education has its origins in the late 1960s/early 1970s when it arose as a specific policy response to the claims of minority groups for greater recognition within education of their ethnic, cultural, religious and linguistic diversity. It has focused predominantly – indeed, almost exclusively – on the needs of ethnic migrants rather than national minorities, the latter including indigenous peoples. The (1978) Galbally Report, which introduced multiculturalism as public policy into Australia, clearly reflects this emphasis when it states: 'We are convinced that migrants have the right to maintain their cultural and racial [sic] identity and that it is clearly in the best interests of our nation that they should be encouraged and assisted to do so if they wish' (cited in Kane, 1997: 550). As we shall see in Chapter 8, Australia's policy toward its indigenous peoples – Australian Aboriginal peoples and Torres Strait Islanders – was (and still is) far less accommodating of their cultural, ethnic and linguistic identities than this multicultural rhetoric might suggest.

The example of Australia highlights that multicultural education is most common and most prominent in those Western nation-states that have regarded themselves historically as 'immigration societies' (Moodley, 1999) or 'polyethnic societies' (Kymlicka, 1995a, 2001; cf. Chapter 3). In addition to Australia, these are most notably the USA, Canada and, to a lesser extent, Britain and Aotearoa/ New Zealand. Multicultural education continues to be widely practiced in these nation-states at local and state level, while multiculturalism has actually come to be adopted as official public policy in both Australia and Canada.[5]

Unlike the two preceding stages in Churchill's typology, multicultural education recognizes that the disadvantages faced by minorities are as much a systemic problem as they are a personal and/or familial one. In other words, we see in multicultural education the first glimmer of recognition concerning the historical role that education has played in the *institutionalized* devaluation and marginalization of minorities within the nation-state. In response, multicultural education offers the concept of 'cultural pluralism', by which the cultural values and practices of minorities come to be specifically recognized and included in the school curriculum. The central aim of this approach is to provide minority students with a positive conception of their social and cultural background in order, in turn, to foster their greater educational success. The early rhetoric surrounding multicultural education in Britain provides us with a representative example of this approach. In the early 1980s, the British Schools Council argued:

In a society which believes in cultural pluralism, the challenge for teachers is to meet the particular needs of pupils from different religions, linguistic and ethnic sub-cultures. ... All pupils need to acquire knowledge and sensitivity to other cultural groups through a curriculum which offers opportunities to study other religions, languages and cultures. ... At all stages this may enhance pupils' attitudes and performance at school through development of a sense of identity and self-esteem. (1982; cited in Crozier, 1989: 67–8)

The subsequent publication in Britain of the Swann Report (DES, 1985) was to solidify this belief in the ability of cultural pluralism to effect educational change for minority students. However, the Swann Report was also to exemplify another central claim of multicultural education, namely the suggestion that cultural pluralism could in and of itself effect a more multicultural and, by implication, less discriminatory society. In this view, multicultural education would be instrumental in achieving 'positive attitudes towards the multicultural nature of society, free from ... inaccurate myths and stereotypes about other ethnic groups' (1985: 321).

These rather grandiose claims on behalf of multicultural education have also been made widely elsewhere, most notably in the USA, Canada and Australia. For example, when Canada adopted multiculturalism as official policy in 1971, the then Prime Minister, Pierre Trudeau, asserted that 'such a policy should help break down discriminatory attitudes and cultural jealousies' (cited in Berry, 1998: 84). But with the passage of time, these claims have come to be regarded by critics as largely illusory. Without wishing to rehearse the already voluminous literature on the merits and demerits of multicultural education, it is worth pointing out briefly two key criticisms that are directly relevant to our concerns here. The first has to do with multicultural education's overemphasis on *lifestyles* at the expense of life *chances*; in other words, that multicultural education overstates the significance of cultural recognition and understates, and at times disavows, the impact of structural discrimination (be it racial, cultural, religious or linguistic) on minority students' lives. Such an approach may in fact serve simply to *reinforce* the current cultural and linguistic hegemonies that multicultural education is concerned, at least ostensibly, to redress. As Kalantzis and Cope assert:

Whilst mouthing good intentions about pluralism ... this sort of multiculturalism can end up doing nothing either to change the mainstream or to improve the access of those historically denied its power and privileges. It need not change the identity of the dominant culture [and language] in such a way that there can be genuine negotiation with 'minorities' about matters social or symbolic or economic.... It need not change education so that diversity might become a positive resource for access rather than a cultural deficit to be remedied by affirmation of difference alone. (1999: 255)

Accordingly, since the 1990s, more critical advocates of multicultural education have consciously distanced themselves from this early focus on a superficial culturalism at the expense of broader material and structural concerns.[6] In so doing, they have acknowledged that the logic of much previous multiculturalist rhetoric failed 'to see the power-grounded relationships among identity construction, cultural representations and struggles over resources'. Rather, it engaged 'in its celebration of difference when the most important issues to those who fall outside the white, male and middle class norm often involve powerlessness, violence and poverty' (Kincheloe and Steinberg, 1997: 17). In contrast, 'critical multiculturalism', as it has come to be known, 'takes as its starting point a notion of culture as a terrain of conflict and struggle over representation ... that may not cease until there is a change in the social conditions that provoke it' (Mohan, 1995: 385). As Mohan proceeds to observe:

> Rather than present culture as the site where different members ... coexist peacefully, [multiculturalism] has to develop strategies to explore and understand this conflict and to encourage creative resolutions and contingent alliances that move [away] from interpreting cultures to intervening in political processes. (Ibid.)

Unlike previous multiculturalist accounts, this more critical approach specifically highlights the ongoing effects of racism, along with its complex interconnections with other forms of discrimination and related inequalities (class gender, sexuality, etc.). In so doing, critical multiculturalism also usefully avoids the vacuous de-ethnicized, apolitical celebration of hybridity or cosmopolitanism discussed in earlier chapters. As I have argued elsewhere with respect to this: 'A critical multicultural approach can thus foreground sociological understandings of identity – the multiple, complex strands and influences that make up who we *are* – alongside a critical analysis of the structural inequalities that still impact differentially on so many minority groups – in other words, what such groups *face* or *experience*' (2009: 42; emphasis in the original).

What critical multiculturalism has not done, or at least not yet, is extend this analysis to include a critical reappraisal of the link between language, identity and education; something it has left to the advocates of bilingual education (see below). Thus, a second key criticism of multicultural education, including critical multiculturalism, is its ongoing unwillingness to engage directly with questions of *linguistic* discrimination, and the continued maintenance of particular linguistic hegemonies within both education and the wider nation-state. This is particularly evident whenever national minorities, including indigenous peoples, agitate for minority language maintenance within education. Multicultural education's tendency to level all groups to the status of 'immigrants' or 'new minorities' most often results in these claims being ruled out of court, since a polyethnic conception of groups does not entail a 'right' to institutional support of a minority language (cf. Chapter 3). Indeed, national minorities and indigenous peoples tend to reject multicultural education precisely because they view it as an educational approach that is employed by the state to dilute or contest their demands for separate educational (and language) provision.[7]

Even where language ostensibly forms a part of multicultural educational policy, as in Australia for example, minority language support does not usually extend much further in practice than the recognition of private minority language maintenance, usually outside the state education system. This assertion might seem strange to some, given that Australia is well known for its significant attempts at language status planning in favor of minority languages, most notably via the National Policy on Languages (NPL), developed by Joseph Lo Bianco in the 1980s (Lo Bianco, 1987). However, the NPL's broad concern with ethnic identity, language rights and language diversity as a social, cultural and economic resource – an admirable exception to much of what has been discussed previously – was quickly eclipsed by a more economically rationalist approach to language within Australia in the early 1990s, exemplified by the Australian Language and Literacy Policy (ALLP) (Dawkins, 1992) and the National Asian Languages Strategy (COAG, 1994).

The ALLP and National Asian Languages Strategy once again peripheralized the issue of minority languages by solely emphasizing their (limited) instrumental value as potential 'trading' languages – excluding, in the process, all minority languages (including indigenous languages) that did not meet this criterion (Ozolins, 1993; Herriman, 1996; May, 1998). The almost sole preoccupation of language education policy since 1997 on improving literacy in English has further retrenched the role and visibility of minority languages in Australia (Lo Bianco, 2004, 2008). Meanwhile, and not surprisingly perhaps, all significant activities conducted in the public domain within Australia remain resolutely monolingual, linguistic shift proceeds largely unabated, and minority language use remains limited to a few restricted (low-status) domains. Suffice it to say, this situation, as with much multiculturalist policy, does little to foster the status and use of minority languages in the longer term. In the end, the essence of the multicultural model is the recognition of the right to be different and to be respected for it, not necessarily to maintain a distinct language and culture.

In contrast, Stage 4 of Churchill's typology does recognize the importance of the link between language, identity and learning – albeit, in an almost solely instrumental way. The promotion of transitional bilingual programs is characteristic of this stage. Such programs use a minority first language in the early stages of schooling so as to facilitate the transition of the minority language speaker to the majority language. In so doing, these programs acknowledge the now-widespread linguistic research consensus that instruction in one's first language is both linguistically and educationally beneficial, and the strongest basis for subsequent second language learning (May, 2008a; García, 2009; Baker, 2011). In this sense, it is a significant advance on the preceding approaches to minority language education. But in other more fundamental respects, transitional bilingualism is little different from its predecessors. Like the latter, transitional bilingual programs continue to hold to a 'subtractive' view of individual and societal bilingualism. In assuming that the first (minority) language will eventually be replaced by a second (majority) language, bilingualism is not in itself regarded as necessarily beneficial, either to the individual or to society as a whole. This in turn suggests that the eventual atrophy of minority languages remains a central objective of transitional bilingualism. The (1968) Bilingual Education Act in the USA exemplifies the key characteristics of this broad policy approach. I will discuss the Act more fully in Chapter 6 in relation to the US 'English Only' movement.

Churchill argues that Stages 1–4 all posit that minority groups should seek the same social, cultural and linguistic outcomes as those of the majority group, or dominant ethnie. In other words, the instrumental objectives of education, as defined by the dominant ethnie, should be the same for *all* ethnic groups within the nation-state. The premise is thus the incorporation of minority groups into the hegemonic civic culture of the nation-state, with minimal accommodation to minority languages and cultures. This in turn is a result of what I described in Chapter 3 as the underlying 'philosophical matrix of the nation-state'. Churchill proceeds to argue that it is only at Stages 5 and 6 that objectives and outcomes also come to incorporate the cultural and linguistic values of minority groups and, by so doing, begin to question the value of a monocultural and monolingual society. Both these stages assume that minority groups can (and should) maintain their language and culture over time, whereas Stages 1 through 4 clearly take the opposite approach. However, significant differences still remain between these latter two policy approaches.

Educating for the minority

Stage 5 of Churchill's typology recognizes the importance of maintaining minority languages and cultures, at least in the private domain. In order for this to be achieved, however, it also recognizes that some measure of *active* protection is required for the minority language if it is not to be supplanted by the dominant (usually, national) language. A maintenance approach to bilingual education is thus the most usual policy response here. In contrast to the 'subtractive' view of bilingualism held in transitional bilingual programs, a maintenance approach regards bilingualism as an 'additive' or 'enriching' phenomenon for the individual.[8] However, as its name suggests, the wider cultural and linguistic benefits of maintaining a minority language are also regarded as central, both for minority groups themselves and for their subsequent contribution to the nation-state. Accordingly, maintenance bilingual education is characterized by 'minority language immersion' programs where school instruction is largely or solely in the minority language. This ensures that the minority language is maintained and fostered, given that the majority language is usually dominant in most other social and institutional domains anyway. Examples of successful maintenance bilingual programs are numerous. They can be found in North America (French and heritage language immersion programs in Canada, and some Spanish language education programs in the USA); in Europe (including Welsh, Basque and Catalan language programs) and among a wide variety of indigenous groups (including Sámi in Norway and Sweden, Māori in Aotearoa/ New Zealand, Inuit in Canada and Native Americans in North, Central and South America).[9]

Stage 5 recognizes that minority languages and cultures may constitute what Margalit and Raz (1995) described in Chapter 3 as an *enduring need* for minority group members; hence the promotion of ongoing language use in the private domain. However, changes to the formal linguistic uniformity of the nation-state are not usually countenanced at this level. The latter in fact is only addressed at Stage 6, the 'language equality' stage of Churchill's typology. At this stage, formal multilingual policies are adopted which require the dominant ethnie to accommodate minority groups and their language(s) in all shared domains (at least in theory), a process which has been described elsewhere as *mutual accommodation* (May, 1994; Nieto and Bode, 2007). By this, Stage 6 assumes that the retention of a minority language and culture is an enduring need *for the majority as well*. A prerequisite for this more plurilingual view of the nation-state is the formal legitimation and institutionalization of minority languages within both the state and civil society, as discussed in the preceding chapter. Examples of this approach remain relatively rare, although this should not surprise us. After all, Stage 6 challenges directly the 'philosophical matrix' of a common language and culture that underlies nation-state formation, and the longstanding 'ideology of contempt' toward minority languages attendant upon it.

The territorial language principle

Where it does occur, the granting of some form of language equality at the level of the nation-state is usually based on one of two organizing principles. The first is the 'territorial language principle', which grants language rights that are limited to a particular territory in order to ensure the maintenance of a particular language in that area (see Colin Williams, 2008, for a useful overview). The most prominent examples of this principle can be found in Quebec, which I will discuss more fully in Chapter 7, as well as in Belgium and Switzerland. In Belgium, for example, there had been linguistic conflict between its two principal language groups – the French in Wallonia to the south and the Flemish in Flanders to the north – since the inception of the Belgian state in 1830. However, much of this had to do with the de facto supremacy of French and the related marginalizing of Flemish (a dialect of Dutch) throughout its history, despite the fact that Flemish speakers (at 60 percent) were a numerical majority. This was, in turn, the result of the early industrialization of Wallonia in the nineteenth century, centered on the coal and steel industries, which meant that French speakers dominated economically and French became associated almost solely with social and economic mobility.

The ongoing conflict that these economic and linguistic disparities invoked led eventually to the adoption of linguistic legislation in 1962–3, which enshrined the territorial language principle in Belgium, thus ensuring equal linguistic status for Flemish speakers. This legislation divided the country into three administrative regions: Flanders and Wallonia, which are both subject to strict monolingualism (Dutch[10] and French respectively), and the capital, Brussels, which is officially bilingual. However, even in Brussels the French/Flemish linguistic infrastructure is quite separate, extending to the workplace as well as to the more common domains of administration and education. This means that throughout the whole country there are only monolingual educational institutions, while administration is also monolingual, even in multilingual regions. The result is that individual bi/multilingualism among Belgians, particularly French speakers, is significantly less than one might expect. In 2000, for example, only 17 percent of the population in Wallonia could also speak Dutch, while only 7 percent identified as trilingual. This was in sharp contrast to Flanders, however, where 57 percent knew both French and Dutch, while 40 percent spoke English as well (Ginsburgh and Weber, 2006).

That said, it is also clear that the territorial principle adopted in Belgium has contributed significantly to its sociopolitical and economic stability by ensuring the maintenance of group language rights (Baetens Beardsmore, 1980; Blommaert, 1996; Nelde, 1997) – that is, at least until recently. In the last five years, this longstanding stability has been progressively undermined, with growing political support for greater devolution and autonomy for Flanders. This was precipitated by a 2005 report, 'A Manifesto for an Independent Flanders within Europe', which argued for the abolition of the Belgian federal system and the independence of Flanders from Wallonia – an argument that, for the first time, gained some purchase beyond the small, far-right, Flemish nationalist party, the Vlaams Belang (Mnookin and Verbeke, 2009).[11] Subsequent federal elections in 2007 and 2010 again brought this issue to the fore – constituting a constitutional crisis of sorts. In the aftermath of both elections, the usual processes of forming a coalition government foundered because the Flemish- and French-speaking political blocs were unable to agree about further state reform. What becomes of Belgian federalism then remains an open question at this point. However, as Mnookin and Verbeke (2009) convincingly argue, a compromise that allows greater autonomy for Flanders within a still-federal Belgium is still a far more likely scenario than secession. This is also broadly in line with recent developments across the European Union for greater linguistic (and related territorial) autonomy at regional level, a trend that I will discuss more fully in Chapter 7 in relation to Wales and Catalonia.

Another much-cited example of successful bi/multilingual federalism can be found in Switzerland. The Swiss confederation is officially multilingual in German, French, Italian and Romansh and, like Belgium, this formal multilingualism is achieved via the territorial language principle – in this instance, through regional cantons. The obvious consequence of this, as in Belgium, is that many Swiss do not actually become multilingual (Watts, 1997; Grin, 1999). There are also significant infrastructural differences between the four official languages. The majority of the Swiss population speak German (63.6 percent), although there are some cantons where it does not constitute the dominant language. French is spoken by 19.2 percent of the population, Italian by 7.6 percent, with the latter being dominant in only one canton (Ticino). Three cantons are bilingual (in French and German) and one is trilingual (German, Romansh and Italian). Meanwhile, Romansh is spoken by only 0.9 percent of the population, approximately 60,000 speakers, and does not constitute a majority language in any Swiss canton, making it clearly the most vulnerable of the four official languages. The consequent difficulties of status and use for Romansh led to an overhaul of Swiss language policy in 1996 and 2000 to provide more support for that language (Grin, 1999, 2003).[12] However, these attempts to further support Romansh also have to contend with the growing presence of English as an additional language in Switzerland, and related calls, most notably by the Swiss National Science Foundation, for it to be made a fifth official language (Davidson, 2010).

The example of Belgium highlights that political federalism and the associated territorial recognition of linguistic rights are not in themselves panaceas for ongoing political stability, although they do provide the basis, at least potentially, for such stability. The example of Switzerland highlights that official language status and supporting linguistic rights at regional level may still not protect the ongoing use of a language, such as Romansh, with now relatively few speakers. Nonetheless official bi/multilingualism based on the territorial language principle clearly does address and, crucially, *redress* the subsumption of other language varieties in the civic realm or public domain. As such, it provides a clear, attested alternative to the still-dominant monolingual nation-state model.

The personality language principle

The second approach to establishing formal language equality is predicated on the 'personality language principle', which attaches language rights to individuals, irrespective of their geographical position. This provides greater flexibility than the territorial language principle in the apportionment of group-based language rights, although it also has its strictures. The most notable of these is the criterion 'where numbers warrant' – that is, language rights may be granted only when there are deemed to be a *sufficient* number of particular language speakers to warrant active language protection and the related use of such languages in the public domain. Canada adopts the personality language principle, where numbers warrant, in relation to French speakers outside of Quebec, via the (1982) Canadian Charter of Rights and Freedoms. A similar approach is adopted in Finland with respect to first language Swedish speakers living there. Swedish speakers can use their language in the public domain in those local municipalities where there are a sufficient number of Swedish speakers (currently, at least 8 percent) for these municipalities to be deemed officially bilingual.

With over 200 language varieties spoken across thirty states and five Union territories, India though provides perhaps the best example of this principle in operation. On the one hand, we have seen in India the longstanding promotion of English, and more recently Hindi, as the state's elite, pan-Indian, languages. On the other hand, there are eighteen languages recognized in India as 'principal medium languages', which, in addition to English and Hindi, include sixteen official state languages. The division of India's states along largely linguistic grounds means that local linguistic communities have control over their public schools and other educational institutions. This, in turn, ensures that the primary language of the area is used as a medium of instruction in state schools (see Pattanayak, 1990; Schiffman, 1996; Daswani, 2001). Indeed, dominant regional language schools account for 88 percent of all elementary schools in India (Khubchandani, 2008). But not only that, the Constitution of India (Article 350A) directs every state, and every local authority within that state, to provide 'adequate' educational facilities for instruction in the first language of linguistic minorities, at least at elementary school level. As a result, over eighty minority languages are employed as medium of instruction in elementary schools throughout India.

The potential to follow the Indian model in the educational provision of minority languages was also evident, at least initially, in post-apartheid South Africa. The then-new 1996 constitution established formal multilingualism, with the existing two official languages (English and Afrikaans) complemented by a further nine African languages. South African Sign Language was subsequently added as a twelfth official language. At the time, it seemed that a wide-ranging bi/multilingual educational approach would result (Heugh et al., 1995; Language Plan Task Group, 1996).

Subsequent developments, however, have proved far less promising. Curriculum revisions over the last fifteen years have focused almost exclusively on English literacy, ignoring the wider multilingual aims of South Africa's language policy (Barkhuizen and Gough, 1996; Heugh, 1997, 2000; Alexander, 2000). There has also been a related trend toward the early transition from African languages to English as medium of instruction in South African schools, delimiting the possibility of more effective maintenance bi/multilingual education options (Heugh, 2002, 2008). Thus, even in overtly multilingual environments, and within a political context at least ostensibly supportive of such multilingualism, the challenge of effectively implementing more plural language education policies still remains formidable.

Minority group responses to language education policies

If we return directly to Churchill's analysis for a moment, while also bearing in mind that any typology is likely to understate significant inter- and intragroup differences, we can also now attempt a broad parallel categorization of minority group responses to minority language education policy (see Churchill, 1986: 48–9):

- *Level 1, the recognition phase*: the minority group seeks to obtain initial recognition of its distinct educational needs and, in many cases, of its very existence as a distinct cultural and/or linguistic group within the nation-state (cf. the distinction made between ethnic categories and groups in Chapter 1).
- *Level 2, the start-up and extension phase*: having obtained some recognition from educational authorities, the minority group seeks to obtain the creation of minority language educational services or, where these already exist, their further legitimation, extension and improvement. At this stage, either transitional or maintenance bilingual education aims can be pursued. As discussed previously, transitional bilingual education aims to expedite successful transference from the minority to the majority language by employing the minority language in the early years of primary schooling. This acts as a bridge for the child to transfer their first language skills to the replacing language and, while educationally sound, remains essentially assimilative in intent. In contrast, maintenance bilingual education aims 'to the maximum extent possible [to] involve use of the minority language as a means of instruction [in order] to resist assimilation pressures outside the school environment' (Churchill, 1986: 49).
- *Level 3, the consolidation and adaptation phase*: If Level 2 is principally concerned with increasing the quantity of minority language programs, this level is

concerned with enhancing their quality. In transitional terms, the emphasis may be placed on greater, more effective social and economic integration of the minority group within the nation-state (including a greater awareness and acceptance of the minority group by the dominant ethnie). In group maintenance terms, emphasis might be placed not only on fostering the minority language as a medium of instruction but also on employing the minority culture as a specific source and context of instruction.

- *Level 4, the multilingual coexistence phase*: At this level, distinct minority educational rights are legally and practically enshrined. Different language groups are accorded formal language and education rights on the basis of the principle of *ethnolinguistic democracy* (Fishman, 1995b). As discussed earlier, this may not amount to actual ethnolinguistic equality, nor does it necessarily imply *a lack of friction* between the groups involved, as the case of Belgium demonstrates. Nonetheless, minority language rights are formally recognized and employed in state and civil society. In this regard, a considerable degree of autonomy is usually accorded to minority groups in relation to the actual control, organization and delivery of minority language education.

The consequences of Level 4 for minority groups bear further discussion here. The granting of a measure of educational control at this level clearly holds considerable symbolic purchase for the minority group concerned. However, three other benefits have also been recognized as a consequence of this process.

- While no causal link can be demonstrated, there appears to be a high correlation between greater minority participation in the governance of education and higher levels of academic success by minority students within that system. As Jim Cummins observed twenty-five years ago, 'widespread school failure does not occur in minority groups that are positively oriented towards both their own and the dominant culture, that do not perceive themselves as inferior to the dominant group, and that are not alienated from their own cultural values' (1986: 22). This conclusion still holds today as subsequent educational research consistently attests (see Cummins 2000; Corson, 2000; Nieto and Bode, 2007).
- The greater the participation in educational decision-making by minority group members, the more likely there is to be a match between minority aspirations and subsequent educational provision (see May, 1994; Corson, 2000; Hinton and Hale, 2001; Skutnabb-Kangas et al., 2009; Menken and García, 2010).
- Direct involvement in the governance of minority education strengthens community links among the members of the minority group themselves. Such involvement may also ameliorate the negative historical experiences

of education held by many within the minority community. Examples of this with respect to community-based indigenous education efforts, for example, can be found in May (1999c); McCarty and Watahomigie (1999); May and Aikman (2003); Hornberger (2011); McCarty (2011).

Bridging the gap between policy and practice

I have chosen Churchill's typology as a useful heuristic device for analyzing policy responses to minority language and education. Of course, it is not the only one of its kind. Another is Ruiz's (1984, 1990) language typology, which is well known within sociolinguistics. In this, he categorizes language policy orientations into three broad areas, each of which can be equated broadly with Churchill's approach. The first is what Ruiz terms *language-as-problem* (comparable with Churchill's Stages 1–4), where the targets of language policy are construed as a social problem to be identified, eradicated, alleviated or in some other way resolved. The second he describes as *language-as-right* (Stage 5), which confronts the assimilationist tendencies of dominant language communities with arguments about the legal, moral and natural right to local identity. The third, and most accommodative, he terms *language-as-resource* (Stage 6) where languages, and the communities which speak them, are viewed as a social resource.

Whatever language typology is employed, it is important to acknowledge their limitations. Perhaps the most important limitation here is the inevitable gap that occurs between policy and practice (see Schiffman, 1996). These discrepancies, which are conceded by Churchill in his own study, occur both among and within nation-states and among and within particular minority groups. In relation to different policy approaches, for example, only the very old bilingual or multilingual states (Belgium, Finland and Switzerland) appear to have reached Stage 6. Sweden is at Stage 5, at least in relation to its Finnish-speaking minority (Skutnabb-Kangas, 1988; Janulf, 1998). In Canada, Article 23 of the (1982) Canadian Charter of Rights and Freedoms enshrines the right of English and French speakers, who represent 90 percent of the country's population, to an education in their first language 'where numbers warrant', while the (1968) Bilingual Education Act ostensibly allows for a Stage 4 approach for Latino (and other) minorities in the USA.

But even here, all is not as it seems. We have already seen that the official multilingualism of Switzerland and Belgium does not necessarily ensure individual multilingualism. Similarly, the actual implementation of a stated language education policy within schools and school systems may be far less frequent than such policy pronouncements suggest. Thus in Canada the actual exercise of minority language rights, including the right to minority language education, varies widely from province to province, ranging from Stage 6 to

Stage 2 for Francophones outside of Quebec. This is a product, in turn, of the federal nature of the Canadian system and the considerable administrative autonomy granted to individual provinces, particularly with respect to education (Coulombe, 1999; Burnaby, 2008). An even more marked disparity between policy and practice can be seen in the USA. Here it is probably safe to say that despite the (1968) Bilingual Education Act, most Latino children continued to be educated in schools that were still at Stages 1 and 2, promoting the merits of an English language submersion approach. This tendency was further entrenched by (2001) No Child Left Behind, which replaced the Bilingual Act, and focused solely on the acquisition of English. This has also been allied/ strengthened significantly over the last 15 years with the rise of the 'English Only' movement and its trenchant opposition to, and successful dismantling of, many existing bilingual education programs (see Chapter 6). Even those that continue to promote bilingual education vary widely between a transitional and group maintenance ethos (Crawford, 2000; Thomas and Collier, 2002; Dicker, 2003). In similar vein, the Indian Constitution, as we have seen, explicitly allows for, and even actively facilitates, the promotion of minority language immersion education. However, there remain strong countervailing pressures in India to learn Hindi and, particularly, English via submersion educational approaches (see Pattanayak, 1985; Tickoo, 1993; Vaish, 2008).

The differences between the delivery of minority language education to different minority groups within the same nation-state can also be quite marked. We will see in Chapter 8 that the indigenous Māori are moving toward Stage 5 with respect to language and education policy in Aotearoa/New Zealand. However, the approach to other (ethnic) minorities in Aotearoa/New Zealand, such as Pasifika groups (those from the Pacific Islands who have since settled in New Zealand), is considerably less well advanced (Benton, 1996; Maxwell, 1998; May, 2010). A similar pattern pertains in Wales, where the Welsh-speaking national minority is now well served by Welsh language education, particularly since Welsh devolution in 1999, but where migrant ethnic groups, and the languages they speak, still are not (Scourfield and Davies, 2005; Williams and De Lima, 2006; Mann, 2007; see Chapter 7).

Canada's approach of 'multiculturalism within a bilingual framework' also illustrates well the discrepancies evident between the various types of language education available to different minority groups. Bearing in mind the caveat of provincial variation outlined earlier, Article 23 of the (1982) Canadian Charter of Rights and Freedoms nonetheless protects the rights of English and French speakers to an education in their first language 'where numbers warrant'. However, the linguistic and educational rights of Canada's indigenous peoples are far less clearly endorsed. This is demonstrated poignantly by their initial exclusion from consideration in the Royal Commission on Bilingualism and Biculturalism (1963–71). The findings of this Commission, known as the Laurendeau-Dunton Commission (see Chapter 7), led to the adoption of English and French as co-official languages in 1969, and significantly influenced the policy of 'multiculturalism within a bilingual framework' two years later (Burnaby, 2008; see also Maurais, 1996). This discrepancy is even more evident in Australia where, as suggested earlier, despite also having an official policy of multiculturalism, its ongoing educational and wider social and political treatment of Aboriginal peoples and Torres Strait Islanders leaves much to be desired (Buchan and Heath, 2006; Robbins, 2007, 2010; see Chapter 8).

Responses to minority language education approaches from within particular minority groups are also extremely varied, as one might expect. In the 1980s, Britain broadly adopted a Stage 3 multicultural approach to education, as exemplified in the Swann Report (DES, 1985), although again actual school practice at the time seldom reflected this, tending toward more assimilative models. However, the responses from within minority groups to even this limited form of multiculturalism ranged from enthusiastic endorsement (Verma, 1989) to outright rejection (Stone, 1981; Chevannes and Reeves, 1987). Key arguments centered on the degree to which multiculturalism mitigated or contributed further to the social and educational marginalization of ethnic minorities in Britain (Goulbourne, 1991a; Modood and May, 2001). Likewise, in the USA some of the most prominent critics of multicultural and bilingual education initiatives are themselves from ethnic minority groups (Rodriguez, 1983, 1993; D'Souza, 1991, 1995).

That said, the current variations in approach, and in their delivery, need not be seen as insurmountable. With regard to issues of delivery, discrepancies between policy formulations and actual practice are increasingly being addressed by the concerted political efforts of minority groups themselves. For all their current inadequacies, minority language education policies *are* being shaped by the growing cultural and linguistic aspirations of minority groups.[13] These aspirations are also, recursively, a product of the growing acceptance of minority rights in the wider social and political arena (cf. Chapter 3).

With regard to variety of educational approach, there is no necessary problem, in my view, with differing policy approaches being directed at different minority groups. Indeed, it is my general position that variations of approach should exist between, for example, national and ethnic minority groups. Thus, while the ideal might be that nation-states provide a Stage 5 (Private Use Language Maintenance) minority education policy approach for *all* minority groups, only national minorities could be reasonably expected to be entitled to a Stage 6 (Language Equality) policy approach. Likewise, all minorities might expect the right to mobilize to at least Level 3 (Consolidation and Adaptation Phase) in terms of their own language and education requirements. However, again, only national minorities could legitimately claim a right to the Level 4 (Multilingual Coexistence Phase).

Minority language and education rights in international law

The broad position that I have outlined accords with recent developments in international law with respect to minority language and education rights. Drawing on the seminal work of the sociolinguist Heinz Kloss (1971, 1977), two broad approaches can be determined here: *tolerance-oriented* rights and *promotion-oriented* rights (see also Macías, 1979).[14] Tolerance-oriented rights ensure the right to preserve one's language in the private, non-governmental sphere of national life. These rights may be narrowly or broadly defined. They include the right of individuals to use their first language at home and in public, freedom of assembly and organization, the right to establish private cultural, economic and social institutions wherein the first language may be used, and the right to foster one's first language in private schools. The key principle of such rights is that the state does 'not interfere with efforts on the parts of the minority to make use of [their language] in the private domain' (Kloss, 1977: 2).

In contrast, promotion-oriented rights regulate the extent to which minority rights are recognized within the *public* domain, or civic realm of the nation-state. As such, they involve 'public authorities [in] trying to promote a minority [language] by having it used in public institutions – legislative, administrative and educational, including the public schools' (ibid.). Again, such rights may be narrowly or widely applied. At their narrowest, promotion-oriented rights might simply involve the publishing of public documents in minority languages. At their broadest, promotion-oriented rights could involve recognition of a minority language in all formal domains within the nation-state, thus allowing the minority language group 'to care for its internal affairs through its own public organs, which amounts to the [state] allowing self government for the minority group' (1977: 24). The latter position would also necessarily require the provision of state-funded minority language education *as of right*.

Both tolerance- and, especially, promotion-oriented language rights, have faced stiff opposition over the years. There are two obvious reasons for this. First, there is the longstanding antipathy toward any notion of minority group-based rights in the post-Second World War era, as discussed in Chapter 3. Second, there remains an ongoing reluctance to include language as a basic human right. The prominent sociolinguist Joshua Fishman ably summarizes the latter position:

> Unlike 'human rights' which strike Western and Westernized intellectuals as fostering wider participation in general societal benefits and interactions, 'language rights' still are widely interpreted as 'regressive' since they would, most probably, prolong the existence of ethnolinguistic differences. The value of such differences and the right to value such differences have not

yet generally been recognised by the modern Western sense of justice ... (1991: 72)

Nonetheless, there is a nascent consensus emerging within international law on the validity of minority language and education rights. This is predicated on the basis that the protection of minority languages does fall within generalist principles of human rights (May, 2011b; cf. Kymlicka, 2001, 2007). Following from this, there is a growing acceptance of differentiated linguistic and educational provision for minority groups, along with the degree of institutional autonomy that such developments necessarily entail. Accordingly, ongoing disputes are increasingly concerned with the degree to which these activities should be state funded, not whether they should exist at all.

The current debates over minority language and education rights within international law can be traced back to approaches adopted toward minority groups in previous centuries. As discussed briefly in Chapter 3, treaties were often employed in the nineteenth century for the protection of minority groups, initially on the basis of religion and later on the grounds of nationality. These practices culminated in the endorsement by the League of Nations of the Minority Protection Scheme (MPS) – a range of bilateral treaties aimed at securing special political status for minority groups within Europe. The MPS – overseen by the League's Permanent Court of International Justice (PCIJ) – was primarily concerned with the protection of 'displaced' minorities in other nation-states, the result in turn of the reorganization of European state boundaries after the First World War. They included two principal types of measures: 1) individuals belonging to linguistic minorities, amongst others, would be placed on an equal footing with other nationals of the state; 2) the means of preserving the national characteristics of minorities, including their language(s), would be ensured.

In the most prominent legal ruling on these provisions – the (1935) Advisory Opinion on Minority Rights in Albania – the PCIJ stated that these two requirements were inseparable. It concluded that 'there would be no true equality between a majority and a minority if the latter were deprived of its own institutions and were consequently compelled to renounce that which constitutes the very essence of its being a minority' (see Thornberry, 1991a: 399–403; Oestreich, 1999: 111). On the basis of this judgment, linguistic minorities were confirmed in their right to establish private schools and institutions, a *minimum* tolerance-oriented right. However, where numbers warranted, another key principle in international law with respect to minority protection, public funding of minority language-medium schools was also advanced, a more promotion-oriented right. In respect of this, and other similar decisions, linguistic minorities were defined purely on a numerical basis – that is, as constituting less that 50 percent of the population. That said, freedom of choice as to membership in a minority also seemed to permeate the treaties, a point to which I will return.

Meanwhile, as we have seen, subsequent developments in international law were rapidly to supersede these treaties and the principles upon which they were based. Minority language and education rights were largely subsumed within the broader definition of human rights adopted by the United Nations since the Second World War. Human rights were thought, in themselves, to provide sufficient protection for minorities, as exemplified in the (1948) UN Declaration of Human Rights.[15] Accordingly, no additional rights were deemed necessary for the members of specific ethnic or national minorities. Nonetheless, even within this more generalist framework of rights, there have been echoes, albeit weak ones, of the principles of minority protection with respect to language and education. The most notable of these has perhaps been Article 27 of the (1966) International Covenant on Civil and Political Rights (ICCPR), which imposes a *negative* duty on nation-states with respect to the protection of the languages and cultures of minority groups:

> In those states in which ethnic, religious or linguistic minorities exist, persons belonging to such minorities *shall not be denied* the right, in community with the other members of their group, to enjoy their own culture, to profess and practise their own religion, or *to use their own language*. (My emphases)

Before proceeding to examine Article 27 in relation to its specific implications for language and education, I should first point out the problematic nature of the initial clause 'In those states in which ethnic, religious or linguistic minorities exist'. Like many other examples of supranational and/or international law (see below), their successful enactment depends in the end on the compliance of nation-states. But even more than this, nation-states have to agree in the first instance that the legislation is applicable to them. Thus, the initial tentative formulation in Article 27 has allowed some nation-states in the past simply to deny that any such minorities exist within their jurisdiction. As we have seen from the previous chapter, France is one such example where this has occurred, but there are many others, including Malaysia, Thailand, Japan, Burma, Bangladesh and many Latin American nation-states (see Thornberry, 1991a, b; de Varennes, 1996a, 2001). This pattern of avoidance has since been addressed by revised guidelines in the General Comment of the Covenant, adopted in April 1994, which stipulate that the state can no longer solely determine whether a minority is said to exist or not within its territory. However, the 'problem of compliance' remains an ongoing one (see below).

Be that as it may, I want to explore what the actual obligations entailed in Article 27 might involve – in particular, to what extent these reflect a tolerance-

or promotion-orientation to minority language rights. Likewise, I am interested in exploring further the degree to which these rights attach to groups and/or to individual members of these groups. Dealing with the latter first, the process of agreeing the particular form of wording in Article 27 provides us with some important clues. As Patrick Thornberry explains, from an initial proposal that 'linguistic minorities shall not be denied the right ... to use their own language', the final wording of Article 27 was arrived at as follows:

> The [UN] Sub-Commission preferred that 'persons belonging to minorities' should replace 'minorities' because minorities were not subjects of law and 'persons belonging to minorities' could easily be defined in legal terms. On the other hand, it was decided to include 'in community with other members of their group' after 'shall not be denied' in order to recognise group identity in some form. (1991a: 149)

The tension evident here between individual and group ascription is reflected in the question of who exactly can claim rights under Article 27. This question has been tackled on two fronts. First, following the precedent set by the earlier minority treaties, 'minorities' in Article 27 have come to be defined strictly in numerical terms. ICCPR defines a minority as a group who share in common a culture, a religion and/or a language and who constitute less than 50 percent of a *state's* population. Thus a minority may be numerically dominant in a particular province (as, for example, are the Québécois in Quebec and the Catalans in Catalonia) but may still be classified as a minority within the nation-state. Second, any person may claim to be a member of a linguistic minority group on the basis of self-ascription. However, to benefit from Article 27 they must also demonstrate that some *concrete* tie exists between themselves and the minority group (cf. the limits of ethnicity discussed in Chapter 1). In relation to a minority language, this would require a real and objective tie with that language. It would not be sufficient, for example, to be a member of a minority ethnic group that is known to speak a particular language if the individual does not speak that language. Nor are particular languages, and the rights associated with them, tied to specific ethnic groups since, as we saw in Chapter 1, more than one ethnic group may speak the same language. Determining that an individual belongs to a particular linguistic minority is thus not an issue of establishing some type of legal or political category, it is principally an objective determination based on some concrete link between an individual and a linguistic community (de Varennes, 1996a).

The definition of what constitutes a linguistic minority for the purposes of Article 27 is important for another reason. It determines whether the rights to minority language and education are tolerance- or promotion-oriented rights. Two opposing schools of thought are clearly evident here. Following the influential review of the scope of Article 27 by Capotorti (1979), some commentators have argued that while the words 'shall not be denied' could be read as imposing no obligation on a state to take positive action to protect those rights, an alternative and equally compelling view 'is that to recognise a right to use a minority language implies an obligation that the right be made effective' (Hastings, 1988: 19). On this basis, Article 27 can be said to encompass a promotion-orientation to language rights, with attendant state support, rather than the more limited tolerance-oriented right that a solely negative duty implies.[16]

This promotion-oriented perspective on language rights can also be linked directly to education. For example, Article 2(b) of the (1960) Convention Against Discrimination in Education specifically provides for the establishment or maintenance, for linguistic reasons, of separate schools, provided attendance is optional and the education meets national standards. Moreover, Article 5 of this Convention recognizes the *essential* right of minorities to carry on their own educational activities and, in so doing, to use *or teach in* their own language. It subsequently qualifies this right, somewhat contradictorily, by making it conditional on a state's existing educational policies, and by ensuring it does not prejudice national sovereignty and the ability of minorities to participate in national life. However, the right to minority language education can nevertheless be established (Hastings, 1988).

The question remains though – to what extent should minority language and education be funded by the state, if at all? Promotion-oriented rights suggest they should but also necessarily impose limits on who is eligible. Capotorti's (1979) review, for example, was predicated on the understanding that Article 27 applied solely to national minorities – immigrants, migrant workers, refugees and non-citizens were excluded. In contrast, tolerance-oriented rights imply no such obligation on the state. While necessarily more limited, such rights may at least have the advantage of being able to apply to a wider range of minority groups.

And this brings us to the opposing school of thought on Article 27. Fernand de Varennes (1996a) argues that Capotorti's interpretation of a more active obligation by the state on behalf of national minorities, and the subsequent commentary which has endorsed this position, does not reflect the actual intentions of Article 27. Indeed, Capotorti admitted as much at the time of his review. In effect, he set aside what the drafters originally meant because of his concern that a negative duty was not sufficient to protect minority language and education rights. In hindsight, de Varennes suggests that Capotorti's pessimism may have been misplaced. After all, the minority treaties of the early twentieth century had already established the long-standing principle of *private* language and education for minorities, without any hindrance from the state. Indeed, there was also recognition that, where sufficient numbers warranted, some form of state-funded minority education could be established. As de Varennes concludes:

> Article 27 thus appears to be part of a long-established and continuous legal continuum that the rights of linguistic minorities to use their language amongst themselves must necessarily include the right to establish, manage and operate their own educational institutions where their language is used as the medium of instruction to the extent deemed to be appropriate by the minority itself. (1996a: 158)

The debates on the merits of Article 27 as an instrument for promotion-oriented rights remain ongoing. Even so, we can at the very least conclude that Article 27 sanctions a clear baseline for tolerance-oriented language and education rights. In this respect, Article 27 allows for the *possibility* of Stage 5 minority language education policy and a Level 3 minority response, as discussed previously, for *all* minorities within the nation-state. This level of protection for minority language and education rights applies to all minority groups on the basis of the strict numerical interpretation of minorities within international law. As such, protection would be extended to include indigenous peoples and immigrant minorities, as well as established national minorities who are more usually the beneficiaries of such measures (cf. Skutnabb-Kangas and Phillipson, 1995; Skutnabb-Kangas, 2000). Indeed, where a minority has sufficient numbers, there remains some additional scope for state-funded language education, although given the emphases of Article 27 this decision remains at the discretion of the nation-states themselves.

Which brings us to the central problem of Article 27 and, indeed, most international law in this area, including more recent developments (see below). In short, much of the implementation of such measures is still dependent on what nation-states *deem appropriate*. The result is thus left to the vicissitudes of internal national politics where the provision of minority rights is viewed principally as one of political largesse rather than a fundamental question of human rights. The consequence of this in turn is, more often than not, the adoption of the bare minimum level of rights required (and sometimes not even that).

Notwithstanding this difficulty, the notion of a more promotion-oriented view of minority language and education rights does appear to be gaining some ground, at least for national minorities. In this respect, there have been a number of recent instruments in international law that, at least in theory, allow for a more promotion-oriented perspective on language and education rights. These instruments are, in turn, a product of a more accommodative approach to minorities in the post Cold War era (Preece, 1998). One of the most significant of these is the United Nations Declaration on the Rights of

Persons Belonging to National or Ethnic or Religious Minorities, adopted in December 1992. This UN Declaration recognizes that the promotion and protection of the rights of persons belonging to minorities actually contributes to the political and social stability of the states in which they live (Preamble). Consequently, the Declaration reformulates Article 27 of the ICCPR in the following way:

> Persons belonging to national or ethnic, religious and linguistic minorities … have the right to enjoy their own culture, to profess and practise their own religion, and to use their own language, in private *and in public*, freely and without interference or any form of discrimination. (Article 2.1; my emphasis)

We can thus see here that the phrase 'shall not be denied' in Article 27 has been replaced by the more active 'have the right'. In addition, and significantly, the formulation recognizes that minority languages may be spoken in the public as well as the private domain, without fear of discrimination. That said, the 1992 UN Declaration, unlike the ICCPR, remains a recommendation and not a binding covenant – in the end, it is up to nation-states to decide if they wish to comply with its precepts. In a similar vein, the actual article which deals with minority language education (Article 4.3) qualifies the more general positive intent of Article 2.1 considerably: 'States *should* take *appropriate* measures so that, *wherever possible*, persons belonging to minorities have *adequate* opportunities to learn their mother tongue *or* to have instruction in their mother tongue' (see Skutnabb-Kangas, 2000: 533–5, for an extended discussion).

Another example where exactly the same question applies can be found in the (2007) United Nations Declaration on the Rights of Indigenous Peoples (UNDRIP). The UNDRIP was formulated over a twenty-five-year period. This included the development over more than ten years of the (1993) Draft Declaration by the Working Group on Indigenous Populations (WGIP), in turn a part of the United Nation's Sub-Commission on the Prevention of Discrimination and Protection of Minorities. The merits of the Draft Declaration were subsequently debated for nearly fifteen years, with many UN member states raising substantive and repeated objections to its promotion of greater self-determination for indigenous peoples. I will have much more to say about the Declaration in Chapter 8, along with the notion of indigenous self-determination, but suffice it to say here that it amounts to a strong assertion of indigenous rights, including promotion-oriented language and education rights. Article 14.1 states, for example, that 'Indigenous peoples have the right to establish and control their educational systems and institutions providing education in their own languages, in a manner appropriate to their cultural methods of teaching and learning.' The key question remains though: given many nation-states' reservations about the document, what likelihood is there of its meaningful implementation within those states?

Other developments in pan-European law also reflect these competing tensions between, on the one hand, a greater accommodation of promotion-oriented minority language and education rights, and on the other, the ongoing reticence of nation-states to accept such a view. The (1992) European Charter for Regional or Minority Languages, which has already been discussed to some extent in relation to France in Chapter 4, is one such example. It provides a sliding scale of educational provision for national and regional minority languages (but not immigrant languages) which ranges from a minimal entitlement for smaller groups – preschool provision only, for example – through to more generous rights for larger minority groups such as elementary and secondary/high school language education. Again, however, European nation-states have discretion in what they provide, on the basis of both local considerations and the size of the group concerned. As discussed previously, these nation-states also retain considerable scope and flexibility over which articles of the Charter they actually choose to accept in the first place. In this respect, they are only required to accede to thirty-five out of sixty-eight articles, although three of the thirty-five articles must refer to education. The process here is twofold. A state must first sign the Charter, symbolically recognizing its commitment to the Charter's values and principles. Following this, states can ratify the treaty – formally recognizing, in this case, which particular regional or minority languages within the state are to be recognized under the treaty's auspices. On this basis, thirty-three European states have since signed the Charter, although only twenty-four of these have actually since ratified it (Grin, 2003; Nic Craith, 2006; Council of Europe, 2008).[17]

A similar pattern can be detected in the (1994) Framework Convention for the Protection of National Minorities, which was adopted by the Council of Europe in November 1994 and finally came into force in February 1998. The Framework Convention allows for a wide range of tolerance-based rights toward national minorities, including language and education rights. It also asserts at a more general level that contributing states should 'promote the conditions necessary for persons belonging to national minorities to maintain and develop their culture, and to preserve the essential elements of their identity, namely their religion, language, traditions and cultural heritage' (Article 2.1). That said, the specific provisions for language and education remain sufficiently qualified for most states to avoid them if they so choose (Gilbert, 1996; Thornberry, 1997; Troebst, 1998; Trenz, 2007).

Developments in international law then are at once both encouraging and disappointing. The principle of separate minority recognition in language and education is legally enshrined at least as a minimal tolerance-oriented right – that is, when restricted to the private domain. However more liberal interpretations of tolerance-oriented rights (involving some state support where numbers warrant), and certainly more promotion-oriented rights, remain largely dependent on the largesse of individual nation-states in their interpretation of international (and national) law with respect to minorities. As a result, there are as yet no watertight legal guarantees for the recognition and funding of minority language and education rights.

However, there *is* an increasing recognition within international and national law that significant minorities within the nation-state have a *reasonable* expectation to some form of state support (de Varennes, 1996a; Carens, 2000). In other words, while it would be unreasonable for nation-states to be required to fund language and education services for all minorities, it is increasingly accepted that, where a language is spoken by a significant number within the nation-state, it would also be unreasonable not to provide some level of state services and activity in that language. In addition, there are strong arguments for extending the strict numerical definition of minorities within international law, on which this notion of reasonableness is based, to include also the particular claims of *national* minorities (irrespective of number). As de Varennes observes of indigenous peoples, for example, although his argument can be extended here to all national minorities:

> Indigenous peoples, in particular, may have a strong argument that they should receive state services such as education in their primary language, beyond what a strictly 'numerical' criterion would perhaps normally warrant. In the case of indigenous peoples [and national minorities more generally], the state may have a *greater* duty to respect their wishes in view of the nature of the relationship between the two, and of the duties and obligations involved. (1996a: 97–8; my emphasis)

The claims of national minorities here are based, as we have seen in Chapters 1 and 2, on their historical rights as ethnies. They also gain credence from the wider political developments in relation to national minorities, including indigenous peoples, discussed in Chapter 3. Given this, nation-states *are* increasingly having to address such arguments in some form or another. This is both a moral and a political choice for these states, since the long-held practice of making no accommodations to minority demands is not so readily defensible in today's social and political climate. Ignoring such demands is also unlikely to quell or abate the question of minority rights, as it might once have done. Indeed, it is much more likely to escalate them, not least because minority groups are far less quiescent about the injustices attendant upon their longstanding cultural and linguistic marginalization as the price of civic inclusion in the (monolingual) nation-state. Under these circumstances, any policy favouring a single language to the exclusion of all others can be extremely risky ... because it is then a factor promoting division rather than unification. Instead of integration, an ill-advised and inappropriate state language policy may have the opposite effect and cause a levée de bouclier. (de Varennes, 1996a: 91)

Nonetheless, one should be under no illusion that establishing the validity of minority rights remains a formidable task. As I have consistently argued, the process of recognizing minority rights contests the hegemonic construction of the nation-state and, by implication, the place of the majority ethnic group, or dominant ethnie within it. By definition, this will engender opposition. Minority language education is particularly contentious in this regard because it may necessitate changes within a given nation-state to the balance of wider power relations between dominant and subordinate groups and the languages they speak. Thus, if significant progress is to be made, the common understanding of the nation-state, deriving from political nationalism, needs to be radically rethought or reimagined. A very few nation-states have already undergone this process, or are presently embarking on such a course, although not without at times considerable difficulty. The remainder though continue to be wedded to the 'philosophical matrix of the nation-state' discussed in Chapters 2 and 3.

For this to change, much still needs to be accomplished. Education *can* play a key role here in promoting more pluralistic and plurilingual aims but it needs to be stressed again that it cannot in itself achieve such change. As Stacy Churchill concludes:

In some cases, the educational response to minorities is in advance of public opinion to a certain extent, but the politicized nature of relations between ethnolinguistic groups and their surrounding societies sets strict limits on how far educational systems can go in responding to minority needs. The root issue is how far societies outside the education system are willing to modify their views of the roles of linguistic and cultural minorities within their countries. Educational systems cannot respond to minority needs unless societies are [also] prepared to respond to those needs. (1986: 163)

This caveat, and the related importance of overcoming adverse majority (and, at times, minority) opinion, are both borne out starkly in the next chapter, which explores the often highly charged debates about the links between education, social and economic mobility, and English as the current world language.

6

MONOLINGUALISM, MOBILITY AND THE PRE-EMINENCE OF ENGLISH

No one speaks English, and everything's broken ...
(Tom Waits: *Tom Traubert's Blues*)

A key reason why plurilingual education programs are still relatively rare internationally was clearly signaled in the last chapter. Given that such programs effectively endorse and promote societal bilingualism, they also necessarily contest existing language hierarchies, particularly the pre-eminence of the state-sanctioned language. It is perhaps little wonder, then, that they are often met with fierce resistance, particularly (but not exclusively) from members of the majority linguistic group. We see this most clearly, as I will outline in this chapter, in the consistently wilful misrepresentation of bilingual education programs.

But first I want to address a parallel debate that is becoming increasingly prominent in academic and popular discourse. In this debate, the nation-state and the languages spoken therein remain a key point of focus. However, the debate itself is cast in ostensibly wider terms. The issue in question is globalization, the aim is cosmopolitanism or global citizenship, and the discussion is framed in relation to how English, as the current world language or lingua mundi, is central to achieving both.

English as global lingua franca

It is indisputable (except perhaps to the French!) that English is the current world language (Crystal, 2003; Graddol, 2007; McCrum, 2011). From an estimated 4 million speakers in 1500 (Jespersen, 1968), limited almost exclusively to the British Isles, English is currently spoken by at least 1.5 billion speakers worldwide. Of these, approximately 400 million use English as a first language, 600 million use English as a second language, and a further 600 million use it fluently as a foreign language (Crystal, 2010). Bolder estimates project the number of English speakers at nearer 2 billion, since this includes those who also increasingly use English to varying degrees as a lingua franca, or language of wider communication, in complex multilingual environments (see V. Edwards, 2004; J. Jenkins, 2006, 2007; Canagarajah, 2007).[1]

While such numbers are undoubtedly significant, they are not the only, or even the principal reason for the current ascendancy of English (Mandarin Chinese still has far more first and second language speakers, for example).[2] David Crystal argues that the ascendancy of English can be demonstrated by its dominance in a wide range of key areas:

English is used as an official or semi-official language in over 60 countries, and has a prominent place in a further 20. It is either dominant or well established in all six continents. It is the main language of books, newspapers, airports and air-traffic control, international business and academic conferences, science, technology, medicine, diplomacy, sports, international competitions, pop music, and advertising. Over two-thirds of the world's scientists write in English. Three quarters of the world's mail is written in English. Of all the information in the world's electronic retrieval systems, 80% is stored in English. English is the dominant language of the Internet (though other languages are catching up...). (2010: 370)

Crystal's observations reflect a wider view of the apparently inexorable 'march to victory' of English in all key language domains. This triumphalist position is most closely associated with the work of Crystal who, via his prolific number of publications, acts as a populist academic champion of English. But even Crystal acknowledges that English has not had it entirely its own way, particularly in recent years (see also Graddol, 2007). For example, in contrast to an earlier presumption that English would completely dominate the internet (Graddol, 1997), the proliferation of new technologies has actually facilitated the growing use of languages other than English on the internet, as well as other forms of social media. Microsoft and Google are now available in multiple languages, including national minority languages such as Catalan, Basque and Welsh, and indigenous languages such as Māori.[3] Internet chat rooms also provide diasporic minority language speakers with dedicated forums for contact and discussion in their languages (Nakamura, 2002; Franklin, 2003).

Be that as it may, Crystal remains correct in highlighting how English is now unquestionably pre-eminent in the majority of *high-status* language domains.

As a consequence of this increasing global ascendancy of English, the language has come to be linked inextricably with modernity and modernization, and the associated benefits that accrue to those who speak it, particularly in developing countries. We have already seen Kay (1993) advocate this position in relation to Africa in Chapter 4, for example. This instrumentalist view of languages is also clearly outlined in recent political theory debates on cosmopolitanism.

The Italian political theorist Daniele Archibugi (2005) argues, for example, that the answer to the 'problem' of increasing linguistic diversity is not the multiculturalist recognition of language rights, as Kymlicka (2001) would have it (cf. Chapter 3), but rather a global cosmopolitanism based on a language of wider communication. This is because, for Archibugi, a democratic politics requires 'the willingness of all players to make an effort to understand each other' and thus a 'willingness to overcome the barriers of mutual understanding, including linguistic ones' (2005: 537). Following from this, he maintains that 'linguistic diversity is an *obstacle* to equality and participation' (ibid., p. 549; my emphasis). While he uses the metaphor of the artificial language, Esperanto, to illustrate his normative arguments,[4] and perhaps also to create some cover for their implications, it is nonetheless still abundantly clear that the 'common language' he has in mind here is English (Ives, 2010). We see this in the case study examples used to illustrate his position. In one – a state school in an increasingly mixed Anglo/Latino[5] neighborhood in California – Archibugi outlines a hypothetical scenario of increasing tension between the two groups with respect to the school's future direction:

> the Hispanic students do not speak English well and their parents speak it even worse. School parents–students meetings end in pandemonium, with the Anglos complaining that their children are starting to make spelling mistakes and the Hispanics protesting because their children are bullied. At the end of a stormy meeting, an Anglo father, citing Samuel Huntingdon, invites the Hispanic community to dream in English. In return, an outraged Mexican slaps him in the face. (2005: 547)

I will revisit two of the bald assumptions made here – that Latinos cannot speak English well and that all Latinos are recent Mexican immigrants – later in the chapter, when I discuss the English Only movement in the United States. Meanwhile, Archibugi also assumes in his scenario that the Anglo parents are middle-class and that most of the Latino parents are 'cleaners', but with aspirations 'to enable their children to live in conditions that will avoid perpetuating the [existing] class division based on different ethnic groups' (ibid., p. 548). In offering potential solutions going forward, he contrasts a multiculturalist response of parallel English and Spanish instruction within the school for the respective groups – bilingual education, in effect – with, in his view, a clearly preferable cosmopolitan solution of English language instruction for all. This cosmopolitan solution is predicated on the basis that 'American citizens with a good knowledge of English have (1) higher incomes; (2) less risk of being unemployed; (3), less risk of being imprisoned and (4) better hopes for a longer life' (ibid., p. 548). As a salve to the Latino population, however, the cosmopolitan proposal also includes compulsory courses in Spanish language and culture for all, while encouraging Latino parents to learn English in night school and Anglo parents 'salsa and other Latin American dances' (ibid.).

In another case study example, Archibugi discusses the European Parliament and its then recognition of twenty (now twenty-three) official languages.[6] The multiculturalist response in this scenario would be to maintain all the official languages, despite the ongoing expansion of the European Union (EU), on the basis of representation and fairness. The favored cosmopolitan response that Archibugi outlines, however, would be to delimit the number of working languages to just English and French. A key basis for the latter is the apparently spiraling costs of translation services and the need for parliamentary debate to be 'more authentic and direct' (ibid., p. 552). Given that English is increasingly predominant over French in the EU (see below), Archibugi once again implicitly endorses here the de facto ascendancy of English.

Abram de Swaan (2001) reaches much the same conclusions in his book-length analysis of the relative reach and influence of languages in the world today,[7] along with their implications for governance and communication. In his analysis of this 'constellation' of world languages, de Swaan distinguishes and ranks languages on the basis of their 'Q value': the higher the Q value, the greater their communicative reach, significance, and usefulness.[8] By this, he identifies 100 or so languages as 'central' (national languages, in effect). Twelve are identified as 'supercentral' (crossing national contexts): English, Arabic, Mandarin, Spanish, French, German, Hindi, Japanese, Malay, Portuguese, Russian, and Swahili; while only one, English, is 'hypercentral'.

Drawing again on the EU as one of his case studies, de Swaan charts the rise of English, at the expense of French and German, as the most commonly spoken lingua franca across Europe, particularly from the time the United Kingdom (UK) joined the then European Community (EC) in 1973. The influence of English increased still further with the fall of the Berlin wall in 1989 and the subsequent opening of Central and Eastern Europe to the West. While German remains a regularly spoken second language in these formerly Soviet controlled areas, English has grown exponentially as an additional language, particularly among young Eastern Europeans. By 1998, de Swaan notes that English had become the second language of choice across Europe and the de facto 'connecting language of the European Union' (2001: 161). These developments are also reflected within the EU itself, with English increasingly dominant as the principal working language of the EU and thus the de facto lingua franca of European administration as well. As with Archibugi, de Swaan notes that these developments may be in response to the burgeoning costs and complexities of translation associated with the EU's multilingual language policy, a regular criticism that has gained even further prominence over the last decade with the subsequent accession of a number of Central and Eastern European countries to the EU.[9]

Neither de Swaan or Archibugi see English as necessarily replacing these other languages – they are not advocating English monolingualism. Rather, their conclusions point to diglossia, where bi/multilingual speakers continue to use their other language(s) in local (low-status) contexts, but English for wider (high-status) purposes, including, of course, those central to the processes of globalization (see also Graddol, 2007). As de Swaan concludes:

> 'globalization' proceeds in English. The attendant emergence of diglossia between English and the domestic language precludes for the time being a stable equilibrium, a solid separation of domains between the two languages.[10] People will have to live with both English and their domestic language, and seek a feasible accommodation between the two. (2001: 186)

Both de Swaan and Archibugi acknowledge, nonetheless, that the adoption of English as global lingua franca may well impact negatively on the retention of other languages over time. They also concede that it may entrench the social and economic advantages enjoyed by existing elites – particularly, those who speak English as a first language (L1) – providing them, in Archibugi's words, with an additional 'linguistic privilege' (2005: 553; cf. Chapter 4). However, both also stress that native English speakers, particularly monolingual ones, may not *necessarily* be automatically advantaged, particularly if, in de Swaan's view, English can be de-anglicized and 'prised loose from its native speakers' (2001: 192; see also Graddol, 2007). Indeed, as first language speakers of other languages (Archibugi, Italian; de Swaan, Dutch), writing in English, their own personal histories would appear to suggest as much.

The normative power of monolingualism

If Archibugi and de Swaan at least continue to see a future for bi/multilingualism, albeit one dominated by English, many other proponents of English do not. These latter commentators likewise laud the multiple benefits of English in a globalized world. However, they add an important corollary: monolingualism in English is the norm to which all should aspire. The argument goes broadly like this:

- English is lauded for its 'instrumental' value, ranking higher than all other languages as the key to social mobility and progress.
- Learning English will thus provide individuals with greater economic and social mobility, particularly in English-dominant countries, and in a globalized world dominated by English.
- Retaining other (minority) languages might (possibly) be important for reasons of cultural continuity, but inevitably delimits individual mobility; in its strongest terms, this may result in 'ghettoization'.
- Accordingly, if minority language speakers are 'sensible' they will opt for mobility and modernity via English.
- Whatever decision is made, the choice between opting for English and/or other languages is constructed as oppositional, even mutually exclusive.

I have already discussed in Chapter 3 the arguments of Arthur Schlesinger Jr. and Brian Barry – particularly their trenchant opposition to Spanish/English bilingual education in the USA. Their position can broadly be said to adhere to the above. Two other important contributions by prominent political theorists – both in Kymlicka and Patten's (2003) collection on political theory and language rights – also explicitly endorse this stance. Thomas Pogge (2003) begins his discussion on the language rights attributable to Latinos in the United States – or, more accurately, in his view, the lack thereof – by asserting unequivocally that English is the predominant language of the US and has been so for much of its (colonial) history. He then proceeds to observe, in close accord with Archibugi's hypothetical example, that many Latinos 'do not speak English well' (2003: 105). Accordingly, in order to best serve the educational interests of Latino children, he specifically endorses an English 'immersion'[11] educational approach so as to ensure that Latino students gain the necessary fluency in English to succeed in the wider society. 'The choice of English as the universal language of instruction is justified', he argues, 'by reference to the best interests of children with other native languages, for whom speaking good English (in addition to their native language)[12] will be an enormous advantage in their future social and professional lives' (2003: 120).

But Pogge doesn't end his arguments there. He also suggests that those parents who opt instead for bilingual education may well be 'perpetuating a cultural community irrespective of whether this benefits the children concerned' (ibid., p. 116). For him, this amounts to an illiberal 'chosen inequality' for those children because it 'consigns' them to an educational approach that, in maintaining Spanish (or other languages), wilfully delimits their longer term mobility in US society. This position is made even starker by Pogge's intimation that such a choice could possibly warrant the same constraints applied to parents as other child protection laws; equating bilingual education, in effect, with child abuse.[13]

Two other political theorists, David Laitin and Rob Reich, argue much the same position in their contribution to Kymlicka and Patten's volume. They assert that 'forcing' bilingual education on children will curtail 'their opportunities to learn the language of some broader societal culture' (2003: 92). Relatedly, they fret that these 'individuals have no influence over the language of their parents, yet their parents' language if it is a minority one ... constrains social mobility'. As a result, 'those who speak a minority (or dominated) language are more likely to stand *permanently* on the lower-rungs of the socio-economic ladder' (ibid.; my emphasis). Indeed, they proceed to observe that, if minority individuals are foolish enough to perpetuate the speaking of a minority language, then they can simply be regarded as 'happy slaves', having no one else to blame but themselves for their subsequent limited social mobility.

Setting aside the patronizing and paternalistic tone of their discussions, what are we to make of these arguments? Surely, as with those who advocate the merits of English as a global language, the argument for the utilitarian ascendancy of English is unassailable? So too is the 'rational choice' (cf. Chapter 1) facing minority language speakers that this seems to entail: opt for English (or another majority language) so as to ensure one's social and economic mobility? Indeed, an increasing number of minority speakers do just that – as the exponential patterns of language shift and loss in the world today clearly demonstrate (cf. Chapter 4). The luxury of arguing for minority language retention on the basis of cultural continuity, educational merit or even the principles of social justice, thus seems wilfully misguided – not least, if minority language speakers have already voted with their feet (or voice) in order to 'get ahead'. Well, not quite. In fact, there are a number of fundamental misinterpretations, along with some wilful misrepresentations, that make these arguments extremely problematic. Let me now turn to a critical examination of these.

The problem with history

First, the argument for English as a neutral, beneficial, and freely chosen language rests specifically upon a synchronic, or ahistorical, view of it. As Pennycook (1994) argues, the view of English as freely chosen, for example, fails to address the wider economic, political and ideological forces that shape and constrain such a choice at both the individual and the collective levels. Likewise, treating English as natural and neutral rests on a structuralist and positivist view of language that (deliberately) ignores the wider historical, cultural and political forces that have led to the current dominance of English; a position we have already seen critiqued by Bourdieu in Chapter 4. And finally, the view of English as beneficial assumes, naively, that people and nation-states deal with each other on an equal footing when clearly they do not.

Consequently, those who advocate the 'benefits' of English largely fail to address the relationship between English and wider inequitable distributions and flows of wealth, resources, culture and knowledge – especially, in an increasingly globalized world. One obvious example of this can be found in the strong evidence that suggests that the adoption of English as an official language by nation-states has little influence on subsequent economic development. The poorest countries in Africa are for the most part those that have chosen English (or French) as an official language. Meanwhile, the majority of the Asian 'tiger economies' have opted instead for a local language, albeit usually in conjunction with English. In short, there is no necessary correlation between the adoption of English and greater economic wellbeing (Pennycook, 1994; Phillipson and Skutnabb-Kangas, 1994; Macedo et al., 2003). As Pennycook (1994; see also 1995, 1998b) concludes, other factors, particularly the relative powerlessness and disadvantage experienced by such states within the wider nation-state system, exert far greater long-term influence.[14]

Globalization has clearly played an important part in the rise of English as the current world language. But it is not the whole story, since the current ascendency of English also clearly has longer historical antecedents (see Graddol et al., 2006; McCrum et al., 2011). Indeed, the rise of English to be the pre-eminent international language has had much to do with the role of Great Britain as the dominant colonial power over the last three centuries. This saw English established as a key language of trade across the globe under the auspices of the expansionist British Empire (Holborow, 1999). With the inexorable decline of Britain as a world power since the mid-twentieth century, this mantle has now passed to the United States. The increasing sociopolitical and socioeconomic dominance of the USA, and its leading position in cutting edge media and telecommunications, has ensured that English remains at the forefront of the world's languages. This has been further entrenched by the collapse of the former Soviet Union, and much of communist Central and Eastern Europe along with it, resulting in the exponential growth of English in these areas over the last two decades as well.

Over the years, the British Council has played a pivotal role in the widespread promotion of English for economic and political purposes, particularly via its central role in English foreign language teaching. In any one year, up to one billion foreign students are learning English (Crystal, 2010), providing the British Council with a significant, seemingly endless, revenue stream. Indeed, the British Council's corporate plan 2008–11 anticipated 'an income of over £100 million from English teaching activities in 50 countries in [its] first year, and an equivalent amount from the administration of British exams' (Phillipson, 2010: 12). The reasons behind this are not hard to ascertain. A press release accompanying the launch of an earlier initiative, *English 2000* (British Council, 1995), states clearly that a key aim of the Council in promoting the 'role of

English as the world language into the next century' was 'to exploit the position of English to further British interests ... Speaking English makes people open to Britain's cultural achievements, social values and business aims' (cited in Phillipson, 1998: 102). Ndebele's observation, made a quarter of a century ago, still holds true it seems: 'the British Council continues to be untiring in its efforts to keep the world speaking English. In this regard, teaching English as a second or foreign language is not only good business ... it is [also] good politics' (1987: 63).

In short, the English language, and the ideology of modernization it conveys, is far from neutral. Indeed, it is simply disingenuous to present English as some kind of tabula rasa, available at no cost and for the benefit of all. Rather, as Phillipson argues, this type of reasoning should be recognized for what it is:

[a] part of the rationalisation process whereby the unequal power relations between English and other languages are explained and legitimated. It fits into the familiar ... pattern of the dominant language creating an exalted image of itself, other languages being devalued, and the relationship between the two rationalised in favour of the dominant language. (1992: 287–8)

Phillipson (1992), in his searing critique of the international English language teaching industry (see also Canagarajah, 2000; Macedo et al., 2003; Phillipson, 2010), summarizes the 'glorification' of English linguistic hegemony, and the related devaluing of other languages, as outlined in Table 6.1.

Without wishing to accept the absolute polarization between English and other languages seemingly implied by Phillipson's analysis (see Holborow, 1999;

Table 6.1 The labeling of English and other languages

Glorifying English	Devaluing other languages
World language	Localized language
International language	(Intra-)national language
Language of wider communication	Language of narrower communication
Auxiliary language	Unhelpful language
Additional language	Incomplete language
Link language	Confining language
Window on the world	Closed language
Neutral language	Biased language

Source: Phillipson, 1992: 282.

Pennycook, 2007; Blommaert, 2010, for useful critiques here), the resonances between these juxtapositions, and those commonly made between national and minority languages, are striking. In effect, the role of English as lingua franca merely extends the latter comparisons to the next level. In Alastair Pennycook's (1994) account of the cultural politics of English as an international language, further aspects of the pre-eminent position of English are highlighted which also resonate closely with our previous discussions. Employing Pennycook's still-excellent analysis as a useful point of departure, these include the following:

1   *The promotion of a continuing English language hegemony.* As we have already seen, this acts to reinforce the dominant economic and political position of nation-states such as Britain and the USA in the modern world. It is also facilitated by the central role that English has come to assume as the language of international capitalism (Holborow, 1999: Macedo et al., 2003). The combined result is the perpetuation of social, economic and political inequality between English and non-English speakers, both within and between nation-states. This process has been termed 'English linguistic imperialism' or, more broadly, 'linguicism' by Phillipson (1992, 2010). As he argues, English linguistic imperialism operates when 'the dominance of English is asserted and maintained by the establishment and continuous reconstitution of structural and cultural inequalities between English and other languages'. Linguicism (of which English linguistic imperialism forms a central part) is the process by which 'ideologies and practices ... are used to legitimate, effectuate and reproduce an unequal division of power and resources (both material and immaterial) between groups that are defined on the basis of language' (Phillipson, 1992: 47). As such, linguicism is also equated directly with other forms of inequality such as racism and ethnicism (see also Skutnabb-Kangas and Phillipson, 1995; Skutnabb-Kangas, 2000). These inequalities continue to apply, even for those who actually speak particular localized varieties of English, such as Indian English, Malay English, etc., in multilingual contexts around the world (Kachru, 2004; Blommaert, 2010). While those who learn these 'world Englishes' might invest in them great hope for enhanced purchase and mobility, they are still most often judged pejoratively in relation to prestigious English language varieties spoken by native speakers elsewhere.[15]

2   *The dominance of English in prestigious domains* – most notably, in academia, electronic information transfer and popular culture. As discussed earlier, English is increasingly the language of science and academia, displacing French and German in the process (see, for example, Ammon, 1998, 2000). And even though the internet does now provide space for other languages, English just as clearly continues to dominate (Maurais, 2003). Likewise, popular culture – in the form of popular music, film and video – is

predominantly in English. Crystal (2003) estimated that in 2002, 80 percent of all feature films were in English, while in the 1990s as much as 99 percent of popular music was written and performed predominantly or entirely in English. Again, more recently, there has been some retrenchment of English here. YouTube and other platforms now provide a space on the internet for the visible presence of films, videos and music in other languages. Meanwhile, the emergence of hip hop as a global phenomenon has also seen the development of localized, hybridized language forms associated with it, combining English with other languages (Pennycook, 2007, 2010). Nonetheless, such is the reach of English still within popular culture that, as we saw in Chapter 4, even nation-states like France are concerned by its impact on French language and culture (Flaitz, 1988; Truchot, 1990; Lamy, 1996). The result is a complex set of relationships between English and other local types of culture and knowledge, usually leading to the diminution in value of the latter. As Pennycook argues, 'access to prestigious ... forms of knowledge is often only through English, and thus, given the status of English both within and between countries, there is often a reciprocal reinforcement of the position of English and the [associated] position of imported forms of culture and knowledge' (1994: 21).

3   *The related threat that English poses to the continuing viability of other languages* – what Skutnabb-Kangas (2000) has termed the potential for 'linguistic genocide'. In this regard, the pattern of English as a 'replacing language' (Brenzinger, 1997) is increasingly evident, particularly among indigenous and other small and less powerful groups (see Chapter 8). Thus, the presumption of stable diglossia that underpins both Archibugi and de Swaan's advocacy of English as global lingua franca, where English can happily and unproblematically sit alongside other languages, simply does not hold. Stable diglossia presumes at least some degree of mutuality and reciprocity among the languages in contact, along with a certain demarcation and boundedness between the languages involved. But when English is accorded a privileged/pre-eminent position, such language contact situations are precisely *not* complementary in these respects. Rather, the normative ascendancy of English specifically *militates* against the ongoing use, and even existence, of minority languages over time. As Dua observes of the influence of English in India, for example, 'the complementarity of English with indigenous languages tends to go up in favor of English partly because it is dynamic and cumulative in nature and scope, partly because it is sustained by socio-economic and market forces and partly because the educational system reproduces and legitimizes the relations of power and knowledge implicated with English' (1994: 132). In other words, if English is consistently constructed as the language of 'wider communication', while other (minority) languages are viewed as (merely) carriers of 'tradition' or

'historical identity', as in Archibugi and de Swaan's accounts, it is not hard to see what might become of the latter. Minority languages will inevitably come to be viewed as delimited, perhaps even actively unhelpful languages – not only by others, but also often by the speakers of minority languages themselves. This helps to explain why speakers of minority languages have increasingly dispensed with their first language(s) in favor of speaking a majority language. Even when not directly threatening linguistic genocide, English may nonetheless contribute significantly to what Pennycook (1994) describes as 'linguistic curtailment'; in effect, the restricting of competing languages to particular (usually low-status) domains. This too does little for the latter's longer term viability.

4   *The extent to which English functions as a gatekeeper to positions of prestige within societies.* Due to the central role that English often assumes within many education systems, it has become one of the most powerful means of inclusion into or exclusion from further education, employment or influential social positions. This pattern is particularly evident in many postcolonial countries where small English-speaking elites have continued the same policies as their former colonizers in order to ensure that (limited) access to English language education acts as a crucial distributor of social prestige and wealth (Holborow, 1999; Heugh, 2008; Ives, 2010). Pattanayak (1969, 1985, 1986) and Dasgupta (1993) describe exactly this pattern in relation to India, where English remained the preserve of a small high caste elite until at least the 1990s.[16] This was also the case in Hong Kong up until its (re)incorporation into China in 1997 (Joseph, 1996; Pennycook, 1998b). However, even with the subsequent attempts by Chinese authorities to legitimate and institutionalize Mandarin Chinese at the expense of English, the latter remains closely aligned to a social elite involved in high-level commerce (Evans, 2000; Berry and McNeill, 2005). A similar scenario is evident in Africa where, despite English being an official or co-official language in as many as fifteen postcolonial African states, the actual percentage of English speakers in each of these states never exceeds 20 percent (Schmied, 1991; Ngũgĩ, 1993; Heugh, 2008). Indeed, Alexandre (1972) has gone as far as to suggest that in postcolonial Africa, social class can be distinguished more clearly on linguistic than economic lines. However, such patterns are by no means limited to postcolonial settings. They are also clearly evident in many so-called developed countries as well, including arguably the 'most' developed of all, the USA. After all, African Americans have been speaking English for over two hundred years and yet many still find themselves relegated to urban ghettos (Macedo, 1994). A similar disjuncture between language and social mobility is evident for Latinos. Twenty-five percent of Latinos currently live at or below the poverty line, for example, a rate that is at least twice as high as the proportion of Latinos who are not

English speaking (Fishman, 1992; Garcia, 1995; San Miguel and Valencia, 1998).

All this points to the fact that the lofty advocacy of English as the basis for a new global cosmopolitanism is significantly overstated. Much like Craig Calhoun's critique of cosmopolitanism itself, discussed in Chapter 3, it is *existing* elites who benefit most from English. For the majority of other minority language speakers, the wider structural disadvantages they consistently face, not least poverty, racism and discrimination, limit, even foreclose, any beneficial effects. Acquiring English is thus more often a palliative than a cure, masking rather than redressing deeper structural inequalities. As Peter Ives concludes:

> Learning English, or any dominant language, is not inherently detrimental in the abstract, but the context in which it occurs often means that it helps to reinforce psychological, social and cultural fragmentation. Thus a 'global language' like English can never fulfil the role cosmopolitanism sets for it, that of helping those marginalized and oppressed by 'globalisation' to be heard. (2010: 530)

The problem with instrumentalism

This conclusion leads to another: that a preoccupation solely with the instrumental benefits of English is itself inherently problematic. Viewing English in relation only to its communicative functions is a key trope of cosmopolitans such as Archibugi and de Swaan, as well as English advocates such as Pogge, and Laitin and Reich. De Schutter (2007), in her discussion of language policy and political philosophy, usefully summarizes this position in Table 6.2.

The normative goals outlined here not only implicitly reflect the ideology of the monolingual nation-state model – with linguistic homogenization the objective – they also all assume that language is largely independent of identity. Following from this, if language is viewed as merely an arbitrary communicative tool, then linguistic diversity is an impediment to easy communication. We saw this clearly in Archibugi's construction of the 'problem' of linguistic diversity, for example. We also see it in the differential functions regularly attributed to minority and majority languages. In the various accounts discussed in this chapter, minority languages are constructed as possibly having some identity but no instrumental value, while English is construed as primarily instrumental with little or no identity value.

However, this is simply wrong (and wrongheaded), since it is clear that *all* language(s) embody and accomplish both identity and instrumental functions for those who speak them (cf. Chapter 4). Where particular languages – especially majority/minority languages – differ is in the *degree* to which they can

Table 6.2   Instrumental language ideology

	Instrumental Language Ideology
Underlying view of linguistic membership (linguistic ontology)	Language as external to who I am (language is a tool or convention for the individual)
Normative conclusion (language policy)	Regulate language(s) in such a way that non-identity goals are realized: 1. communication, democratic deliberation 2. efficiency 3. equality of opportunity 4. mobility 5. social cohesion or solidarity
Outcome	Language homogenization

Source: Adapted from de Schutter (2007: 11).

accomplish each of these functions, and this in turn is dependent on the social and political (not linguistic) constraints in which they operate (Carens, 2000; May, 2003). Thus, in the case of minority languages, their instrumental value is often constrained by wider social and political processes that have resulted, as we have seen, in the privileging of other language varieties in the public realm. Meanwhile, for majority languages, the identity characteristics of the language *are* clearly important for their speakers, but often become subsumed within and normalized by the instrumental functions that these languages fulfil. This is particularly apparent with respect to monolingual speakers of English, given the current global dominance of English. After all, if English is the instrumental norm or benchmark against which all other languages are judged, it is hardly surprising that its monolingual speakers seldom, if ever, think of their language in identity terms. Much like discussions of ethnicity and whiteness (cf. Chapter 1), English simply constitutes the unmarked (linguistic) category.

On this basis, the limited instrumentality of particular minority languages at any given time *need not always remain so*. Indeed, if the minority position of a language is the specific product of wider historical and contemporary social and political relationships, as I have consistently argued, changing these wider relationships positively with respect to a minority language should bring about both enhanced instrumentality for the language in question, and increased mobility for its speakers. This is precisely what is happening in regions such as Quebec, Catalonia and Wales, as we will see in the next chapter. But, contra the likes of Pogge, and Laitin and Reich, this can also apply to Spanish in the USA. With the continuing rise of Spanish speakers in the USA, the result in turn of ongoing immigration patterns (see below), it is clear that a knowledge of Spanish in the US context, alongside English, *is* of increasing importance. Indeed, as we shall shortly see in the discussion of the English Only movement, a key catalyst for this movement is precisely a visceral fear of the increasing growth and influence of Spanish. And what of the fact that Spanish, of course, is also a world language, and a majority language in Spain and many Latin American states (Mar-Molinero, 2000)? Certainly, in those contexts, it is seen as highly useful instrumentally – again, why not then in the US?

This highlights another key problem with the regular unfavorable juxtaposition of minority languages vis-à-vis English and other dominant languages – the problem of consistency. On the one hand, we have the construction of minority languages in these accounts as essentially anti-instrumental, as merely 'carriers' of 'identity', and yet on the other, when such languages do become useful instrumentally in the public realm, this is held against them as well! Let me return to the arguments of Brian Barry, first encountered in Chapter 3, to illustrate this point.

When Barry discusses language, he focuses predominantly on bilingual education in the US. However, he does turn his attention at various points to Wales, and the revival of Welsh, to illustrate his opposition to language rights more generally. Specifically, he uses Wales as an example of a context where 'representatives of a group defined by a certain minority language ... may [as in Wales] press for that language to be taught in schools as a major compulsory subject', even though this is in his view at the inevitable expense of 'other subjects (including other languages) that *would better equip* [students] for the job market' (2001: 215; my emphasis). And yet, at the same time, Barry also specifically bemoans the labor market advantages that a knowledge of Welsh provides because local authorities in Wales increasingly require this as a condition of employment. For him, bilingual Welsh/English speakers are unfairly advantaged over monolingual English speakers by this entirely 'artificial creation' (ibid.). As he concludes, 'unless knowledge of Welsh can be shown to be related to the effective discharge of duties of the job ... it is clearly unfair discrimination' (ibid., pp. 106–7).

This is a clear double standard. After all, Barry accepts unequivocally the need for English as a key criterion of employment in English-dominant contexts (and never applies the critique of artificiality to dominant national languages, or to English as a global language). Why then not Welsh in a context where Welsh is a key language of public administration? Proponents of English simply can't have it both ways – deriding minority languages for their lack of utility, and then opposing their utility when it proves to be politically inconvenient. Although, of course, it doesn't stop them trying. Barry also complains, for example, that Welsh language requirements in education may amount to 'discrimination' against (monolingual) English speakers, delimiting their individual language rights. As he laments:

> it has to be recognized that the great majority of the people of Wales do not speak Welsh at home, and for them learning Welsh in school from scratch is in direct competition for time with learning *a major foreign language*. It is therefore scarcely surprising that compulsory instruction in Welsh schools has aroused opposition from English-speaking parents … (2001: 105; my emphasis)

However, cries of discrimination on this basis are similarly spurious, since the assertion is not based on any perceived threat to English, but rather upon the implicit, sometimes explicit, wish of English language speakers to remain monolingual (May, 2000). Certainly, the requirement to be bilingual in English and Welsh does not at any point threaten the individual's ability and scope to use English within Wales; quite the reverse, in fact, since English remains dominant in all language domains (cf. Chapter 7). Indeed, this is true in almost all cases where a minority language is formalized in the public realm since what is being promoted is not a new monolingualism in the minority language – indeed, this is usually neither politically nor practically sustainable – but merely the *possibility* of public bilingualism or multilingualism. In other words, the majority language (English, in this instance) is not being precluded from the public realm, nor proscribed at the individual level, nor are majority language speakers actually penalized for speaking their language.[17] Rather, monolingual majority language speakers are being asked to *accommodate* the ongoing presence of a minority language and to recognize its status as an additional language of the state (cf. my discussion in Chapter 5 of 'mutual accommodation').

Dismantling the identity-instrumental opposition between minority and majority languages also immediately brings into question the idea of incommensurate linguistic identities on which it is based. In other words, the distinctions often made with respect to majority languages such as English, and minority languages, are themselves predicated on a singular, exclusive and oppositional notion of linguistic identity. We must have one linguistic identity *or* the other, we cannot have both. In contrast, a more nuanced sociological understanding of the complex links between language and identity can instead allow for the possibility of, or potential for holding multiple, complementary cultural and linguistic identities at both individual and collective levels. On this view, maintaining a minority language – or a dominant language, for that matter – avoids 'freezing' the development of particular languages in the roles they have historically, or perhaps still currently, occupy. Equally importantly, it questions and discards the zero-sum language replacement approach that commentators like Pogge and Laitin and Reich espouse. Linguistic identities – and social and cultural identities more broadly – need not be constructed as irredeemably oppositional. Narrower identities do not necessarily need to be traded in for broader ones. One can clearly remain, for example, both Spanish-speaking and American, Catalan-speaking and Spanish, or Welsh-speaking and British. The same process applies to national and international language identities, where these differ. To insist otherwise reveals both a reductionist and an essentialist approach to language and identity (cf. Chapter 4).

Adopting this more complementary approach to languages also allows for another possibility. If majority language speakers realize that their own languages fulfil important identity functions for them, they may be slightly more reluctant to require minority language speakers to dispense with theirs. Or to put it another way, if majority languages do provide their speakers with particular and often significant individual and collective forms of linguistic identity, as they clearly do, it seems unjust to deny these same benefits, out of court, to minority language speakers. This does not preclude cultural and linguistic change and adaptation – all languages and cultures are subject to such processes. But what it does immediately bring into question is the necessity/validity of the unidirectional movement of cultural and linguistic adaptation and change *from* a minority language/culture *to* a majority one.

The problem with bilingual education

A third key problem with the advocacy of English at the specific expense of other languages is that it is inconveniently contradicted by incontrovertible research evidence in support of bilingual education. This research clearly demonstrates that long-term or 'late-exit' bilingual programs are the most effective educationally for bilingual students, followed by short term or 'early-exit' bilingual education programs.[18] Monolingual or English-only programs for bilingual students are consistently the *least* effective programs on *all* educational measures – including, crucially, the long-term educational success of bilingual students in these programs. The academic literature supporting these conclusions is voluminous and I am not able to explore it in detail here (see May, 2008a; García, 2009; Baker 2011, for useful recent overviews). But I will discuss briefly, by way of example, two major studies, both conducted in the United States, which clearly support these general conclusions.

Ramírez et al. (1991) compared English-only programs with early-exit and late-exit bilingual programs, following 2,352 Spanish-speaking students over four years. Their findings clearly demonstrated that the greatest growth in mathematics, English language skills and English reading was among students in late-exit bilingual programs where students had been taught predominantly in Spanish (the students' L1). For example, students in two late-exit sites that continued L1 instruction through to grade 6 made significantly better academic progress than those who were transferred early into all-English instruction. Ramírez et al. conclude that:

> Students who were provided with a substantial and consistent primary language development program learned mathematics, English language, and English reading skills as fast or faster than the norming population in this study. As their growth in these academic skills is atypical of disadvantaged youth, it provides support for the efficacy of primary language development facilitating the acquisition on English language skills. (1992: 38–9)

The Ramírez study also confirmed that minority language students who receive most of their education in English rather than their first language are *more* likely to fall behind and drop out of school. In fact, it is important to note here that the English-only programs used for comparison in the Ramírez study were not typical to the extent that, while the teachers taught in English, they nonetheless understood Spanish. This suggests that in the far more common situation where the teacher does not understand the students' L1, the trends described here are likely to be further accentuated.

In the largest study conducted to date, Thomas and Collier (2002) came to broadly the same conclusions. Between 1996 and 2001, Thomas and Collier analyzed the education services provided for over 210,000 language minority students in US public schools and the resulting long-term academic achievement of these students. As with the Ramírez et al. study, one of Thomas and Collier's principal research findings was that the most effective programs – 'feature rich' programs as they called them – resulted in achievement gains for bilingual students that were above the level of their monolingual peers in English-only classes. Another key conclusion was that these gains, in both first language (L1) *and* second language (L2), were most evident in those programs where the students' L1 was a language of instruction for an extended period of time. In other words, Thomas and Collier found that *the strongest predictor of student achievement in L2 was the amount of formal L1 schooling they experienced*: 'The more L1 grade-level schooling, the higher L2 achievement' (2002: 7). Thomas and Collier also found that students in English-only 'submersion' classes performed far less well than their peers in late-exit bilingual programs, as well as dropping out of school in greater numbers. Students in early-exit, transitional, bilingual programs demonstrated better academic performance over time, but not to the extent of late-exit bilingual programs. In both these major longitudinal studies, then, length of L1 education turned out to be more influential than *any* other factor in predicting the educational success of bilingual students, *including* socioeconomic status.

Suffice it to say, these findings stand in direct contradiction to Barry, Pogge, and Laitin and Reich's conclusions about bilingual education for Latino students, discussed earlier. English-only instruction neither ensures 'fluency in English' (Pogge) nor participation in 'broader societal culture' (Barry; Laitin and Reich). Indeed, it is most often the *cause* of, rather than the solution to, the educational failure of bilingual students. Two conclusions can be drawn from this: one is about due diligence, the other about consistency. First, while political theorists may feel that they can comment with impunity on other areas of academic research (and they regularly do), they should at least take the time to read the relevant literature first. Second, these political theorists need to apply one of their own key normative principles – that of generalizability – to their arguments against bilingual education. After all, we do not see them argue that 'elite' bilingualism – say, learning English and French – is injurious to one's involvement in and grasp of 'broader societal culture'. Quite the reverse in fact – Barry specifically argues against Welsh on the basis that a language such as French would be more useful. So, why should it be different for any other language? As Jim Cummins (2000) has pointedly asked, why should bilingualism be good for the rich but not for the poor?

What we need to separate out here then are the educational and linguistic factors in learning other languages (including learning *in* other languages), and the broader social and political issues concerning the perceived status of the particular languages involved. In so doing, we can begin to deconstruct and critique the rhetorical move employed in these accounts – that is, to attempt to discredit the educational and linguistic merits of bilingual education on the basis of the *political* challenge it presents for a monolingual conception of the nation-state.

This perhaps also helps to explain why the copious educational research highlighting the efficacy of bilingual education surfaces so seldom in wider academic, policy and public debates. Research evidence that appears to contradict the dominance of English and/or the related ideology of public monolingualism is not a welcome feature for those wishing to buttress or ensure them. As Thomas Ricento observes of the US context, for example, in spite of an impressive amount of both qualitative and quantitative research now available on the merits of bilingual education, 'the public debate (to the extent that there is one) [still] tends to focus on perceptions and not on facts' (1996: 142). Or as Joshua Fishman despairingly asks of the same context, 'why are facts so useless in this discussion?' (1992: 167). This laissez-faire approach to the facts is no more starkly demonstrated than in the ideology and political advocacy of the so-called 'Official English' movement in the United States – or, as I prefer to term it, the 'English Only' movement.[19]

'Doesn't anyone speak English around here?' The US 'English Only' movement

I want to begin, by way of background, with three revealing vignettes. The first concerns the New York State constitutional convention in 1916 where, during a debate on an English literacy requirement for voting, a proponent of the measure traced the connection between the English language and democratic values *directly* back to the Magna Carta: 'You have got to learn our language [English] because that is the vehicle of the thought that has been handed down from the men in whose breasts first burned the fire of freedom' (cited in Baron, 1990: 59). Irrespective of the merits of these sentiments (and there are not many), the obvious point to be made here is that the Magna Carta was actually written in Latin! As I discussed in Chapter 4, English did not assume any formal prominence in Britain until the fifteenth century.

The second occurred in the mid-1920s. In opposing the teaching of Spanish as a foreign language in Texas schools at that time, the first female governor of Texas, Miriam (Ma) Ferguson was reputed as saying 'If the King's English was good enough for Jesus, it's good enough for the children of Texas!' One might possibly forgive these idiocies on the basis that both were mooted nearly a century ago. However, a variation of Ma Ferguson's statement, perhaps apocryphal, is regularly attributed to an unnamed US congressman outlining on talkback radio in 1997 why he supported English Only legislation in the USA.

Another recent example, which *is* documented, concerns a 1995 court case in Amarillo Texas, between a monolingual English father and a bilingual Spanish/ English mother over custody of their daughter. In this case, the judge ordered that a key condition of awarding custody to the mother was that she was not to speak Spanish to her child at home on the grounds that this was equivalent to a form of 'child abuse':

> If she starts [school] with the other children and cannot even speak the language that the teachers and others speak, and she's a full-blooded American citizen, you're abusing that child ... Now get this straight: you start speaking English to that child, because if she doesn't do good in school, then I can remove her because it's not in her best interests to be ignorant. (Cited in de Varennes, 1996a: 165–6)

The only ignorance demonstrated here appears to be the judge's. As de Varennes observes, the reasoning behind the judgment is bizarre, to say the least. However, what is most concerning is that it obviously never occurred to the judge that it may have been the state's school system which was 'abusive' for not meeting adequately the linguistic and educational needs of its large Spanish-speaking population. Instead, he simply places the blame on the parent – and, by extension, the child – for their 'wilful' failure to assimilate.

These examples illustrate clearly the three broad areas that I have already discussed in this chapter. The first is the historical inaccuracy, even amnesia, that characterizes many of the arguments in support of English. The second is the explicit link that is made between a lack of English language facility and subsequent educational failure. The third is the related misrepresentation of bilingual education. But, if this were not enough, two further disturbing features are evident in the English Only movement. One is the inherent nativism of much English Only rhetoric; language is used, in effect, as a convenient proxy for maintaining racialized distinctions in the USA. The final feature is the assumption that speaking English is a unifying force, while multilingualism is by definition destructive of national unity. Before examining each of these dimensions in turn, let me briefly sketch the origins of the English Only movement in its current form.

The genesis of a movement

In April 1981, Senator Samuel Hayakawa of California proposed an English Language Amendment (ELA) to the Constitution of the United States that would make English, for the first time, an official rather than a de facto national language. In his initiating speech, the senator gave the following reasons for his ELA (see Marshall, 1986: 23):

- 'a common language can unify; separate languages can fracture and fragment a society';
- learning English is the major task of each immigrant;
- only by learning English can an immigrant fully 'participate in our democracy'.

Hayakawa's proposal was to set the tone and the broad parameters of much of the subsequent English Only debates in the USA in its assertion of the unifying power of a common language, its (convenient) elision of ethnic and national minorities – treating all such groups as if they were immigrants or new minorities (see Chapter 2) – and its faith in the role of English as the principal agent of social mobility. On this basis, Hayakawa proceeded to argue that his principal concern in making English the official language of the USA was to help clarify the 'confusing signals' being sent to 'immigrant' groups over the preceding decade. Such signals included the provision of bilingual (voting) ballots which he considered 'contradictory' and 'logically conflicting' with the requirements of naturalized citizens to 'read, write and speak' English. Late-exit maintenance bilingual education programs were also regarded as 'being dishonest with linguistic minority groups'. Accordingly, he was determined that only early-exit transitional forms of bilingual education should be allowed, if that, in order to 'end the false promise being made to new immigrants that English is unnecessary to them'.

The themes expressed by Hayakawa at the beginning of the 1980s were to spawn a movement. While his ELA failed, the publicity that it garnered led Hayakawa to join forces with Dr John Tanton to establish the organization 'US English' in 1983. US English is not the only organization of its type ('English First' is another[20]) but it is certainly the most prominent, having grown rapidly in both number and profile from the time of its inception.[21] During the 1980s, a further five ELAs were tabled under the auspices of the English Only movement, a pattern that has continued to the present. In 1996, the House of Congress accepted an ELA, but the Senate declined to enact it. In 2006 and 2007, proposals to make English the national language were incorporated in amendments to immigration reform bills in the Senate, although these were also not subsequently enacted.

A key reason why none of these proposals has been successful thus far is largely due to the care and caution with which constitutional amendments are treated (see Marshall, 1986). However, the English Only movement has continued to lobby vigorously for restrictionist language policies at the federal level, while also increasingly focusing on changing state-level language policies (Nunberg, 1989; Ruiz, 1990). As Daniels observes of the latter, 'the overall strategy [here] seems to be to get some official-English law on the books of a majority of states and to continually fan public resentment over schooling policies that "degrade English" and "cater" to immigrants' (1990: 8). In this regard, they have been far more successful. Using their considerable organizational, lobbying and media skills, the English Only movement has effectively used the vehicle of popular state referenda (originally, implemented as a progressive measure to avoid the special interest lobbying endemic to US politics) to endorse and implement restrictionist language policies. The first of these, California's Proposition 63, was passed in 1986 by a majority of 73 percent to 27 percent – albeit on a very low voter turnout – and included a significant degree of Latino voter support (MacKaye, 1990). Since then, over thirty states have adopted English as their official language; the latest (in 2010) being Oklahoma and Utah.[22]

Many of these statutes and amendments are largely symbolic, although some states have implemented specific punitive measures against bilingual education, as we shall see shortly. Nonetheless, all are concerned to declare English as the official language of the state and most are aimed at ensuring that English is the only language of government activity (see Adams and Brink, 1990; Crawford, 2000, 2008). In summary, the key objectives of the English Only movement, which have remained constant since its inception, are to:

1   Adopt a constitutional law establishing English as the official language of the United States
2   Repeal laws mandating multilingual ballots and voting materials
3   Restrict federal funding of bilingual education and, if possible, eliminate all forms of bilingual education
4   Strengthen the enforcement of English language civic and immigration requirements for naturalization.

It should be stressed that these concerns are not particularly new in themselves. The primacy of English and the links with nativist concerns about immigration were also clearly evident in the 'Americanization Movement', which arose in the late nineteenth century and culminated with the First World War (Higham, 1963).[23] However, what is distinct about the present English Only movement is its national profile and organization (previous debates about language were usually confined to local or state arenas) and, relatedly, the increasingly wide support that it seems to have garnered among the American public (A. Padilla, 1991; Donahue, 1995). Much of the success of the English Only movement here has been in its ability to articulate forcefully a particular view of the USA as a resolutely monolingual, English-speaking country, currently threatened by the (recent) rise of multilingualism. This multilingualism is also linked implicitly, and sometimes explicitly, with the growing number of Spanish-speaking Latino communities within the US who, despite comprising a wide range of disparate groups, including national minorities (e.g. Puerto Ricans), are conveniently viewed as a homogeneous mass of (often illegal) recent 'immigrants'. The often alarmist rhetoric promulgated by the movement is thus endemically racist, as I will also proceed to argue in due course. Here I want to explore further the historical amnesia that attends so much of this rhetoric. As we saw Ernest Renan observe in Chapter 2, 'forgetting, I would even go so far as to say historical error, is a crucial factor in the creation of a nation' (1990: 11). The nationalist myth-making of the English Only movement certainly bears this out.

Historical amnesia: the 'forgotten' languages of the USA

The English Only movement makes three principal claims in relation to the language history of the United States. The first is that the USA is a monolingual, English-speaking country *and always has been*. The second is that the English language is a central and indispensable symbol of American national identity; a view, moreover, that has been consistently supported by historical language policy and practice. The third is that English is under serious threat for the first time as a result of the recent rise of bilingual voting and bilingual educational developments. Each of these propositions is demonstrably wrong.

First, it is clear that English is, and has been historically the dominant language in the USA. This point is not in doubt. However, to extrapolate from this the myth of English *monolingualism* is another story entirely (cf. Silverstein, 1996). And story it is, for the USA is not and never has been a monolingual country. Indeed, multilingualism has been a feature of US society since the colonial times of the eighteenth century (Kloss, 1977), a feature which should not surprise us given the USA's much vaunted status as the largest immigrant country of them all. In American colonies between 1750 and 1850, non-English-speaking European settlers made up one quarter of the white population and Dutch (New York), Swedish (Delaware) and German (Pennsylvania) were widely spoken. Indeed, in 1790 German speakers comprised 8.7 percent of the total US population (Zentella, 1997). Native Americans, and their languages, were also still numerous and widespread at this time (see below). And Black Americans – mostly slaves, and with their many African languages – numbered more than one-fifth of the total population (Shell, 1993). Moreover, outside of the early colonies, Spanish and French language speakers predominated. Many of these language speakers were eventually incorporated into the United States as it expanded. For example, the (1803) Louisiana Purchase saw this territory, which included a majority of French speakers, acquired from France. Likewise, the (1848) Treaty of Guadalupe Hidalgo saw Mexico cede nearly half of its predominantly Spanish-speaking territory to the US, including areas of present-day New Mexico, Texas, Arizona, Colorado and California.

To take just one example of the historical language diversity apparent in the United States, the case of Native American languages bears closer examination. When the Spanish first arrived on the North American continent in the early sixteenth century (See Conklin and Lourie, 1983), it is estimated that at least 500 Native American languages were spoken (Leap, 1981). The subsequent impact of European colonization on Native Americans – along with its usual corollaries of introduced diseases, land dispossession and genocide – were to change all that. By 1920, the Native American population reached a nadir of 400,000, having fallen from an estimated 30–40 million at time of contact (see McKay and Wong, 1988). An educational policy over this period of actively repressing Native American languages, and replacing them with English, also contributed significantly to the related decline and extinction of many Native American languages.

One notable example of this assimilationist and also clearly racialized approach can be seen in the US Congress's passing in 1887 of the General Allotment and Compulsory Education Acts. This amounted to a policy of forced assimilation, aimed at transforming Native Americans into yeoman farmers by dividing their lands, while schooling their children in English *specifically* for the trades and domestic service (McCarty, 2002; for comparable examples elsewhere, see Chapter 8). As a federal commissioner of Indian Affairs,

J. D. C. Atkins observed in his annual report at the time: 'schools should be established, which [Native American] children should be required to attend, [and where] their barbarous *dialects* should be blotted out and the English *language* substituted' (1887; reprinted in Crawford, 1992b: 48; my emphases). Note here, the deliberate relegation of Native American language varieties to mere 'dialects' in contradistinction to the English 'language', along with all this implies about language hierarchy (see the discussion on language and dialects in Chapter 4). Although the Bureau of Indian Affairs formally rescinded this assimilationist education policy in 1934, punishment for native language use in schools continued through to the 1950s (Crawford, 1989).[24] Notwithstanding this sorry history, Native American languages are still spoken today in the USA, although they are seldom commented upon. In the 1990 census, 1,878,275 people identified as Native Americans, of whom 331,600 over the age of five years reported speaking a Native American language (Ricento, 1996). In the 2000 census, however, the number who identified as still speaking a Native American language had fallen below 300,000 in total, with 71.8 percent of all Native Americans speaking only English at home (Ogunwole, 2006).

'We have room for but one language here': English and other languages in the USA

So much for the myth of a monolingual USA. But what of the pivotal role of English in US society, and the language policies and practices that have supposedly *consistently* supported this? Again, all is not as it seems. There are actually two clear countervailing tensions apparent historically in the USA's approach to status language policy and planning. On the one hand, there has certainly been a clear drive toward English linguistic uniformity at various times in US history. This drive has been characterized most often by a prominent advocacy of the role of English as a central organizing symbol of American identity. In this context, much has been made of John Jay's assertion at the time of America's independence 'that Providence has been pleased to give this one connected country, to one united people; a people descended from the same ancestors, *speaking the same language*, professing the same religion' (cited in Shell, 1993: 103; my emphasis). Likewise, Theodore Roosevelt's famous appeal 'The Children of the Crucible' in 1917 is often invoked: 'we have room for but one language here, and this is the English language, for we intend to see that the crucible turns our people out as Americans, of American nationality, and not as dwellers in a polyglot boarding house' (cited in J. Edwards, 1994: 166).

Like Hayakawa's more recent English Only arguments, Roosevelt's notion of the American crucible assumes that *all* Americans are *willing* immigrants. At the risk of repetition, this completely ignores the subjugated status of African Americans, and the various national minorities – including Native Americans and

Puerto Ricans – who have been incorporated by conquest into the United States. Be that as it may, such sentiments accord with a strong emphasis historically in American federal policy on fostering English as the language of administration, education and the legislature, a feature the English Only movement is only too willing to point out. In effect, from the time of the Louisiana Purchase, English has been promoted as the language of government, voting and the courts, often in the face of strong local opposition. English has also been the recognized language of instruction in schools since the Constitution of 1868 (Hernández-Chávez, 1995). The example of the trenchant assimilationist language and education policies directed toward Native Americans, described earlier, would also seem to bear out the general significance attributed to English in the educational domain.

On the other hand, there have also been significant examples where minority language rights – albeit limited ones – have been specifically accommodated. These examples are simply ignored by the English Only movement (as they were by Roosevelt before them) but they cannot just be wished away, much as some might want them to be. The historical language context of the USA is thus far more complex than English Only advocates would care to admit. For a start, one of the principal reasons that the English Only movement places such store in a constitutional amendment is because of the *deliberate* ambiguity of the Declaration of Independence and the Constitution in relation to the role of English in US society. Although the documents were written in English, neither the Declaration of Independence nor the Constitution specified an official language for the United States. This was not an oversight, as the English Only movement argues, but a planned political strategy (Heath, 1977, 1981; Pavlenko, 2002). Underpinning this decision of the 'Founding Fathers' was the centrality of the principle of individual choice. This was exemplified in the notion of free speech, and the related adoption of a laissez-faire language policy, deriving from the British model, which specifically eschewed the legislative formality of granting 'official status' to English (see Marshall, 1986; Nunberg, 1992). Coupled with the widespread multilingualism described earlier, 'the intellectual climate of the times, which depended upon communication across language groups ... supported maximum flexibility in language use' (Heath, 1977: 270).

This 'flexibility of language use' was also reflected in the well-established practice of granting limited minority language rights to (some) minority language speakers in the USA. The territory of Louisiana is a case in point. When Louisiana was annexed from France to the US in 1803, the then President, Thomas Jefferson, initially made few accommodations to the territory's Francophone majority. His first act, in fact, was to appoint a territorial governor who spoke no French and who proposed that English be the official language of the local government (Leibowitz, 1969). In the face of strong opposition, this policy was subsequently modified. After Louisiana joined the Union in 1812,

Louisiana's laws and other public documents were printed in French, and the courts and legislature operated bilingually. These concessions, along with the right to bilingual schooling, survived in Louisiana law until 1921 (Crawford, 1992a). However, despite the relatively liberal language policy adopted over this time, the eventual demise of French as a public language was seldom in any doubt (Ricento, 1996).

The German-speaking minority in the USA was also accorded a measure of minority language protection, both prior and subsequent to the country's declared independence in 1776. Indeed, the strength of the German language in Pennsylvania led the essayist and publisher Benjamin Franklin to complain bitterly in 1750: 'Why should *Pennsylvania*, founded by the *English*, become a colony of *Aliens*, who will shortly be so numerous as to Germanize us instead of our Anglifying them, and will never adopt our Language or Customs' (cited in Crawford, 1992a: 37).[25] Official proclamations were published in German until 1794 and at least thirty-two German-language newspapers were published between 1732 and 1800 (Crawford, 1992b; for a wider account of the multilingual nature of American literature, see Sollors, 1998). While the process of Anglicization and assimilation had reduced the influence of German in public life by 1815, the language remained a strong, unofficial presence throughout the nineteenth century, both in Pennsylvania and elsewhere. The ongoing strength of the German language was attributable here largely to a new influx of German migrants, beginning in the 1820s, who settled in cities such as St Louis, Milwaukee and Cincinnati as well as in the rural heartlands (Daniels, 1991). The German language dominated cultural and educational institutions in these areas and resulted in the widespread establishment of German-language schools, both private *and* public. Beginning in 1839, a number of states passed laws allowing German as the language of instruction in public schools, where numbers warranted, a clear tolerance-oriented language right (Dicker, 2003; cf. Chapter 5).

The growing acceptance of German-language education may have continued well into the twentieth century had it not been for two events. From the 1880s, state legislation was passed in several states mandating English as the only language of public (and even private) education. These clearly restrictionist policies were directed principally against German-language schools and formed part of a wider anti-immigration 'Americanization movement' that emerged at this time (Pavlenko, 2002). Although many of these laws were subsequently rescinded by the courts, the deleterious effects on German bilingual schooling were reinforced by the subsequent anti-German hysteria surrounding the First World War. The most (in)famous case of language restrictionism at this time occurred in Nebraska. A 1913 state law required public schools to provide instruction in any European language if fifty or more parents requested it; German was the only language ever requested. In 1918 the law was repealed on the basis that it was pro-German and thus un-American. The legislation that replaced it went so far as to prohibit any public or private school teacher from teaching a subject in a foreign language or, indeed, from teaching a foreign language *as a subject* (Dicker, 2003). The severity of the approach is not dissimilar to those adopted in totalitarian regimes such as Franco's Spain. The new law was overturned in the Supreme Court in 1923 in the *Meyer v. Nebraska* case (see below). However, by then, the damage was done. By the 1930s, bilingual instruction of any type in German had all but disappeared in the United States, while the study of German as a foreign language had fallen from 24 percent of secondary school students nationally in 1915 to less than 1 percent in 1922 (Crawford, 1989).

One further example of the formal recognition of minority language rights can be explored with regard to the use of Spanish in the state of New Mexico. New Mexico currently uses both Spanish and English as languages of the state government. As with Hawaii's official recognition in 1978 of the indigenous Hawaiian language, the de facto endorsement of bilingualism in New Mexico acknowledges that Spanish is the language of a historical ethnie, not (simply) an immigrant language. When the area was ceded to the United States by Mexico at the end of the Mexican-American war, via the (1848) Treaty of Guadalupe Hidalgo, over half its population were Spanish-speaking. As with the incorporation of French speakers in Louisiana before it, local language use was at first ignored. However, Spanish soon came to play a more prominent role within the territory when the US Congress in 1853 authorized the New Mexico Assembly to hire translators and interpreters to conduct its affairs. Subsequent funding was provided in 1884 for the translation and publication of the Assembly's proceedings into Spanish (Marshall, 1986) and a school law passed in that year permitted either Spanish or English as the language of instruction (Hernández-Chávez, 1995).

With the eventual granting of statehood in 1912,[26] these provisions were further formalized in New Mexico's constitution. All laws could be published in both English and Spanish on a twenty-year 'trial basis' and thereafter 'as the legislature may provide'. Given the relatively hostile climate toward minority languages at that time, as a result of the Americanization movement, the ensuing decades saw the gradual ascendancy of English. Nonetheless, provisions for training teachers in both languages were established for the purposes of better serving Spanish-speaking pupils. Likewise, guarantees were provided to ensure that Spanish-speaking children were not discriminated against or segregated in schools. State statutes also called for the use of Spanish in a wide range of governmental activities, including elections, the posting of legal notices, and bilingual/multicultural education (Dicker, 2003). Needless to say, as a result, Spanish is still widely spoken in New Mexico, *alongside* English, in a wide range of language domains.

Before examining the English Only movement's third claim in relation to the language history of the United States – that bilingual practices such as these threaten for the first time the ascendancy of English in the US – I want to refer briefly to two key Supreme Court cases in the twentieth century which also support some accommodation of minority rights. The first has already been mentioned, *Meyer v. Nebraska* (1923). It challenged the restrictionist language policies adopted by Nebraska at the end of the First World War – one of many states to do so at the time. The US Supreme Court ruled in this case that the state *was* able to restrict the language of instruction to English in state-funded schools but could not do so for private schools. The Court based its argument on the due process clause of the 14th Amendment, which protects certain substantive individual liberties from restrictive state policies. The relevant part of the 14th Amendment reads: 'No states shall make or enforce any law which shall abridge the privileges or immunities of citizens; nor shall any state deprive any person of life, liberty, or property, without due process of law; nor deny any person within its jurisdiction to equal protection of laws.'

Since language is not specifically mentioned in this clause, an important precedent was thus established with regard to the protection of private minority language education.[27] That said, the judgment was also clearly sympathetic to the general tenor of the state language policy in question, with its strong emphasis on the centrality of English: 'Perhaps it would be highly advantageous if all had ready understanding of our ordinary speech, but this cannot be coerced by methods which conflict with the Constitution – a desirable end cannot be promoted by prohibited means' (cited in Marshall, 1986: 15). Thus, the decision upholds only the most minimal interpretation of tolerance-oriented language rights, although this in itself remains an important guarantee in the US context.

Another landmark decision was *Lau v. Nichols* (1974) where the US Supreme Court ruled in a case brought by Chinese-American parents that the English-only education policy in the San Francisco Unified School district effectively excluded Chinese-speaking children from meaningful participation in the education system. The Court concluded that this constituted a violation of equality of treatment under the (1965) Civil Rights Act: 'Under these state-imposed standards there is no equality of treatment merely by providing students with the same facilities, textbooks, teachers, and curriculum; for students who do not understand English are effectively foreclosed from any meaningful education' (cited in de Varennes, 1996a: 197). Proponents and opponents alike interpreted the decision as at least tacit endorsement of bilingual education. However, the Court specifically refrained from ordering any particular educational remedy. As the judgment clearly states: 'No specific remedy is urged upon us. Teaching English to the students of Chinese ancestry who do not speak the language is one choice. Giving instructions to this group in Chinese is another. There may be others. Petitioners ask only that the Board of Education be directed to apply its expertise to the problem and rectify the situation' (cited in Crawford, 1989: 36). Thus Macías has observed that while 'it is tempting to say that somehow the *Lau* decision created some [minority] language rights ... it did not. The plaintiffs sought no specific remedy [from] the School District and the Court demanded none' (1979: 92; see also Schiffman, 1996: 269–70). In effect, the court did not make it a legal requirement for schools to provide bilingual education but simply ruled on the illegality of excluding minority language students from such programs.

The ambiguity of the *Lau* decision has since been exploited by citizens-initiated referenda (including in California) proposing the retrenchment, even elimination, of bilingual education (see below). Nonetheless, there is still clearly some precedent in both law and state policy and practice for a limited recognition of minority language and education rights in the USA. But this might appear to confirm the fear expressed by the English Only movement that such concessions, along with the provision of bilingual voting ballots, threaten the ascendancy of English in the USA (see, for example, Bikales, 1986: 84–5). Not so. If it is not already apparent by now, such an assertion is simply nonsense. Linguistic shift *from* minority languages *to* English – what Gorlach (1986) has described as 'reduced multilingualism' – is the dominant pattern in the USA. The number of people who spoke a language other than English at home did grow by 47 percent in the 1990s. However, in the 2000 census, a combined total of 77 percent still reported they spoke English 'well' (22 percent) or 'very well' (55 percent) (Shin, 2003). Immigrants are actually currently shifting to English at a faster rate than was true of European immigrants at the turn of the twentieth century (Baron, 1990). Indeed, 75 percent of all Latino immigrants – who cause the most 'concern' for English Only advocates – speak English frequently each day (Veltman, 1983, 1988; Portes and Hao, 1998). The only variation for Latino communities to this general pattern of language shift is that it takes perhaps one further generation to occur fully – that is, four as opposed to two or three – given the continued influx of monolingual Spanish speakers (Fishman, 1992). As Veltman sensibly concludes, the only languages that are threatened in the USA are languages *other* than English.

Bilingual education and its discontents

The historical fictions perpetuated by the English Only movement in relation to minority language policy and practice are thus plain to see. However, it does not end there. English Only advocates also *actively* misrepresent the educational (and psychological) merits of bilingual education; an approach which has been aptly described by Cummins (1995) as a deliberate 'discourse of disinformation' (see also Krashen, 1996, 1999). This strategy can now be examined.

A key tenet of much English Only rhetoric, echoing our earlier discussions, is that English is essential for social mobility in US society, or rather, that a lack of English *consigns* one inevitably to the social and economic margins. As Linda Chávez, a former President of US English, has argued: 'Hispanics who learn English will be able to avail themselves of opportunities. Those who do not will be relegated to second-class citizenship' (cited in Crawford, 1992c: 172). Guy Wright, a prominent media supporter of English Only policies, takes a similar line in a 1983 editorial in the *San Francisco Examiner*, asserting that 'the individual who fails to learn English is condemned to semi-citizenship, condemned to low pay, condemned to remain in the ghetto' (cited in Secada and Lightfoot, 1993: 47). A more recent example can be found in US English advertising in 1998: 'Deprive a child of an education. Handicap a young life outside the classroom. Restrict social mobility. If it came at the hand of a parent it would be called child abuse. At the hand of our schools ... it's called "bilingual education"' (cited in Dicker, 2000: 53).

This has also been the leitmotif of Ron Unz, a prominent software entrepreneur and conservative public figure, and his organization 'English for the Children'. Targeting four key US states that allow for citizens-initiated referenda, Unz has successfully promoted public propositions delimiting or dismantling bilingual education in three of these states. The most prominent of these is California's Proposition 227 (1998), which effectively ended bilingual education programs in the state (with some exceptions), replacing them with rapid one-year 'Structured English Immersion' programs. Sixty-one percent supported the measure overall, *including* 37 percent of Latino voters. However, Unz was also successful in sponsoring similar measures in Arizona (2000; 63 percent) and Massachusetts (2002; 68 percent). Only in Colorado (2002; 44 percent) was a comparable measure defeated, although, controversially, this was because those opposing the measure played on the fears of Anglo parents that this would result in the reintroduction of too many Latino students into mainstream classrooms (Crawford, 2007). Suffice it to say, in none of the referenda did evidence in support of the educational efficacy of bilingual education inform wider public debate. Prior to the Arizona referendum (Proposition 203), for example, the *New York Times* ran a front-page story in August 2000 strongly supporting the efficacy of its precursor, Proposition 227. Subsequently, it was revealed that the claims made in the article simply repeated key talking points in Unz's campaign, although, not surprisingly, it still had a powerful effect on strengthening public support for Proposition 203 (Wiley and W. Wright, 2004; Schildkraut, 2005; W. Wright, 2005).

In these wider debates, proponents of bilingual education are often constructed as being 'anti-English' and/or dismissing the value of learning standard English in the USA.[28] But no serious bilingual education proponents ever do this. For example, Donaldo Macedo, a trenchant critic of English Only, has argued, following Gramsci, that bilingual 'educators should understand the value of mastering the standard English language of the wider society. It is through the full appropriation of the standard English language that linguistic-minority students find themselves linguistically empowered to engage in dialogue with various sectors of the wider society' (1994: 128; see also Ives, 2010). If nothing else, this highlights the inherent intellectual dishonesty of the English Only movement, an intentional dishonesty that is also reflected in their highly effective dismissal of the merits of bilingual education. The strategy adopted here is threefold. First, English Only advocates imply that, given sufficient motivation, anyone can master English in an English-only environment, a position which is usually tied to the related lament that bilingual education has replaced the beloved 'sink or swim' approach (see Imhoff, 1990; Porter, 1990). In effect, the argument is that 'children of normal intelligence' are sure to learn English if they are exposed to it. As Donahue (1985) argues, this position conveniently blames the victim and, in so doing, masks a deeply racist attitude to non-English speakers (see also Zentella, 1997). Second, the English Only movement deliberately ignores and/or ridicules the widely attested research in support of bilingual education. Drawing on Chomsky (1987), Cummins observes that this is because the 'threat of the good example' must be neutralized. And finally, it specifically deploys to great effect the limited and highly questionable research that does cast (some) doubt on bilingual education. I will explore briefly two key examples of the latter.

The first of these, the American Institutes for Research's (AIR) evaluation of bilingual education programs, was commissioned in the 1970s by the United States Office of Education (Danoff, Coles, McLaughlin and Reynolds, 1978). It provided an overview of US federally funded bilingual programs operating at the time and found that such programs had no significant impact on educational achievement in English, although they did enhance native-like proficiency. It furthermore suggested that pupils were being kept in bilingual programs longer than necessary, thus contributing to the segregation of such students from 'mainstream' (English-only) classes.

Despite significant concerns about its methodology (see below), the conclusions of the AIR study were seemingly replicated by a second piece of US federally commissioned research by Baker and de Kanter (1981, 1983; see also Rossell and Baker, 1996). These authors reviewed the literature and likewise concluded that bilingual education was not advancing the English language skills and academic achievements of minority language students, predominantly Spanish-speaking first language (L1) students. In short, Baker and de Kanter argued that students in bilingual programs demonstrated no clear educational advantages over those in English-only programs.

Given the increasingly skeptical political climate of the time, this research generated enormous publicity and exerted even more influence on subsequent federal US policy. However, as Crawford (1989) observes, while the Baker and de Kanter (1983) report is easily the most quoted US federal pronouncement on bilingual education, it is probably the most criticized as well. As with its predecessor, much of this criticism had to do with the methodology that was employed. For example, as with the AIR study, Baker and de Kanter specifically rejected the use of data gathered through students' first languages. They also failed to account for the fact that two-thirds of the comparison group in English-only education programs *had previously been in bilingual programs* where, presumably, they had benefited from first language instruction (Crawford, 1992a). Moreover, both reports consistently failed to differentiate between early- and late-exit bilingual programs in their analysis. As we saw earlier, early-exit programs, where bilingual instruction is usually only pursued for one to two years before 'transitioning' to the majority language, are less effective than late-exit programs (usually four to six years). Given that early-exit programs constituted the majority of the programs under review, this inevitably subsumed the better educational results of the late-exit programs (Cummins, 2000).

Overall, the inadequacy of Baker and de Kanter's findings has been confirmed by Willig's (1985, 1987) subsequent meta-analyses of their data. Willig controlled for 183 variables that they had failed to take into account. She found, as a result, small to moderate differences in favor of bilingual education, even when these were predominantly early-exit programs. Willig's conclusions were also replicated in the two major longitudinal bilingual education research studies by Ramírez et al. (1991) and Thomas and Collier (2002), discussed earlier (see also Hakuta et al., 2000).

This pattern of deliberate misrepresentation and obfuscation by proponents of English Only continues to the present largely unabated. For example, George W. Bush's flagship educational policy *No Child Left Behind* (NCLB; 2001) saw the revocation of the (1968) Bilingual Education Act on the premise that English language instruction and assessment is best for all students.[29] Subsequent advocacy of NCLB has touted its positive effects for bilingual students. However, research evidence suggests, not surprisingly, that the opposite is true. Kate Menken (2008) has documented the clearly negative educational effects that NCLB testing policies are having on bilingual students. In New York City, for example, she found that as a result of NCLB's requirement to be assessed in English, with no recourse to one's first language, bilingual students ranged from 20 to 50 percentage points below native English speakers.

Insisting on the merits of English only education for bilingual students in the face of research evidence that clearly suggests otherwise demonstrates a remarkable degree of cynicism. But this cynicism becomes breathtaking when measured against another variable: the funding of these English only programs. In this respect, the English Only movement is again clearly found wanting.

Many who supported the establishment of official state-level English policies, for example, including the Unz-led referenda against bilingual education, logically assumed that a principal concern of the legislation was to expand the opportunities for immigrants to learn English. However, logical or not, this has proved not to be the case. While US English spent lavishly to get ELA measures on the ballot, in 1988 it declined to support legislation creating a modestly funded federal program for adult learners of English (Crawford, 1992c). As a result of public criticism, US English did make some subsequent effort to fund similar ventures, but these efforts have remained largely desultory and continue to constitute only the barest minimum of their total funding efforts (Dicker, 2000). The attitude adopted here appears to be that English language programs should be the sole responsibility of Spanish-speaking volunteers! Guy Wright, whom we have already encountered, wrote somewhat wistfully along these lines in his media column in 1986, suggesting that a grassroots volunteer movement was by far the best solution since 'the legislature will balk when it realizes how much it would cost to hire enough credentialed teachers and professional administrators to cope with the waiting lists for English classes'. Taking the latter route was also not necessary in his view since 'the immigrant doesn't need to learn perfect English ... [only] survival English'. Accordingly, 'volunteers will need some guidance from the state. But not too much. A simple briefing and a handbook that set out the lessons should do' (cited in Tollefson, 1991: 124).

Wright's ruminations contradict (albeit unwittingly) a central tenet of the English Only movement – that non-native English speaking immigrants (particularly Latinos) are *unwilling* to learn English. This is flatly contradicted by the facts, as Wright's comments on 'waiting lists' implicitly suggest (see Dicker, 2000, 2003, for further details). His sentiments concerning 'survival English' also clearly illustrate the underlying racism and indifference toward minority language speakers that are evident in so much of English Only rhetoric (see below). As James Crawford concludes:

> One thing is clear. Rather than promote English proficiency, 99 percent of the [US English] organization's efforts go toward restricting the use of other languages. Certainly there is nothing in Official English legislation to help anyone learn English. On the other hand, there is much to penalize those who have yet to do so ... English Only is a label that has stuck, despite the protests of US English, because it accurately sums up the group's logic: That people will speak English only if they are forced to. That the crutch of bilingual education must be yanked away or newcomers will be permanently handicapped. That immigrants are too lazy or dim-witted to accept 'the primacy of English' on their own. (1992c: 176)

The return of the nativist

If US English and like-minded proponents like Ron Unz are not actually concerned with extending opportunities to minority language speakers to learn English, despite all their rhetoric proclaiming just that, there must be another, more sinister agenda at work. In this respect, it is interesting to note that all previous movements that advocated English-only policies did so as part of a wider nativist and anti-immigrationist agenda. The current English Only movement, despite its disavowals, is no exception to this trend – in effect, it provides us with a modern variant of the Americanization movement of the late nineteenth/early twentieth century. The links that the organization US English has with anti-immigrationist groups would appear to confirm this, not least because the co-founder of US English, John Tanton, was also previously the founder of a smaller anti-immigration organization, Federation for American Immigration Reform (FAIR: see Schmidt, 2008).

The principal concern of Tanton, and other anti-immigrationists involved in the English Only movement, if it is not already apparent, is the rapidly rising Latino population in the United States. In the 2000 census, of the nearly 47 million aged over 5 who speak a language other than English at home, 28 million were Spanish speakers (Wiley, 2005). By 2009, the population of Latino Americans had grown to 48.4 million or 16 percent of the total population, overtaking African Americans to become the largest minority in the USA. It is further suggested that by the year 2050 Latino communities will have increased to 30 percent of the total population, outnumbering the combined total of African Americans, Asian Americans and Native Americans (US Census Bureau, 2010). This will coincide with a concomitant decline in the number of white Americans. It is this population growth – what Tanton has termed 'the Latin onslaught' on the USA – which is the real concern of many English Only advocates. Zentella (1997) has coined the term 'Hispanophobia' to describe it.

Tanton's own Hispanophobia was exposed when an internal memorandum he wrote in 1986 was made public two years later, causing his resignation from US English. In it, he discusses a range of cultural threats posed by 'Spanish-speaking immigrants', including a lack of involvement in public affairs, Roman Catholicism, low 'educability', high school dropout rates and 'high fertility'. Among a range of questions he raised in relation to these concerns were: 'Perhaps this is the first instance in which those with their pants up are going to get caught with their pants down'. 'Will the present [white] majority peaceably hand over its political power to a group that is simply more fertile?' 'As whites see their power and control over their lives declining, will they simply go quietly into the night? Or will there be an explosion?' (cited in Crawford, 1992c: 173). A number of notable public supporters of the organization also resigned at the time because of the anti-Latino and anti-Catholic sentiments expressed, including Linda Chávez, the then President of US English.

Despite this setback, US English has continued to garner increasingly wide support. And this is where the present English Only movement differs from its predecessors. In short, it cannot *simply* be a nativist movement – or, rather, it cannot just be a simple (transparent) nativist movement – since, one would expect, it would not have generated the broad following that it has. This would appear to be confirmed by the extent of the movement's appeal to many minority language speakers themselves, as we saw previously with the support for California's Proposition 227 among Latino voters. Indeed, its prominent minority supporters have been regularly paraded by the movement as the epitome of the 'good alien' (Tarver, 1994): the success stories of immigration and the embodiment of the American dream. These have included Hayakawa himself – although, as Donahue (1985) points out, he actually came from British Columbia – Gerda Bikales, Linda Chávez and Richard Rodrigeuz, among others.

How is the movement able to generate this wide appeal, among both majority and minority language speakers? One way it does so is by *inverting* the usual immigration and language axis. Where previous movements concentrated primarily on concerns over immigration, from which arose (subsequent) language policies, the English Only movement attempts the reverse, thus making it far more politically palatable. In short, it concentrates almost solely on the status of the English language in the USA as a convenient proxy for a more overtly racialized politics. The approach adopted here is similar to the 'new racism' which substitutes (at least ostensibly) culturalist arguments about 'race' for biological ones (see Chapter 1). Deutsch has observed that 'language is an automatic signalling system, second only to race, in identifying targets for privilege or discrimination' (1975: 7; see also Chapter 4). James Crawford argues along more specific lines:

> The English Only movement, an outgrowth of the immigration-restrictionist lobby, has skillfully manipulated language as a symbol of national unity and ethnic divisiveness. Early in [the twentieth] century, those who sought to exclude other races [sic] and cultures invoked claims of Anglo-Saxon superiority. But … explicit racial loyalties are no longer acceptable in political discourse. Language loyalties, on the other hand, remain largely devoid of associations with social injustice. While race is [supposedly] immutable, immigrants can and often do exchange their mother tongue for another. And so, for those who resent the presence of Hispanics and Asians, language politics has become a convenient surrogate for racial politics. (1989: 14)

Certainly, this could explain why states such as California, where Latinos currently comprise 37 percent of the state's population (Pew Hispanic Center, 2011), appear so enamored with the English Only movement's agenda.[30]

The 'curse' of multilingualism

Which brings us to the final dimension of the English Only movement that I want to examine here, its argument that multilingualism and minority language rights are inherently destabilizing to the nation-state. As we saw in Chapter 3, this is a view that is widely shared by both liberal and conservative commentators. Given its commonsense assumptions, it also finds considerable support among the wider public, providing another reason for the English Only movement's wide appeal. Thus, Kathryn Bricker, former executive director of US English, can assert:

> Language is so much a part of our lives that it can be a great tool either for unity or disunity. And we are getting close to the point where we have a challenge to the common language that we share ... We are basically at a crossroads. We can reaffirm our need for a common language, or we can slowly go down the road of division along language lines. (Cited in Secada and Lightfoot, 1993: 46)

Other assertions are even more apocalyptic – emphasizing the potential nightmares of separatism and civil strife apparent in prominent 'ethnic conflicts' elsewhere in the world. Gary Imhoff, for example, baldly states that 'language diversity has been a major cause of [international] conflict ... Any honest student of the sociology of language should admit that multilingual societies have been less united and internally peaceful than single-language societies' (1987: 40). Likewise, Hayakawa has argued:

> For the first time in our history, our nation [sic] is faced with the possibility of the kind of linguistic division that has torn apart Canada in recent years; that has been a major feature of the unhappy history of Belgium, split into speakers of French and Flemish; that is at this very moment a bloody division between the Sinhalese and Tamil populations of Sri Lanka. (Cited in Nunberg, 1992: 492)

However, as I have already indicated in the preceding chapter, the position painted here is simply wrong – in both its historical and comparative dimensions. Historically, the principal cause of most language-based conflicts has been the *denial* of legitimate minority language rights rather than their recognition. This is true of Canada, Belgium and Sri Lanka. We have already seen this to be the case with respect to Belgium, and I will outline in the next chapter why the Canadian context, with particular reference to Quebec, can also be regarded in the same light. The conflict in Sri Lanka between the Sinhalese majority (comprising 75 percent of the population) and the Lankan Tamils (who comprise 12.5 percent of the remaining Tamil-speaking population) was also largely precipitated by, but not limited to, the language question. In 1956, eight years after independence, Sinhala was made the sole official language, replacing English. This language law created much discontent among Tamil speakers who, with limited access to land, had previously looked to the civil service for employment. With the implementation of the official language law, this option was increasingly denied to them also. Moreover, the language measure was the first of many that restricted the rights and opportunities of Tamil speakers. The subsequent Tamil Tigers independence movement, which emerged formally in 1976 and was only finally quelled in 2009, thus draws its grievances from this wider background of the apparent denial of minority Tamil aspirations by the majority Sinhalese (Fishman and Solano, 1989; see also Little, 1994).

In short, attempting to enforce linguistic homogeneity – the central aim of the English Only movement – is far more likely to foster disunity than to ameliorate it. Indeed, of all possible scenarios, this one is likely to be the most divisive, the most contentious and fractious (Donahue, 1985). As Donahue asserts: 'The final irony of [the English Only] approach to the matter of language use is that by ... aligning itself with a theory which holds that all ethnic intergroup behaviour is inevitably conflict producing, [it] forecloses itself from the possibility of unifying American society' (1985: 107). In contrast, a 'language competent society' (A. Padilla, 1991) – where all minority language speakers are able to learn English, while also retaining their first language – is far more likely to result in both social mobility for minority speakers and a more flexible and less contentious national language policy overall. As Marshall and Gonzalez conclude, 'it is not multilingualism itself that is disruptive, but denying a group that speaks a different language from participating in greater social mobility' (1990: 33).

In addition to their historical inaccuracy, the English Only movement's critique of other, multilingual, contexts is also wrong comparatively. In Canada and Belgium, for example, minority language claims center on the rights of historical ethnies who are formally recognized, at least ostensibly, in the bicultural and bilingual frameworks of the countries concerned. The question is thus not about the eventual linguistic assimilation of these minority language speakers, and the best way(s) this might be achieved, as in the USA. Rather, it concerns how separate language recognition as befits their status as ethnies can be established, and how past injustices that have militated against such recognition can be rectified. Although there are also historical ethnies within the USA, notably Native Americans and some Spanish speakers, the principal concerns of the language debates there remain focused on immigrants or new minorities. Likewise, the erosion and infringement of existing *constitutional* minority language rights, leading to the threat of conflict and secession, has no precedent in the USA, not even with the Louisiana Purchase or the Treaty of Guadalupe Hidalgo.

Bearing these important distinctions in mind, I want to turn in the next two chapters to specific examples where language rights for minority ethnies have been successfully implemented. In Chapter 7, I will explore three areas – Quebec, Catalonia and Wales – where national minority language rights have been realized via the 'territorial language principle', as discussed in Chapter 5. In Chapter 8, I will focus on examples where indigenous language rights have been successfully implemented, most usually via the 'personality language principle'. Suffice it to say, the examples from both cases bluntly belie the apocalyptic scenarios so often attributed to them by opponents of language rights.

7

THE RISE OF REGIONALISM

REINSTATING MINORITY LANGUAGES

The debates about globalization, discussed in the previous chapter, highlight the changing nature of our world and, particularly, the reconfiguration of flows of people, capital, technology, information and ideas (Appadurai, 1990). Some suggest from this, that the era of the nation-state is already on the wane.[1] I do not share this sense of inevitability (cf. Chapter 1). Of course, nation-states *are* clearly subject to wider trends toward greater economic and political interdependence in this age of late capitalism. To suggest otherwise would be foolish. But the idea that this is an entirely new phenomenon, the recent product of globalization in effect, would also appear to be misplaced. After all, nation-states have always been subject to wider economic and political forces of one form or another. As Hinsley observes, the idea of complete economic and political sovereignty is a 'situation to which many states may have often aspired, but have never in fact enjoyed' (1986: 226).

We also see this tension reflected in the rise of supranational organizations, such as the European Union (EU). On the one hand, the EU's influence contributes to a reinforcement of global trends, such as the increasing use of English, and the retrenchment of formal multilingualism, as discussed in the previous chapter.[2] On the other hand, it can be argued that, far from undermining nation-states, supranational organizations such as the EU may serve, at least in some key respects, to reinforce them. Certainly, the two countervailing political views on European integration that have been promoted over the last two decades – the idea of the federal European 'super state' versus the national 'opt out' – both perpetuate the notion of nationhood. The former simply transfers nationhood to a wider entity, adopting in the process much of its key political apparatus and symbols (territorial boundaries, immigration controls, parliament, currency and an electorate). The latter continues to define membership of the EU in terms of existing nation-states and national boundaries (Billig, 1995; Anthony Smith, 1998). Indeed, some have gone so far as to argue that the EU has been a key bulwark of the nation-state. As Milward asserts, 'it has been its buttress, an indispensable part of the nation-state's post-war construction. Without it, the nation-state could not have afforded to its citizens the same measure of security and prosperity which it has provided and which has justified its survival' (1992: 3).

Thus, the impending demise of nation-states is overstated (cf. Heller, 2011). So too is the reach or influence of supranational organizations over them. But supranational organizations remain influential for other reasons, not least their role as both catalysts and intermediaries in the promotion of other forms of identity – particularly at the local and regional level (see Jones and Keating, 1995; D. Smith and S. Wright, 1999; Keating, 2009; Fitjar, 2010). Supranational organizations have been central to developments in international law facilitating the greater recognition of promotion-oriented language rights for minorities, as discussed in Chapters 4 and 5. These developments have also been closely allied with the emergence over the last decade of stronger regional administrations, via processes of greater devolution and regional control. Cumulatively, both provide considerably more scope and institutional space for the fostering of minority languages.

In Europe, for example, the process of 'Europeanization' (Trenz, 2007; Keating, 2009) has allowed national minority groups to operate independent of (or at least in conjunction with) the nation-states in which they are currently subsumed in order to achieve greater cultural and linguistic recognition in the civic realm, or public domain. As Esteve noted in the early 1990s, 'the dynamics of the present-day situation suggest that Europe may evolve into a complex association of autonomous communities in which the supranational unifying process is accompanied by a reinforcement of … regional autonomies' (1992: 259). The intervening period would appear to confirm this observation, with the growing influence of the Europe of the Regions and, in particular, the Council of Europe's Congress of Local and Regional Authorities (Trommer and Chari, 2006; Likhachev, 2009). Indeed, minority language groups have been particularly adept at using this 'intermediary space of contention' in the multilevel European system to facilitate and diffuse 'common orientations and particular policy models of minority protection' (Trenz, 2007: 161).

Catalonia and Wales are two clear examples in Europe where this has already successfully occurred. In both these contexts, the move toward greater devolution in the once highly centralized states of which they are a part has facilitated the (re)legitimation and institutionalization[3] of Catalan and Welsh, respectively. In so doing, a long history of derogation, proscription and neglect of these historically associated languages has begun to be redressed. This has led to their current revival after many years of language shift and loss and, just as significantly, to their re-entry into, and re-establishment within the civic realm. Having said that, and given all that I have discussed thus far, it should perhaps not come as too much of a surprise that these developments have also generated their fair share of controversy. I will discuss Catalonia and Wales more fully shortly. First, however, let me return to North America in order to focus briefly on one of the other most cited examples of growing regional linguistic autonomy, Quebec.

Quebec: safeguarding French in a sea of English

Francophones in Quebec at the time of the 2001 census constituted a clear majority (81.4 percent) in the province, and a considerable minority (22.9 percent) throughout the whole of Canada (Dumas, 2007). This makes French a 'regional majority language' in the area of Quebec (Maurais, 1997; Lisée, 2007), although it still clearly remains a minority language throughout Canada as a whole. Along with the historical status of Francophones as one of the two colonial charter groups of Canada, the apparent strength of French, particularly in Quebec, might suggest a measure of cultural and linguistic security for the language. Not so.

The history of Francophones in Canada conforms broadly to the experiences of minority language speakers elsewhere. Since the defeat of the French in 1759 in what was then called New France, and with its subsequent incorporation into the Canadian Confederation in 1867, Francophones have clearly been the minority partner in Canadian institutional life. In short, they have been subject to the political, cultural, and economic dominance of English speakers (Anglophones) throughout Canada and, until recently, in Quebec itself. Consequently, it has only been within the last sixty years that significant linguistic accommodations have been made toward Francophones. For example, it was only in 1958 that simultaneous translation became available for the first time in the Canadian House of Commons. It was not until 1969 that bilingualism in the Canadian federal civil service was formalized with the passing of the first Official Language Act (revised in 1988 and again in 2005).[4] And it was not until 1982 that the right to minority language education in French outside of Quebec was entrenched via the Canadian Charter of Rights and Freedoms (Réaume, 1999).

However, it is true to say that Francophones, at least in Quebec, have also consistently achieved, and been able to maintain a considerable degree of institutional autonomy over time (Colin Williams, 1994, 2008). This measure of institutional autonomy was initially based upon their status as French Canadians or 'Canadiens', which in turn was perceived in primarily ethnic and religious terms, rather than in language terms (Juteau, 1996). Identification via the French language was only to come much later (see below). Nonetheless, in carving out an institutional niche for themselves in Quebec, French

Canadians were also able to safeguard an ongoing role for French within the civic realm, albeit indirectly at first. That said, developments immediately after the conquest of New France by the British suggested a far less promising picture. This was because the first significant piece of legislation – the (1763) Royal Proclamation – was specifically punitive toward the French Canadian majority in the region. The Proclamation imposed English law and effectively barred French Canadians from public office by requiring them first to abjure, or formally renounce, their Catholicism. A more accommodative approach, however, quickly replaced this punitive one in the actual practice of provincial administration. The latter tendency was further confirmed by the (1774) Quebec Act, which, in attempting to ensure the loyalty of French Canadians at the time of the American War of Independence, reinstated civil laws and institutions (including the right for Catholics to hold public office) and indirectly recognized the use of French alongside English in their application.

The process of linguistic accommodation was furthered by the (1791) Constitutional Act, which recognized the regional majority rights of French Canadians by dividing the territory into Upper and Lower Canada (corresponding today to the southern portions of Ontario and Quebec respectively). In the latter, French Canadians were able to exercise considerable autonomy in political and civil administration, while French was also able to continue in its de facto role as the language of that administration. After rebellions in the late 1830s in both areas, Britain attempted to reimpose a more overtly assimilationist approach. Following a report by Lord Durham in 1839, which situated the problems of the region in the continued cultural and linguistic existence of the French Canadian community, the (1840) Union Act was implemented. This reunited the two areas of Upper and Lower Canada and specifically proscribed French as a language of public record or of debate in the new legislative assembly. However, actual practice again proved to be more accommodative, leading to a reunified Anglo and French Canadian political administration in 1847, and the reinstatement of French as an administrative language in 1848 (Magnet, 1995). This accommodation of bilingualism was subsequently to be reflected in the (1867) British North American Act, which established Canada in its modern form and which in Section 133 recognized a limited administrative and judicial role for French/English bilingualism. While Canadian courts were subsequently to delimit the provisions of Section 133 even further (see Réaume, 1999), it nonetheless provided an important precedent, leading to the eventual extension of minority language rights in the (1982) Canadian Charter of Rights and Freedoms.

'The Québec we wish to build will be essentially French'

The institutional autonomy carved out by the French Canadian community in Quebec was aided, until the 1950s, by the relative geographical isolation of

Quebec, by its predominantly rural outlook and, primarily, by its Catholicism. Indeed, from the time of the conquest of New France until the 1950s, it was the Catholic Church rather than the provincial administration that was most concerned with defending French language and culture (Guibernau, 1999; Heller, 1999). However, with the emergence of the 'Quiet Revolution' in the 1960s – which saw the transformation of Quebec into a modern Western economy – the role of the church faded rapidly. In its place, a new territorial conception of 'Québécois' identity as a 'distinct society' was established, thus excluding French Canadians from outside Quebec, while Quebec French came to be seen as its principal marker (Handler, 1988: 163–6; see also Balthazar, 1990; McRoberts, 1999). This new Québécois identity adopted a modernist political outlook centered on the economic political, cultural and linguistic liberation of Quebec (Juteau, 1996; Heller, 1999), a process that equates closely with cultural nationalism, as discussed in Chapter 2.[5]

The establishment of the Office de la langue française in 1961, whose primary function was to protect and standardize the use of French within Quebec, reinforced the growing identification of the language with Québécois identity. Two important commissions at that time also reaffirmed the significance of language. The Parent Commission of 1966 recommended that the major responsibility of the provincial government was to protect the French language, regulate its use, encourage its improvement and ensure the fullest possible development of the culture it expressed (Mallea, 1989). The Laurendeau-Dunton Commission, which first reported in 1967, found that the wider principle of French/English language equality enshrined in the Canadian Confederation could only realistically be achieved within Quebec, let alone elsewhere in Canada, when the marked economic and educational disparities between Francophones and Anglophones were addressed. In Quebec, for example, a cultural division of labor was clearly apparent in which an Anglicized elite dominated the economy, and where English had accordingly become inextricably associated with social mobility. Indeed, the Laurendeau-Dunton Report found that, on the basis of average income, monolingual Anglophone males in Quebec constituted the most economically privileged group in all of Canada. In contrast, their Francophone counterparts earned 35 percent less in comparison (Barbaud, 1998). French was further threatened by a declining birth rate among the Francophone population, by increased emigration to other provinces and by an increasing pattern of new minorities in Quebec choosing to send their children to English-speaking schools, given the higher status of English within Canada. In this last respect, it was found that in 1971–2 fully 85 percent of new minorities were being educated in English-language schools, while in 1973 even 25,000 French-speaking students were enrolled in such schools (Maurais, 1997).

The immediate concerns over the fate of the language were also framed within a wider skepticism toward the Canadian federal government's bilingual policy, which seemed to be doing little to redress the decline of French throughout Canada (Heller, 1999). Indeed, given the predominance of English elsewhere in Canada, and in prestigious institutional domains within Quebec, only an active promotion-oriented language policy in favor of French could redress the balance. This was the conclusion of the Laurendeau-Dunton Commission since, in its view, 'the life of the French-Canadian culture necessarily implies the life of the French language' (cited in Coulombe, 1995: 75).

As a result of this increasing focus on language as the core of Québécois identity, a range of significant language legislation actively promoting French was enacted in the 1970s. These legislative developments were also facilitated by the rise of the nationalist and social democratic party, the Partí Québécois (PQ), to provincial government for the first time in 1976. The most prominent of the language laws passed at this time, Bill 101 (Charte de la langue française, 1977), has also been the most controversial. The Charte de la langue française aimed to address the historical cultural division of labor in Quebec by formalizing French in economic, educational and political domains. As its architect, Camille Laurin, argued:

> The Québec we wish to build will be essentially French. The fact that the majority of its population is French will be clearly visible – at work, in communications and in the countryside. It will also be a country in which the traditional balance of power will be altered, especially in regard to the economy ... this will accompany, symbolise and support a reconquest by the French-speaking majority in Québec of that control of the economy that we ought to have. (Laurin, 1977; cited in Colin Williams, 1994: 196)

Specifically, the Charte de la langue française entailed that all children in state education, except those whose parents had themselves been taught in English *in Quebec*, attend Francophone schools – requiring, in effect, all Francophones, new minorities and other Canadians to be educated in French. Freedom of choice with respect to language of instruction would now be available only at the Cegep (pre-university) and university levels (Maurais, 1997). In addition, all commercial signs were required to be solely in French. And all businesses with over fifty employees had to undertake 'francization' programs so as to ensure the right of any Quebecer to be able to work in French, in both the public and the private sectors. The process of francization, in particular, provided Francophones with significant linguistic capital in business and commerce while, in so doing, opening up higher status occupations to them – both of which had been, until then, traditionally denied them (Keating, 1997; Heller, 1999). The Office de la langue française was given responsibility for the application and enforcement of the Charte de la langue française and was subsequently supported by two related organizations, the Commission de toponymie du Québec, responsible for approving and disseminating place names, and the Conseil supérieur de la langue française, which advises the government on all matters related to the French language in Quebec (Dumas, 2007).

Needless to say, the requirements of the Charte de la langue française, and its enforcement, initially generated considerable opposition, particularly from the Anglophone minority in Quebec and the Anglophone majority elsewhere in Canada. Subsequently, aspects of it were ruled unconstitutional. The educational restrictions were deemed by the Canadian Supreme Court in 1984 to contravene Article 23 of the (1982) Canadian Charter of Rights and Freedoms protecting the rights of minority language speakers (although Quebec had not actually been involved in its endorsement; see below). Thus, the Supreme Court ruled that, in addition to the exemptions outlined in the Charter, children whose parents had received elementary instruction in English *anywhere in Canada*, and the siblings of a child who had received, or was receiving elementary or secondary instruction in English in Canada, could also attend English-language schools in Quebec. The commercial signage restrictions were also deemed discriminatory by the Supreme Court in the *Ford v. Québec* (1988) case, although a comparable case brought before the United Nations Human Rights Committee (UNHRC) the following year, *Ballantyne, Davidson and McIntyre v. Canada*, was more favorable toward the policy. In this respect, the UNHRC acknowledged that, under Article 27 of the International Covenant on Civil and Political Rights (ICCPR; see Chapter 5), the Quebec government could validly seek to protect French within Quebec as long as such a policy was not used to limit the use of other minority languages in the private domain. Similarly, the UNHRC ruled that the litigants, who were Anglophones living in Quebec, were *not* a linguistic minority under Article 27, as they claimed, because 'English-speaking citizens *of Canada* cannot be considered a linguistic minority' (cited in de Varennes, 1996a: 142; my emphasis).

In response to the contested legal nature of their language policy, the Quebec provincial government initially disregarded the Canadian Supreme Court's rulings by invoking the 'notwithstanding clause'[6] of Canada's Constitution, arguing that the Charte de la langue française was in the best interests of Québec's distinct character (Tully, 1995; Coulombe, 1999). However, over time, and in light of the actual success of the francization program in cementing French within the civic and commercial domains (see below), language restrictions were gradually relaxed. For example, most of the machinery for enforcing francization was subsequently abolished in 1993, along with the legislation restricting non-French advertising (Keating, 1997).

The tensions between the francization program of the Quebec government and the rest of Canada (ROC) have nonetheless remained ongoing. The general skepticism in the ROC toward the arguments employed in defence of the Charte de la langue française was, for example, to result in the eventual failure of the (1987) Meech Lake Accord. The Accord had attempted to reconcile Quebec's aspirations as a 'distinct society' with the federalism of the Canadian state as represented by the Canadian Charter of Rights and Freedoms. This was regarded as extremely important by both sides, not least because the provincial Quebec government had never formally agreed to the latter, viewing it as too weak on the question of French language rights. However, the Meech Lake Accord lapsed when Manitoba and Newfoundland failed to sign it over concerns about the 'distinct society' clause. The Accord's failure, and the subsequent failure of a similar attempt, the (1992) Charlottetown Accord, highlighted the contested question of Quebec's relationship with the ROC, fueling calls among Quebec nationalists, particularly members of the Partí Québécois (PQ), for independence. This culminated in the October 1995 referendum on Quebec sovereignty, which was lost by only 54,288 votes, or 1.6 percent (Guibernau, 1999), although since that time support for sovereignty has receded significantly.[7] Lest the issue of secession be given too much prominence, however, one further caveat can be added here. Even at its most strident, the PQ's vision of a sovereign Quebec was (and continues to be) highly attenuated, emphasizing ongoing close economic and political partnership with Canada (Keating, 1996, 1997). Moreover, the principal concerns of the PQ, *in practice*, have focused primarily on questions of cultural nationalism – notably, on the question of language – rather than on secession as such.

Developments over the last decade bear this out, with an ongoing focus on ensuring the status of French as a langue publique commune (common public language) in Quebec for all those in the region. This has involved a further entrenching of French as the key to Québécois identity, rather than ethnicity or religion, and a related highlighting of the centrality of Québécois (regional) citizenship, *alongside* Canadian citizenship (Oakes, 2004; Oakes and Warren, 2007). These emphases are most apparent in the Larose Commission, which was set up in June 2000 to ensure the continued use, expansion and quality of French in the region. When it reported back in 2001, the Commission concluded that 'French is now a language for everyone' in Quebec (Gouvernement du Québec, 2001; cited in Oakes, 2004: 540).

The Quebec language laws have thus largely achieved their intention of raising the public profile of French within Quebec (Larrivée, 2003). In effect, the previously marginalized status of French within the economy and within education has been reversed. French now features as both a functional and legitimate language in commerce and industry (Colin Williams, 1994, 2008), while there is a pattern of increasing enrolment in French-language schools, even by those eligible for English-language education (Coulombe, 1995; MacMillan, 2003). But these results have only been achieved, it seems, at the expense of certain individual freedoms with regard to language choice. In relation to Will Kymlicka's distinction between external protections and internal restrictions, discussed in Chapter 3, it is clear that the Quebec language laws are *primarily* an external protection. In other words, they relate to *inter*group relations where a national minority group seeks to protect its distinct identity by limiting the impact of the decisions of the larger society. However, they necessarily involve some internal restrictions on members of that community as well, particularly with respect to the children of new minorities who can now only be schooled in French.

These apparent restrictions have caused ongoing controversy in the English-language Canadian media and in the wider political sphere, particularly in the ROC. French language laws are regularly compared with tribalism, ethnic cleansing, racism and apartheid (Venne, 2000; Oakes, 2004; Oakes and Warren, 2007).[8] But there are three problems with these criticisms. The first is that, much like the arguments of the English Only movement in the USA discussed in Chapter 6, they are often spectacularly ill informed. For example, critics regularly suggest that the public school system is only in French and that Anglophones thus have to attend private or bilingual schools. In contrast, the Anglophone minority in Quebec has a guaranteed right to its own publicly funded schools, a right that also applies at the post-secondary level. Similarly, health care provision provides Anglophones with the guaranteed right to access services in English, if they so choose (Dumas, 2007).

The second problem is one of consistency, similar to that already discussed in Chapter 6. Those opposing Quebec's language laws seldom, if ever, apply a comparable critique of linguistic hegemony to English, or other majority languages, in existing nation-states. It only becomes problematic, it seems, when a minority language is promoted as a language of the civic realm. But even here, they get it wrong because the third rejoinder is that French language laws in Quebec specifically do not replicate the monolingual nation-state model and its exclusionary tendencies – simply replacing English, in effect, with French; quite the reverse, in fact. For a start, Québécois identity is always situated in conjunction with Canadian identity, and so too, necessarily, then are French and English as the two charter languages of the Canadian federation. Following from this, access to English is not being denied in Quebec, not least because it clearly remains the majority language of Canada and because Francophones are thus invariably bilingual in English as well. Moreover, as the earlier examples of educational and health provisions for Anglophones reveal, the English language minority in Québec actually has stronger language rights than do French minority speakers in most other Canadian provinces (Kymlicka, 2007). Rather, it is ongoing monolingualism *in English* that is being circumscribed within Quebec. We have already seen that 'unfettered' language choice inevitably results in the loss of minority languages, grounded as it is in wider asymmetrical sociopolitical and socioeconomic power relations. Consequently, advocates of the Charte de la langue française argue that the only way that individual bilingualism can be maintained and fostered is by, counter-intuitively, setting strict limits on the extent of institutional bilingualism (Maurais, 1997).

More significantly even than this, however, is that other language speakers in Quebec retain distinct, inviolate language rights of their own (Carens, 1995). Indigenous peoples in Quebec are accorded distinct language rights on the basis that they are also, along with Francophones, historical ethnies in the territory. The architect of the Charte de la langue française, Laurin, admitted as much when observing: 'the Amerindians and the Inuit are the only ones who ... can consider themselves as peoples separate from the totality of Québécois and in consequence [can] insist on special treatment under the law' (cited in Coulombe, 1995: 119). To be sure, this has not stopped French acting as a 'replacing language' with respect to indigenous languages in Quebec, in much the same way as English has elsewhere in Canada (Maurais, 1996). Nor are the broadly comparable rights claims of French and indigenous languages without their tensions (see Salée, 1995). Nonetheless, Quebec's approach does specifically allow for the ongoing *active* protection and promotion of indigenous languages, particularly via education.

The intent of the Quebec language legislation is thus *not* to curb the use of other minority languages – unlike the English Only movement for example, or, for that matter, in France itself (cf. Chapter 4). Indeed, the (1975) Quebec Charter of Rights and Freedoms specifically recognizes that persons belonging to new minorities – who are termed 'cultural communities' in Quebec – have the right to continue to maintain and develop their own languages and cultures. This was followed by a 1978 White Paper, 'La politique québécoise du développement culturel', which stipulated a clear and active role for the state in support of minority languages and cultures. It was further formalized by the 1981 Quebec government publication *Autant de façons d'être Québécois* which promoted the notion of 'interculturalism' as a stronger form of multiculturalism, specifically stating that its central aim was 'to ensure the survival and development of [Quebec's] cultural communities as well as their individuality' (cited in Handler, 1988: 178; see also Gagnon, 2000).

In other words, the specific protections set in place for other language speakers within Quebec specifically allow for the legitimation and institutionalization of French, the majority language *within Quebec*, alongside the promotion of wider cultural and linguistic pluralism (Larrivée, 2003; Kymlicka, 2007). One might add here that this formal promotion of French in the civic realm also constitutes a central part of the wider political question raised by Francophones' *minority* position within Canada – a position confirmed by the UNHRC case, discussed earlier. As such, it is entirely consistent with the granting of promotion-oriented rights in international law to minority language speakers, where numbers warrant (cf. Chapter 5). In this respect, the questions raised here are inevitably related to the broader issue of the degree to which Francophone speakers in Quebec (and elsewhere in Canada) can maintain their autonomy, and the language and cultural rights attendant on this, as a legitimate part of the historical power-sharing agreement with Anglophone Canadians. Any ongoing discontents concern the *failure* adequately to ensure these protections; a failure, moreover, that continues to be evidenced in Canada by the ongoing decline of French in the majority of those provinces that do not accord French civic status. As a result, nearly one-third of Francophones (that is, those of French Canadian ancestry) outside of Quebec no longer speak French. Indeed, rates of assimilation in some areas are as high as 75 percent (see Joy, 1992; Cardinal, 1999, 2005, 2007).

Catalonia: the quest for political and linguistic autonomy

Catalonia presents us with another example of the successful reinstantiation of a minority language in the civic realm. Since 1979, Catalonia has first successfully re-established and then entrenched its minority Catalan cultural and language rights as one of the seventeen 'autonomías' (autonomous regions) of the post-Franco multinational Spanish state. The Catalonian Generalitat (regional government) has achieved this via the multilateral recognition afforded different regions by the (1978) Spanish Constitution (see below). But it has also been a leading supporter of Europeanization and, within the narrow constraints of the intergovernmental system of policy-making, has participated as fully as possible in the formal workings of the EU (Keating, 1996, 1997, 2009). These developments at the regional or sub-state level have thus provided considerable scope and institutional space for the re-emergence of Catalan as the language of the civic or public realm in Catalonia, after its long-standing proscription under the Franco regime, albeit, as we shall see, not without opposition still from the wider Spanish state. Indeed, as with Quebec, the often-strident opposition to these developments also illustrates clearly the unevenness with which minority nationalisms are treated in comparison with their majoritarian counterparts.

Catalan is a regional majority language in the area of Catalonia (Catalunya in Catalan), which currently boasts over 9 million speakers in Catalonia and throughout Europe. It is currently spoken outside of Catalonia in Valencia, the Balearic Islands, Andorra, the city of l'Alguer in Sardinia, and the French Departement of Pyrénées-Orientales (also known as the French Roussillon) (see Fishman, 1991). However, it also clearly remains a minority language in relation to the wider Spanish state in which it is situated. Strubell (1998) argues in fact that Catalan is unique within Europe because it is the only language of that size that has managed to survive the last three centuries of nation-state ideology – what I termed in Chapter 3, the 'philosophical matrix of the nation-state' – without actually having a state to back it. It is also the only language in that circumstance that has also not entered into an irreversible demographic decline (although, as we shall see, it has clearly suffered periods of decline). A large part of the reason for the resilience of Catalan has to do with its prominent role in the long history of Catalonia that can trace its roots back to before the tenth century (Castells, 1997). This history, in turn, is characterized by a repeated quest for greater political and linguistic autonomy for Catalonia, often in the face of highly centralist policies that actively repressed Catalan political institutions, and the Catalan language along with it.

The rise and fall of Catalunya

In the tenth century, the territory now known as Catalonia gained de facto independence from the Franks (Miller and Miller, 1996), while the actual name of 'Catalunya', as a political entity with its own language, was first recorded in 1176 (Hoffmann, 1999). By the thirteenth and fourteenth centuries, Catalonia, as part of the Kingdom of Aragon, had established itself as a maritime and Mediterranean region of some considerable influence and power. In the process, it had incorporated Mallorca (1229), Valencia (1238), Sicily (1282), Sardinia (1323) and Naples (1442), as well as parts of Greece (including Athens) and Roussillon beyond the Pyrénées in modern-day France. Catalan had also become well established by that time, having emerged from the fragmentation of Latin to become one of the original Romance languages, along with, among others, Galician and Castilian (Spanish). Indeed, by the thirteenth century, Catalan had already replaced Latin as the language of record within the Catalonian region – providing us with the first European feudal code in a vernacular language, the oldest European maritime code, and the first Romance language to be used in science and philosophy (Fishman, 1991).

Catalonia, and Catalan, began to decline in power and influence, however, from the time of the 1412 Compromiso de Caspe between Catalonia and Castile. The process of political convergence the agreement initiated was meant to see the language, customs and institutions of each region respected. However, this did not prove to be the case. Guided by the power and wealth of the Spanish Crown, and the fundamentalist Catholic Church of the Counter-Reformation, Castile quickly adopted a centralist approach to governance. This led eventually to the rebellion of Catalonia and Portugal in 1640 against the then Spanish King Philip IV. While Portugal, supported by the English, succeeded in gaining its independence, Catalonia was defeated, with the consequence of the loss of most of its political freedoms (although it retained Catalan as its official language). The defeat inevitably fueled further discontent, and Catalonia again attempted to regain greater autonomy via the Spanish War of Succession (1705–14), siding with the Austrians against Philip V. But Catalonia was again defeated, following the siege of Barcelona in 1714. As a consequence, it lost all its political institutions of self-government – established as we have seen, since the early

Middle Ages – with Philip V abolishing the Catalan Parliament (the Corts) and government (Diputació Generalitat) of the time (Strubell, 1998). At the same time, a history of 500 years of Catalan as the official language of Catalonia was brought unceremoniously to an end. The ensuing period thus saw Catalonia's first experience of active institutional, cultural and linguistic repression from a centralized Spanish state. It was not to be its last. In this period, the wider Spanish state attempted to replace Catalan with Castilian, progressively proscribing Catalan as the language of administration, the language of commerce and the language of education. In the end, the only domains left to Catalan were the family and the church (Castells, 1997). Consequently, the nobility, higher clergy, military and civil servants quickly became completely 'Castilianized'. The middle classes retained spoken Catalan for informal use and only the illiterate rural population remained monolingual in Catalan (Hoffmann, 1999). Catalan thus experienced the usual processes of stigmatization and peripheralization associated with the 'minoritization' of a language by a hegemonic state (cf. Chapter 4).

These setbacks were ameliorated somewhat in the nineteenth century, when Catalonia successfully industrialized, one of the few areas of Spain to do so. Industrialization contributed to the rise of a strong middle class and established a pattern that was to characterize Catalonia's position within the wider Spanish state until well into the twentieth century. In effect, while Catalonia remained politically marginalized, it increasingly became the economic powerhouse of Spain. Meanwhile, though Catalan continued to be formally banned from the civic realm, it (re)gained credence as the preferred language of a highly educated and economically successful Catalan bourgeoisie. The nineteenth-century Catalan language movements, Renaixença and Modernista, also reaffirmed the status of Catalan. These cultural nationalist movements emphasized the long (and strong) historical links of the language with a cosmopolitan political administration, and a high-status culture, and promoted the widespread use of Catalan in literary fields, journalism and education. Catalan thus came to be increasingly viewed as the focal point, and principal medium of expression, of Catalan cultural nationalism (Miller and Miller, 1996). This emphasis was further bolstered at the beginning of the twentieth century when, as a result largely of this cultural nationalism, the language was standardized and modernized (Yates, 1998; DiGiacomo, 1999).

From Franco to federalism

If the nineteenth century saw Catalan regain some of its lost cultural and linguistic status, the early twentieth century saw Catalonia re-establish its political status on two occasions, albeit briefly in both instances. In 1914–25, Catalonia was granted a degree of home rule under the presidency of Enric Prat de la Riba. However, the first of Spain's twentieth-century dictators, Primo de Rivera, who led a successful military coup in 1923, quickly returned Catalonia to centralized Spanish control. The Second Republic (1931–6) restored a degree of political autonomy to Catalonia – granting it a Statute of Autonomy in 1932, while at the same time granting Catalan co-official language status. But this was also to be short-lived. With the success of Franco in the Spanish Civil War (1936–9), Catalonia was subjected once again to absolute political, cultural and linguistic repression – this time for a period of nearly forty years. Catalonia's political autonomy was annulled and the region was divided into four provinces administered by the central government in Madrid. As I have already briefly discussed in Chapter 5, Franco's years of repression also included the official proscription of Catalan in all public domains – administration, commerce, education, the media and even, this time, the church – and the ruthless enforcement of these linguistic strictures. Even Catalan names and toponyms were banned and replaced by Spanish equivalents. Catalan itself was declared a 'mere dialect' and official propaganda of the period described its speakers as 'barking like dogs' or as 'non-Christian' (Fishman, 1991). Only after some twenty years were these restrictions eased, at least to a degree, with some latitude allowed for the use of Catalan within the church. By 1970 an education law permitting the teaching of (but not in) Catalan was also proposed, but was not actually implemented until 1975, the year of Franco's death (Fishman, 1991). These late and limited concessions aside, Franco's 'glorioso Movimiento nacional' was clearly a centralist Spanish nationalist movement that had as a key aim the repression of Catalan, and its replacement with Castilian Spanish or 'la lengua del Imperio' (Strubell, 1998).

One consequence of Franco's years of repression, and his centralist Spanish nationalism, was the further strengthening of Catalan cultural nationalism, with the Catalan language its leitmotif and point of resistance. Anti-state nationalism was also a feature of the Basque Country, which was similarly oppressed by Franco. However, Basque nationalism has been preoccupied primarily with the question of secession, seen most prominently in the longstanding terrorist activities of the ETA movement (Euzkadi 'ta Askatasuna). Catalan nationalism, in contrast, has always sought greater political autonomy *within* Spain, rather than secession as such, in line with the key tenets of cultural nationalism discussed in Chapter 2 (see also Conversi, 1997; Grugel and Rees, 1997; Guibernau, 2004).

Despite the growing strength of Catalan cultural nationalism, and the fact that the language continued to be spoken privately by a wealthy middle class, Catalan did inevitably suffer at the hands of Franco. There was an undeniable negative impact on Catalan use, and even Catalan competence, among native Catalan speakers (Fishman, 1991). Generations of Catalans were taught to be literate only in Castilian Spanish, while the scope and functions of Catalan were inevitably delimited, preventing the language from adapting to new situations and communicative requirements (Hoffmann, 1999). The influx of Spanish-speaking migrants from other areas of Spain over this period, who came seeking work in Catalonia's prosperous industries, was also to have a major impact on the health of the Catalan language. Since the rise of industrialization, in-migration from other areas of Spain had always been on a much smaller scale, with the result that most in-migrants were able to adopt successfully dual Catalan and Spanish identities. This was particularly the case during the two previous periods of political autonomy in the twentieth century, where the Catalan language was actively promoted, principally via education, and was seen by in-migrants as the language of social mobility. The combination of Franco's repression, which meant in-migrants had no incentive to learn Catalan, and the sheer scale of in-migration, particularly during the period 1950–75, was to change all this. Thus, the number of Catalan speakers in Catalonia fell from 90 percent in 1939 to 60 percent in 1975 (Miller and Miller, 1996). The period also saw the establishment of linguistic differences along broadly class lines, as the in-migrants who spoke Castilian Spanish were predominantly working class, while Catalan remained a language of prestige closely associated with the economically prosperous middle class. This ongoing association of Catalan with economic dominance, even during the years of its political marginalization, is certainly a key factor in its survival – amounting, in effect, to a form of reverse diglossia within Catalonia (although, of course, not within Spain itself). But the class-based juxtaposition of Catalan and Castilian Spanish was also to have its own deleterious consequences in the subsequent re-establishment of Catalan within Catalonia post-Franco, as we shall see.

After the death of Franco, democracy was quickly restored to Spain and a new Constitution agreed by all the main political parties that emerged from the first democratic election, a not inconsiderable achievement in itself. But more radically still, the (1978) Spanish Constitution moved away, to some considerable extent, from the centralist and overtly assimilationist policies that had dominated Spanish politics for so much of the preceding two centuries – most starkly under Franco. In this respect, the Constitution accomplished a delicate balancing act. On the one hand, it continued to emphasize the ongoing unity and social cohesion characteristic of the traditional centralist conception of the (Spanish) nation-state, what I described as 'civism' in Chapter 3. This was most notable in its proclamation of Spanish as the sole official language of Spain, to be spoken by all its citizens. On the other hand, the Constitution also specifically recognized Spain's cultural and linguistic pluralism – granting specific cultural and linguistic rights, as well as a considerable degree of political autonomy, to the different historical ethnies within the Spanish state. The latter moved Spain much closer to the model of a multinational (and multilingual) state. Article 2 of the Constitution encapsulates both these features:

The Constitution is founded upon the indissoluble unity of the Spanish nation [sic], the common and indivisible patria of all Spaniards, and recognizes and guarantees the right to autonomy of all the nationalities and regions integrated in it and the solidarity among them. (Cited in Guibernau, 1997: 93)

On this basis, the seventeen Spanish 'autonomías' were subsequently established, with varying degrees of devolution and autonomy. Those granted the greatest degree of political autonomy – termed 'autonomías históricas' – included Catalonia, the Basque Country and Galicia. These three regions were regarded as having the strongest historical claims to a separate identity, based centrally on their language and culture. They had also enjoyed political autonomy (in the case of Catalonia) in the Second Republic (1931–6), or would have (in the case of the Basque Country and Galicia) had the Spanish Civil War not intervened. Consequently, Catalonia was the first of the autonomías to be so recognized when it was granted its Statute of Autonomy in 1979, while the Basque Country and Galicia followed in 1980.[9]

The 1979 Catalan Statute of Autonomy is significant for its stress on the historical origins of Catalonia, particularly its language and culture, *coupled with* their restoration within a specifically modern and modernizing democratic political project. These are both key attributes, as I argued in Chapter 2, of cultural nationalism. Thus the Preamble states: 'In the process of regaining their democratic freedom, the people of Catalonia also recover their institutions of self-government' (cited in Guibernau, 1997: 94). The Statute is also significant for its specific recognition of collective identity and freedom – or more accurately, group-differentiated rights, as envisaged by Kymlicka (cf. Chapter 3) – a recognition that is implicit in the following:

The *collective freedom* of Catalonia finds in the institutions of the 'Generalitat' [government] a link with a long history of emphasis on and respect for the fundamental rights and public freedoms of individuals *and peoples*: a history which the people of Catalonia wish to continue, in order to make possible the creation of a forward-looking democratic society. (Cited in Guibernau, 1997: 95; my emphases)

A concrete example of just such a group-differentiated right is the right to speak Catalan within Catalonia. Here the 1979 Statute is unequivocal, asserting that Catalan is 'la llengua pròpia de Catalunya' (Catalonia's own language) and that 'Catalan is the official language of Catalonia as Castilian is the official language of the whole of the Spanish state' (Art. 3.2; cited in Artigal, 1997: 135; Guibernau, 1997: 96). But as we already know, the legitimation of a language (though important) is one thing, its institutionalization quite another (cf. Chapter 4). The Statute thus also stipulates a specific plan of action:

> The Generalitat ... will guarantee the normal and official use of both languages, adopt whatever measures are deemed necessary to ensure both languages are known, and create suitable conditions so that full equality between the two can be achieved as far as the rights and duties of the citizens of Catalonia are concerned. (Art 3.3; cited in Strubell, 1998: 163)

As Strubell proceeds to observe, this amounts to a clear social contract between Catalan and Spanish speakers – a process of mutual language accommodation that is evident only in Stage 6 of Churchill's typology, as discussed in Chapter 5. The task of bringing this about was given to the center-right nationalist coalition Covergencia i Unio (CiU), led by Jordi Pujol and elected to lead the Generalitat in the first post-democratic regional elections in 1980. The CiU remained in power continuously from 1980 to 2003, and regained power in 2010.[10] It insists on the distinct political character of Catalonia, but emphasizes that this can be effectively maintained within the multinational Spanish state, rather than by secession (see Guibernau, 1997, 2004, for extended discussion). The CiU also places considerable store on the importance of fostering and maintaining a distinct Catalan identity. Its definition of who is Catalan includes all those who live and work in Catalonia – no ethnic, religious or racialized distinctions are made. But the CiU does add the key caveat 'and wants to be Catalan', and the sign of 'wanting to be' Catalan is to learn to speak the language (Castells, 1997).[11] As Pujol, the former longstanding leader of CiU, asserted: 'our identity as a country, our will to be, and our perspectives for the future depend on the preservation of our language' (cited in Guibernau, 1997: 101). Much like the efforts of the Partí Québécois in Quebec to establish French as a 'langue publique commune', the subsequent political focus of the CiU has been on both maximizing Catalonia's political autonomy within Spain and re-establishing Catalan fully as the language of the state and civil society.

The quest for greater political autonomy is demonstrated by the considerable (opponents would say, disproportionate) influence that the CiU has wielded at the level of Spanish national politics over the last thirty years. For example, the CiU formed a coalition with the Spanish Socialist (PSOE) government in 1993, and then with the conservative Partido Popular (PP) when they first came to power in 1996, after both had failed to gain a working majority on their own. In both instances, Pujol was able to extract significant concessions that further bolstered Catalonian autonomy – for example, being granted direct control of 30 percent of its income taxes, as well as exclusive control of education, health, environment, communications, tourism, culture social services and most police functions (Castells, 1997). The granting of these further concessions to Catalonian autonomy was all the more remarkable in the latter instance, given that the conservative PP initially campaigned for the retrenchment of devolution, and against the perceived 'nationalisms' of autonomous regions.

With the fall of the CiU as the ruling party in Catalonia in 2003, their influence on Spanish national politics has obviously been far more attenuated over the last ten years. However, having regained regional control in 2010, and with national elections scheduled for 2012, their national influence may again become more significant. The success of the CiU over the years might also explain why the civic culture of Catalonia leaves little room for extremism. In this respect, separatist groups continue to have only a small following in Catalonia, in sharp contrast to the Basque Country (Conversi, 1997). Indeed, as a 1982 survey found, Catalans self-identify most often as 'equally Catalan and Spanish' (Stepan, 1998), seeing no necessary contradiction between the two forms of identity (see my discussion of multiple identities in Chapter 2). This was also confirmed by a subsequent survey in 1990, which indicated that Catalans continued to remain largely skeptical of independence as a feasible or necessary political option for Catalonia (Strubell, 1998).[12]

The re-establishment of Catalan as a civic language, which I will focus upon in what follows, has been achieved by embarking on an extensive language status-planning program within Catalonia itself. The principal instrument of this program, at least initially, was the (1983) Llei de Normalització Lingüística (Law of Linguistic Normalization), also known as the 'Charter of the Catalan Language'.

Linguistic normalization

Linguistic normalization in the Catalonian context was first described by the Congress of Catalan Culture (1975–7) as 'a process during which a language gradually recovers the formal functions it [has] lost and at the same time works its way into those social sectors, within its own territory, where it was not spoken before' (cited in Torres, 1984: 59). In this light, and following Fishman (1991), the process of linguistic normalization subsequently embarked on in Catalonia can be described as having three broad initial aims:

1   to achieve the symbolic promotion and functional institutionalization of Catalan in all key public and private language domains;
2   to redress illiteracy in Catalan, and any remaining sense of inferiority attached to Catalan, both legacies of the Franco years; and
3   via a 'policy of persuasion' (Woolard, 1989), to gain the commitment of first language Spanish speakers to Catalan, while at the same time countering any hostility toward Catalan as a perceived 'threat' to Spanish as the language of the Spanish state.

Over the course of the last thirty years, Catalonia has been largely successful in achieving the first two objectives, although, as we shall see, the third still remains contested. Today Catalonian citizens have the right to use Catalan on all (public and private) occasions, while virtually all written and oral work in the Generalitat and local authorities is now undertaken in Catalan. For example, a 1991 census found that 94 percent understood, 68 percent spoke and 40 percent could write in Catalan (Artigal, 1997), a considerably more favorable position for the language than in 1975 (see above).[13] Of course, these changes did not happen overnight and the most prominent feature of Catalan language planning, particularly in its early stages, was its graduated approach. Education provides us with a representative example here (see Miller and Miller, 1996; Artigal, 1997; Mar-Molinero, 2000).

Catalan language education

Catalan was legally reinstated as a language that could be taught in schools in 1978, although this was largely limited, at least initially, to teaching Catalan as a subject (in 1978, only 3.3 percent of schools actually taught in Catalan). Nonetheless, this initial development acknowledged the possibility in the longer term of extending teaching in Catalan – that is, the more widespread adoption of group maintenance bilingual programs. The latter possibility was further solidified in the (1983) Law of Linguistic Normalization which stated categorically: 'Education centres are obliged to make Catalan the normal vehicle of expression' (cited in Webber and Strubell, 1991: 34). Thus, from 1983 to 1993, Catalan was given priority in education. Three models were available at preschool and elementary schools, described by Artigal (1997) as 'predominantly Catalan-medium', 'bilingual instruction' and 'predominantly Spanish-medium'. The first approach was encouraged wherever possible, although schools always had the final choice of which language education approach to adopt (at secondary level, the choice of language medium remained entirely open). Nonetheless, nearly 90 percent of preschools and elementary schools did in fact opt for predominantly Catalan-medium programs, not least because of the wide and careful dissemination of their educational advantages to both parents and teachers. Drawing in particular on the experiences of Canadian French-immersion programs, the Catalonian Department of Education argued that the formal promotion of Catalan within schools, as the still socially weaker language, would allow Spanish speakers to become bilingual, given that Spanish remained dominant in the wider social setting. This obviated the (misplaced) fear of many Castilian Spanish-speaking parents that immersion in Catalan might have led to their children losing their Spanish. These developments were supported by an extensive program of in-service language support for teachers (itself part of a wider program within the civil service), given the initial lack of Catalan-speaking teachers. Bilingual textbooks and other supporting curriculum materials were also developed over this period, along with training in the theory and methodology of bilingual/immersion language education.

These developments were consolidated in 1993 by the implementation of a single model of Catalan immersion for all schools at preschool and elementary/ primary levels (although at secondary level free choice continued). This extension of Catalan immersion programs was predicated, in turn, on the demonstrable success of such programs over the preceding decade in teaching Spanish-speaking students Catalan, particularly in the industrialized, predominantly Spanish working-class areas where Catalan had very little social presence. There remained some element of choice within the preschool/elementary program, as Spanish-speaking parents could demand that the first stage of teaching (from 3 to 7 years old) be in Spanish, with only the minimum of Catalan required by law. This provision was limited to individual families, however, and involved individual, rather than classroom-based, instruction. Subsequently, the unified nature of the Catalan immersion system was reinforced by the implementation of the (1998) Catalan Linguistic Policy Act – although, as we shall see, not without controversy.

The Catalan Linguistic Policy Act: controversy and contention

The (1998) Catalan Linguistic Policy Act had three main objectives. The first was to support the legal consolidation of Catalan language policies in schools and the wider civil service, the former by fully implementing the unified Catalan immersion education approach, the latter by further strengthening formal Catalan language requirements for civil servants working in the Generalitat and in local authorities. The second objective was to increase the presence of Catalan in the media and commerce fields (in which Spanish remained dominant), principally via the introduction of minimum Catalan language quota systems in the media, and the requirement of bilingual service provision in the commercial sector (Costa, 2003; Pujolar, 2007). With respect to business, for example, the Act specifically called for private companies to implement programs and measures in support of the further use of Catalan at work. The third objective of the Act was a more broad-based one, to achieve full equality or comparability between Catalan and Spanish in all formal language domains. This included not only the devolved areas of administration regarded as the responsibility of the Generalitat but also those areas that still remain under the jurisdiction of the Spanish central government, notably the judicial system, law and order, and tax administration (Costa, 2003).

'Igual que Franco pero al revés: persecución del castellano en Cataluña'

While the (1993) Law of Linguistic Normalization was primarily concerned with the extension of the knowledge of Catalan within Catalonia, particularly within education and the wider civil service, the (1998) Catalan Linguistic Policy Act focused on the further extension of its legal status and institutional reach. These measures constituted, in effect, the 'next stage' of the legitimation and institutionalization of Catalan within Catalonia – adopting a more promotion-oriented language right for Catalan. This involved, in turn, a movement away from the previous gradualist, 'politics of persuasion' approach to one much closer to the Quebec model of legislative enforcement, à la Bill 101 (Charte de la langue française, 1977). Inevitably, such a 'change of pace' generated controversy and opposition, despite the widespread acceptance of Catalan language measures up to that point. However, a significant feature of this opposition was that it was largely initiated and fostered from elsewhere in Spain, rather than from within Catalonia itself. It also tended to be firmly located within a broader conservative political agenda advocating the return of a traditional centralist Spanish nationalism, and a related retrenchment of regional autonomy (DiGiacomo, 1999; Guibernau, 2004). Thus Catalan language laws, as the most visible manifestation of an alternative Catalan nationalism, and as a demonstrable example of the wider federalism of Spain, have become something of a bête noire for these traditional Spanish nationalists. Before proceeding to a brief analysis of their campaign, I should point out that these Spanish nationalists almost never actually see themselves as such – their avowedly 'anti-nationalist' stance with respect to regional nationalisms obviously does not extend to a critique of their own (DiGiacomo, 1999; Mar-Molinero, 2000). The subsumption of majoritarian forms of nationalism at work here is a process we saw Billig describe in Chapter 2 as 'banal nationalism' where the nationalism of the dominant ethnie 'not only ceases to be nationalism ... it ceases to be a problem for investigation' (1995: 17). There are none so blind, it seems, as those who cannot see.

The campaign mounted against Catalan language laws was a key feature of the political rhetoric of the right-wing PP when it was in power from 1996 to 2004. Opposition to regional nationalisms has continued to form part of its political platform in opposition since that time (see below). And it was also reflected in the presumption, regularly trumpeted in the Spanish media, that the ongoing promotion of Catalan constituted a direct threat to the primacy of Castilian Spanish, and of the language choices of Spanish speakers. The general tenor of this campaign is captured well by the banner headline in a national Spanish paper, the right-wing ABC daily, in 1993: 'Igual que Franco pero al revés: persecución del castellano en Cataluña' [The same as Franco but the other way round: the persecution of Castilian [Spanish] in Catalonia] (quoted in Mar-Molinero, 2000: 163). The inference here is abundantly clear – minority language rights constitute 'special treatment' and may well be illiberal (cf. Chapter 3). Consequently, much of the subsequent vocal and often vituperative debates on Catalan language laws have focused on the supposed threat they pose to the right to speak the majority language, Spanish. In this respect, opponents of the Catalan language laws have termed themselves, without any degree of irony it seems, 'bilingüistas' (see Strubell, 1998). I say without any degree of irony because, as with the comparable campaigns in North America, these critics are specifically *not* arguing for bilingualism at all but, rather, for the right of majority Spanish speakers to remain monolingual.

Thus, when the single model of Catalan immersion education was first adopted in 1993, opponents took the Catalonian government to the Spanish Constitutional Court, arguing that the measure contravened the individual language right to speak Spanish, enshrined within the Spanish Federal Constitution. Unfortunately for the plaintiffs, the Constitutional Court ruled in December 1994 that the Catalan immersion education model *was* constitutional, given that its stated aim was the acquisition of both Catalan and Spanish, and given that this goal is clearly reached because of the broad presence of Spanish in the wider social milieu (see Artigal, 1997: 140). This particular decision was broadly congruent with a previous one reached by the same Court in February 1991, concerning the formal requirement of a working knowledge of Catalan within the civil service in Catalonia. Catalan language opponents had also argued before the Court on that occasion that such a requirement discriminated against Spanish speakers on the grounds of language, while limiting the freedom of movement that the Spanish Constitution guarantees all its citizens. However, the Constitutional Court ruled that the command of an official language within a given autonomous region was neither an unreasonable nor disproportionate requirement (Miller and Miller, 1996). Returning to Kymlicka's distinction, discussed in Chapter 3, internal restrictions imposed by Catalan language laws were deemed not to be so great as to render those laws, and their basis as an external protection, illiberal.

These early legal setbacks, however, have not stopped opponents of the language laws from relitigating these whenever they could. The most notable recent example of this ongoing contest has centered on the revision and replacement of the 1979 Statute of Autonomy with the 2006 Catalan Statute of Autonomy. The 2006 Statute of Autonomy consolidated and extended key areas of regional autonomy, including Catalan language and education. It grew out of an influential 'Report on the Reform of the Statute of Catalonia' in 2004 by the Institut d'Estudis Autonomics, which highlighted a range of limitations in relation to the regional autonomy allowed by the original 1979 Statute. These included an ongoing lack of recognition of Catalonia as a 'nation' and a lack of bilateral negotiation over regional funding, particularly taxation.

Throughout 2004 and 2005, intense, often controversial, negotiations occurred between Catalan regional political parties and the central government, by then led by the Spanish Socialist Party (PSOE) under Prime Minister Rodriguez Zapatero (for an extended discussion and analysis, see Colino, 2009).

Much of the controversy focused on the inclusion of 'nation' in the new statute, which was eventually deemed unconstitutional, as well as proposed bilateral relationships and the new funding arrangements. However, a compromise was duly fashioned between the Catalan parties and the central government, and adopted in March 2006. Up to 2010, seven other statutes of autonomy throughout Spain have been similarly revised, while Catalonia itself has implemented over forty new laws in relation to the newly revised Catalan Statute.

The key aspects of the 2006 Catalan Statute emphasize a separate regional identity, distinct from the Spanish state, with notions of national identity included (by way of compromise) in the Preamble rather than the text itself. This wider reassertion of regional autonomy further entrenched the language policy developed by Catalonia over the last thirty years. As Colino summarizes it:

> Following the notion that Catalan is Catalonia's only 'proper' language, considering Spanish as simply the official state language, the new statute establishes Catalan as the language of preferential use in public administration bodies, in the public media and as the language of normal use for instruction in the education system, now extending this to university education. … [it requires citizens] to know the regional language … thus equalizing its status with that of Spanish in the constitution. It also introduces the so-called obligation of linguistic availability, which imposes the obligation for businesses and establishments of answering its users or consumers in the language of their choice. (2009: 275)

The new Statute also fueled ongoing debate about the rights of Spanish speakers in Catalonia. For example, a longstanding criticism of opponents of Catalan language laws is that they specifically 'disenfranchise' Spanish-speaking in-migrants to the region by delimiting access to Spanish as the wider language of the state (much like the arguments vis-à-vis French and English in Quebec). This argument is also linked specifically to class as well as linguistic discrimination, given that, as we have seen, the majority of in-migrants are working-class and the majority of Catalan speakers are middle-class and economically prosperous.

But the clear weight of evidence in debates on Catalan language laws suggests that the arguments of these oppositionalists are almost entirely invalid. For a start, most in-migrants still actively accept and support 'Catalanization' policies (Keating, 1997; Strubell, 1998; Guibernau, 2004). Meanwhile, the formal promotion of Catalan does *not* threaten either the position of Spanish or the rights of Spanish speakers. Unlike Quebec's formal exclusion of English in commerce and advertising for example, Spanish has never been officially proscribed in Catalonia in any domain (not least because the Spanish Constitution forbids it), nor for that matter has any other language. Indeed, Spanish is specifically enshrined as the *only* official language of the *whole* Spanish state, while Catalan only has co-official rights within the autonomous region of Catalonia. And Spanish still remains the dominant language in the media, as well as in fields such as justice, commerce and taxation within Catalonia. As Yates sensibly concludes, 'by any objective standards, Catalan is still a subordinate language in a process of "reverse shift", with a long way to go towards normalization in key areas' (1998: 207) – an observation that still holds true today.

If there is a valid point to be made in relation to the language claims of 'immigrants' within Catalonia, it is not one made by opponents of the Catalan laws, nor is it about Spanish. Rather, it is that, prior to the 2006 Statute of Autonomy, the promotion of Catalan did not extend to the *active* recognition of other minority languages and cultures within Catalonia, 'where numbers warrant'. This is equivalent to Stage 5 of Churchill's minority language typology, as discussed in Chapter 5. In this respect, there have been long-settled communities of Roma in Catalonia, and more recent migrants from North Africa (Yates, 1998; Hoffmann, 1999; Pujolar, 2007), whose languages and cultures were almost entirely ignored in the language debates of the 1980s and 1990s. There had been a few 'compensatory' (Stage 2) educational programs aimed at Roma during this period, but nothing more (Tarrow, 1992).

However, the 2006 Statute of Autonomy has begun to address this lacuna – at least in principle – by granting specific language rights to speakers other than Catalan. For example, the Statute extends promotion-oriented language rights within the region to the Aranese variant of Occitan, spoken in the subregion of Val d'Aran, and to Catalan sign language, both of which are elevated to co-official languages alongside Catalan and Spanish. The new statute also directly addresses the rights of other language speakers, particularly the growing number of Arabic and Urdu speakers who have migrated to the region in increasing numbers over the last decade. Specific tolerance-oriented language rights are now provided so that other language-speakers can maintain these languages privately, if they so choose, as well as ensuring access to key services and opportunities to learn the official languages of the region (París, 2007). While the institutional support attendant upon these rights is still limited, this clearly constitutes a significant development in broadening language rights and support mechanisms in Catalonia.

Be that as it may, the overall legitimacy and reach of the 2006 Statute of Autonomy remains an open question. As recently as July 2010, the Spanish Constitutional Court, in response to an appeal in 2006 from the Partido Popular, the right-wing opposition party, has overturned key aspects of the previously agreed 2006 Catalan Statute of Autonomy. The Court ruling, mired in four years of controversy and dominated currently by conservative (Spanish nationalist) judges, has revised aspects of the Statutes such that *any* notion of nationhood for Catalonia, even in conjunction with the Spanish state, is specifically excluded (Pericay, 2010). The Court acknowledges that Catalonia as a separate nation 'is a perfectly legitimate idea', but the judges still deemed it to have no legal basis (Krumova, 2010). Rather, the court asserts, 'Catalonia is a nationality' within 'the only and indissoluble Spanish nation [sic]'. Moreover, the recognition of Catalan as the official language of Catalonia is somewhat retrenched. The Catalan linguistic model has been retained (there were initial fears that even this would be dismantled). But in the end, the Court rejected the notion that Catalan was the region's 'only proper language', reducing the Catalan language to 'the main' language used by the public administration and by public media (Pericay, 2010).

These recent developments in Catalonia highlight, once again, that the validity of promotion-oriented language rights for national minorities remains controversial and contested, *even when* they are already well established. As with Quebec, ongoing opposition to promotion-oriented language rights is often couched in terms of individual rights – most usually, the right of majority language speakers (Spanish, in this case) to remain monolingual. Similarly, opposition is likely to become more intense when an initially gradualist consensus approach is superseded by a more legislatively enforceable one. But critics of the latter also presuppose that consensus, left to its own devices, will achieve the same result, albeit much more slowly (cf. Hoffmann, 1999, 2000). This is simply naive, not least because it ignores, or at least significantly underplays the ongoing powerful influence of the 'philosophical matrix of the nation-state' (see Chapter 3) to undermine and subvert such attempts. Similarly, the criticism of potential 'illiberality' needs to be applied equally to majoritarian language policies, and not just minority ones. After all, if Spanish speakers in Spain can regard the formal recognition of their language, within their own historic territory, as an inalienable right (with no question of illiberality), why cannot Catalans as well? All of these issues, and related controversies, are also clearly evident in the final case study that I want to examine here: the re-establishment of Welsh as a civic language of Wales.

Wales: the development of a bilingual state in a 'forgotten' nation

> The Welsh, as a people, were born disinherited.
>
> (Gwyn Williams, 1985: 45)

Wales is one of the three constituent nations of the multinational British state, alongside England and Scotland. If one adds Northern Ireland to this triumvirate we also get the United Kingdom (UK). But of these constituent members, Wales is the one most often overlooked. The difficulties in Northern Ireland dominated the British political landscape throughout the latter half of the twentieth century, as did the concerns of Ireland as a whole and 'Irish Home

Rule' in the nineteenth century. Scotland, though united by treaty with England in 1707, has since retained intact much of its civil society (including its own legal, church and education systems). Consequently, it has enjoyed a far greater degree of institutional autonomy, and therefore maintained a considerably higher profile within both British politics and the corpus of British history itself. And England, of course, has been the dominant partner – or simply, dominant – for much of the modern history of the British state. Which leaves Wales; unremarked and, to many, unremarkable.[14] As Kenneth Morgan, the noted Welsh historian, poignantly observes in an essay written in 1971 on the origins of Welsh nationalism: "'For Wales – see England". This notorious directive in the early editions of the *Encyclopaedia Britannica* crystallises all the emotion, the humiliation, and the patronising indifference which helped to launch the national movement in Wales' (1995: 197).

That these attitudes still linger on in Britain is clearly illustrated by the controversial English literary critic and columnist, A. N. Wilson. Writing in the London daily paper the *Evening Standard* in 1994, he commented disparagingly on the cultural contribution of the Welsh (or lack thereof) to British life:

> The Welsh have never made any significant contribution to any branch of knowledge, culture or entertainment. Choral singing – usually flat – seems to be their only artistic achievement. They have no architecture, no gastronomic tradition and, since the Middle Ages, no literature worthy of the name. Even their religion, Calvinistic Methodism, is boring. (Cited in Moss, 1994: 26)

The misplaced attempt at humor aside, Wilson's comments are simply wrong. The one thing, above all else, that *has* distinguished the Welsh from their other British partners has been their cultural distinctiveness; most significantly, their language. The fault lies then not so much with a lack of Welsh cultural expression, as Wilson speciously suggests, but with the failure historically to recognize and accord value to it. A key reason for this failure resides in the long history of political and institutional incorporation of Wales within the British state – a history that has only begun to change significantly with the advent of Welsh devolution in 1999.

Incorporating Wales

The degree of Welsh political incorporation into the British state is clearly illustrated by the administrative term 'England and Wales', employed to describe a wide range of shared institutions and programs. It is also exemplified by the fact that Wales was not recognized as a constituent nation of Britain until the late nineteenth century, the last of the constituent nations of Britain to be so.

Prior to this time, Britain was regarded for formal purposes as comprising only England, Scotland and Ireland. There simply was no 'Welsh question' in British politics comparable to the question of Irish Home Rule, for example, and the reiterated litany of British Westminster politicians was that 'there was no such place as Wales' (Morgan, 1995). Even the eventual recognition of Wales as a nation, in 1886, had its origins elsewhere, being precipitated by the Irish crisis of 1885–6. In the wake of the Irish crisis, Gladstone – the then British Prime Minister – was led to re-examine his assumptions and publicly recognize Welsh nationality for the first time (E. Williams, 1989).

The reasons for this reticence are not hard to find – long regarded as a 'non-historic nation', Wales was simply not seen as having a necessary, sufficient or legitimate claim to independent statehood. To this end, Friedrich Engels – whose views on non-historic nations we have already encountered in Chapter 1 – avers:

> The Highland Gaels and the Welsh are undoubtedly of different nationalities to what the English are, although nobody will give to these remnants of people long gone the title of nations [nation-states] ... [To do so would mean] the Welsh ..., if they desired it, would have an equal right to independent political existence, absurd though it be, with the English! The whole thing is absurdity. (1866; cited in Fishman, 1989e: 14)

Setting aside the clearly pejorative tone of Engels's assertions, there is some basis for this view. Wales was brought increasingly into the ambit of English rule from the time of the Norman King Edward I (1239–1307). The subsequent colonization of Wales in the fourteenth and fifteenth centuries led to the area's increasing Anglicization, particularly with respect to trade (Kearney, 2006). Relatedly, while much of Wales continued to speak Welsh – a language spoken since the sixth century and for which written records exist from the eighth century[15] – Welsh/English bilingualism became an increasing feature in these areas (P. Jenkins, 1992). These developments were the prelude to the region's formal incorporation within the British state in the sixteenth century. The (1536) Act of Union, and the related Act of 1542, instigated by Henry VIII (1491–1547), firmly situated Wales within the political, legal and administrative jurisdiction of the British Crown and Parliament. As a result of these Acts, the Welsh language was banned from the courts, and from all official domains, in favor of English, while virtually all separate Welsh institutions were eliminated (see also below).

The instructions of the Acts of Union directly affected only a small number of the Welsh elite – those who held or sought property or position. However, with the dismantling of any separate institutional focus, the establishment of a political norm soon became a powerful social norm as well (Butt Philip, 1975). As we saw Iris Marion Young observe in Chapter 3, if particular groups 'have greater economic, political or social power, their group related experiences, points of view, or cultural assumptions will tend to become the norm, biasing the standards or procedures of achievement and inclusion that govern social, political and economic institutions' (1993: 133). This describes well the English–Welsh relationship. In effect, the Welsh elite became assimilated into the English class and political system – adopting both the latter's mores and its language. Concomitantly, Welsh language and culture – still strongly evident among the peasantry (Y Werin) – were deemed of little value, both by the Welsh elite themselves and by the English political system to which they were increasingly beholden. As Morgan concludes of this: 'Wales continued to be regarded as a remote tribal backwater, economically backward, adhering obstinately to its antique language in the face of the "march of intellect"' (1995: 198).

It was not until the rise of religious Nonconformity in the early half of the nineteenth century, and the industrialization of Wales in the latter half, that this state of affairs was to change significantly. These two developments provided the basis for a new Welsh nationalist movement, which had as its principal focus the *re-establishment* of separate Welsh institutions and legislative measures. These were primarily cultural, religious and educational – reflecting the particular emphases of the nationalist movement of the time.[16]

Yet, despite these advances, the basic political and social organization of Wales still remained largely indistinguishable from England's. For example, it was not until 1956 that a Welsh capital (Cardiff) was officially designated. Indeed, it was only after the Second World War that a specifically Welsh institutional framework was to emerge. As Charlotte Davies (1989) argues, this development was tied principally to the expansion of the British welfare system, which saw many government departments reorganized on a regional basis. In most cases, Wales came to be treated as a single administrative unit, resulting in the steady growth of Welsh bureaucracy and, for the first time, a degree of coordinated economic planning in Wales. That said, such developments still fell well short of the idea of regional government in the wider European sense (Jones and Keating, 1995).

Easily the most prominent of the newly emergent regional organizations was the Welsh Office, established in 1964 and headed by a Welsh Secretary of State within the British cabinet. The Welsh Office was initially regarded as a symbolic rather than a substantive bearer of Welsh interests by the still highly centralist British government of the day. However, once established, it gradually began to aggrandize power (Charlotte Davies, 1989). This gradual enlargement of the Welsh Office's administrative responsibilities led, in turn, to the introduction of a range of legislative measures specific to Wales and, in particular, the Welsh language. These measures, which began to lay the basis for a bilingual state, included: the (1967) Welsh Language Act, offering 'equal validity' for English and Welsh in Wales; the (1988) Education Reform Act which incorporated a specifically Welsh (and Welsh language) dimension into the newly established National Curriculum for England and Wales; and the (1993) Welsh Language Act which extended the 1967 Act considerably in its support for Welsh in the public domain.

These developments were also initially supported, and expedited, by the emergence in the 1960s of Cymdeithas yr Iaith Gymraeg (the Welsh Language Society), an organization that employs non-violent direct action in support of the extension of Welsh in the civic realm (see Butt Philip, 1995; Gwyn Williams, 1985; Colin Williams, 1994). The activities of Cymdeithas yr Iaith Gymraeg contributed, at least in some measure, to the normalization of bilingual public signs, the establishment of Welsh-language media (notably, the Welsh-language television channel, Sianel Pedwar Cymru, S4C) as well as a Welsh Language Board, and to an increasing demand for public services available in Welsh.[17]

From the 1960s to the 1990s, the combination of top–down institutional infrastructure, via the Welsh Office, and the grassroots activism of Cymdeithas yr Iaith Gymraeg, resulted in the Welsh language becoming an increasing point of focus in debates about civic administration in Wales. This language focus has been further sharpened, and extended, over the last decade with the advent of Welsh devolution. In 1997, as part of a wider program of constitutional change implemented by the then newly elected British Labour Government, Wales, along with Scotland, voted in a referendum about devolution. While Scotland voted overwhelmingly for devolution (74.3 percent to 25.7 percent), Wales only did so by the narrowest of margins (50.3 to 49.7 percent; an actual majority of only 6,000). The closeness of the Welsh referendum notwithstanding, both institutions were formally established in 1999.[18]

The closeness of the Welsh referendum vote perhaps highlighted the ongoing consequences of the long history of political and institutional incorporation of Wales within Britain, with many within Wales still ambivalent at that time about the need for greater political autonomy. Another key issue, however, was the difference in what was on offer in terms of devolved government – again, a consequence of the different institutional histories of Wales and Scotland. Devolution saw Scotland establish a 129-seat Parliament, compared with only sixty seats for the National Assembly for Wales. More significantly, the Scottish Parliament could enact primary legislation and vary taxes. In contrast, while the National Assembly for Wales did assume responsibility for the administrative powers previously exercised by the Welsh Secretary of State, it had no legislative and tax varying powers beyond the enactment of secondary legislation. In short, the British Westminster Parliament still had the final say.

The relatively limited functions of devolved government in Wales at the time of devolution have since changed considerably. An independent review of the Assembly's functions, known after its chair as the Richard Commission (2003–4), recommended the extension of the Assembly's legislative remit and a more parliamentary-like structure. These recommendations were enacted via the (2006) Government of Wales Act, which transferred responsibility for the devolved (albeit, still secondary) legislation to the Welsh Assembly Government (WAG). Most significantly, however, has been the recent 'yes' vote in another referendum in March 2011, which provides the WAG with the authority to enact *primary* legislation in the areas in which it has devolved responsibilities, as with the Scottish Parliament.[19]

Thus, the long history of Wales's incorporation within Britain may finally be coming to an end – or, at least, has been put into reverse – as Wales (re)gains a significant degree of institutional autonomy within the British state for the first time since the sixteenth century. But this four-century history of incorporation has not always been disadvantageous to Wales. Indeed, it can be argued that its *political* incorporation has actually facilitated the *cultural* distinctiveness of the Welsh – principally, through the maintenance of their language and cultural traditions. Richard Jenkins (1991) argues, for example, that Welsh incorporation within the British state may have actually *created* the social and economic space within which the Welsh language and culture could survive. The Welsh language may have been formally proscribed from the civic realm from the time of the (1536) Act of Union, and may have been regarded, along with its culture, as antediluvian. However, it was not viewed as a threat to the state. In contrast, the far more problematic and contested political incorporation of Scotland and Ireland – and the close association of Gaelic language and culture in these areas with Catholicism – contributed, most likely, to the more rapid and widespread decline of the latter within the (Protestant) British state.

Vitiating Welsh

Be that as it may, the Anglicization of Wales remains a prominent feature of the nation's history. In this respect, the Welsh nationalist R. S. Thomas despondently observes of the English language: 'this is the major language, spoken by hundreds of millions of people with enormous resources devoted to it, that our small, bullied and embattled nation is called upon to maintain itself in the face of. And that is the way of it' (1992: 15). Although perhaps not entirely, since, at least prior to the twentieth century, the *spread* of English was not the crucial factor in the Anglicizing of Wales. Indeed, Wales remained 90 percent Welsh-speaking in the sixteenth and seventeenth centuries and as late as 1880 three out of four Welsh people still spoke the Welsh language by choice (Morgan, 1981). This compared dramatically with the mere 10 percent in Scotland who still spoke Gaelic (P. Jenkins, 1992) and, as we saw in Chapter 4, the even lower percentage in Ireland who still used Irish regularly by the end of the nineteenth century.

Rather, it has been the diminution of the status of Welsh and its restriction to private, low-status language domains which has proved to be more debilitating historically (cf. Chapter 4). It was this, more than anything else, which led to the rapid loss of the Welsh language over the course of the twentieth century. During this period, the once strong Welsh-speaking heartland (Y Fro Gymraeg) retreated in the face of English into the western and northern rural margins of Wales. This retreat was also reflected in the overall percentage of Welsh speakers in Wales. In 1911, 43.5 percent of the population spoke Welsh. In the 1991 census this had diminished to only 18.7 percent – approximately 600,000 speakers – although the 2001 census saw an improvement to 21 percent (Aitchison and Carter, 2004). Even so, Welsh monolingual speakers – who, in 1911, still constituted 8.5 percent of the population – have now all but disappeared. As one might expect, virtually all Welsh speakers today are bilingual in English as well.

The attrition of the Welsh language, however, is by no means a recent historical phenomenon, beginning as early as the Norman colonization of Wales in the late eleventh century. During that time, the prestige languages were Latin and French and to speak a local vernacular language such as Welsh was seen as a mark of bondage (Kearney, 2006). Consequently, Latin and French quickly acquired the status of formal languages of administration and documentation in Wales, a mantle that English would assume by the fourteenth century. This marked the first significant restriction of Welsh within formal language domains, since previously Welsh had been used as the language of customary law. Thus, with the emasculation of legal and administrative systems in Welsh, such as they were, only the literary tradition remained as a formal linguistic indicator of Welshness (Aitchison and Carter, 1994).

The (1536) Act of Union formalized the complete exclusion of Welsh from the public realm, making English the sole language of government. In so doing, the Act was unequivocal about the obstacle that Welsh presented to the successful incorporation of Wales within Britain:

> because the people of [Wales] have and do daily use a speech nothing like … the natural mother tongue used within this Realm [England] … to reduce them to perfect order notice, and knowledge of the laws of this, his Realm … *and utterly to extirpate all and singular the sinister usages and customs differing from the same* … bringing all the citizens of this Realm to amiable concord and unity. … From henceforth, no person or persons that use the Welsh speech or language shall have or enjoy any manor, office or fees … unless he or they use and exercise the speech or language of English. (Acts of Incorporation of Wales with England, 1536, cited in Williams and Raybould, 1991: 2; my emphasis)

The effect of the Act was to exclude Welsh from the public realm for the next four centuries. The only formal arena where the Welsh language continued to be recognized was the church. Ironically, this was because Henry VIII's successor,

Elizabeth I, had authorized a Welsh translation of the Bible in 1563. While this authorization of the Welsh translation of the Bible might appear contrary in intent to the preceding Act of Union it was not actually so. The principal reason for the concession – as for the Act – had to do with facilitating integration of the Welsh into Britain. More pertinently, the authorization was *not* an endorsement of the Welsh language but was, again, specifically assimilationist in intent. The provisions for the authorization state clearly that its purpose was 'such as do not understand the said Language [Welsh] may be conferring both Tongues together, the sooner attain to the Knowledge of the English Tongue' (cited in Jones, 1997: 15). In this it was to some extent successful, since bilingualism became an increasing feature of life in Wales from this time. However, it also had the effect of maintaining the Welsh language in the face of English – something not countenanced by its proposers. Indeed, the translation, which was to emerge subsequently in 1588, became the 'sheet-anchor' of the language (Gwyn Williams, 1985). Crucially, it allowed Welsh to remain a standardized literary language, with the *capacity* to be used in any domain (even if it was not so used). The literary standard provided by the 1588 translation thus prevented the language from diverging into mutually incomprehensible dialects and/or atrophying altogether (Morgan, 1981).

That said, the Welsh language continued to face considerable opposition and consistent negative attribution as a perceived low-status language. While Wales remained predominantly Welsh-speaking up until the advent of the twentieth century, the Welsh landed gentry were the first to adopt English as first an additional and then a substitute language. This pattern was well established by the eighteenth century (P. Jenkins, 1992). Concomitantly, the use of Welsh was invariably equated with backwardness and inferiority (Morgan, 1995; Miles, 1996). This pejorative view of the Welsh language (not to mention, the Welsh themselves) is ably demonstrated by William Richards, in his *Wallography* of 1682:

> The Native Gibberish is usually prattled throughout the whole of Taphydome, except in their Market Towns, whose inhabitants being a little raised, and (as it were) pufft up into Bubbles, above the ordinary scum, do begin to despise it ... 'Tis usually cashier'd out of Gentlemen's Houses ... the Lingua will be Englishd out of Wales. (Cited in Aitchison and Carter, 1994: 27)

These sentiments continued to be echoed in succeeding centuries. In 1866, *The Times* newspaper thundered that 'The Welsh language is the curse of Wales' (Mayo, 1979). Likewise, the nineteenth-century English educationalist and literary critic, Matthew Arnold, while paying tribute to the Welsh literary classics in his *Study of Celtic Literature*, could also state:

The fusion of all the inhabitants of these islands into one homogeneous, English-speaking whole, the breaking down of barriers between us, the swallowing up of provincial nationalities, is a consummation to which the natural course of things irresistibly tends. It is a necessity of what is called modern civilisation ... *The sooner the Welsh language disappears as an instrument of the practical, political, social life of Wales, the better; the better for England, the better for Wales itself.* (Cited in Griffith, 1950: 71; my emphasis)

Similar views on the Welsh language were also clearly apparent in an influential nineteenth-century review of the state of education in Wales. Published in 1847 as *Reports of the Commissioners of Enquiry into the State of Education in Wales*, it has since come to be known as 'Brad y Lyfrau Gleision' (The Treachery of the Blue Books). Compiled by three young English, Oxford-educated lawyers, their initial terms of reference were to conduct 'an inquiry ... into the state of education in ... Wales, especially into the means afforded to the labouring classes of acquiring a knowledge of the English language' (cited in Jones, 1997: 14–15). To this end, they made some well-merited criticisms of the limited and variable educational provision of the church-based schools in Wales at that time (Morgan, 1995; Jones, 1997). However, they then also proceeded to blame Welsh language and culture as the principal cause of these inadequacies. Indeed, all the social, cultural and economic disadvantages the three commissioners saw in Wales were, in one way or another, attributed to the language: 'His language keeps him under the hatches, being one in which he can neither acquire nor communicate the necessary information.' They concluded: 'The Welsh language is a vast drawback to Wales, and a manifold barrier to the moral progress and commercial prosperity of the people.' This is because '[i]t dissevers the people from intercourse which would greatly advance their civilisation, and bars the access of improving knowledge to their minds' (cited in E. Evans, 1978: 14).

The *Reports'* conclusions with respect to Welsh were to provide the intellectual background and rationale for the (1870) Education Act. This Act, which established the joint state elementary system in England and Wales, formally excluded Welsh from the pedagogy and practice of Welsh schools. The subsequent valorization of English within state education, along with the specific proscription of Welsh, continued well into the twentieth century. It has been only in the last seventy years that Welsh has effectively re-emerged as a school language (see below). In this respect, the educational policy of Welsh language proscription was itself merely a reflection of the wider, long-established hierarchizing of English over Welsh, along with the accompanying belief that in the English language lay the route to social and economic mobility. However, a monolingual English educational policy was also to entrench the view among many that the very *retention* of Welsh itself was actively *dis*advantageous (cf. Chapter 4).

Thus, where previously Welsh monolingualism and de facto bilingualism had been the norm, English monolingualism was increasingly to replace them both. Many Welsh-speaking parents, for example, while continuing to speak Welsh among themselves, stopped speaking it to their children. The result at the individual level, as for so many other minority language speakers, was a generational loss of the language. As Gwyn Thomas poignantly observes of this process: 'My father and mother were Welsh-speaking, yet I did not exchange a word in that language with them. The death of Welsh ran through our family like a geographical fault' (quoted in Osmond, 1988: 149).

To many this decline was viewed as a positive trend – English was perceived as the language of progress, equality, opportunity, the media and mass entertainment (Colin Williams, 1990; cf. Chapter 6). Even today, the practice of unfavorably comparing the utility and status of Welsh to English remains commonplace. We have already seen Brian Barry outline such a view in Chapter 6. Christie Davies, a Welsh sociologist, provides us with another recent example:

> English became a world language ... as part of a *spontaneous* order emerging from the *free* interaction of individuals and corporations. Men and women have *voluntarily* learned to speak English because there are gains to them as individuals. ... The ancestors of today's Welsh people shifted from speaking Welsh to speaking English, not because of external political pressure, but in order to take advantage of economic and educational opportunities. English and Welsh are, in a quite objective sense, not equal languages. Welsh people who become fluent in English gain enormously, whereas English people learning Welsh gain very little. (1997: 42; my emphases)

I do not want to deconstruct Davies's arguments further since I have already dealt at length in previous chapters with the misconceptions and misrepresentations within them as they relate to minority languages in general: notably, the unquestioned primacy of a homogeneous, unilingual nation-state, the equation of majority languages – particularly, English – with modernity, progress and social mobility, and the notion of 'free', 'spontaneous' language choice. What I do want to highlight again briefly here is the process of symbolic violence, as described by Bourdieu (see Chapter 4), which has occurred historically in relation to Cymraeg – the Welsh language. In effect, the English language came to be seen by the Welsh as a form of cultural and linguistic capital, an escape from primitivism, and a demonstration of having embraced the 'modern' way of life (Miles, 1996). Meanwhile, a Welsh linguistic habitus was increasingly regarded as having little cultural, social and economic value. As Bourdieu argues, to understand the nature of symbolic violence, it is crucial to see that it presupposes a kind of active complicity, or implicit consent, on the part of those subjected to it. This is clearly the case historically in Wales where Welsh speakers themselves came to 'collaborate in the destruction of their [own] instruments of expression' (Bourdieu, 1991: 49).

This is not to apportion blame in any way. After all, as Joshua Fishman has argued, the choice facing minority language speakers like the Welsh has often been presented as an intractable one: 'either to remain loyal to their traditions and to remain socially disadvantaged (consigning their own children to such disadvantage as well), on the one hand; or, on the other hand, to abandon their distinctive practices and traditions, at least in large part, and, thereby, to improve their own and their children's lots in life via cultural suicide' (1991: 60; see Chapter 4). R. S. Thomas echoes this analysis, in relation to class, when he observes: 'A Welshman or woman was faced with a partial choice. He [sic] could, by remaining loyal to his or her native speech, be dubbed a member of an inferior class, or by assiduously imitating the English upper class could be admitted to it, generally at the expense of Welsh' (1992: 13). Given the long historical vitiation of Welsh, that so many adopted this latter option should not surprise us. It certainly helps to explain the process of rapid language loss that occurred throughout the twentieth century. What *is* surprising is that it took so long for them to do so and that, despite it all, Welsh remains a living language, still spoken today as a language of everyday life by 20 percent of the Welsh population. This encouraging counter-trend is a direct result of the reinstantiation of Welsh as a civic language over the last thirty years.

Relegitimating and reinstitutionalizing Welsh

Welsh is currently experiencing a remarkable renaissance, in both public and private language domains. In the 1991 census, for example, there was a *reduction* in the decline of Welsh speakers over the previous ten-year intercensal period for the first time in nearly a century. In the 2001 Census, there was actually a 2 percent increase of Welsh speakers over the intercensal period, rising to 21 percent of the total population. The proportion of those who could speak, read and write Welsh also increased from 13.6 percent in 1991 to 16.3 percent in 2001 (Aitchison and Carter, 2004; Colin Williams, 2007).[20]

As well as the reversal of Welsh language decline in the total population, a second key feature of recent language trends has been the growing urban base of the Welsh language. Much like Ireland's Gaeltacht (see Chapter 4), the traditional Welsh-speaking areas within Y Fro Gymraeg have continued to decline, although they still remain proportionately the strongholds of the language. However, the majority of Welsh speakers, in absolute terms, are now to be found in urban and suburban areas. Most notable among these is the capital city, Cardiff, which has become the administrative center of the Welsh language. The growing urbanization of the Welsh language is a direct product of the growing institutionalization of Welsh, particularly in the public sector where the ability to speak Welsh is beginning once again to be viewed as a form of linguistic and cultural capital. As Aitchison and Carter observe of this, while the long demonstrated detraction of the language is still extant, 'it is by no means as powerful as it was, and there is [now] a widespread awareness of the advantages of a knowledge of Welsh, especially in public employment' (1994: 115). Also significant is the rapid growth in the Welsh language among the 3–15 year age group. The burgeoning use of the Welsh language in this age group is largely attributable to the influence of Welsh-medium education, particularly in the Anglicized areas of south and northeast Wales. Accordingly, many of these speakers are second language learners of Welsh, a feature that is increasingly evident in the adult population as well, where adult language courses are growing in popularity (Mann, 2007).

As a result, the prospects for the Welsh language itself, and the possibilities of successfully developing a bilingual Welsh state, have never looked better. A national survey in the mid-1990s on attitudes to the language, for example, found widespread support across Wales (71 percent) for the use of Welsh. Similarly strong support (75 percent) was found for making Welsh co-equal in status with English in Wales, while almost nine out of ten (88 percent) agreed that the Welsh language is something to be proud of (NOP, 1995). The last decade, post-devolution, has further strengthened this remarkable turnaround in the fortunes of the Welsh language, and for the prospects of state bilingualism. Key legislation that has underpinned these developments can now be examined.

The (1993) Welsh Language Act

Writing in the early 1990s, Colin Williams argued in relation to Wales that, 'if a fully functional bilingual society [is to be achieved], where choice and opportunity are the twin pillars of individual language rights, then clearly that possibility has to be constructed through both the promotional and regulatory powers of the state' (1994: 162). The last fifteen years have proved his case. A significant step in establishing such rights in Wales occurred with the (1993) Welsh Language Act (Mesur yr Iaith Gymraeg). The Act replaced its more limited 1967 predecessor and repealed all previous legislation to do with the Welsh language, including the original Acts of Union. In the 1993 Act, Welsh was treated for the first time as having 'a basis of equality' with English within Wales, although it qualified this equality as being that which is appropriate within the circumstances and 'reasonably practicable'.

The Act also importantly provided a statutory basis to Bwrdd yr Iaith Gymraeg (the Welsh Language Board). Bwrdd yr Iaith had originally been established in July 1988, although merely as an advisory body on the language, with little status and power. In this respect, it was not too dissimilar initially to its Irish equivalent, Bord na Gaeilge (Irish Language Board; cf. Chapter 4). Under the 1993 Act's aegis, however, Bwrdd yr Iaith was authorized not only to promote and facilitate the use of the Welsh language but also to ensure its adoption within the public sector. The latter was to be achieved via formal language schemes provided by public organizations to the Board, which specified the measures each organization would take in order to provide effective bilingual public services in Wales. Again, the caveat was invoked that such bilingual services would be provided 'so far as is both appropriate in the circumstances and reasonably practical'. However, the Board attempted to overcome this limitation, albeit not always successfully (see below), by insisting that they, not the organizations, would determine the parameters of reasonableness and practicality. Likewise, the Board insisted that organizations should not rely on the *current* demand for services in Welsh, on the premise that once more effective bilingual services become available, demand for such services would also increase.

The Board also highlighted the need for organizations to recruit more Welsh-speaking staff, particularly in historically Anglicized areas of Wales. As with comparable debates in Quebec and Catalonia, this position has proved to be controversial. Indeed, the question of whether a knowledge of Welsh could be stipulated as a requirement of employment faced a number of legal challenges in Wales. In one prominent case, *Jones v. Gwynedd County Council* (1985), two monolingual English-speaking applicants from Liverpool, England, took Gwynedd county council in the northwest of Wales to court when they failed to secure a council position working with senior citizens (many of whom were Welsh-speaking). They argued that the Welsh language requirement for the position was discriminatory under the British (1976) Race Relations Act. The initial industrial tribunal upheld the complaint on the basis that Welsh speakers formed a 'sub-ethnic' group, thus suggesting that differentiation on the basis of ethnicity had occurred. This was later overturned on appeal, with the final ruling concluding that language differences within an ethnic group were not applicable under the Race Relations Act.

The eventual resolution of this case confirmed the legitimacy of requiring Welsh language qualifications in the labor market for specific forms of employment where bilingualism and/or multilingualism are a functional necessity. But in other areas, promotion of the Welsh language under the 1993 Act has met with less success. While over 350 Welsh Language Schemes were subsequently agreed between 1993 and 2008 (Colin Williams, 2008), these have been predominantly with public bodies in Wales. Both Crown bodies (those that operate across Britain) and the business sector were exempted from complying with the 1993 Welsh Language Act. The Welsh Language Board, reporting ten years later to the Richard Commission, catalogued the numerous difficulties it had experienced in gaining any traction in either sector over the intervening period. Crown bodies, for example, were reluctant to implement Welsh language requirements in the delivery of their services and often prevaricated about, or simply obstructed implementation (Roddick, 2007).[21] Meanwhile, businesses could remain largely untouched by Welsh language requirements, if they so chose, often citing practicality and profitability as the means of avoidance.

Be that as it may, the 1993 Welsh Language Act, and the related functions of Bwrdd yr Iaith Gymraeg, did provide a significant statutory basis for further developments post-devolution in support of Welsh. The establishment of the National Assembly for Wales, and subsequently the Welsh Assembly Government (WAG), highlighted the importance of bilingual provision at the governmental level. The Assembly transacts its daily business bilingually, a development that has also since extended to the judiciary. And for the first time in its history, bilingual legislation of equal status in English and Welsh is being enacted (Roddick, 2007).[22] In its first term, the Assembly adopted a formal strategy, Iaith Pawb (Everyone's Language; 2003), aimed at establishing a fully bilingual society. It too suffered from a lack of binding legislation and related enforcement mechanisms (Dunbar, 2007; Colin Williams, 2007) but was an important statement of intent, nonetheless. But by far the most significant development has been the replacement of the Welsh Language Board with an Official Language Commissioner in February 2011, via the 2011 Welsh Language (Wales) Measure. The Commissioner's role will be precisely to address the longstanding weaknesses of statutory compliance in relation to the provision of Welsh language services to the public, a welcome development that has been strongly advocated by Welsh language proponents (Colin Williams, 2007, 2008).

Welsh-medium education

The move to greater compliance with respect to bilingual delivery in Wales is also evident within education. Welsh-medium education has been available in Wales since 1939, when the first (initially) private Welsh-language elementary school was established in Aberystwyth by local Welsh-speaking parents. From this, the Welsh-medium school movement was born. The Aberystwyth school was incorporated into the state education system in 1951 and other Ysgolion Cymraeg (Welsh-medium schools) were also established at that time. Since then, the development of Welsh-medium education has been nothing short of spectacular. By 2009, there were 438 such schools at both primary/elementary and high school level throughout Wales.[23] As a result of this expansion, more than a fifth of elementary-aged pupils are now in classes where Welsh is the main medium of instruction. One quarter of all school students in Wales are taught through Welsh (Williamson, 2010). Many of these students come from English-speaking families. This is because a key feature of the Welsh-medium movement has been its ability to convince non-Welsh speaking parents, the majority of whom are also middle-class, of its academic merits (Charlotte

Davies, 1989). Subsequently, the greatest growth of Welsh-medium education – and, by extension, of Welsh speakers – has occurred in the historically Anglicized areas of Wales. Welsh-medium education has even generated demand from parents across the border in England (C. Hill, 2004). So much for Barry's views, discussed in Chapter 6, that students in Wales would be better served by 'a major foreign language'.

But the path of Welsh-medium education has not always run so smooth. In the early years, parents took much more convincing about the educational benefits of schooling in Welsh, not least because of the longstanding pejorative positioning of the language within the wider society. Welsh-medium education thus remained dependent on sufficient local parental demand and/or the beneficence of individual local headteachers for its successful enactment (Rawkins, 1987; Baker, 1985, 1995). Welsh only became a compulsory subject in Wales as a result of the (1988) Education Reform Act, albeit accidentally. The Act, a notable feature of the Conservative Thatcher administration, established a National (sic) Curriculum for England and Wales. The deliberate qualification in the title of the 'National' Curriculum is important here. Like all previous major educational reform affecting 'England and Wales', the whole thrust of the Act was actually concerned with the needs of the English (national) curriculum (Jones, 1997). However, the formal recognition of Welsh throughout all schools in Wales occurred because, at the time of the drafting of the National Curriculum in the mid-1980s, there were a sufficient number of Welsh-medium schools to ensure that the British government could not define the core language component of the National Curriculum (at least in Wales) as solely English. Conceding that Welsh was now the language of instruction and initial study for a significant minority of schools in Wales meant that Welsh had to be recognized as a 'core subject' in these schools under the Act. Following from this, Welsh was also given the status of a 'foundation subject' within all other schools in Wales, to be compulsorily studied as a second language (L2) by all students.

The Education Reform Act thus laid the initial basis for the normalization of Welsh-medium education, and of Welsh as an L2 within education in Wales.' Over the last decade, the Welsh Assembly Government (WAG) has continued this process, given that education is one of its key devolved areas of responsibility. This culminated in 2010 with the WAG's Welsh-medium education strategy, aimed at ensuring that local councils are more responsive to increasing parental demands for the provision and further expansion of Welsh-medium education. The strategy also stressed the need to improve the teaching of Welsh as an L2, so that all students in Welsh education might be able to use the language effectively upon leaving school (Williamson, 2010). A recognition that the latter is not always easy to achieve reflects the wider limitations of the role of education in language revitalization, as discussed in Chapter 4. Education cannot compensate for society, or remediate, at least on its own, longstanding language loss (Fishman,

1991). Welsh-medium education is no exception here, not least because even now it still only reaches approximately 25 percent of the school population of Wales. Similarly, the strength of Welsh-medium schools in Anglicized areas of Wales is both a benefit and a curse. Such schools may well have contributed to the creation of a new generation of Welsh speakers in the post-Second World War period. However, they also epitomize the growing fragmentation of the wider bilingual community within Wales, since these schools often provide the only significant domain where a predominantly Welsh-medium milieu can be experienced (Colin Williams, 2008).

Ongoing challenges and possibilities

Developments in Wales over the last thirty years, and particularly in the last decade, augur well for the reconstruction of a Welsh national identity that once again includes the Welsh language as an important (but not necessarily pre-eminent) component. As David Miller, writing on national identity, observes: 'a national identity helps to locate us in the world; it must tell us who we are, where we have come from, what we have done' (1995: 165). He proceeds to argue that this

> must then involve an essentially historical understanding in which the present generation are seen as heirs to a tradition which they then pass on to their successors. Of course the story is continually being rewritten; each generation revises the past as it comes to terms with the problems of the present. Nonetheless, there is a sense in which the past always constrains the present: present identities are built out of materials that are handed down, not started from scratch. (Ibid.)

Bhikhu Parekh argues, along similar lines: 'A community's identity is subject to constant change ... Every community must wrestle with it as best it can, and find ways of reconstituting its identity in a manner that is both deeply sensitive to its history and traditions and fully alive to its present and future needs' (1995: 267). These positions have a close resonance with my discussion of habitus in Chapter 1. They also appear to encapsulate what is occurring in Wales as it moves to cement a formal bilingual state. The construction of a bilingual Wales, based on a new set of urban Welsh identities, rejects both a narrow language-based conception of Welshness *and* its opposite, the disavowal of any public role for Welsh within contemporary Wales. Writing in the early 1990s, Fiona Bowie observed that 'Wales is increasingly looking out, towards Europe, as well as within, at its own mixed population, its bilingualism, and its cultural roots.' From this, she argued, those living in Wales must 'forge a Welsh identity which builds on all these disparate groups and experiences. It will be different from the Wales of the imagination and from the Wales of the past, but it will also be distinctively and assertively Welsh' (1993: 191). Nearly fifteen years later, Coupland and Bishop reach a remarkably similar conclusion:

> It is the moment for Wales to build an openness of perspective around who we are in terms of 'community' and 'communities' (perhaps diverse, welcoming, loyal, quarrelsome and inconsistent) and around what makes us legitimately and distinctively Welsh in the domain of language – perhaps multi-valenced, combative, performative, and impossibly and irreverently multilingual. (2006: 49)

But that is not to suggest that there is nothing more to be done. As with Catalonia, the new conception of Welshness apparent in Wales has, despite its rhetoric of inclusion and respect for differences, not yet adequately recognized the cultural and linguistic histories of its various ethnic minorities (see Tarrow, 1992; Charlotte Williams, 1995; Williams and De Lima, 2006). These ethnic minorities, primarily Black British or of South Asian ancestry, comprised only 1.7 percent of the Welsh population at the time of the 2001 British census (Office for National Statistics, 2003) but their linguistic needs and rights still need to be addressed. Relatedly, while the formal development of Welsh/English bilingual education is no bar necessarily to the recognition and use of other minority languages within Welsh education, such languages have to date received little formal recognition. Indeed, even at the ostensibly more superficial level of multiculturalism, there has been little actual progress made in establishing a consciously multicultural curriculum in Wales. Norma Tarrow argued in the early 1990s, for example, that the major barrier to implementing effective multicultural policies 'is the widely held belief that there is little representation in Wales of groups other than English, Welsh and long-standing assimilated ethnic minorities' (1992: 502). Not much has changed since.

Meanwhile, the attitudes of English speakers in Wales toward these changes cannot be taken for granted, *despite* the apparent widespread support for them at a general level (cf. NOP, 1995). For example, in a language survey that I conducted in the late 1990s among nearly 500 teacher trainees in Wales (May, 2000; see also Chapter 9), I found, alongside this widespread support of Welsh at a general level, a more complex and contested picture. In particular, more specific questions of language compulsion in education, or the requirement to be bilingual for certain employment positions, continued to elicit considerable skepticism, and at times outright opposition, from majority language speakers. Indeed, in this respect, the survey demonstrated a remarkable congruence with anti-Catalan language discourses, with many non-Welsh speakers articulating a discourse of individual language rights, or 'language choice' as a means of *opting out* of bilingual requirements. Pejorative attitudes about minority languages more generally, particularly in relation to their 'adequacy' in and 'relevance' to the modern world, were also clearly apparent, as was the notion that bilingual requirements for employment were somehow in themselves 'racist' and illiberal.

I have already discussed at length how the discourses of individual language rights, illiberality and relevance are regularly deployed to buttress the monolingualism of majority language speakers. I won't belabor this point again here except to say that these ongoing frictions point (if we need reminding) to the contest and conflict that necessarily attach to *any* attempt to legitimate and institutionalize a minority language. In this sense, while much *has* clearly been accomplished by the recent institutional changes in Wales, much more still needs to be achieved if the significant progress made thus far in legitimating and institutionalizing Welsh is not to be undone within the crucible of majority language speakers' attitudes. I return to this point, more generally, in Chapter 9, when I discuss the notion of 'tolerability'.

8

INDIGENOUS RIGHTS

SELF-DETERMINATION, LANGUAGE AND EDUCATION

> We were ghost peoples, hidden, like our languages and cultures, by the concept of the nation-state.
>
> (James Youngblood Henderson)

This chapter begins with a brief review of the debates surrounding the rights and standing of indigenous peoples within national and international law, with particular emphasis on issues of self-determination, language and education. I will then proceed to discuss the example of Māori in Aotearoa/New Zealand in specific relation to these issues.

Indigenous peoples – who number more than 370 million in some ninety countries (United Nations, 2009) – are at the forefront of international developments regarding the recognition of group-differentiated minority rights. A key catalyst for this central involvement is their highly problematic and contested status within modern nation-states. After all, indigenous peoples have, in nearly all cases, a long history of colonization which has seen such groups faced with systematic disadvantage, marginalization and/or alienation in their own historic territories (Tully, 1995; cf. Chapter 2). As a result, they have been undermined economically, culturally and politically, with ongoing, often disturbing, consequences for their individual and collective life chances (United Nations, 2009).

At the same time, indigenous peoples have been viewed extremely pejoratively in relation to modernization – as 'primitive' or premodern. Consequently, they have been subjected in many cases to forced assimilation, on the misplaced assumption that this was the only viable option for their social and cultural survival and/or 'advancement'. The shocking case of the 'stolen generations' in Australia illustrates the extremes of such a position all too starkly. For sixty years, from 1910 to 1970, the Australian authorities enforced a systematic policy of 'resettlement' which saw up to a third of Aboriginal and Torres Strait Island children forcibly removed from their families and adopted by white families or, more often, simply fostered or institutionalized. In the process, original family records were deliberately destroyed because, it was thought, any life was better than a traditional aboriginal one (see Edwards and Read, 1992; Andrea Smith, 2009; Tatz, 2011).[1]

Thus, indigenous peoples have not had access, in many instances, to even the most basic rights ostensibly attributable to all citizens in the modern nation-state. Aboriginal peoples and Torres Strait Islanders, for example, were only granted full citizenship rights in Australia in 1967 – some two hundred years after the advent of European colonization. Indeed, it was only at this time that they were granted the distinction of being human in Australian law, having previously been classified under the Flora and Fauna Act. Where indigenous peoples have had access to citizenship rights, they have, more often than not, been treated solely as a disadvantaged ethnic minority group rather than as a national minority ethnie within the nation-state (Kymlicka, 1989; May, 2002).

That said, indigenous peoples have been granted, in certain circumstances, some 'special privileges' and protection not afforded 'regular' citizens. Traditional systems of social order, for example, including the right to very limited forms of governmental autonomy (e.g. tribal or band government on Native American reservations) have been preserved in some cases in order to *allow* indigenous peoples to exercise a modicum of control over their traditional territories and ways of life (Kymlicka, 1989; Carens, 2000). However, it is perhaps not surprising that protectionism in this form has also simply been used as a variant of assimilation. As Hartwig argues, concerning Māori in Aotearoa/New Zealand and Aboriginal and Torres Strait Islanders in Australia: 'whatever the differences between "amalgamationist" and "protectionist" strategies, the ultimate aim of the state for long periods in both countries was the disappearance of Aboriginal and Māori societies as distinguishable entities' (1978: 170; cited in Harker and McConnochie, 1985). Joshua Fishman is also particularly critical of this kind of 'protectionism'. As he argues, 'even in such settings, indigenous populations are robbed of control of the natural resources that could constitute the economic bases of a more self-regulatory collective life and, therefore, robbed also of a possible avenue of cultural viability as well' (1991: 62).

The extremely limited nature of these concessions has also tended to place indigenous peoples in a double bind. On the one hand, such concessions have done little, if anything, to redress the extreme marginalization facing indigenous peoples in modern nation-states. On the other hand, the granting of even very limited local autonomy to indigenous peoples is usually viewed with a good deal of suspicion, and often with outright opposition, because it may infringe on the individual rights of majority group members. Again drawing on Australia as an example, the influence in the late 1990s of the populist and overtly racist politician Pauline Hanson, with her 'One Nation' Party and her specifically anti-Aboriginal policies, illustrates the extreme antagonisms that such a position can promote. While her political ascendancy was brief,[2] her key achievement was to normalize an overtly anti-Aboriginal agenda in Australian politics (Robbins, 2007, 2010; see also below).

Given this historical background of colonization, and the ongoing reticence of many nation-states to recognize its legacy, indigenous groups have become increasingly disaffected with their treatment by national majorities and have sought the right to greater *self-determination* within nation-states. Where nation-states have ignored or derided their claims, indigenous peoples have turned instead to supranational organizations, and international law, with surprisingly successful results (see Kymlicka, 1999c; Feldman, 2001; Stavenhagen and Charters, 2009). In this respect, the definition of what constitutes an indigenous people becomes important. However, as we saw in Chapter 2, such definitions are not entirely unproblematic and indigenous groups themselves, like all broad groupings, exhibit a range of significant inter- and intragroup differences. This caveat of heterogeneity notwithstanding, the International Labor Organization's (ILO) Convention 169, formulated in 1989, may serve as a useful starting point:

a) tribal peoples in independent countries whose social, cultural and economic conditions distinguish them from other sections of the national community, and whose status is regulated wholly or partially by their own customs or traditions or by special laws or regulations;

b) peoples in independent countries who are regarded as indigenous on account of their descent from the populations which inhabited the country, or a geographical region to which the country belongs, at the time of conquest or colonization or the establishment of present state boundaries and who, *irrespective of their legal status*, retain some of their own social, economic, cultural and political institutions. (Art 1.1; my emphasis)

Lest objectivist definitions be accorded too much weight, however, Article 1.2 adds the rider that 'self-identification as indigenous or tribal shall be regarded as a fundamental criterion for determining the groups to which the provisions of this Convention apply' (cf. Chapter 1). Suffice it to say at this point, that self-identification, along with the qualification 'irrespective of their legal status' highlighted previously, are both central to any discussion of indigenousness since not all nation-states are willing to recognize indigenous groups in their territories. Indeed, governments in Malaysia, India, Burma and Bangladesh have at various times claimed that everyone in their territory is indigenous and that no one is thus entitled to any special or differential treatment (de Varennes, 1996a). This unwillingness on the part of national governments to recognize indigenous peoples is also extended to minorities more generally, as we saw in the discussion of Article 27 of the (1966) International Covenant on Civil and Political Rights in Chapter 5.

The ILO Convention 169 is also significant for another reason. It replaces an earlier convention (107), drawn up in 1957, which exhibited a much more paternalistic approach to indigenous peoples. These differences are reflected in both the wording and the general intent of the two conventions. With regard to wording, for example, Convention 107(a) uses the phrase 'tribal populations' whereas 169(a) employs 'tribal peoples'. This is significant, given the connotations of the term 'peoples' in international law (see below). Convention 169(a) also states that the social, cultural and economic conditions of tribal groups are *distinguished* from other sections of the national community whereas 107(a) employs the more pejorative phrase 'at a less advanced stage'. Likewise, where Convention 169(b) states that indigenous peoples 'retain some of their own social, economic, cultural and political institutions', 107(b) specifically equates these institutions with premodern practices and contrasts them with 'the [modern] institutions of the nation to which they belong'. These differences are not simply semantic ones. More broadly, Convention 107 clearly views indigenous culture as a temporary obstacle to modernization. As Patrick Thornberry observes of this: 'In reading the earlier Convention, it is impossible to avoid the feeling that [indigenous] peoples were regarded as a relic of the past to be "developed" or "integrated" out of existence' (2002: 520). As such, it is as much concerned with the assimilation of indigenous peoples as with their protection. In contrast, Convention 169 reflects a far more positive view of indigenous cultures and is specifically anti-assimilationist in intent. As Patrick Thornberry concludes:

> There is a remarkable shift in perception between the ILO conventions of 1957 and 1989 ... [Convention 169] is a radical document that recognizes the presence of indigenous peoples, their historicity and cultural indelibility. It evinces respect for their societies, their characteristic modes of existence and holistic social constructs, and is characterized by the affirmation of *collective as well as individual rights*. (2002: 520–1; emphasis in original)

The ILO Convention 169 is also significant because it remains the only internationally *binding* instrument aimed specifically at protecting the rights of indigenous peoples. That said, only twenty nation-states (as of July 2010) have subsequently ratified the convention. This has inevitably limited its global impact, not least because many indigenous peoples are still unable to rely on its legal framework for protection (Barelli, 2010).

Indigenous peoples, self-determination and international law

The distinctions between the two ILO Conventions do nonetheless illustrate the different status that has come to be accorded to indigenous peoples in international law over the intervening forty-year period, and subsequently to the present day (see Anaya, 1996; Xanthaki, 2007 for full reviews). Central to this change has been the argument of indigenous groups themselves that they are not simply one of a number of ethnic minority groups, competing for the limited resources of the nation-state, and therefore entirely subject to its largesse, but are *peoples*, with the associated rights of self-determination attributable to the latter under international law (cf. Chapter 2). This argument first began to be articulated in the 1970s by a nascent international network of indigenous scholars and activists. As James Youngblood Henderson, a Canadian First Nations peoples' representative, observes of these early developments:

> We sought to understand why the [International] Labour Conventions, the Human Rights Covenants or the [Universal] Declaration and conventions of UNESCO had never been used to protect us [indigenous peoples]. In these international systems we found we were invisible; we were neither minorities nor peoples. We were ghost peoples, hidden, like our languages and cultures, by the concept of the nation-state. (2008: 35–6)

Growing pressure and advocacy from indigenous peoples led in 1982 to the formal establishment of the Working Group on Indigenous Populations (WGIP), a United Nations Sub-Commission on the Prevention of Discrimination and Protection of Minorities. The WGIP was particularly influential in these early years in solidifying a growing tendency to regard indigenous peoples 'as a separate issue [from other minority groups] in international and constitutional law' (Thornberry, 1991b: 6). The WGIP consulted widely with over 100 indigenous organizations in the initial drafting of the United Nations Declaration on the Rights of Indigenous Peoples (UNDRIP). Indeed, the active participation of indigenous groups ranged from 'issue setting and agenda creation' through to 'influence on institutional procedures' (Corntassel, 2007: 137; see also Stavenhagen and Charters, 2009). This was a highly unusual development, given that such UN consultations usually occurred between member states and a restricted number of officially recognized delegations. As a result of this decade-long dialogue between indigenous peoples and the UN legal representatives on the WGIP subcommittee, the draft Declaration, when it was published in 1993, clearly articulated the key legal and political demands of the indigenous organizations involved. Two key principles stood out. The first centered on the 'collective and individual right' to maintain and develop distinct indigenous identities, 'including the right to identify themselves as indigenous and to be recognized as such' (Art. 8). The second, which I will return to more fully below, unequivocally asserted the right of indigenous self-determination (Arts. 3 and 4).

Not surprisingly perhaps, the Draft Declaration did not sit well with UN member states at the time, with many viewing it with overt skepticism, and some with outright hostility. The controversial and contested nature of the UNDRIP was clearly borne out by the subsequent process of revision of the draft for final acceptance by the United Nations (UN). After its initial publication in 1993, a Working Group on the Draft Declaration (WGDD) was established with the sole purpose of reworking the text, in (further) consultation with indigenous organizations and member states. The first session of the WGDD was convened in November 1995. Unlike the previous consultative process, however, the WGDD was to be dominated once again by the interests of states, with only a restricted number of attested non-government organizations allowed to contribute. As a result, many indigenous groups involved in the formulation of the earlier Draft Declaration were excluded while, at least theoretically, any state could veto an objectionable element of the draft under review. In this latter respect, state representatives on the WGDD did endorse the WGIP text as a 'sound basis' for future drafting. However, subsequent proceedings saw many substantive objections raised by states about specific principles outlined in the Draft Declaration. Indeed, some states, notably Japan and the United States, contended that the text as a whole was 'not a reasonable evolution of human rights law' (Barsh, 1996: 788). The full range of contentions raised by the various states need not concern us here (see Barsh, 1996; Xanthaki, 2007, for further discussion). Rather, in what follows, I want to concentrate solely on the most important issue raised in these debates – that of self-determination.

Despite the more favorable view adopted toward indigenous peoples over the last forty years, there remains, even now, considerable reticence about the right of self-determination being accorded to them. Much of this reticence has to do with the specific meaning of self-determination in international law. As we saw in Chapter 3, the right of minority national groups (including indigenous peoples) to self-determination is not actually inconsistent with international law, since the (1945) United Nations Charter clearly states that 'all peoples have the right to self-determination'. However, the UN Charter does not define the term 'peoples' and the injunction has tended to be interpreted only in relation to the recognition of postcolonial states (the 'salt water thesis') rather than to national minorities within existing nation-states, even though the latter may have been subjected to broadly the same processes of colonization. Self-determination has thus been limited *in practice* to existing states in the post-Second World War era (Clark and Williamson, 1996; Thornberry, 1991a, 2002).

This widely accepted practice has been further reinforced by the implicit assumption that any claim to self-determination by indigenous peoples (the term 'peoples' rather than 'people' being, in itself, an indication of this) carried with it an implication of secession. On this basis, the potential threat of secession that self-determination implied could simply not be accepted by many states (although, interestingly, international law nowhere says that 'peoples' have the right to secede from existing states by virtue only of the right to self-determination; see Scott, 1996). However, in the course of the WGGD's discussion, some states argued for a more restricted view of self-determination, termed by some as 'internal self-determination', and by others as 'autonomy'. Thus, Chile argued that the idea of internal self-determination allowed:

[a] space within which indigenous peoples can freely determine their forms of development, [including] the preservation of their cultures, languages, customs and traditions, in a manner that reinforces their identity and characteristics, in the context and framework of the States in which indigenous peoples live. (Cited in Barsh, 1996: 797)

Similarly, Australia argued that the right of indigenous peoples to self-determination could be accepted, 'subject to the understanding that the exercise of this right should [remain] within existing State boundaries, that is not [including] a right to secession'. Nicaragua agreed that 'autonomy' captured the 'sense and meaning of the concept of self-determination, without affecting the unity of the State' (both cited in Barsh, 1996: 799). An earlier observation by the New Zealand government on the conclusions of the WGIP provides us with a useful summary of this position:

There is no indication at present that governments will recognise a right of *external* self-determination for indigenous peoples, that is, including the right to secede from a state. Any 'right of self-determination' for indigenous people would therefore have to be understood differently from its traditional meaning in international law if it were to be acceptable to governments. [In this regard] international law may be moving towards recognition of an 'aboriginal right to self-determination' or autonomy which does not include the right of secession. (Te Puni Kōkiri, 1994: 9; my emphasis)

In effect then, we see in these initial WGDD discussions the first tentative emergence of an intermediate position in international law with respect to self-determination which acknowledges the right to greater *autonomy* within the nation-state for indigenous peoples but which does not necessarily include the right to secession (Clark and Williamson, 1996; Barelli, 2010). This form of 'internal self-determination' emphasizes *negotiated* power-sharing, both through constitutional reform and within existing institutions, and extends well beyond the desultory measures of local autonomy previously established for some indigenous groups. As Madame Daes, the UN rapporteur for the WGIP had earlier observed of this:

> [T]he existing state has the duty to accommodate the aspirations of indigenous peoples through constitutional reforms designed to share power democratically. It also means that indigenous peoples have the duty to try and reach an agreement, in good faith, on sharing power within the existing state and to exercise their right to self-determination by this means to the [fullest] extent possible. (Cited in Te Puni Kōkiri, 1994: 11)

More broadly, Craig Scott has argued that rethinking the notion of self-determination has required us 'to begin to think of self-determination in terms of people existing *in relationship with each other*' (1996: 819; my emphasis; see also Anaya, 1996). This view echoes the relational aspects of ethnicity, discussed in Chapter 1, and Iris Marion Young's arguments with respect to the relational basis of group-differentiated rights, discussed in Chapter 3.

But this nascent view on 'internal self-determination' or 'autonomy' for indigenous peoples was still adamantly contested by some member states during the WGGD negotiations. For example, France, Japan and the USA continued to oppose any notion of self-government for indigenous people, *in principle*, for much of the negotiations. Meanwhile, other states, notably an African confederation led by Namibia, consistently tried to dilute the principle of indigenous self-determination, albeit to no avail. This consistent opposition helps to explain why it took over ten years for the WGGD to agree a final text of the UNDRIP, even though the broad principle of self-determination eventually remained intact, as reflected in Articles 3 and 4 in the final agreed text of the UNDRIP (2007):

> Indigenous peoples have the right to self-determination. By virtue of that right they freely determine their political status and freely pursue their economic, social and cultural development. (Art. 3)

> Indigenous peoples, in exercising their right to self-determination, have the right to autonomy or self-government in matters relating to their internal and local affairs, as well as ways and means for financing their autonomous functions. (Art. 4)[3]

The reason why the final version of the UNDRIP retained the central principle of indigenous self-determination, despite member states' attempts to exclude or dilute it, was because of other caveats added in the final text that made it explicit that indigenous self-determination did not entail a right to secession. Article 46.1, for example, states:

> Nothing in this Declaration may be interpreted as implying for any State, people, group or person any right to engage in any activity or to perform any act contrary to the Charter of the United Nations or construed as authorizing or encouraging any action which would dismember or impair, totally or in part, the territorial integrity or political unity of sovereign and independent States.

But even these caveats ensuring the ongoing 'territorial integrity' of nation-states were not enough to satisfy all. Thus, while the vote in favor of adoption of the UNDRIP in 2007 was overwhelming (143 in favor), there were eleven abstentions and, most significantly, four major nation-states which still voted against the UNDRIP's adoption. These four were Australia, Canada, New Zealand and the United States. Each of these states unabashedly championed its treatment of indigenous peoples at the national level – if nothing else, a significant demonstration of Renan's maxim: 'forgetting, I would even go so far as to say historical error, is a crucial factor in the creation of a nation' (1990: 11; cf. Chapter 2; see also below). But none could endorse UNDRIP. Even though it is a non-binding international treaty, Canada and New Zealand could not reconcile it with their domestic law. The United States criticized the transparency of the drafting process and the final recommendations, despite unprecedented access and consultation over a twenty-five-year period. The US also argued that the UNDRIP was not a 'consensus text' despite the overwhelming vote in favor of its adoption. But it was Australia, under the then conservative administration of John Howard (1996–2007), which stated its ongoing opposition to UNDRIP most clearly, again focusing directly on the notion of indigenous self-determination:

> Australia's representative said his Government had long expressed dissatisfaction with the references to self-determination in the Declaration ... The [Australian] Government supported and encouraged the full engagement of indigenous peoples in the democratic decision-making process, but did not support a concept that could be construed as encouraging action that would impair, even in part, the territorial and political integrity of a State with a system of democratic Government.[4]

Even these four nation-states were subsequently to endorse UNDRIP, albeit reluctantly, with the USA the last to do so in December 2010. Thus, while it may have been an arduous and contested process, the acknowledgment of indigenous self-determination in the UNDRIP does clearly mark a major shift in international law. Indeed, as Barelli observes, 'the UNDRIP is the first international human rights instrument to expressly recognize the right to self-determination to a sub-state group' (2010: 959). Whether it provides the basis for a *sustainable* consensus on this issue remains to be seen.

Indigenous peoples and national law

> No doubt most states owe their existence to some combination of force and fraud. However, the issue is not simply a matter of how a state came to be, but of how it can become 'morally rehabilitated'. (Ivison et al., 2000: 3)

Meanwhile, the essentially contested nature of debates about indigenous rights is even more apparent in national contexts, not least because they shape and influence so clearly the daily lives of indigenous peoples, their affordances and constraints. The precedents of international law with respect to the rights and representation of indigenous peoples are important here too, of course. But as we saw in Chapter 5, such laws are still dependent in the end on the willingness of nation-states to accede to them in the first instance, and to implement them effectively in the next (Ivison et al., 2000; Kuppe, 2009). Neither is guaranteed. Nor can advances in indigenous rights in one era necessarily be ensured in another.

Examples of significant advances in indigenous rights and representation at the level of the nation-state are increasingly numerous, but so too are setbacks and/or subsequent periods of retrenchment. In Brazil, for example, the adoption in 1988 of a new Constituição (constitution) recognized for the first time 'povos indígenas no Brasil' (the indigenous peoples of Brazil), of whom there are over 400,000. Article 231 specifically endorses indigenous social organization, customs, languages, beliefs and traditions, along with the right of native title to their lands (Brazil, 1996; see also Hornberger, 1997). Article 67 of the constitution also ordered the demarcation of all indigenous territories within Brazil within five years. But despite the significance of this constitutional development, subsequent progress toward actualizing indigenous rights in Brazil has been variable, to say the least. Writing a decade later, Borges and Combrisson (1997) comment despairingly on how little indigenous land had been demarcated in the intervening period. A decade later again, disputes over indigenous lands in Brazil are still proliferating. Indigenous peoples have become increasingly militant in the face of numerous legal setbacks over land, as well as the use of strong-arm tactics, including murder, by mining companies and other major landholders against them (Osava, 2006).

Norway provides us with a somewhat more hopeful example. After a century of enforcing a stringent 'Norwegianization' (read: assimilationist) policy toward the indigenous Sámi, their languages and their culture, Norway also moved in 1988 to revise its constitution in order to grant greater autonomy for Sámi. As the amendment to the Constitution stated: 'It is incumbent on the governmental authorities to take the necessary steps to enable the Sámi population to safeguard and develop their language, their culture and their social life' (cited in Magga, 1996: 76). The effects of this new amendment are most apparent in the regional area of Finnmark, in the northernmost part of Norway, where the largest percentage of the Sámi peoples live. The formal recognition accorded to Sámi led to the subsequent establishment of a Sámi Parliament in Finnmark in 1989, while the Sámi Language Act, passed in 1992, recognized Northern Sámi as its official regional language. The Sámi Language Act saw the formal promotion of the language within the Sámi Parliament, the courts of law and all levels of education (see Corson, 1995; Huss, 1999).[5] In addition, a separate Sámi curriculum was introduced in Finnmark in 1997, and in 2000 the Sámi Parliament took responsibility for some aspects of the Sámi school system, previously controlled by the central Norwegian Government (Todal, 2003). Both these latter developments, along with the passing of the (2005) Finnmark Act, have further entrenched regional autonomy and indigenous control for Sámi in the area (Semb, 2005).

The precedent of regional autonomy for indigenous peoples set by Finnmark has also been evident in Canada over the last fifteen years. In December 1997, the Canadian Supreme Court ruled in a landmark decision, subsequently referred to as the Delgamuukw Decision, in favor of the recognition of aboriginal title, or indigenous land rights. This ruling coincided with an initiative entitled 'Gathering Strength, Canada's Aboriginal Action Plan', developed by the then Canadian Liberal government of Jean Chrétien. The Action Plan aimed to redress and, crucially, make actual restitution for the colonial appropriation of the lands and resources of Canada's indigenous peoples. Both developments have formed the basis for the subsequent extension of aboriginal title claims and indigenous regional control in Canada over the last decade.

For example, in April 1999, the new Arctic province of Nunavut was established, the first formal subdivision of territory in Canada for fifty years. Its establishment was the end result of a twenty-year negotiation process with the 22,000 Inuit of the region (out of a total regional population of 25,000). In return for ceding wider claims to their traditional territories across the north of Canada, the indigenous Inuit were granted 22,000 square kilometers of territory to the immediate northwest of Hudson Bay and a comparable degree of autonomy to Canada's other provinces. The provincial administration is Inuit-led, and the local Inuit language, Inuktitut, is co-official with English and French in the region, as well as being the first working language of the provincial government (Légaré, 2002).[6] Given the scale of these developments, it is perhaps surprising that so little controversy has actually attended them – although, no doubt, the remoteness of the territory, and the relatively sparse non-indigenous population within it, have played a part here. These geographic features also contribute, however, to the ongoing socioeconomic weakness of the region and a related over-reliance on the Canadian Federal government to address adequately socioeconomic needs. Both militate against the further extension of self-government in Nunavut over time, despite all that has been achieved thus far (Légaré, 2008).

Another key recent development in Canada with respect to indigenous rights is the Nisga'a Agreement. Also following a twenty-year period of negotiation, the Agreement was eventually reached in August 1998 between the regional government of British Columbia and the Native Canadian Nisga'a band (who describe themselves as a 'nation'). The Agreement was ratified by the Canadian federal government in the following year although, as we shall see shortly, not without difficulty. The Agreement called for the transfer of nearly 2,000 square kilometers of land to the 5,500 strong Nisga'a in Northern British Columbia. Central features of the agreement also included restitution amounting to $C330 million, and the granting of substantial powers of self-government – including an autonomous legislature responsible for citizenship and land management. The Agreement was based, in turn, on a longstanding claim – first raised in the nineteenth century – against the colonial appropriation of Nisga'a lands (Rynard, 2000).

However, the subsequent ratification of the agreement in the Canadian Parliament was characterized by strong and vituperative opposition from the Reform Party, a conservative, Anglocentric 'one nation' party that had also been prominent in opposing any separate recognition of Quebec (cf. Chapter 7). The Reform Party claimed that the Agreement would give the Nisga'a too much power over local businesses and non-indigenous peoples and that it would set a precedent for the establishment of similar treaties with Canada's fifty other Native Canadian bands. Consequently, it tried to derail the legislation by tabling 471 amendments and required the then Liberal-led Canadian Parliament to sit in session for over forty-two hours before managing to pass the Agreement in its original form (*Guardian*, 11 Dec. 1999: 23). Setting aside the clear inconsistency that seems to have escaped the Reform Party – that non-indigenous control of indigenous peoples is regarded as legitimate without question, whereas the reverse is not – this opposition highlights, once again, the strong antipathy to any notion of group-differentiated rights within modern nation-states. The effects of the latter are also graphically illustrated by the successes, and subsequent reverses, in policy toward Aboriginal land rights in Australia over the last twenty years.

In 1992 the High Court of Australia ruled in favor of Koiki Mabo and four other plaintiffs over their claims that a common law property right of 'native title' had existed prior to European colonization and the subsequent annexation of their lands by the Queensland government (see Patton, 1995). The Mabo Decision (*Mabo v. Queensland* (no. 2), 1992) set a major new precedent since, as we saw in Chapter 2, up until that time European colonization of Australia had been predicated on the convenient legal fiction of terra nullius (empty land). Consequently, indigenous land rights were never acknowledged and did not evolve as part of Australian land and property law – in contrast to Aotearoa/New Zealand, for example (see below). The consequence of the Mabo decision was the belated recognition that Australia's indigenous peoples could lay claim to native title on the 25 percent of Australia that remained Crown or public land (Webber, 2000). The (1993) Native Land Act, implemented by the Australian Labor Party, the government of the day, formalized and clarified this position. The Mabo Decision also required that indigenous peoples had to demonstrate a continued (and continuous) association with their traditional lands. However, this caveat was modified somewhat by the Wik Decision in the Australian High Court in 1996, which ruled that, where land had been given to white farmers under a colonial pastoral lease scheme, native title was not *automatically* extinguished.[7]

The response to these decisions, particularly the latter, can be seen in the high-profile campaign of 'white hysteria' (Perera and Pugliese, 1998) that was subsequently waged. This was most apparent in the aforementioned rise of Pauline Hanson's 'One Nation' Party, with its overtly anti-Aboriginal policies, and in the orchestrated opposition of the National Farmers Federation (NFF) to the Wik Decision. With respect to the latter, the NFF argued disingenuously that it would give carte blanche to Australia's indigenous peoples to make claims on private land – although what was actually at stake was the land granted under the colonial pastoral lease scheme. At the same time, the NFF campaign continued to promote the 'myth' of the centrality of the white pioneers to Australia's 'national' (read: colonial) heritage and identity. As a result of this often-vitriolic campaign, and with the subsequent election of the conservative Howard government in 1996, a significantly delimited Native Title Act was implemented in 1998, retrenching most of the gains achieved for Australian Aboriginal peoples in the Mabo and Wik decisions.

There were to be many more examples of the retrenchment of Aboriginal rights over the next decade. While Hanson's One Nation Party rose and fell relatively quickly, its major political achievement was perhaps to so normalize political opposition to Aboriginal rights that the conservative Howard government (1996–2007) could then champion this opposition as its own. The Howard government's success in doing so can also be attributed to the way it cloaked its arguments against Aboriginal rights within the discourse of social unity and identical treatment, rather than overt racism (Robbins, 2006, 2010). Australian Aboriginal peoples were accordingly repositioned as just one of many competing interest groups, rather than as a national minority, or ethnie, with specific rights and representation. This allowed the Howard government to dismantle many of the mechanisms that had already been established for separate indigenous representation. For example, in 2005 the government disbanded the Aboriginal and Torres Strait Islander Commission, ending a tradition of elected indigenous representation established since the 1970s. In 2007, it also implemented a state-enforced 'national emergency response' in the Northern Territory aimed ostensibly at addressing alcoholism and sexual abuse among rural Aboriginal communities. This was particularly controversial because, while it was addressing real social concerns, it was also overtly paternalistic and punitive, with no meaningful consultation or partnership with Aboriginal peoples.

Meanwhile, Howard consistently refused to make any links between the current plight of many Australian Aboriginal peoples, including abject poverty and widespread social disintegration, and their history of forced resettlement, marginalization, racism and genocide. Throughout his eleven-year tenure, he refused point blank, for example, to offer an official apology for the 'stolen generations', dismissing it as a 'black armband' view of Australian history. It was only after the Howard government finally fell in November 2007, that such an apology was eventually forthcoming. The then new Australian Labor Prime Minister, Kevin Rudd, offered an official apology about the stolen generations to the Australian Aboriginal peoples on 13 February 2008.[8]

It is clear from the above examples that recent developments toward greater 'internal self-determination' for indigenous peoples, both at national and international levels, have been significant, yet also contested and highly uneven. As de Varennes comments of these developments: 'Whilst there is certainly no unanimity, both international and national law appear to be heading towards increased recognition of the special position which indigenous peoples occupy within a [nation-state's] legal and political order' (1996a: 274). But just as clearly, these gains remain fragile and subject to ongoing, often debilitating, opposition. This is despite the fact that indigenous claims are not principally concerned with the politically contentious question of secession. Indeed, internal self-determination bears a remarkable resemblance to the concept of cultural nationalism, discussed in Chapter 2, with its emphasis on the transformation of national communities from *within* the nation-state, rather than with secession per se. Indigenous peoples are not consumed with questions of secession since, generally, their limited socioeconomic, demographic and political strength precludes such an option. Rather, indigenous peoples are advocating a right to separate representation, *alongside* national majorities, on the basis that they constitute a distinct ethnie in the nation-state. Indeed, as we have seen, many nation-states already acknowledge as part of their internal law, however begrudgingly, that indigenous peoples have either retained some degree of inherent sovereignty that has not been extinguished by conquest and/or colonization, or have a continuing legal status that sets them apart (de Varennes, 1996a, b; Thornberry, 2002; Xanthaki, 2007).

These national minority claims thus contrast with the usual polyethnic concerns of (immigrant) ethnic minority groups for the abolition of barriers that lead to disadvantage and preclude greater integration into the nation-state (see Chapter 2). This is not to say, of course, that indigenous peoples do not also share these concerns – they clearly do. However, polyethnic claims are not their *principal* preoccupation. Thus, state policies that address only these concerns, on the basis that indigenous peoples are simply one of many disadvantaged ethnic minority groups, do little to allay their specific demands. The Howard government's actions in Australia from 1996–2007 illustrate this point all too clearly.

Indigenous language and education rights

The cultural nationalist emphases of indigenous claims are also significant for our purposes because, in addition to questions of land restoration and the granting of greater political autonomy, they often have, as a central concern, issues of language and education. In this respect, Articles 14 and 15 of the UNDRIP are most pertinent. Article 14 reads:

1   Indigenous peoples have the right to *establish and control their educational systems* and institutions *providing education in their own languages*, in a manner appropriate to their cultural methods of teaching and learning.
2   Indigenous individuals, particularly children, have the right to all levels and forms of education of the State without discrimination.
3   States shall, in conjunction with indigenous peoples, take *effective* measures, in order for indigenous individuals, particularly children, including those living outside their communities, to have access, when possible, to an education in their own culture and provided in their own language. (My emphases)

Article 15:

1   Indigenous peoples have the right to the dignity and diversity of their cultures, traditions, histories and aspirations, which shall be appropriately reflected in education and public information.
2   States shall take effective measures*, in consultation and cooperation with the indigenous peoples concerned*, to combat prejudice and eliminate discrimination and to promote tolerance, understanding and good relations among indigenous peoples and all other segments of society.[9] (My emphasis)

The clear desire of indigenous peoples for greater linguistic and educational *control* apparent in these articles is, in turn, a product of colonial histories of cultural and linguistic proscription, particularly within education, that must be regarded as being at the most extreme end of such practices. These extremes were reinforced by the wider historical attempts at the 'resocialization' of indigenous children (of which education formed a key part), discussed at the beginning of this chapter. The result, not surprisingly, has been not only the loss of indigenous languages but also a long history of educational 'failure' for indigenous students within education (see Shields et al., 2005; Hornberger, 2011; McCarty, 2011).

Given this history, it is thus also not surprising that education has now come to be seen as a key arena in which indigenous peoples can reclaim and revalue their languages and cultures and, in so doing, improve the educational success of indigenous students. As a result, we have seen over the last thirty years the emergence internationally of numerous indigenous community-based education initiatives where indigenous community control and a central role for indigenous languages and cultures are prominent features (see McCarty and Zepeda, 1995; Henze and Davis, 1999; May, 1999c; May and Aikman, 2003). While still in many cases small-scale, and while still facing considerable odds, these initiatives *are* beginning to have a positive effect on the specific educational futures of indigenous students and, more broadly, the retention of indigenous language and cultures. In the process, the normalization and valorization of European languages and cultures, and their representation within education, are being critiqued and contested. In particular, indigenous language education proponents argue that the long historical dominance of European norms and values in schooling has nothing to do with their greater intrinsic value or use, but rather with the exercise and legitimation of unequal power relations which privilege such languages and cultural practices over all others, indigenous ones in particular. There is clearly potential in these arguments for the reinforcement of a static, reified view of (indigenous) languages and cultures, and their unhelpful juxtaposition with dominant 'European' cultural and linguistic practices (see, for example, Hornberger and King, 1999; Patrick, 2004, 2007). But emergent practice has tended to demonstrate a more contextual, relational approach – one that incorporates a dynamic and ongoing process of 'cultural negotiation', rather than a simple return to, or retrenchment of past practices.

An exemplar of the latter can be found in Aotearoa/New Zealand, [10] which has seen, in the last thirty years, the successful revitalization of the indigenous Māori language. This development, based primarily on the (re)establishment of Māori-language education, is both a product and illustration of a wider repositioning of identity and minority rights' issues within this once 'British settler society' (see May, 2002; Walker, 2004; Spoonley et al., 2004).

Aotearoa/New Zealand: a tale of two ethnicities

When one significant section of the community burns with a sense of injustice, the rest of the community cannot safely pretend that there is no reason for their discontent. (Waitangi Tribunal, 1986: 46)

Until the 1960s, Aotearoa/New Zealand had regarded itself, and been regarded by others, as a model of harmonious 'race' relations; a rare success story of colonization. Pākehā (European)[11] New Zealanders, in particular, looked back with pride at a colonial history of mutual respect, cooperation and integration with the indigenous Māori iwi (tribes). This colonial history began with Pākehā settlement of Aotearoa/New Zealand in the late eighteenth century, although prior to the arrival of the first Pākehā, Māori had been resident in Aotearoa/New Zealand for at least 500, perhaps as many as 1,000 years (King, 2003).

The British Crown subsequently formalized colonial relations between Māori and Pākehā in the nineteenth century, most notably via the foundational colonial document, the Treaty of Waitangi – Te Tiriti o Waitangi – signed on 6 February 1840 between the British Crown and Māori chiefs. A surprisingly progressive document for its time, the Treaty specifically attempted to establish the rights and responsibilities of both parties as a mutual framework by which colonization could proceed. Captain Hobson, the Crown's representative, was instructed to obtain the surrender of Aotearoa/New Zealand as a sovereign state to the British Crown, but only by 'free and intelligent consent' of the 'natives'. In return, Māori were to be guaranteed possession of 'their lands, their homes and all their treasured possessions (taonga)'. Consequently, the Treaty had come to be commemorated as the central symbol of this apparently benign history. The words 'he iwi tahi tātou' (we are all one people) – spoken by William Hobson, at the Treaty's signing – provided its leitmotif. In short, while undeniably a white settler colony in origin (Larner and Spoonley, 1995), the emergence of Aotearoa/New Zealand as a nation-state was seen to have avoided the worst excesses of colonialism. Māori were highly regarded, intermixing and miscegenation were common, and Māori language and culture were incorporated, at least to some degree, into New Zealand life. Or so the story went.

From the 1970s, a quite different story emerged into the public domain. A generation of young, urban and educated Māori articulated a history of continued conflict and oppression of Māori by Pākehā (Sharp, 1990), a theme that was to be taken up in subsequent revisionist histories of the country (see especially Sinclair, 1993; Belich, 1996, 2001; King, 2003). It was a history that had been consistently told by many Māori over previous generations but one that had seldom actually been *heard* before. In this view, the Treaty of Waitangi was a fraud; an inconvenient document that had been quickly and ruthlessly trivialized by Pākehā settlers in their avaricious quest for land.

The issue of legitimacy centers on the question of whether the informed consent of Māori was ever obtained at the signing of the Treaty. Much of this has to do with the discrepancies between the English language version of the Treaty and the Māori language version that the Chiefs actually signed. The Treaty comprises three articles. In Article 1, for example, there is a distinction between the ceding of 'all the rights and powers of *Sovereignty*' in the English version – equating to the term 'tino rangatiratanga', or absolute Chieftainship, in Māori – and the actual use in the Māori text of the lesser term 'kāwanatanga', or governorship. In Article 2 this discrepancy is reinforced. In the official English translation Māori are granted 'exclusive and undisturbed possession of their Lands and Estates, Forestries, Fisheries and other properties which they may individually and collectively possess'. In the Māori translation this becomes 'the absolute Chieftainship (tino rangatiratanga) of their lands, of their homes and all their treasured possessions'. The Chiefs are thus likely to have understood Article 2 as confirming their own sovereign rights in return for a limited concession (granted in Article 1) of Pākehā 'governorship'. Article 3 – the least contentious – extends to Māori the rights of British citizens, although the Māori version talks again of governance, rather than sovereignty – reinforcing the previous emphases (see Orange, 1987; Kawharu, 1989). In short for Māori, power was to be shared under the aegis of the Treaty and its central principle (so they thought) of partnership. But for the British colonizers, it was simply to be transferred (Fleras and Spoonley, 1999).

And that was not the only thing that was to be transferred, since any considered reading of New Zealand history unequivocally supports the subsequent ruthless quest for land by Pākehā settlers. While a period of prosperity and relative stability between Māori and Pākehā followed the signing of the Treaty, this ended with the land wars of the 1860s in which the Settler Government, established in 1852, invaded the Taranaki and Waikato districts of the North Island of New Zealand. The ostensible aim of these campaigns was to move against iwi (tribal) supporters of Kīngitanga (the King movement) – a confederation of tribes under the Māori king, Te Wherowhero – who supposedly posed a threat to law and order. The actual aim was to remove the opposition of Kīngitanga to the expropriation of Māori land for the rapidly growing numbers of Pākehā settlers (Belich, 1986; Walker, 2004). When military means proved inconclusive, the government resorted to legislation, which transformed communally owned Māori land into individual titles – as in English law – in order to expedite the further sale of the land. This proved so successful that by the turn of the twentieth century almost all New Zealand territory was in European hands. Meanwhile, the Pākehā population had risen from 1,000 in 1838 to 770,000 by 1900, while the Māori population had fallen from an estimated 100,000–200,000 at the time of European settlement to the nadir of 45,549 in 1900 – in effect, a 75 percent population collapse of Māori over the course of the nineteenth century (Stannard, 1989). As Claudia Orange concludes: 'In many respects New Zealand, in spite of the treaty, has been merely a variation in the colonial domination of indigenous races [sic]' (1987: 5).

Indeed, the degree to which Treaty obligations came to be overtaken by 'events' is reflected by the New Zealand Chief Justice, Sir James Prendergast, who in 1877, in *Wi Parata v Bishop of Wellington*, could declare the treaty 'a simple nullity'. This legal view was to hold sway until the 1980s. As Orange's previous comment suggests, what resulted for Māori were the usual deleterious effects of colonization upon an indigenous people – political disenfranchisement, misappropriation of land, population and health decline, educational disadvantage and socioeconomic marginalization. The cumulative weight of this historical process, allied with the rapid urbanization of Māori since the Second World War,[12] had seen their economic and social incorporation into a metropolitan-based cultural division of labor, usually at the lowest point of entry, that of surplus unskilled labor (Miles and Spoonley, 1985; Pearson, 1990; Spoonley, 1996). The economic downturn precipitated by the international oil crisis in the 1970s, and the neoliberal economic agenda of successive New Zealand governments from the 1980s onwards, exacerbated further the disparities between Māori and Pākehā on most social and economic indices. Thus, while Māori comprised 14.6 percent (565,329) of New Zealand's population of 4 million at the time of the last (2006) census, they are disproportionately located in social and economic 'at risk' categories when compared with the rest of the population. Māori workers, for example, are heavily under-represented in high-income, high-skilled and growing sectors of the economy. Conversely, they are over-represented in low-paid, low-skilled, declining occupations, and among beneficiaries and those not in paid employment. The emasculation of low-skilled, semi-skilled occupations over the last three decades, under the neoliberal economic agenda, has also resulted in a disproportionately high level of unemployment for Māori; 11 percent of all Māori over fifteen years, compared with 5.1 percent for the total population at the time of the 2006 census. Median annual income for Māori also compares unfavorably, being $NZ5000 less than the national average (Statistics New Zealand, 2009).

These ongoing disparities in employment and income are also apparent in other economic, social and educational indices. For example, in 1991, 56 percent of Māori aged between 15 and 59 years were receiving some form of income-support benefit and Māori were also proportionately over-represented on all other welfare benefits, except for the pension. With respect to the latter, 4.3 percent of the Māori population received a pension compared with 17.1 percent of non-Māori. While some of this has to do with the younger age structure of the Māori population, it is also because, quite simply, too few Māori live long enough. Health indicators here present a disturbing picture. Māori live eight years less, on average, than non-Māori (Statistics New Zealand, 2010).

The immunization rates of Māori children – less than 60 percent compared with 90 percent for most other 'developed' countries – see Māori children suffer disproportionately from preventable diseases. Half of all Māori over 15 smoke (compared with about a quarter of the non-Māori population). This includes 45 percent of men and 57 percent of women, with Māori women having one of the highest lung cancer rates in the world (McLoughlin, 1993).

Educational status completes the picture of comparative disadvantage for Māori. In 1991, for example, 60 percent of Māori aged more than 15 still held no formal educational qualifications. This compared with 40 percent for non-Māori. At the same time, Māori were nearly half as likely as the total population to hold a tertiary qualification. This low level of educational attainment was also a key factor in the disproportionate location of Māori in the lowest levels of the labor market (Davies and Nicholl, 1993).

While school retention rates for Māori have improved since that time (Chapple et al., 1997), more recent data suggest that these negative educational patterns continue to persist. The proportion of Māori students leaving school with little or no formal attainment in 2007 (10.1 percent) was still 2.9 times higher than the corresponding percentage for Pākehā students (3.5 percent) (Education Counts, 2008). The latest (2006) PISA results for New Zealand for reading literacy also indicate that 15-year-old Māori students are disproportionately represented in the lowest levels of reading achievement (9 percent, compared with 2 percent for Pākehā; see Marshall et al., 2008). Meanwhile, Māori adults are also over-represented in the lowest levels of reading achievement. The (1997) International Adult Literacy Survey found, for example, that 70 percent of Māori adults were situated below Level 3, the minimum level required for functional literacy in English (New Zealand Ministry of Education, 2001).

In light of these longstanding unfavorable indicators, Māori activists have since the 1970s increasingly rejected the assimilationist tenets upon which colonization, and much public policy toward Māori, had historically been based. Drawing initially on contemporary notions of ethnic nationalism (Mulgan, 1989) and subsequently on the right as indigenous peoples to self-determination (Wilson and Yeatman, 1995; Durie, 1998), they have argued, instead, for the separate recognition by the state of Māori political culture and social organization, and for the recognition of the cultural and linguistic *distinctiveness* of Māori.

Again, these claims have proved to be controversial, particularly among the Pākehā majority in Aotearoa/New Zealand (Fleras and Spoonley, 1999). As elsewhere, there were the usual proclamations of 'special treatment' and/or 'reverse apartheid' that accompany oppositional majoritarian discourses toward the recognition of group-differentiated rights (cf. Chapter 3). However, such was their momentum that by the early 1980s Māori claims to indigenousness had set the platform for a significant realignment of Māori–Pākehā relations.

This realignment took the form of a constitutional revolution that saw the Treaty of Waitangi return to center stage in New Zealand public life after more than a century of neglect. As a result of increasing Māori advocacy and political protest, greater emphasis was placed on pursuing legal and constitutional redress for Māori in relation to the Treaty. In this regard, the key constitutional vehicle for arbitrating Māori claims has been the quasi-legal body, the Waitangi Tribunal. Originally set up in 1975, with limited powers to hear Māori grievances, it was invested in 1984 with the retrospective power to settle Māori claims against the Crown, dating back to 1840 when the Treaty was first signed. While land issues have been the principal focus of the Tribunal's subsequent deliberations, the Tribunal has also ruled on the status of, among other things, the Māori language (see below). The Waitangi Tribunal has thus been central to reinvesting moral and legal authority in the Treaty of Waitangi and this has led, both directly and indirectly in recent years, to considerable restitution by the Crown to Māori claimants.

As a result of the Treaty's return to prominence, the concept of biculturalism has also come to the fore in Aotearoa/New Zealand (Durie, 1998; Walker, 2004; O'Sullivan, 2007). The concept has a twofold meaning in the New Zealand context. First, it highlights ongoing Māori sovereignty, or 'tino rangatiratanga', something Māori argue they never ceded as a result of signing the Treaty of Waitangi. As such, it accords with wider notions of indigenous self-determination within international law, as discussed earlier in this chapter. While retaining an emphasis on some degree of separate development and/or autonomy for Māori, biculturalism has also been employed to describe a *partnership* between Māori and Pākehā, under the Treaty's auspices, rather than separation of one group from the other (see, for example, New Zealand Ministerial Advisory Committee, 1986). This clearly accords with Iris Marion Young's emphasis on the relational nature of group-differentiated rights, discussed in Chapter 3, as well as reflecting accurately the close and symbiotic relationship between Māori and Pākehā since the time of colonization. Second, the partnership model emphasizes the Crown's *active* commitment to redressing past injustices toward Māori, and its commitment to the inclusion of Treaty 'principles' within the constitutional and administrative framework of the modern New Zealand nation-state. Again, the active requirement of the Crown's commitment accords with recent interpretations in international law in relation to indigenous rights, which highlight that laissez-faire policies toward indigenous peoples do little, if anything, to remediate historical injustices (for further discussion, see Anaya, 1996; Thornberry, 2002; cf. Chapter 5).

Where the New Zealand government has balked at its own rhetoric, it has been kept to its task by the judiciary. In June 1987, for example, the New Zealand Court of Appeal, in a landmark judgment, ruled against a key piece of government legislation – the State Owned Enterprises Act – which would have seen the transfer of Crown land to semi-privatized 'state owned enterprises' (SOEs). The central legal point of the case concerned the Treaty of Waitangi. Section 9 of the SOE Act stated that nothing in the Act shall permit the Crown to act in a manner inconsistent with the principles of the Treaty. Accordingly, the five appeal judges were unanimous that the Treaty of Waitangi prevented the Crown from transferring land without first entering into proper arrangements to protect Māori rights. It was a historic judgment. As Ranginui Walker observes, in the space of just a few years, the Treaty had been transformed 'from "a simple nullity" to the level of a constitutional instrument in the renegotiation of the relationship between Māori and Pākehā in modern times' (2004: 266). In short, the doctrine of biculturalism had become established in political and public discourse by the late 1980s, and increasingly institutionalized in law from that time on.

As a result, Māori have made significant advances over the last twenty years with respect to their wider political claims to indigenous self-determination. The 1990s saw the New Zealand government begin to provide reparation for raupatu, the illegal appropriation of Māori land during the colonial period. As part of the Waitangi Tribunal process, individual iwi (tribes) were granted significant land settlements, beginning in 1995 with the Tainui iwi (the central tribe of the Kīngitanga movement, discussed earlier). These settlements have continued to the present day on a case-by-case basis. Other significant developments include the establishment of the Māori Television Service (MTS) in March 2004. This built directly on developments in Māori-language radio over the previous two decades. While there was some initial political ambivalence to establishing MTS on the ostensible grounds of costs and audience reach, consistent advocacy from Māori groups saw the eventual enactment of the legislation, and related funding.[13]

However, as with the other contexts discussed above, there have also been ongoing contention and opposition to these developments, particularly among the Pākehā ethnic majority. In 2004, the then leader of the conservative National opposition party, Don Brash, delivered a 'state of the nation' speech decrying the politics of 'race-based legislation' and the Treaty 'grievance industry'. Its tone and intent were strikingly similar to Pauline Hanson's rhetoric against Aboriginal peoples in Australia and generated considerable public controversy and a growing backlash against Māori political gains (Walker, 2004).

So much so that the New Zealand Labour Government, under then leader Helen Clark, reneged on a number of key commitments to Māori in a blatant attempt to retain political power.[14] The most notable of these was its failure to support a legal ruling allowing Māori to test the issue of customary rights to the foreshore through the court system. Instead, the Labour Government used its legislative powers to rush through Parliament the Foreshore and Seabed Bill (2004). The Bill specifically precluded the possibility of Māori seeking such redress – denying Māori due legal process in so doing. This political timidity in the face of growing public opposition to biculturalism is also likely to have influenced the New Zealand Government's subsequent decision not to support the final version of UNDRIP (see above). Ongoing debates and controversies over the politics of biculturalism continue to the present day, albeit in somewhat more muted tones in recent years. Having said that, not all areas of indigenous self-determination for Māori have proved to be contentious. One such area is Māori language and education policy, where significant gains over the last thirty years are clearly apparent and have not been retrenched – or at least, not yet.

Māori language and education policy

As with many other colonial contexts, New Zealand's early colonial history was characterized by a resolutely assimilationist approach to the education of Māori. Accordingly, the teaching of English was considered to be a central task of the school, and te reo Māori was often regarded as the prime obstacle to the progress of Māori children (Benton, 1981). In particular, Māori have historically had very little meaningful influence in educational policy decision-making (G. Smith, 1990a). As Linda Tuhiwai Smith (1999) observes, schooling came to be seen as a primary instrument for taming and civilizing the 'natives' and forging a nation which was connected at a concrete level with the historical and moral processes of Britain. Ironically, in this process, Pākehā were not only to repudiate and replace Māori language and knowledge structures within education but were also to deny Māori full access to European knowledge and learning.

This was not always so. Prior to the arrival of Pākehā, Māori had practiced a sophisticated and functional system of education based on an extensive network of oral tradition, and with its own rational and complex knowledge structure (G. Smith, 1989). Moreover, upon European colonization in the early nineteenth century, Māori actively sought to complement their own educational knowledge, and their long-established oral tradition, with 'Pākehā wisdom'. Largely for these reasons they turned to the early mission schools which, while teaching only the standard subjects of the English school curriculum, did so through the medium of te reo Māori. As a result, the period in which these schools were most influential – 1816 to the mid-1840s – saw a rapid spread of literacy among Māori *in both Māori and English*. The initial aim for Māori in incorporating Pākehā learning was one of enhancing their traditional way of life. However, from the 1840s this outlook was increasingly modified as Māori came to perceive European knowledge as a necessary defence against the increasing encroachment of Pākehā society upon Māori sovereignty and resources (J. Williams, 1969). As Ward observes of this:

> the Maori response to Western contact was highly intellectual, flexible and progressive, and also highly selective, aiming largely to draw upon the strengths of the West to preserve the Maori people and their resources

from the threat of the West itself, and to enjoy its material and cultural riches co-equally with the Westerners. (1974: p. viii)

The growing fear among Māori of Pākehā encroachment was, as already evidenced, well founded. It was also to coincide in the 1840s with a change to a much more overtly assimilationist policy toward Māori in education. As Barrington and Beaglehole argue: 'Education was to be deliberately out of touch with the Maori environment in the belief that formal schooling could transform the Maori and fit him [sic] for a different environment. The Maori was to be lifted from one society to another' (1974: 4). The (1844) Native Trust Ordinance stated, for example, that the 'great disasters [that] have fallen on other uncivilised nations on being brought into contact with Colonists from the nations of Europe' would only be avoided by 'assimilating as speedily as possible the habits and usages of the Native to those of the European population'. The (1847) Education Ordinance Act reinforced this sentiment by making state funding of mission schools dependent on English being the medium of instruction, effectively ending teaching through te reo Māori. As the Auckland Inspector of Native Schools Henry Taylor was to argue in 1862, echoing the sentiments of J. D. C. Atkins about Native Americans in the USA (see Chapter 6):

> The Native language itself is also another obstacle in the way of civilisation, so long as it exists there is a barrier to the free and unrestrained intercourse which ought to exist between the two races [sic], it shuts out the less civilised portion of the population from the benefits which intercourse with the more enlightened would confer. The school-room alone has power to break down this wall of partition ... (AJHR, E-4, 1862: 35–8)

This position was further formalized in 1867 when the state established a system of village day schools in Māori rural communities, ten years prior to the establishment of a parallel public system. While some privately funded Māori schools remained independent, Māori schooling was now effectively controlled by the state. The Native School system, as it came to be known, operated a modified public school curriculum, with a particular emphasis on health and hygiene. Initially, teachers were expected to have some knowledge of the Māori language, which was to be used as an aid in teaching English. However, by the turn of the twentieth century the Māori language had all but been banned from the precincts of the schools; a prohibition, often enforced by corporal punishment, that was to continue until the 1950s (Simon and Smith, 2001).

But this was not all. Another theme which came to dominate state educational policy for Māori over this time was their supposed unsuitability for 'mental labour'. The aim of assimilation was ostensibly 'to lift Māori from one society to another', but only as long as they were not lifted *too* high. A key objective of native schooling thus came to be the preparation of Māori for laboring-class status, an objective that was rationalized largely through racial ideologies (Simon and Smith, 2001). As the Director of Education, T. B. Strong, observed in 1929, Māori education should 'lead the Maori to be a good farmer and the Maori girl to be a good farmer's wife'. Barrington has argued that such views 'included the assumption that Maori rural communities should be preserved and that Maori should stay within them, a biological and racist assumption that the "natural genius" of Maori lay in manual labor, and a strategy to reduce competition for expanding bureaucratic, commercial and professional positions in urban areas by putting impediments in the way of Maori students' (1992: 68–9). That Māori were to become largely proletarianized after the Second World War, as the needs of industry drew them to the urban areas in rapidly increasing numbers, must be seen as the logical outcome of these education policies, along with those directed at land alienation (Simon, 1989). It certainly goes some considerable way to explaining the current unfavorable socioeconomic and educational indices of Māori.

Education and language loss

Assimilationist policies in education also contributed significantly to the rapid decline of the Māori language over the course of the twentieth century. This was despite the fact that the English-only policy of Native schools was not initially seen as in any way threatening the Māori language and culture, and was strongly supported by some Māori (Simon and Smith, 2001). Since the 1940s, however, there has been a growing concern among Māori about the state and status of the Māori language, a concern compounded by the rapid urbanization of Māori since the Second World War. While the Māori language had long been excluded from the realms of the school, it had still been nurtured in largely rural Māori communities. Urbanization was to change all that. Thus, in 1930, a survey of Māori children estimated that 96.6 percent spoke only Māori at home. By 1960, only 26 percent spoke Māori. By 1979 the Māori language had retreated to the point where language death was predicted (R. Benton, 1979, 1983; see also N. Benton, 1989).

With this growing realization came an increased advocacy of the need for change in educational policy toward Māori. New approaches to language and education were sought. Assimilation was replaced in the 1960s by a brief period of 'integration'. Heralded by the 1961 Hunn Report, integration aimed 'to combine (not fuse) the Maori and Pakeha elements to form one nation wherein Maori culture remains distinct' (see Hunn, 1961: 14–16). While an apparently laudable aim, integration proved little different in either theory or practice from its predecessor. It was less crude than assimilation in its conceptions of culture but a distinct cultural hierarchy continued to underpin the model. Hunn, for example, clearly regarded those aspects of the Māori culture that were to 'remain distinct' as 'relics' of a tribal culture of which 'only the fittest elements (worthiest of preservation) have survived the onset of civilisation'. Compared with this 'backward life in primitive conditions', he argued that 'pressure [should] be brought to bear on [Māori] to conform to ... the pakeha mode of life' (ibid), which he equated with modernity and progress. This deficit view simply reinforced the previous assimilationist agenda and resulted in the continued perception of Māori as an educational 'problem' (Bishop and Glynn, 1999; Shields et al., 2005). As such, it corresponds with Stages 1 and 2 of Churchill's typology, discussed in Chapter 5.

In the face of mounting criticism from Māori, integration was replaced in the 1970s and 1980s by multicultural education. This latter approach – representing Stage 3 of Churchill's typology – came to be known as taha Māori (literally, the Māori side). In what was, by now, an integrated state education system, taha Māori approaches to teaching attempted to incorporate a specifically Māori dimension into the curriculum that was available to *all* pupils, Māori and non-Māori alike. As its official definition outlines: 'Taha Māori is the inclusion of *aspects of* Māori language and culture in the philosophy, organisation and the content of the school ... It should be a normal part of the school climate with which all pupils should feel comfortable and at ease' (New Zealand Department of Education, 1984a; my emphasis). While the emphasis here was clearly on biculturalism, this was also seen as a first step to the incorporation of other cultures within the curriculum along similar lines. As a related publication states: 'an effective approach to multicultural education *is through* bicultural education' (New Zealand Department of Education, 1984b: 31; my emphasis).

But many Māori were wary of multiculturalism in the form of taha Māori. One key criticism was that the process of limiting biculturalism to support for 'aspects of Māori language and culture' within schools fell far short of the biculturalism that many Māori sought; a biculturalism concerned primarily with institutional transformation and social change (see also below). In this sense, multiculturalism was also seen as a useful ideology for *containing* the conflicts of ethnic groups within existing social relations rather than as the basis for any real power-sharing between Māori and Pākehā and, from that basis, other ethnic groups. Second, the peripheral and selective treatment of Māori language and culture did little, if anything, to change the cultural transmission of the dominant group within schooling, a criticism that has been directed at multicultural education more widely (May, 1994, 1999a; cf. Chapter 5). And third, the control of the policy, as with all previous educational approaches, remained firmly with Pākehā educationalists and administrators (Bishop and Glynn, 1999). The very process of cultural 'selection' highlights this lack of control for Māori in educational decision-making. However well intentioned, cultural 'selection' is a paternalistic exercise – inevitably reflecting more the interests and concerns of

Pākehā than those of Māori. This irony is illustrated by the conclusion of many Māori educationalists at the time that the main beneficiaries of taha Māori were actually Pākehā students (Irwin, 1989; G. Smith, 1990b).

None of these educational approaches ameliorated the issue of Māori language shift and loss. Consequently, by the 1990s, only one in ten, 50,000 people in all, were adult native speakers of Māori, and the majority of these were middle-aged or older (Te Taura Whiri i te Reo Māori, 1995). In the 2006 Census, 131,613 (23.7 percent) did identify as Māori speakers (New Zealand Ministry of Education, 2007), although this figure is likely to encompass a wide range of language proficiency. To reinforce this point, the National Māori Language Survey, undertaken in 2001 (Te Puni Kōkiri, 2001), found that among Māori adults, there were as few as 22,000 *highly fluent* Māori speakers, many of whom (73 percent) were 45 years of age or older, with a further 22,000 with medium fluency levels. More worryingly, 58 percent of Māori adults could not speak Māori beyond a 'few words or phrases'. The most recent report to date continues to highlight the risk of endangerment for te reo Māori, particularly in relation to the ongoing decline of fluent speakers and limited intergenerational transmission (Waitangi Tribunal, 2010). However, these figures would be even worse if it had not been for two key developments in New Zealand language and education policy in the last twenty-five years.

Language reversal

The first occurred in 1985/6, when a legal decision by the Waitangi Tribunal concerning the recognition and role of Māori as a language of the state concluded that te reo Māori could be regarded as a taonga (treasured possession) and therefore had a *guaranteed* right to protection under the terms of the Treaty of Waitangi (Waitangi Tribunal, 1986). In the ruling, the term 'guarantee' was defined as 'more than merely leaving Māori people unhindered in their enjoyment of the language and culture'. It also required 'active steps' to be taken by the guarantor [the state] to ensure that Māori have and retain 'the full exclusive and undisturbed possession of their language and culture' (Waitangi Tribunal, 1986: 29), a clear promotion-oriented language right. As a result, in 1987, the Māori Language Act was passed, legitimating for the first time Māori as an official language of Aotearoa/New Zealand. This legal recognition of the language is still somewhat limited. In particular, the right to use or to demand the use of Māori in the public domain does not extend beyond the oral use of the language in courts of law and some quasi-legal tribunals. Nonetheless, it still stands as one of the few examples where the first language of an indigenous people has been made an official state language.[15] The Act also provided for the establishment of a Māori Language Commission, Te Taura Whiri i te Reo Māori. Closely modeled on the Irish Bord na Gaeilge (cf. Chapter 4), the

Commission's role is to monitor and promote the use of the language, although its number of staff and resources are limited.[16]

More significant still have been developments in Māori-language education, most prominently since the 1980s, of which more in a moment. However, these developments had their genesis, in turn, in the 1960s, when a formal review of the education system, the Currie Commission, included in its recommendations the teaching of Māori as an optional subject at high school level. This first tentative step to reintroduce te reo Māori into the school curriculum initiated a period of renewed debate on the merits of bilingual schooling in Aotearoa/New Zealand. It was to culminate, in 1977, with the first officially sanctioned English/Māori bilingual primary school at Ruatoki – one of the last predominantly Māori-speaking communities in the country. Other schools were to follow – providing, primarily, a 'transition' approach to bilingualism (Stage 4 in Churchill's typology; see Chapter 5). By 1988, twenty such bilingual schools had been established, predominantly in Māori rural communities. These developments led in turn to the rapid expansion of bilingual programs across New Zealand schools. By 1996, the overall number of students in bilingual programs had expanded exponentially to 33,438, the vast majority of whom were Māori (New Zealand Ministry of Education, 1998). The numbers have held relatively constant since then (New Zealand Ministry of Education, 2007).

Given the developments in bilingual education that the Currie Commission precipitated, it is no doubt ironic that the Commission itself remained deeply ambivalent about any greater role for the Māori language in the educational process (Benton, 1981). It certainly did not envisage the development of Māori/English bilingualism in schools in the ways just described. In a close echo of the Swann Report (see Chapter 5), the Commission stated that the school 'is not, nor can it ever be the prime agency in conserving the Māori cultural heritage'. This is, of course, true to a point. However, it begs a question – if the school clearly performs this function, at least to some degree, for Pākehā children, why not also for Māori?

The Currie Commission may well have been surprised by the subsequent development of bilingual programs in light of its own, far more tentative recommendations. However, it would surely have been agog at the subsequent development of whole-school, full-immersion, Māori-language schools from the 1980s onwards, which have formed the vanguard of Māori-language revitalization in Aotearoa/New Zealand. This began with the establishment of Te Kōhanga Reo – full-immersion Māori-language preschool programs, initially run independently by parents. It has since developed to all levels of education and has subsequently been incorporated into the state education system, thus spearheading the beginnings of what Christina Paulston (1993: 281) has described as 'language reversal'; a process by which 'one of the languages of a state begins to move back into more prominent use' (see May, 2004, for an extended discussion).

Kōhanga reo (preschool 'language nests')

To gauge the significance and impact of these developments, one only has to look at the growth of the Māori-language education movement. In 1982, the first kōhanga reo was established – by 1993, at its high point, there were 809 kōhanga catering for over 14,500 Māori children (New Zealand Ministry of Education, 1998). Numbers have declined somewhat since then but continue to remain significant. In 2009, 9,288 children were attending 464 kōhanga reo, a quarter of all Māori children in preschool education (Waitangi Tribunal, 2010).

The kaupapa (philosophy, set of objectives) of Te Kōhanga Reo combines an emphasis on Māori language revitalization with indigenous control of education, consonant with the key principles of UNDRIP. Its key philosophical principles can be summarized as follows:

- total immersion in te reo Māori at the kōhanga reo;
- the imparting of Māori cultural and spiritual values and concepts to the children;
- the teaching and involvement of the children in tikanga Māori (Māori customs and cultural practices/protocols);
- the complete administration of each center by the whānau (extended family; see below);
- the utilization of many traditional techniques of child care and knowledge acquisition (Sharples, 1988).

From this, three aspects can be highlighted as key organizing principles (see Kā'ai, 1990).

Te Reo (language)

'He kōrero Māori' (speaking in Māori) is a central organizing principle of Te Kōhanga Reo. An environment where only Māori is spoken is seen as the best means by which 'language reversal' can be achieved. Only this can contest the current dominance of English in almost every other domain in New Zealand life. Culturally preferred styles of pedagogy – such as tuakana/teina roles (peer tutoring) and collaborative teaching and learning – also feature prominently in the ethos and practice of kōhanga (see Metge, 1990).

Whānau (extended family)

Te Kōhanga Reo has been, from its inception, a parent-driven and resourced initiative based on whānau (extended-family) principles. Kōhanga are typically staffed by fluent Māori-speaking parents, grandparents and caregivers, often working in a voluntary capacity, and are supported by the wider whānau associated with the preschool. Whānau are usually constituted on traditional kinship grounds but have also come to include, in urban centers, a more generic concept in which criteria for affiliation has moved from kinship ties to that of commonality of interests and/or residence. The latter amounts to a contemporary form of cultural adaptation. The significance of kaumātua (elders) is also highlighted in the whānau structure. Kaumātua are regarded as active participants in the educational process. They are used not just as repositories of knowledge but also as teachers who can model the language, and other forms of cultural practice and behavior, to kōhanga children (L. Smith, 1989).

Mana motuhake (autonomy)

The central involvement of whānau in Te Kōhanga Reo has meant that Māori parents have been able to exert a significant degree of *local* control over the education of their children. The whānau approach is characterized by collective decision-making and each whānau has autonomy within the kaupapa (philosophy) of the movement (Irwin, 1990). Meaningful choices can thus be made over what children should learn, how they should learn and who should be involved in the learning (L. Smith, 1989). Individual whānau are also supported at a national level by the Kōhanga Reo Trust, which was established in the early 1980s to develop a nationally recognized syllabus for the purposes of gaining state funding. This latter objective was achieved in 1990. Prior to this, kōhanga had been almost entirely funded by whānau.

Kura Kaupapa Māori

Te Kōhanga Reo thus represents a major turning point for Māori perceptions and attitudes about language and education. Its success has also had a 'domino effect' throughout the education system, as kōhanga graduates have worked their way through the school system over the course of the last twenty-five years. This is particularly evident at the elementary (primary) level, with the emergence in the 1980s of full-immersion Māori-language schools, Kura Kaupapa Māori (literally: Māori philosophy school). The first Kura Kaupapa Māori, entirely privately funded, opened in February 1985. Five years of political advocacy by Māori followed before a pilot scheme of six Kura Kaupapa Māori was approved for state funding in 1990. By the end of that decade, fifty-nine Kura Kaupapa Māori had been established, serving approximately 4,000 students (New Zealand Ministry of Education, 1998). By 2007, the number of kura kaupapa Māori had grown to seventy-three, and 6,144 students (New Zealand Ministry of Education, 2007).[17]

The development of Kura Kaupapa Māori is largely attributable to the success of Te Kōhanga Reo and the increasing demand that it created for Māori-language education at the elementary level. A principal concern of kōhanga parents was to maintain the language gains made by their children. Kura Kaupapa Māori, in adopting the same language and organizational principles as Te Kōhanga Reo, could thus continue to reinforce these language gains within a Māori cultural and language environment. More broadly, the importance of 'relative autonomy' and 'community control' featured prominently in the advocacy of Kura Kaupapa Māori during the 1980s and 1990s (see G. Smith, 1990a, 1997). Te Kōhanga Reo had served to politicize Māori parents with regard to the education of their children (L. Smith, 1989, 1992; G. Smith, 1990b) and the advocacy of Kura Kaupapa Māori was the natural extension of this. In 1984, for example, the Māori Education Conference brought together Māori teachers, community leaders and educationalists from across the political spectrum to discuss Māori educational concerns. The consensus from the conference was that only significant structural reform of the state education system could change the educational circumstances of Māori children. If this did not occur, the Conference urged 'Māori withdrawal and the establishment of alternative schooling modeled on the principle of Kōhanga Reo'. In 1988, another hui (conference) produced the Mātawaia Declaration, which states:

> our children's needs cannot be met through a continuation of the present system of Pākehā control and veto of Māori aspirations for our children. It is time to change. Time for us to take control of our own destinies. We believe this development is both necessary and timely.

These calls from Māori for greater autonomy, and structural change, within education were to coincide with the reorganization of the state education system in 1988/9. The reforms emphasized parental choice, devolution and local school management. While many of the changes that resulted can be seen as problematic (Dale and Ozga, 1993), the reforms did provide Māori with a platform to argue for separate recognition of Kura Kaupapa Māori. Initially, the government responsible for the reforms was reticent in applying its own rhetoric of local control to the Kura Kaupapa Māori case. However, after a considerable degree of prevarication, and as a result of consistent and effective lobbying by Māori, Kura Kaupapa Māori was eventually incorporated into the (1990) Education Amendment Act as a recognized (and state-funded) schooling alternative within the New Zealand state education system. The principles that have since come to characterize it can be summarized as follows (see G. Smith, 1997; Bishop and Glynn, 1999).

1   *Rangatiratanga (relative autonomy principle)* A greater autonomy over key decision-making in schooling has been attained in areas such as administration, curriculum, pedagogy and Māori aspirations.

2   *Taonga Tuku Iho (cultural aspiration principle)* In Kura Kaupapa Māori to be Māori is taken for granted. The legitimacy of Māori language, culture and values is normalized.

3   *Ako Māori (culturally preferred pedagogy)* Culturally preferred forms of pedagogy such as peer tutoring and collaborative teaching and learning are employed. These are used in conjunction with general schooling methods where appropriate.

4   *Kia piki ake i ngā Raruraru o te Kainga (mediation of socioeconomic difficulties)* While Kura Kaupapa Māori (or education more generally) cannot, on its own, redress the socioeconomic circumstances facing Māori, the collective support and involvement provided by the whānau structure can *mitigate* some of its most debilitating effects.

5   *Whānau (extended-family principle)* The whānau structure provides a support network for individual members and requires a reciprocal obligation on these individuals to support and contribute to the collective aspirations of the group. It has been most successful in involving Māori parents in the administration of their children's schooling.

6   *Kaupapa (philosophy principle)* Kura Kaupapa Māori 'is concerned to teach a modern, up to date, relevant curriculum (within the national guidelines set by the state)' (G. Smith, 1990b: 194). The aim is not the forced choice of one culture and/or language over another but the provision of a distinctively Māori educational environment that is able to promote effectively bilingualism and biculturalism.

Some caveats

A number of caveats need to be outlined at this point. First, it needs to be reiterated that education cannot compensate for society (cf. Chapter 4), a reality also recognized by those directly involved in Māori-language education. The developments in Māori-language education must thus be situated clearly within the much wider social, economic and political framework of change that has occurred in Aotearoa/New Zealand over the last thirty years. This has had, at its heart, the restoration of Te Tiriti o Waitangi to its central role in mediating Māori/Pākehā relations and the related institutionalization of biculturalism in public policy and law.

But this then raises a second concern. The promotion of biculturalism as public policy may simply entrench essentialized conceptions of Māori ethnicity and culture, along with the (unnecessary) bifurcation of Māori and Pākehā identities. Critics of biculturalism in the New Zealand context repeatedly stress this point (see, for example, Hanson, 1989; Rata, 2000, 2005; Rata and Openshaw, 2006).[18] There are two responses to this critique. The first is that, despite consistent skepticism toward the legitimacy of Māori ethnicity in these accounts, there is nonetheless still a real sense in which Māori ethnicity and culture *can* be regarded as distinct from Pākehā. For example, in the *April Report* (Royal Commission on Social Policy, 1988), the following values were held to be representative of Māori culture: Te Ao Tūroa (guardianship of the natural environment), Whanaungatanga (the bonds of kinship), Manaakitanga (caring and sharing), Mana (authority and control among themselves), Kotahitanga (an emphasis on group commitment rather than individualism), Taonga-tuku-iho (cultural heritage) and Tūrangawaewae (a place to stand, a piece of land inalienably one's own). Even skeptics and critics broadly accept this description. As Andrew Sharp argues, in relation to the Commission's summary, 'irritating, unsubtle, simplifying, romantic, and naive as such a summary gloss of any culture must be ... [this] nevertheless does capture much of the way things were' (1990: 53).

In this sense, current Māori identity has inevitably been constructed out of colonialism and a symbiotic interaction with Pākehā. Following Anthony Smith's formulation of an ethnie (see Chapter 1), Māori may be said to have drawn on shared historical memories, myths of common ancestry and a growing sense of solidarity, in order to develop a common ethnic and cultural parlance in the face of a colonizing power. Indeed, the construction of a pan-Māori identity, where previously none had existed, was the principal means by which Māori came to distinguish themselves from Pākehā. A pan-Māori ethnic identity has not, however, replaced previous forms of identity formation among Māori, notably whānau (family), hapū (subtribe) and iwi (tribal) affiliations. Rather, it has emerged as an additional form of identity that both accommodates and is in tension with more particularistic and traditional affiliations (Pearson, 2000a, b). The continued interaction – and, at times, discontinuities – between these different levels of identity for Māori highlight the multifaceted nature of identity formation.

Despite these various tensions, Māori also clearly have a sufficient basis and claim to be recognized as a separate ethnie or nation within Aotearoa/New Zealand. Their political assertiveness is based on some form of unity, implied or actual, and the claims to resources and rights have been made on the basis of their rights as indigenous peoples. The politicization of Māori ethnicity then can perhaps be best described by the aphorism 'old symbols, new meanings' – the phenomenon of going into the future by way of reclaiming the past (Greenland, 1991). This process has also inevitably involved the (re)mobilization and (re)articulation of Māori identities – in a dynamic and changing combination of traditional, new and hybrid forms – as a basis for their claims to greater self-determination (O'Sullivan, 2007). This is a feature that is characteristic of the wider international indigenous rights movement as well. As Alice Feldman observes of this:

In international contexts, indigenous peoples have sought to articulate a unifying and politically operational identity emanating from their shared experiences of colonialism and goals of self-determination, as well as the diversity of their localized experiences and immediate needs. They have drawn upon cultural traditions, both intact and fragmented, to construct and empower an overarching 'indigenousness' that is simultaneously hybrid. Recognition of their identity as peoples and nations who have legitimate claims to the rights and means of sovereignty and self-determination constitutes the foundation of this collective consciousness and the claims it animates, and serves as a central vehicle for change. (2001: 149–50)

And this provides us with the second response to this concern. Nothing in the assertion of indigenous rights – or, as I have argued throughout this book, minority rights more generally – precludes the possibilities of cultural change and adaptation. The specific aim of Māori-language education, for example, is to accomplish this very process, *but on its own terms*. The crucial question then becomes one of control rather than retrenchment or rejection. Te Kōhanga Reo and Kura Kaupapa Māori provide the opportunity for Māori parents, working within national curriculum guidelines, to 'change the rules' that have previously excluded Māori language and culture from recognition as cultural and linguistic capital in schools, and beyond (cf. Chapter 4). Māori knowledge and language competencies thus come to frame, but do not exclude, those of the dominant Pākehā group, and they are themselves the subject of negotiation and change. The stated outcomes of Kura Kaupapa Māori clearly highlight this process of mutual accommodation with their emphasis on bilingualism and biculturalism (see Chapter 5). As Graham Hingangaroa Smith argues, 'Kura Kaupapa Māori parents ... want for their children the ability to access the full range of societal opportunities' (1990b: 194; see also May and Hill, 2008). Moreover, Kura Kaupapa Māori remains only one option among many and still very much a minority one. Proponents of Kura Kaupapa argue that the crucial point is that Māori-language education *is made available* as a legitimate schooling choice, not that it is the answer to everything.

The third caveat has to do with the regular juxtaposition of biculturalism and multiculturalism in Aotearoa/New Zealand. As we saw earlier, many Māori remain overtly skeptical toward multiculturalism, which necessarily involves or includes the claims of other minority groups. For Māori, the key point of concern with the politics of multiculturalism is its potential leveling effect – relegating Māori to the status of a single group among many (albeit a large and influential one). Many Māori argue that multiculturalism, in practice, would simply work in favor of the numerically dominant Pākehā group. Minority groups would be encouraged to fragment and to compete with one another for limited resources, thus maintaining current Pākehā dominance in Aotearoa/ New Zealand (Spoonley, 1993).[19] Specifically, relegating Māori to the status of a single group among many (albeit a large and influential one) disadvantages Māori in two ways:

> it denies Māori people their equality as members of one among two (sets of) peoples, and it also tends to deny the divisions of Maoridom their separate status while exaggerating the status of other immigrant groups. In the end, Māori interests become peripheral, combined with other special problem areas. (Benton, 1988: 77)

The Waitangi Tribunal is equally clear on this point:

> We do not accept that the Māori is just another one of a number of ethnic groups in our community. It must be remembered that of all minority groups the Māori alone is party to a solemn treaty made with the Crown. None of the other migrant groups who have come to live in this country in recent years can claim the rights that were given to the Māori people by the Treaty of Waitangi.

> Because of the Treaty, Māori New Zealanders stand on a special footing reinforcing, if reinforcement be needed, their historical position as the original inhabitants, the tangata whenua [people of the land] of New Zealand ... (1986: 37)

Biculturalism thus emphasizes the right of Māori to exist and persist as a distinct and unique people, on equal terms with Pākehā (Sharp, 1990). This position is also reinforced by an awareness that support for multiculturalism amongst some Pākehā arises less out of a valuing of diversity, and/or a concern for the interests of minority groups, than from a fear of the possible fulfilment of Māori bicultural aspirations (Simon, 1989). I will return in the final chapter to the potential tension between a recognition of indigenous or national minority rights on the one hand and the rights attributable to ethnic minorities on the other hand. By way of example, I will discuss there the position of Pasifika peoples in Aotearoa/New Zealand.

Meanwhile, it is enough to conclude for the purposes of this chapter that much has clearly been achieved for Māori over the last thirty years, particularly via the central role of Māori-language education. However, remembering our discussion in Chapter 4 of the limits of education, this is also a key weakness, since the over-reliance on education has meant that ongoing Māori language use is increasingly limited to this domain. Intergenerational family transmission remains weak, while wider public policy in support of te reo Māori continues to be largely symbolic (De Bres, 2008; Waitangi Tribunal, 2010). These concerns are reflected in a recent review of Māori Language Strategy, *Te Reo Mauriora* (Te Paepae Motuhake, 2011), which proposes that intergenerational family transmission and a wider public policy infrastructure in support of te reo Māori be the two central priorities in Māori language policy over the next twenty years.

In short, the gains for te reo Māori are significant, but still fragile and easily usurped, not least because of the pervasive national and international dominance of English. Despite the advances in indigenous language and education rights for Māori, the latter continues to militate against the revitalization of te reo Māori, as well as the further development of public bi/multilingualism within New Zealand society.[20] The key question for Aotearoa/New Zealand, as for other many other nation-states, thus still remains. How can the language and education rights that majority language speakers simply take for granted be extended *meaningfully* to minority groups as well? This ongoing challenge is a key focus of the final chapter.

9

REIMAGINING THE
NATION-STATE

> If, despite the evidence of our senses, we accept the premise that we or our
> forebears created the state, then we must also accept its entailment: that we or
> our forebears could have created the state in some other form, if we had chosen;
> perhaps, too, that we could change it if we collectively so decided.
>
> (J. M. Coetzee, *Diary of a Bad Year* (2007: 3))

It is clear that nation-states remain the bedrock of the international inter-state
system and look likely, despite many predictions to the contrary, to be around
still for some time to come. Like Mark Twain's famous retort to the premature
media report of his death, the imminent demise of nation-states is obviously
greatly exaggerated. But if this is the case, it certainly does not necessarily follow
that the traditional organization of nation-states should remain unchanged.
Indeed, the forces of economic and political globalization, and the related rise
of multinational companies and supranational organizations, have already had a
considerable effect in renegotiating the parameters of the economic and political
sovereignty of nation-states.

This is all well and good. But my argument is that, if we accept this process
of change for the nation-state from above, so to speak, there is no reason why we
should not accept pressure for change from below as well. In this latter respect,
the principle of nation-state congruence, and the allied notion of cultural
and linguistic homogeneity – both of which are the specific products of the
political nationalism of the last three centuries – have been brought increasingly
into question by national and ethnic minorities within nation-states. What
such minorities are asking is simple and direct – why should the notion of a

homogeneous national identity, represented by the language and culture of the dominant ethnie, invariably *replace* cultural and linguistic identities that differ from it? This 'intolerance of difference' (Billig, 1995: 130) embedded within the structural organization of nation-states has resulted in the historical subjugation and, at times, evisceration of the traditional languages and cultures of minority groups. For centuries this process has been 'validated' on the basis that it is necessary for establishing social and political cohesion, or 'civism' (Bullivant, 1981) within the nation-state (see Chapter 3). But it is a cost that many minority groups are simply no longer prepared to pay.

When this is recognized, it becomes clearer why alternative ethnic, linguistic and/or national identities and affiliations – what Castells (1997) has called 'resistance identities' – continue to be a source of identity and mobilization for many minority groups, confounding the 'liberal expectancy' (Fenton, 1999, 2003) that they would atrophy in the face of modernity. In this respect, my central contention throughout this book has been the reverse of much academic and popular commentary (cf. Chapter 1). It is not the cultural, linguistic and political expression or mobilization of minority ethnicities and nationalisms which are the cause of so much contemporary mayhem in the modern world, but their *disavowal*. We ignore their ongoing influence and purchase at our peril.

Addressing constructionism

In adopting this position, I want to reiterate that we do not need to abandon the social constructionist consensus on ethnic and national identities. Clearly, all collective forms of identity – indeed, *all* forms of identity – are permeable, fluid and subject to change. They vary in salience depending on the individual, the immediate context, their complex articulation with other identities, and the wider vicissitudes of history. There is certainly nothing inherent about them – the constructionist case has clearly won the day here. But there are two crucial caveats to this position. The first is that while identities may well be constructed, they are no less meaningful for all that. Thus it is clear that particular ethnic and/or linguistic identities continue to exert considerable influence, both individually and collectively, in the world today. I have argued that this apparent conundrum can be explained by the fact that such identities, constructed though they may be, are also at the same time an embodied set of dispositions, or habitus (Bourdieu, 1990a). In this sense, they are not simply representations of some inner psychological state, nor even particular ideologies about the world. Rather, they are social, cultural and political *forms of life* – material ways of being in the world today (see Chapter 1).

The second caveat is that, if all identities are constructed, then this recognition must apply equally to majoritarian forms of ethnic and national identity, and not just to minority identities. The tenacity with which majoritarian conceptions of national identity, and the language(s) historically associated with them, are defended, suggests as much (think: the English Only Movement in the USA, for example). And yet, in much of the literature on ethnicity and nationalism, as well as media and popular commentary, it is usually only minority identities and/or languages that are the subject of such critical scrutiny. This unidirectional analysis needs to be challenged and rethought. There is no reason, for example, why we cannot rethink nation-states, and the ethnic and national identities therein, in more plural and inclusive ways (cf. Parekh, 2000; Kymlicka, 2001, 2007). Indeed, doing so is congruent with the allied recognition that individuals have access to, and value, a wide range of different identities, often simultaneously (cf. Chapter 1). Given this, advocacy of group-differentiated minority rights need not lead inevitably to cultural reification and essentialism, as its many critics suggest, but can actually lead to its opposite, the central recognition of the significance of plural or multiple identities, including linguistic ones.

But advocates of minority rights are quick to point out that a recognition of multiple identities does not necessarily entail the postmodernist view that such identities are equal and interchangeable – one may still retain a primary or 'encompassing group' identity (see Chapter 3). They also make the important point that these identities need not always be in conflict, although inevitably there will be times when they are. As I argued in Chapter 4, narrower identities do not necessarily need to be traded in for broader ones since one can clearly remain, for example, Welsh-speaking and British, Catalan-speaking and Spanish, or Spanish-speaking and American.

What we see here is simply the opportunity or potential for holding multiple, complementary cultural and linguistic identities at both individual and collective levels. On this view, maintaining a minority language – or a majority language, for that matter – avoids 'freezing' the development of particular language varieties in the roles that they have come to occupy. Equally importantly, it questions and discards the requirement of a singular and/or replacement approach to the issue of other linguistic identities, which, as I have argued, arises specifically from the nationalist principle of linguistic and cultural homogeneity. To insist otherwise, as many critics of minority rights do, betrays both a reductionist and an essentialist approach to language and identity. This is a significant irony, given that many of these same critiques are explicitly couched in terms of the supposed essentialism of minority identities and the related reification of minority languages (cf. Makoni and Pennycook, 2007; Edwards, 2010; Wee, 2010).

Recognizing and acknowledging the constructedness of all ethnic and national identities is also important for a related reason. It requires us to consider critically why it is that the constructedness and contingency of majoritarian forms of ethnic and/or national identity (and the languages that are associated with them) tend so often to escape such recognition. In this sense, ethnicity and nationalism do not simply lurk *out there* – the sole preserve of 'extremist' nationalists or malcontented national or ethnic minorities, although they are often painted as such. Rather, they inhabit the very structures of the civic societies in which we live. In effect, both the political and administrative structure of the state and its civil society are *ethnicized*. As I have argued throughout this book, this is achieved principally via the artificial establishment of a 'common' civic language and culture. This supposedly common language and culture in fact represents and is reflective of the *particular* cultural and linguistic habitus of the dominant ethnie, or Staatsvolk. It is a majoritarian particularism masquerading as universalism (see Taylor, 1994; see Chapter 3).

This recognition leads in turn to another. We need to examine and critique the specific historical processes by which particular ethnic and/or national identities, and their historically associated languages, have come to be legitimated and normalized in the first place. As I have argued, the rise of political nationalism and the 'philosophical matrix of the nation-state' (Churchill, 1996) that is its product are the principal catalyst and agent in this process of selective identity construction. Following from this, the valorization of national languages and the stigmatization of minority languages can be seen for what they are – a move in the wider politics of nationalism and ethnicity (of which the politics of language forms a part), nothing more. Consequently, the unfavorable juxtaposition of majority national languages and minority languages is neither inevitable nor inviolate.

And this brings us to one further key issue that we need to consider. We must never lose sight of the central importance of (unequal) power relations, and the means by which these have come to be articulated within modern nation-states – particularly with respect to language. A critical perspective of power relations helps to explain why, for example, in Bourdieu's terminology, the cultural and linguistic habitus of majority group members are accorded cultural and linguistic capital, while those of minority groups specifically are not. It also helps to explain why the principal consequence for many minorities – at both the individual and collective level – has been the enforced loss of their own ethnic, cultural and linguistic habitus as the necessary price of entry to the civic realm of the nation-state. As we saw Peter McLaren (1995) observe in Chapter 3, a prerequisite of 'joining the [national] club' is to become denuded, de-ethnicized (or, rather, *re*-ethnicized) and culturally stripped. There are numerous examples where this act of defenestration has been achieved by state coercion – Wales and Catalonia provide us with two clear historical examples here (see Chapter 7). But there are also more contemporary examples of these coercive processes, with the overt proscription of Kurdish in Turkey up to the 1990s, and Tibetan in Chinese-controlled Tibet to the present day. If the US English Only movement has its way, as discussed in Chapter 6, such will also be the case for Spanish-speaking Latino communities in the USA.

However, it is via civil society that the marginalization and stigmatization of minority languages have been most widely and effectively achieved (although, it must be said, often in conjunction with more coercive measures). Language and education play pivotal roles here. Indeed, the construction of national languages and their reinforcement via mass education have become a sine qua non of modern nation-states. These linguistic and educational processes have also linked dominant language varieties inexorably to modernity and progress, while consigning their minority counterparts to the realms of primitivism and stasis. The cultural and linguistic capital ascribed to dominant language varieties also inevitably leads to the view that they are of more *value* and *use* in the world today. Such associations operate on the international stage as well – with the dual status of lingua franca and world language currently ascribed to the English language being a reflection largely of the sociopolitical dominance of those Western nation-states (notably the USA) with which it is most closely associated (see Chapter 6).

It is perhaps not surprising then that, in light of all of the above, many minority group members have come to accept and internalize the view that their own cultural and linguistic habitus have little or no value. This, in turn, leads many to become active participants in the jettisoning of their traditionally associated languages and cultures. Bourdieu (1991) describes this process as one of méconnaissance (misrecognition) – assuming the greater value accorded the dominant language and culture to be a 'natural' rather than a socially and politically constructed phenomenon. As Bourdieu argues, the resulting 'symbolic violence' that is visited upon particular minority languages and cultures is often sustained by an active complicity, or implicit consent, on the part of those subjected to it.

So how can we change this state of affairs? Not easily is the simple answer. But the examples discussed in this book demonstrate that real progress *can* be made on behalf of minority languages and their speakers. The nation-state can be reconfigured – reimagined, in effect – to accommodate greater cultural and linguistic diversity. Or rather, as Homi Bhabha argues, it can be reimagined in order to accommodate greater cultural and linguistic *difference*. The distinction Bhabha makes is crucial here. The former, most evident in the rhetoric of multiculturalism, treats culture as an *object* of empirical knowledge – as static, totalized and historically bounded, as something to be valued but not necessarily *lived*. The latter is the process of the *enunciation* of culture as 'knowledgeable', as adequate to the construction of systems of cultural identification. This involves a dynamic conception of culture – one that recognizes and incorporates the ongoing fluidity and constant change that attends its articulation in the postmodern world (May, 2009).

A formal recognition of cultural and linguistic difference along these lines is what is presently occurring in the likes of Quebec, Catalonia, Wales and Aotearoa/New Zealand, as I have outlined in detail in previous chapters. In each of these examples, minority languages are in the process of being legitimated and institutionalized in the public domain – after centuries of proscription, derogation and neglect – *alongside* the majority national language. These developments are often allied with, and framed within a wider cultural nationalism that aims to build on, and where necessary transform, the minority language and culture in question in order more adequately to meet the demands of modernity. However, as we have also seen, this process remains a highly contested one, and the contest is perhaps most virulent at the intersection of group-differentiated and individual rights.

Tolerability and the crux of majority opinion

Minority language rights will always be controversial, it seems, no matter how valid are the arguments in their favor. As Stacy Churchill has observed, this is because responding to 'the needs of linguistic and cultural groups outside the majority group ... often poses a serious threat to the status quo' (1986: 33). More skeptically, John Edwards asserts: 'The brutal fact is that most "big" language speakers in most societies remain unconvinced of either the immediate need or the philosophical desirability of officially-supported cultural and linguistic programs for their small-language neighbours' (1994: 195–6). The issue of majority opinion thus remains a crucial one for minority language rights' initiatives. In effect, the long-term success of such initiatives may only be achieved, or be achievable, if at least some degree of favorable majority opinion is secured. This has been discussed elsewhere as the problem of ensuring greater 'tolerability' (Grin, 1995; May, 2000; de Bres, 2008) for minority languages or, more positively, a climate of 'socially enlightened self-interest' (Secada and Lightfoot, 1993).

But tolerability is not always easy to come by, even when minority language rights are already well established. A key flashpoint often occurs with the shift from a general affirmation of the value of minority languages to policies that require individuals to change their actual language practices. Thus, there might be positive support among the wider population of a given territory for the ongoing use of a minority language. However, this support often dissipates when an individual is required to speak that language for the purposes of employment, for example. Clear evidence of these differences in tolerability can be seen in the language survey, briefly mentioned in Chapter 7, which I conducted among nearly 500 teacher trainees in Wales (May, 2000). As one monolingual English-speaking respondent observed there:

> A bilingual requirement for public service employment is by no means a fair system, it promotes cultural insularity, is divisive and fails to recognize individual merit. It is, in effect, an expression of the Welsh 'ghetto' mentality that predominates in many levels of society. (Quoted in May, 2000: 120)

Another English-speaking respondent could similarly assert:

> I would have thought it does turn out to be a racial issue if you can prove that a job where you're forced to speak both Welsh and English, say, doesn't really require that skill.
>
> *Interviewer:* What about jobs that do require it?
>
> I would have thought that it's a very subjective issue, being able to prove that ... *You're always going to have people that want to speak English.* I would have thought that it's going to be very difficult to prove that satisfactorily in law. (Quoted in May, 2000: 122; my emphasis)

I have already argued that this assertion of continued monolingualism has no real or legitimate basis – certainly, at least, not under the auspices of individual rights, since the opportunity and right to continue to speak the dominant language is in no way threatened by such minority language recognition. Nonetheless, the problem of tolerability remains a significant one. In light of this, how might we proceed? First, by reiterating that the question of the granting of minority language rights is not about a neutral, disinterested state responding to the claims of vociferous, 'politically motivated' minorities. It is about a *contest* in which *all* players are culturally and politically *situated* and one in which much is at stake on all sides. Specifically, it is a contest for recognition, for resources and for justice, fairness and equity. As such, it is perhaps not surprising that many monolingual majority language speakers are unwilling to renegotiate the terms of agreement that have served them so well in the past. However, do so they must. Otherwise, the greatest fear of many opponents of minority language and education rights will be realized: the eventual break-up of the nation-state that they are so intent on defending. This is simply because national and ethnic minority groups are increasingly unwilling to settle for the degree of marginalization and cultural and language evisceration which have historically characterized their incorporation into modern nation-states.

Second, we also need to recognize that these issues are never likely to be entirely resolved. More significantly, it is not necessary that they should be. As Bhabha (1994) again observes, an alternative minority discourse amounts to a strategy of intervention, which is similar to what the British parliamentary procedure recognizes as a supplementary question. A supplementary strategy suggests that *adding 'to' need not be the same as adding 'up'*. In other words, what we may have here in the end are *incommensurable* discourses – 'abseits designating a form of social contradiction or antagonism that has to be negotiated rather than sublated' (1994: 162). We cannot, and perhaps should not, evacuate tension and conflict from these negotiations about minority language rights (and minority rights more generally), since real and substantive differences continue to underlie the various positions involved.

Indeed, the continuing debates around individual and group-differentiated rights may help to guard against the possibility of and potential for social and political closure – of simply substituting one kind of totalizing and exclusionary (national, ethnic and/or linguistic) discourse for another. After all, the world is replete with examples of minority groups who, on attaining greater sociopolitical and sociocultural status for themselves, promptly deny it to others.[1] The tenets of international law with regard to minority groups are pivotal here. With regard to language, for example, three key tenets can be highlighted. The first principle, which is widely accepted, is that it is not unreasonable to expect from national members some knowledge of the common public language(s) of the state. On this basis, it is clearly possible to argue for the legitimation and institutionalization of the languages of national minorities within nation-states, affording to them at least some of the benefits that national languages currently enjoy.

A second principle is that in order to avoid language discrimination, it is important that where there is a sufficient number of other language speakers, these speakers should be allowed to use that language as part of the exercise of their *individual* rights as citizens. That is, they should have the *opportunity* to use their first language if they so choose. As de Varennes argues, 'the respect of the language principles of individuals, *where appropriate and reasonable*, flows from a fundamental right and is not some special concession or privileged treatment. Simply put, it is the right to be treated equally without discrimination, to which everyone is entitled' (1996a: 117; my emphasis).

The third principle arises directly from the previous one – how to determine exactly what is 'appropriate and reasonable' with regard to individual language preferences. The distinction between national minority and polyethnic rights (see Chapter 3) is useful in this respect. I have consistently argued that only national minorities – as historical ethnies – can demand *as of right* formal inclusion of their languages and cultures in the civic realm – that is, promotion-oriented language rights. But contrary to the way my argument has been interpreted subsequently by some commentators (see, for example, Skutnabb-Kangas, 2000), I am *not* endorsing language rights for national minorities *at the expense* of other minorities. Rather, I am simply highlighting the difference in the basis of entitlement. Let me illustrate this by returning to Aotearoa/New Zealand and the example of Pasifika peoples therein.

Polyethnic language and education rights

In the last chapter, I discussed the gains that Māori have made over the last thirty years in Aotearoa/New Zealand with respect to promotion-oriented language and education rights. The gains have been secured on the basis of their status as indigenous peoples, endorsed by an official policy of biculturalism, and demonstrated via the not inconsiderable successes of Māori language education. These developments do not preclude, in principle at least, the extension of promotion-oriented language and education rights to other minority groups in Aotearoa/New Zealand. However, they have led, in *practice*, to a convenient lack of interest by the New Zealand state in *substantively* addressing the language and educational entitlements of other minority groups. This is most evident in relation to the long-settled Pasifika population in Aotearoa/New Zealand, a key pan-ethnic migrant group comprising peoples from the principal Pacific Islands of Samoa, Tonga, Cook Islands, Niue, Tokelau, Tuvalu and Fiji, who have since settled in New Zealand.

In the 2006 Census, 265,974 people, approximately 6.9 percent of the total New Zealand population, identified themselves as Pasifika. Of this broad Pasifika ethnic grouping, nearly half (131,100) identified in the Census as being Samoan. The next largest grouping, Cook Islands Māori, was considerably smaller at 58,011 (22 percent), with Tongan following at 50,478 (19 percent) and Niuean at 22,473 (8 percent) identified members. All other New Zealand Pasifika communities have less than 10,000 members: Fijian 9,861, Tokelauan 6,819 and Tuvaluan 2,625 (Statistics New Zealand, 2007).

The migration of Pasifika communities to Aotearoa/New Zealand began immediately after the Second World War, although the most intensive period of migration occurred in the 1960s and 1970s. Pasifika migrants were treated as a source of cheap and ready manual labor and initially found work primarily in the expanding manufacturing and service sectors of the post-war New Zealand economy (Macpherson, 1996; Macpherson et al., 2001). Subsequent Pasifika migrants have also experienced similarly delimited work and employment patterns. Consequently, Pasifika communities remain disproportionately represented in the lowest socioeconomic indices of work and employment. Pasifika settlement patterns are similarly circumscribed, with the majority to be found in South Auckland, one of the poorest urban areas in New Zealand.

While there has been some economic improvement in recent years, particularly for younger Pasifika peoples (New Zealand Ministry of Pacific Island Affairs, 2002), the social, economic and educational indicators for many Pasifika remain poor. Taking education as one such key indicator, Pasifika students, many of whom still speak a Pasifika language (see below), are consistently and disproportionately represented in the lowest levels of English literacy proficiency in international literacy surveys. Indeed, until recently, New Zealand was identified as having the largest 'home-language gap' in relation to literacy achievement of any OECD country – that is, it had the greatest gap in achievement between those students for whom the language of the school was also their first language (English in the New Zealand context) and those for whom it was not (Wilkinson, 1998). This pattern of differential achievement continues, not surprisingly, into adulthood.

The International Adult Literacy Survey (IALS), conducted in 1996–7, found that adult literacy levels in English are consistently lower overall for Pasifika adults when compared to the New Zealand population as a whole. While adult literacy levels across the population were comparable with other developed countries, 75 percent of Pasifika adults failed to meet minimum levels in English literacy (New Zealand Ministry of Education, 2001).

Pasifika language and identity

The 2006 Census indicates there are now over 100,000 speakers of Pasifika languages in Aotearoa/New Zealand, the vast majority of whom are Samoan speakers (77,109). In addition, 28,816 identified in the Census as being Tongan speakers, 9,075 as Cook Islands Māori speakers and 5,190 as Niuean speakers.[2] These figures point to important differences both within and among specific Pasifika groups with respect to Pasifika language retention and attendant attitudes toward Pasifika languages.

New Zealand Samoan and Tongan groups have the greatest level of Pasifika language retention, with over 60 percent in each community still able to hold an everyday conversation in their respective Pasifika languages, although high levels of fluency are concentrated in a diminishing number of older speakers. In contrast, other Pasifika groups exhibit far lower Pasifika language retention rates. For example, only 28 percent of the New Zealand Niuean community still speak Niuean, while for the Cook Islands Māori community, the percentage is even lower, with only 18 percent still able to speak Cook Islands Māori (Bell et al., 2000; Davis et al., 2001).

The reasons for these markedly varying language patterns are likely to be complex. However, there are two key contributory factors that can be readily identified. The first concerns the role of the church within particular Pasifika communities. Where that role is still central – as it is for New Zealand Samoan and Tongan groups – it provides an important domain for ongoing Pasifika language use. Where it is less central, as is the case for the Cook Islands Māori and Niuean communities, that language domain is not so readily available.

The second relates to the percentage of New Zealand-born Pasifika within individual communities. For Samoan and Tongan communities, there is a growing percentage of New Zealand-born members, but this is counterbalanced by ongoing migration to New Zealand from Samoa and Tonga and related intergenerational language use. For the Cook Islands Māori, Tokelauan, and Niuean communities, however, the New Zealand-based population now far outnumbers those in their original homelands, with a concomitant shift to English, particularly among younger members (Macpherson, 2004).

Despite these, often marked, variations in Pasifika language retention and shift, the link between Pasifika language and identities is still an important one for many Pasifika peoples. Davis et al.'s study of Pasifika language patterns in South Auckland 'emphasised the importance of their language in relation to their identity as members of [particular] Pasifika communities' (2001: 12). Likewise, Fetui and Malaki-Williams's study on Samoan language use concluded that the maintenance of Samoan is important for 'the self esteem, confidence and identity of Samoan youngsters [in New Zealand], as well as making them appreciative and aware of their cultural heritage' (1996: 234).

But highlighting the importance of language for identity purposes does little to address or subvert ongoing negative attitudes toward Pasifika languages in the wider New Zealand society. These attitudes are most evident in relation to the regular positioning of Pasifika languages as low-status 'minority' or 'community' languages, and thus of little value or use for educational and wider social mobility. The result is a still-widespread presumption in Aotearoa/New Zealand that maintaining bilingualism in a Pasifika language and English is somehow educationally detrimental. Indeed, such is the pervasiveness of these negative attitudes toward Pasifika languages that many in the Pasifika communities have come to internalize them.

This is most evident in sharply differing views among Pasifika parents on whether Pasifika languages should have any formal role in education. For example, a 1995 survey of Māori and Pacific language demands for educational services found that over half of the 550 Pasifika respondents wanted their children to be able to speak fluently both their first (Pasifika) language and English by the time they finished elementary school. Like other parents, they also wanted their children to succeed academically (Coxon et al., 2002). However, it has also been documented elsewhere that migrant Samoan parents have not always considered Samoan as having any educational value within the context of schooling. Parents often thought that English was the key to academic success and that speaking Samoan to their children, even at home, would be a serious disadvantage to them (Fetui and Malaki-Williams, 1996; Hunkin-Tuiletufuga, 2001).

Pasifika language and education policy

Meanwhile, the New Zealand Ministry of Education has used this lack of consensus among Pasifika parents as an excuse for their own ongoing inaction and inertia with respect to the provision of Pasifika-language education. This is despite the poor educational achievement that Pasifika students have consistently experienced to date – almost wholly in English-only education contexts (cf. Chapter 6). It is also despite an earlier assurance by the New Zealand Ministry of Education that 'students whose mother tongue is a Pacific Islands language or a community language will have the opportunity to develop and use their own language as an integral part of their schooling' (1993: 10).

The result is a still-paltry provision of Pasifika-language programs across Aotearoa/New Zealand. Moreover, those that have been developed are almost always a product of individual school-based and/or local community initiatives. In 2001, just over 2,500 early childhood students were in Pasifika-language nests, modeled on kōhanga reo, although this figure was also the lowest for ten years, and well down from a mid-1990s peak of nearly 4,000 (Peddie, 2003). As for the school population, Pasifika students comprise 6 percent of all New Zealand school students, about half being Samoan. However, as Roger Peddie observes:

> In 2001, and in [only] 20 [elementary and high] schools, just over 1600 students were in Pacific language education, with almost three-quarters of these students learning at least some of the time in Samoan. However, this total represents only 2.8 per cent of all Pasifika students. Furthermore, fewer than 5 per cent of Pasifika students in schools were learning a Pasifika language. While the figures are a little better for Samoans, the numbers are still well under 10 per cent, with fewer than 1000 students learning Samoan in secondary schools. (2003: 22)

There have been some recent encouraging developments in related policy areas, notably, the establishment of a website for teachers – LEAP (Language Enhancing the Achievement of Pasifika) – that draws on relevant bilingual and second language acquisition research to highlight how best to teach bilingual Pasifika students (see http://leap.tki.org.nz).[3] However, the wider relative inaction with respect to Pasifika-language education reflects a distinct lack of political will, a product in turn of the highly marginalized status of Pasifika peoples within Aotearoa/New Zealand. In this respect, Pasifika are specifically constructed *by the state* in quite different terms to Māori – as a 'migrant' minority group, with no right of recourse to minority language and education provisions.

I have spent some time on the example of Pasifika in Aotearoa/New Zealand because their marginalized position illustrates, writ large, the experiences of a wide range of ethnic migrant groups the world over. The key point is that, in the end, it is the nation-state that has the responsibility for the recognition (or lack thereof) of any promotion-oriented language and education rights for these groups. This is *irrespective* of whether such rights have already been accorded to national minority and/or indigenous peoples. Thus, granting minority language and education rights to national minorities and/or indigenous peoples does *not* obviate the individual state's responsibility to address the language and education needs of other ethnic groups, where it can, and to the degree possible. I have outlined in Chapter 5 how at least some promotion-oriented language and education rights can be extended to groups such as Pasifika on the principle within international law of 'where numbers warrant'.[4] This principle also, importantly, allows us to address the inevitable criticism that often arises at this point: namely, if we grant rights to one minority group, where will this all end? (What this usually means, of course, is that no rights will be accorded to any minority groups.) Thus, while continuing to recognize the rights attributable to other minorities, this distinction allows us to avoid the problem of cultural relativism. In short, greater ethnolinguistic *democracy* is not necessarily the same as ethnolinguistic *equality*.

The challenge of multiculturalism

Distinguishing between ethnolinguistic democracy and equality also addresses the question, to which I have alluded on a number of occasions, of the role of multiculturalism. In this respect, a common argument has been that bicultural/ bilingual policies privilege one particular minority group over others and are therefore both disadvantageous and discriminatory toward the latter. In this view, differential treatment of minorities is illiberal – either all minority groups should be so recognized, or none should be.

However, this argument can be challenged on a number of grounds. First, as with much discussion of minority rights, no distinction is made in a multiculturalist approach between the differing rights attributable to national and ethnic minorities. National minority rights are thus treated as merely equivalent to the rights of all other competing groups. What is being advocated, in effect, is the applicability of *polyethnic* rights (and only these) to *all* minorities. In the process, and this is my second point, the demands of multiculturalism come to be articulated as an *alternative* to national minority rights – that is, as a means of *avoiding* biculturalism/bilingualism. This suggests, in turn, the distinct possibility that the articulation of multiculturalism along these lines is not seriously countenanced by at least some of its proponents. Remembering Bhabha's earlier distinction, the rhetoric of cultural and linguistic *diversity* is used as a spoiling device against the articulation of cultural and linguistic *difference*. Pierre Coulombe makes this point forcefully in relation to Canada's official policy of French/English bilingualism:

> Those who object to bilingualism often do so because they fear differences and are unable to reconcile themselves with the loss of their hegemony over society. Needless to say, it is an attitude that is not receptive to multiculturalism and the maintaining of differences. There is no way that the cultural imperialists who wrap themselves in the language of moral outrage in denouncing bilingualism will open their arms to multiculturalism. ... They will, in other words, profess their tolerance towards a diversity of languages and cultures, so long as that diversity is consigned to the private sphere. Ethnic minorities ought to be cautious

when they too oppose official bilingualism, for they may be unwillingly
supporting an attitude that will turn against them. (1995: 104)

As such, we should treat the competing claims of multiculturalism with
considerable skepticism. But having said that, it is clearly unwise to dismiss
multicultural claims out of hand, as Coulombe comes close to doing.
Multiculturalism may still have an important, perhaps essential part to
play as an *addition* or *complement* to bicultural/bilingual policy. Certainly, the
example of Pasifika suggests that much still needs to be done in order to
address adequately the cultural and linguistic needs and rights of other ethnic
minority groups, even within those territories where minority language rights
are already recognized. The examples of Quebec, Catalonia and Wales also
clearly bear this out. In short, the development of formal bilingualism *must*
remain sensitive to and accommodating of other ethnic minority groups and
the languages they speak.

Likewise, there is a continuing necessity to guard against essentialism
and reification in the articulation of minority cultural and language rights.
Multiculturalism may thus usefully ensure against the objectification of ethnicity
and the hardening of ethnic and national boundaries, while contributing at the
same time to ongoing debates about a more open, evolving conception of ethnic
and national identities. Bourdieu argues, to this end, that one needs 'to keep
together what go together in reality: on the one hand the objective classifications
... and, on the other hand, the practical relation to those classifications, whether
acted out or represented, and in particular the individual and collective strategies
... by which agents seek to put these classifications at the service of their material
or symbolic interests, or to conserve or transform them' (1991: 227).

Toward a more pluralist conception of language rights

And this brings me to my final point. It has been my argument throughout this
book that in order to rethink or reimagine the nation-state along more plural and
inclusive lines we must first, and somewhat counter-intuitively, acknowledge
the cultural-historical dimensions of the ethnic and national identities that
comprise it. As Stuart Hall argues, a positive conception of ethnicity must begin
with 'a recognition that all speak from a particular place, out of a particular
history, out of a particular experience, a particular culture, *without being contained
by that position*' (1992b: 258; my emphasis). Moreover, if a particular language has
played an important part in that historical positioning, there is no reason why it
cannot continue to do so.

However, Hall's qualification points to the second key aspect of my argument
here – that the recognition of our cultural and historical situatedness should not
set the limits of ethnicity and nationality, nor act to undermine the legitimacy of

other, equally valid forms of identity. This requires a reflective, critical approach to ethnic and national identity, and the role of languages within them. Such an approach would have to engage with the present and the future as well as the past, and would have to remain open to competing conceptualizations, diverse identities and a rich public discourse about controversial issues (Calhoun, 1993b).[5] As Peter McLaren observes, echoing Renan's conception of the 'will to nationhood' (see Chapter 2): 'rather than searching for the origins of our identities as historical agents of struggle, we need to focus more on what we can achieve together. What we might become takes precedence over who we are' (1995: 109). Likewise, Terry Eagleton asserts: 'Any emancipatory politics must begin with the specific ... but must in the same gesture leave it behind. For the freedom to question is not the freedom to be [this or that particular identity], whatever this might mean, but simply the freedom now enjoyed by certain other groups *to determine their identity as they wish*' (1990: 30; my emphasis).

Such a position recognizes the ongoing interspersion of groups, the complex interconnections between ethnic and national identities and other forms of identity, and the ambiguities, tensions and competing demands that inevitably arise as a result. But even more importantly, it recognizes that these can be outworked from within (or centrifugally), rather than always being determined from without (or centripetally). Or, to put it another way, they can be negotiated on one's own terms, rather than the terms set by others, as has so often been the case historically for minority groups. Thus, the arguments of minority groups for the retention of their ethnic, cultural and linguistic identities are most often *not* characterized by a retreat into traditionalism or cultural essentialism but, rather, by a more *autonomous* construction of group identity and political deliberation (Kymlicka, 1995a). After all, as Kymlicka has pointedly observed: 'leaving one's culture [and language], while possible, is best seen as renouncing something to which one is reasonably entitled' (1995a: 90).

It is thus about time – indeed, it is long overdue – that we started paying much closer attention to these arguments, and their emancipatory possibilities. Without it, the vast majority of the world's minority languages will not see the dawn of a new century. Even more importantly, minority language speakers will continue to be marginalized and discriminated against in the various interconnected arenas, or 'fields' in Bourdieu's terms, in which they live and work. This is an urgent political imperative that we should not sidestep in the name of academic 'disinterestedness'. After all, as I argued in the original preface to this book (see also Chapter 4), those that make this claim tend simply to reinforce the existing status quo of the linguistic inequalities currently facing minority language speakers, along with the wider social and political inequalities of which invariably they are a part. The dismissal of minority language rights, or the significance of particular language varieties to individuals and groups, amounts, in effect, to a post-hoc argument legitimating inequality. This is demonstrably not disinterested but simply a specific 'move' in the wider politics of language – nothing more, nothing less.

If the challenge of addressing these inequities directly remains an unpalatable prospect for some, there are also more straightforward intellectual reasons for taking far greater cognizance of the arguments for minority language rights. While acknowledging the constructedness of all language varieties, we also have to explain *why* questions of language, and language rights, continue to remain so important for so many individuals and groups. And why, when it matters, it seems to *really* matter. As Adrian Blackledge has observed (see Chapter 4): 'We can hardly argue theoretically that for students who died protesting the right to establish Bengali as the national language of East Pakistan in 1952, language was not a key feature of identity' (2008: 33). And yet, this is precisely what many social constructionist and postmodernist commentators on language still do, including those within critical sociolinguistics who increasingly question the reified nature of formal language varieties (see Introduction).

I do not demur entirely from these critical observations, as should be clear from my own discussion of the contingency of language and identity and the overtly sociopolitical processes underpinning the construction and ongoing constructedness of languages. However, I do demur from the unidirectional critique of minority languages that usually attends these accounts, as if, oddly, the question of linguistic diversity and its challenge to essentialism and reification are problems peculiar to/for minorities. As I hope I have shown clearly, they are just as significant, if not more so, for majoritarian language discourses. And as I also hope to have demonstrated, developments in minority language rights, while not immune to essentialism and reification, are at least more cognizant of their dangers – arguing for public bi/multilingualism in the first instance being a case in point.

Language diversity on the ground will always deconstruct standardized conceptions of languages, to be sure. But this shouldn't ipso facto preclude the possibility of the public legitimation and institutionalization of minority languages, alongside majority languages. It may well be a 'pluralization of monolingualism' rather than its absolute deconstruction, as Makoni and Pennycook (2007) and Pennycook (2010) have argued. But one has to start somewhere, not least because it is in the public, or civic, realm that the effects of linguistic inequality are most marked. A sole focus on linguistic hybridity in the micro sociolinguistic practices of bi/multilingual speakers does little to address these inequalities. Nor, as I argued in the Introduction, does it recognize the recursive effects of public recognition on individual language use. And anyway, the associated celebration of hybridity, linguistic or otherwise, in constructionist and postmodernist accounts, including within critical sociolinguistics, invariably masks the fact that it is usually only elite cosmopolitans who experience its full 'benefits'.

In short, we need to explain more adequately than we have to date why the ongoing differential positioning of language varieties still has such significant negative, stratified, implications for minority language speakers, particularly in the civic realm. And why too, of course, it still contributes so prominently to many of the political disputes in the world today. Addressing these issues seriously means balancing the, at times, countervailing demands of individual and group rights. It requires broadening the conception of what constitutes social, cultural and linguistic capital, and how these may be defined and used in the private and public realms. And it requires jettisoning the language replacement ideology of the nation-state for one of public linguistic complementarity.

At stake here are questions of individual and collective social mobility – what we can already do and, more importantly, *what we might actually be able to do* via the languages we speak. Also at stake are wider questions of minority inclusion and exclusion within nation-states, as well as in relation to an increasingly globalized world dominated by English. The historical power relations that have disadvantaged minority language speakers in relation to both remain formidable. I am certainly not suggesting that reimagining the nation-state, or globalization, in more plurilingual terms will be an uncontested and unproblematic task – or, indeed, a panacea if accomplished. But if the obstacles are complex and daunting, and the implications remain uncertain, the possibilities that inhere in such a task – for *both* minorities *and* majorities – are nonetheless significant enough to warrant a serious attempt. The stakes are high but the potential rewards of a more just, inclusive and pluralist conception of language rights are even more so.

NOTES

Introduction

1 In what follows, I use the distinction between 'majority' and 'minority' languages not in relation to numerical size or number of speakers but rather to highlight the differential status, power and influence of particular language varieties (although the two are often related). In so doing, I acknowledge that the majority/minority language dichotomy inevitably understates the complex situatedness of particular language varieties with respect to power relations (Coulmas, 1998; Pennycook, 1998a). Nonetheless, the distinction remains useful because, as I will show, it highlights the sociohistorical and sociopolitical processes that inevitably underlie the privileging of certain language varieties over others.

2 There are various challenges associated with what actually constitutes a language and, following from this, the enumeration of languages (see Makoni and Pennycook, 2007; Pennycook, 2010, for further discussion). However, the general trend of language loss, and its current exponential rate, is not in doubt.

3 A well-known alternative formulation of this process, which also usefully charts a minority language's private and public functions in relation to the nation-state, is found in Joshua Fishman's 'Graded Intergenerational Disruption Scale' (GIDS) (see Fishman, 1991: 81–121). In this eight-point scale, Stage 1 is seen as the most secure position for a minority language while Stage 8 is seen as the least secure. The various stages may be paraphrased as:

Stage 1: some use of the minority language (henceforth ML) in higher level educational, occupational, governmental and media realms

Stage 2: ML used in lower governmental and media spheres

Stage 3: use of the ML in the work sphere, involving (informal) interaction between ML and other language speakers

Stage 4: ML use as medium of instruction in education

Stage 5: informal maintenance of literacy in the home, school and community

Stage 6: intergenerational family transmission of the ML

Stage 7: while the ML continues to be spoken, most speakers are beyond childbearing age

Stage 8: remaining speakers of an ML are old and usually vestigial users

4 See e.g. Mühlhäusler (1996, 2000); Maffi (2000, 2001). See also Nettle and Romaine (2000); Dalby (2003); Harrison (2007).
5 For recent critiques along these lines, see Blommaert (2001); J. Edwards (2001); Brutt-Griffler (2002); May (2003a); Pennycook (2004).
6 Skeptics of minority language rights often view the term 'linguistic genocide' as highly problematic – as too emotive and conspiratorial. Skutnabb-Kangas argues, in response, that terms such as 'language death' and 'language loss', which many of these skeptics prefer, have significant problems of their own – not least the notable absence of agency or responsibility. Language 'loss' or 'death' does not just happen, nor is it natural and/or inevitable. Rather, it is always socially, culturally and politically situated within a wider nexus of (often highly unequal) power relations between, and within, language groups.
7 As we shall see in Chapter 4, the process of stigmatizing minority languages often involves their equation with, or more accurately, relegation to dialects – i.e. a view that they are not 'really' languages.
8 I use the term 'nation-state' advisedly throughout this account, since the confluence of one nation and one state (hence, nation-state), though a major aspiration of political nationalism, has seldom ever occurred. In short, as Anthony Smith observes, there are very few nation-states 'in the strict sense of the term' (2001: 286). Smith's alternative is to use 'national states', since, as he argues, this highlights better the aspiration of many states to achieve congruence between country and culture. Using Smith's alternative might potentially undermine what Wimmer and Schiller (2002) have termed 'methodological nationalism', i.e. the naturalization of the nation-state form in much social science commentary. However, given its widespread usage, I have stuck with the term, albeit, as with other commentators (see e.g. Guibernau, 2001), clearly recognizing in so doing that the second word is the dominant or motive force. I will discuss the distinctions between nation and state, and the problems attendant upon political nationalism, in more detail in Chapter 2.
9 See e.g. Skutnabb-Kangas and Phillipson (1995); Phillipson (1992, 2000); Skutnabb-Kangas (2000, 2008).
10 See e.g. Blommaert (2010); Pennycook (2007, 2010); Wee (2010). See also: Canagarajah (2007); Makoni and Pennycook (2007); Heller (2008).
11 There is no reason why this principle cannot also be extended to encompass intra-language varieties, a key concern of these critical sociolinguistic accounts (see, especially, Wee, 2010). For example, new localized forms of English, or 'world Englishes' (see Chapter 6), are minoritized in very similar ways. As with minority languages, this results in often sharply differing views as to the 'worth' of these language varieties.
12 Essentialism is taken to mean here the process by which particular groups come to be described in terms of fundamental, immutable characteristics. As a result, the relational and fluid aspects of identity formation are ignored and the group itself comes to be seen as autonomous and separate, impervious to context and to processes of internal as well as external differentiation (Werbner, 1997b).
13 Following Gramsci (1971), hegemony is taken to mean here the diffusion and popularization of a particular view of the world – that of the dominant group – as if it was representative of all other groups. In other words, so effective and widespread is the promotion and promulgation of a particular (dominant) point of view, that even those who may not initially share such a view come to accept it and internalize it as normative, as simply the commonsensical 'way of seeing things'.
14 I return to this issue again in Chapter 9.

1 The denunciation of ethnicity

1 There are two points at issue here. Just because so-called 'ethnic groups' are involved does not mean that the conflict is driven by ethnicity (Fenton, 2003). Second, such conflicts are not exclusive to ethnic groups or to postcolonial and/or 'less stable' states with which they are usually associated. As Andreas Wimmer observes, '[what] we nowadays call ethnic cleansing or ethnocide ... have in fact been constants of the European history of nation-building and state formation' (2004: 44). I will return to this often-overlooked history in Chapter 2.

2 Britain is not a nation; it is a multinational state. For a fuller discussion of these distinctions, see Chapter 2.

3 There are important exceptions to this position within liberal ideology, as Will Kymlicka (1989, 1995a, b, 2001, 2007) has consistently exemplified. I will return to this point, and its implications, in Chapter 3 when I discuss the question of the legitimacy of group-based minority rights within modern nation-states.

4 For representative examples, see Nairn (1981); Hroch (1985); Balibar (1991); Hechter (1975, 2000); Wallerstein (1983, 1991, 2001).

5 In a still central text on globalization, Held et al. (1999: 15) describe it thus: 'Globalization can be taken to refer to those spatio-temporal processes of change which underpin a transformation in the organization of human affairs by linking together expanding human activity across regions and continents.' Given its rise to prominence in the late twentieth century, some globalization theorists limit its genesis to the current era (e.g. Cox, 1996). Other globalization theorists, however, acknowledge that its origins emerge from, or out of, previous forms of social and political organization, notably the nationalism of the previous few centuries (Held et al., 1999; Robertson, 1992, 1995; Hobsbawm, 2008). Blommaert (2010) usefully bridges this apparent dichotomy by distinguishing between what he terms 'geopolitical globalization' and 'geocultural globalization'. The former, he argues, has clearly emerged from earlier historical antecedents such as capitalist expansion in the nineteenth century. The latter is linked to the more recent features of late capitalism, such as new technologies, business process outsourcing (e.g. establishing multinational company call centers in developing countries) and related changes in migration patterns, the division of labor and wider social and economic inequalities.

6 See e.g. Hall (1992a, b); Bhabha (1994); Featherstone (1995); Kraidy (2002, 2005); Hobsbawm (2008); Pieterse (2009).

7 Advocates of cosmopolitanism within political theory share a similar preference for global identities, as seen e.g. in Martha Nussbaum's (1997) notion of 'citizen of the world'. I return to a detailed discussion of cosmopolitanism, and its critique, in Chapter 3.

8 Kaufmann's (2004) focus on ethnic majorities, or 'dominant ethnicities', is a useful corrective to this historical pattern.

9 As Fishman (1997) observes, this largely negative semantic association derives from the biblical Hebrew distinction between *goy* and *'am*, the former denoting an ungodly people and the latter a godly people. In the third-century Greek translation of the Hebrew Bible (the Septuagint), the Greek word 'ethnos' was used for 'goy', hence its subsequent association with heathenism.

10 Eller and Coughlan (1993) develop a strawman argument against primordialism, asserting that it is 'unscientific', 'unsociological', even 'racist', while at the same time both misrepresenting and traducing Geertz's contribution as a supposed exemplar of these various sins. As I have argued, any serious or close reading of Geertz would demonstrably suggest otherwise.

11 This process of equating group differences on 'racial' grounds is now considered to be scientifically invalid (see e.g. Gould, 1981; Fenton, 2003; Miles and Brown, 2003); hence, the use of quotation marks around the term 'race'.

12 Cornell and Hartmann (2007) describe this process as one of 'racial assignment'. See also Song (2003); Wimmer (2008).

13 The longevity of this view within both sociology and anthropology is demonstrated by the following representative examples: Cohen (1974); Glazer and Moynihan (1975); Rex and Mason (1986); Roosens (1989); Nagel (1994); Sandall (2001); Chandra and Wilkinson (2008).

14 No one else describes the golfer, Tiger Woods, by his preferred self-description 'Calibasian'.

15 In unranked, polyethnic states – i.e. those states where ethnic groups are represented across the social strata – ethnically aligned parties, rather than class-based parties, invariably predominate. Examples include, among many others, Sri Lanka (Sinhalese, Tamils), Nigeria (Ibo, Yoruba, Hausa), Malaysia (Malay, Chinese) and Fiji (Fijian, Chinese, Indian).

16 For examples of the application of habitus to ethnicity, see Bentley (1987); Smaje (1997); Wimmer (2004, 2008); May (2003a, 2011a).

17 The material dimension of habitus outlined here is broadly consonant with Fishman's (1980) articulation of ethnicity as a matter of 'being', 'doing' and 'knowing'. I will explore in more depth Fishman's arguments about ethnicity, particularly with respect to language, in Chapter 4.

18 Examples include: Calhoun et al. (1993); D. Robbins (1991, 2000); R. Jenkins (2003); Albright and Luke (2008); Grenfell (2011).

19 In arguably his most influential publication, *Distinction* (1984), Bourdieu specifically asserts that practices can neither be reduced to habitus nor field but rather develop from their 'interrelationship'. He summarizes this as follows: '(habitus) (capital) + field = practice' (p. 101).

2 Nationalism and its discontents

1 See Anthony Smith (1986, 1991, 1995a, 1998, 2004b, 2008, 2009, 2010). See also Hutchinson (1994, 2000, 2005, 2008).

2 I will distinguish further between ethnies and nations later in this chapter where I discuss ethno-symbolic accounts of nationalism.

3 Walker Connor's argument, linking notions of kinship directly to nation-building, is similar/comparable to Shils (1957) and Geertz's (1973) observations of the 'ineffable significance' of the link in relation to ethnicity (Horowitz, 2002; see Chapter 1).

4 Essentialism is taken to mean here the process by which particular groups come to be described in terms of fundamental, immutable characteristics. In so doing, the relational and fluid aspects of identity formation, as discussed in Chapter 1, are ignored and the group itself comes to be seen as impervious to context and to processes of internal as well as external differentiation and/or change (Werbner, 1997b). A much more succinct explanation is offered by John Joseph: '[e]ssentialism, a pejorative term, consists of whatever constructionists do not like' (2004: 89–90).

5 That said, the political objectives of Herder and Fichte did differ significantly. While Herder, as I have already suggested, was clearly not immune to anti-French sentiment, his general view of the direct links between language and 'national' communities led him to adopt a pluralist and egalitarian stance toward other ethnocultural/ ethnolinguistic groups (see Fishman, 1989d: 570–1). This can be contrasted directly with Fichte's subsequent hierarchizing of these same communities; principally, via his application of Herder's views on language to the tenets of political nationalism.

6 Renan is now regularly touted as one of the earliest modernist commentators on nationalism for taking this position. However, as John Joseph (2004: 114–15) observes, there is not a little irony here, since his early work on the nature of language, as preformed and irreducible, was in fact remarkably similar to the views of the German Romantics.

7 I am not suggesting here that religious sectarianism is absent in Scotland (see e.g. McCrone, 1992), simply that, unlike Northern Ireland, it is not the principal factor in questions of Scottish nationalism and national identity.

8 For a representative sample of modernist accounts of nationalism, see Kedourie (1960); H. Kohn (1961); Deutsch (1966); Nairn (1981); Gellner (1983); Hobsbawm and Ranger (1983); Giddens (1984); Anderson (1991); Hobsbawm (1990, 1995); Breuilly (1993, 2005a, b).

9 The inherent Eurocentrism of the majority of these accounts, however, has been challenged by the likes of Blaut (1993) and Mignolo (1995, 2000), who argue that the colonialism of the sixteenth and seventeenth centuries, particularly in the Americas, may also have been a key precursor to the subsequent rise of nationalism.

10 The historical recency of nationalism is highlighted by the term 'nationalism' itself which, as Connor (1978) points out, only gained a permanent place in dictionaries in the nineteenth century. Likewise, it was probably Lord Acton (1907) who first coined the term 'nationality' (J. Edwards, 1985).

11 See e.g. Calhoun (1997); McCrone (1998); Grosby (2005), James (2006); Anthony Smith (2010).

12 The main difference here between Gellner's theory and most Marxist perspectives (see e.g. Nairn, 1981; Hroch, 1985; Hobsbawm, 1990) is that Gellner sees nationalism as the concomitant of industrialization (in any form) whereas Marxist analyses link nationalism more specifically to capitalism.

13 See e.g. Armstrong (1982); Fishman (1989b); Hutchinson (1994, 2005); R. Jenkins (1995, 2007); Anthony Smith (1986, 1998, 2004b, 2009).

14 Smith argues that there are two principal types of ethnie: lateral, which develop round a centralized state and are confined to a social and political elite; and vertical, which are usually subordinated status groups that are sustained by cultural and religious institutions and values that act to unify the population (see Smith, 1986: ch. 4). In either case, however, the pre-existing profile serves to shape the contours of the modern nation-state.

15 It should be noted, however, that Gellner never accepted this widely made criticism of his work. In response, he argued that his account was causal rather than teleological. The development, diffusion and related discontents associated with industrial society, in his view, caused nationalism (see Gellner, 1996).

16 Parekh does not adopt an ethno-symbolic position in the way described here. Nonetheless, his description of national identity lends itself well to a comparison with habitus and field.

17 This is the point that Geertz (1973) was also making in relation to ethnic identification; see Chapter 1.

18 Anthony Smith has argued that the different historical and organizational trajectories of statist and cultural nationalisms relate to the distinction between lateral and vertical ethnies (see n. 10); a position that Hutchinson (1994, 2005), in his formulation of cultural nationalism, also implicitly accepts. However, I am inclined to agree with Richard Jenkins's (1995) conclusion that this perpetuates the 'ethnic' and 'civic' divide within nationalism and that, rather, all nationalisms should be regarded as in some sense 'ethnic' (see also Brown, 2000: ch. 3). If there is a more appropriate distinction to be drawn then, perhaps it is between those nationalisms which claim territory on the basis of putative ethnic commonality and those which attempt to construct ethnic

commonality within an already occupied territory (see R. Jenkins, 1995: 387). The latter, in my view, are more often associated with cultural forms of nationalism.

19 For further discussion, particularly in relation to Europe, see Joppke and Lukes (1999); Modood (2007); May (2001, 2008a); Joppke (2004, 2010).

20 Although see my previous provisos in relation to economistic accounts of the spread of ethnonationalisms.

21 See e.g. Churchill (1986); Ogbu (1987); Gibson and Ogbu (1991); Kymlicka (1995a); Fenton (1999).

22 In Chapter 8, I will explore more fully these developments in national and international law with respect to indigenous peoples.

3   Liberalism and multiculturalism

1 As Gramsci argues, in order to understand any nation-state as a whole, one must always distinguish between its 'state' or political and administrative structure, and its 'civil society'. The latter comprises e.g. its principal non-political organizations, its religious and other beliefs, and its specific 'customs' or way of life. In making these distinctions, there are inevitably features that do not fit easily under either category. However, as Nairn summarizes it: 'that is relatively unimportant. What matters is that they are distinguishable, and that the singular identity of a modern society depends upon the relationship between them' (1981: 131).

2 The term multiculturalism is thus used here to encompass a wide range of policies aimed at providing some level of public recognition and/or distinctive provision for minority groups. The latter include a range of sociological minorities, as discussed in Chapter 2 – national minorities, indigenous peoples and immigrants, among others. The policy implications for these different minority groups vary widely (see Kymlicka, 2007, for further discussion), depending on their sociohistorical and sociopolitical positioning with nation-states and their associated rights claims. However, as we will see, this does not stop many critics of multiculturalism from deliberately failing to make any meaningful distinctions among minority groups; treating all as equally illegitimate.

3 This is certainly the position of Gordon and Glazer in their respective analyses of the two approaches (see also Glazer, 1998), although Walzer adopts a more sympathetic stance toward pluralism, most notably through his (1994) attempt to distinguish between Liberalism 1 and Liberalism 2. Other examples of this rejection of a more pluralist perspective are wide-ranging. They include: Rawls (1971); Dworkin (1978), (1983); Rorty (1991); Barry (2001); Levy (2001); Waldron (1993, 1995, 2000, 2002). I will discuss Brian Barry and Jeremy Waldron's important and controversial contributions in more detail later in this chapter.

4 See e.g. Goulbourne (1991a, b); Joppke and Lukes (1999); Waldron (1995, 2000); Barry (2001); Pieterse (2007, 2009); J. Edwards (1985, 1994, 2010).

5 All languages are linked to one's ethnic habitus, not just so-called minority languages, which are usually accorded the moniker 'ethnic' (as here). I briefly introduced this point in Chapter 1, in my discussion of Bourdieu's notions of habitus and field, and I will return to it more fully in Chapter 4 when I explore directly the links between language and identity.

6 For other examples of this broadly articulated position, see Bloom (1987); Hirsch (1987); Schlesinger (1991); Hughes (1993); D'Souza (1991, 1995); Lind (1995); Glazer (1998); Ravitch (1992, 2001); Huntingdon (2005).

7 For two useful, critical overviews of Afrocentrism, see S. Howe (1998); Adeleke (2009).

8 Latino communities in the USA are not a single category, as so often described in the literature. Rather they comprise a diverse range of groups, including Spanish-speaking national minorities (Puerto Ricans and Chicanos), various Spanish-speaking immigrants from Latin America, Cuban refugees and often-illegal Mexican migrant workers (Kymlicka, 1995a: 15–17; see also Gracia, 2007).

9 This concern also extended into the political and policy arenas. His last major book, *Why Social Justice Matters* (2005), was a bracing critique of new right economic policies in Britain and the US and the exacerbation of social and economic inequalities that resulted from them.

10 This is not to say that all theorists advocating a liberal egalitarian approach are as dismissive of culture as Barry; for a more sympathetic account of cultural claims within liberal egalitarianism, see e.g. Caney (2007); Levy (2007).

11 There are clear echoes here of the skepticism inherent in situational accounts of ethnicity, as discussed in Chapter 1.

12 Barry also specifically discusses Welsh language education in Wales in similar terms. I will return to both examples, and the wider argument underpinning them, in Chapter 6, when I explore issues of language and education in relation to English, bilingual education and social mobility. I also discuss the Welsh context in more depth in Chapter 7.

13 Barry does allow that the acquisition of a new identity may not require completely dispensing with the old one. He describes this process as one of 'additive assimilation' (2001: 81). However, he tends to associate this with overtly multinational states, such as Switzerland or Britain. And certainly, from his subsequent discussion (pp. 81–90), it remains for him the exception, rather than the rule.

14 Communitarians believe that we discover our ends embedded in a social context, rather than choosing them ex nihilo. Their principal objection in this regard is thus to the idea of a self divorced from, or stripped of, the social features of identity (Coulombe, 1995).

15 This approach can be regarded as even more problematic when one considers e.g. that indigenous and other non-Western groups tend to place greater emphasis on shared communal values *as ends in themselves* than does the more individualistically oriented West (Corson, 2000; May, 1999c, 2002; see Chapter 8).

16 For examples of these wide-ranging critiques of communitarianism, see Mouffe (1993); Burtonwood (1996); Ellison (1997); Carter and Stokes (1998); Bielefeldt (2000); Dalacoura (2002).

17 The links between social, political and wider economic disadvantage are most evident among indigenous peoples, as I will discuss further in Chapter 8. But as Will Kymlicka (2007: 81–2) notes, while economic disadvantage is a factor in many minority rights claims, there are groups that are culturally and politically disadvantaged and/or excluded while still remaining economically privileged. The latter include Chinese minorities in various South Asian countries (Indonesia, Philippines, Malaysia, Thailand) and in the Pacific (Fiji). As we will see in Chapter 7, the Catalans under Franco's fascist regime in Spain were a historical example of the same.

18 Barry discusses and summarily dismisses a wide range of commentators who countenance any accommodation with multiculturalism, describing them all as either communitarians and/or multiculturalists rather than liberals. This is so even when those, such as Will Kymlicka, continue to endorse liberalism specifically. Kymlicka argues that minority claims can be accommodated within a more broadly conceived liberalism, as I will discuss further shortly. But Barry has no truck with this. Kymlicka, whatever he might have to say about his own position, supports multiculturalism so, ergo, he is clearly not a liberal! As David Miller concludes,

'Barry at times seems to want to invert the old Groucho Marx joke by refusing to join any club that would let anyone besides himself in as a member' (2002: 262; see also Squires, 2002).

19 For a discussion and critique of this instant dismissal of multiculturalist accounts on the basis of the apparently unforgivable sin of essentialism, see Mason (2007).

20 I will return to the issues attendant upon bilingual education at various points in Chapters 5–6. In Chapter 5, I will explore the links between educational provision and the wider pluralism of society. In Chapter 6, I will address more fully the specific charges invoked by liberals against bilingual education in relation to both parental choice and wider social mobility. In this chapter, I will also examine and critique the arguments of the English Only Movement, which campaigns against all forms of bilingual education in the USA, particularly those directed at Latino students.

21 In her later work (see especially Young, 2007), Young tries to clarify two major strands of the 'politics of difference'. One is primarily focused on positional difference – one's location in the social/economic/political arena – and the structural inequalities that ensue from such positioning. This, she argues, is the predominant focus of her own work, as will become evident in my discussion below, although she also clearly incorporates cultural differences as well. The other is focused primarily on cultural difference, as exemplified most clearly in the work of Charles Taylor and Will Kymlicka. Her 2007 essay, published just after her untimely death, argues that the two are, or at least can be, complementary but need to be conceptually distinguished.

22 The adoption of a formal Swiss Language Act in 2010, while not addressing immigrant languages directly, does nonetheless encourage their use as medium of instruction in schools in major urban areas (cf. Chapter 5).

23 For representative examples of these concerns, particularly in relation to the impact on women, see: Yuval-Davis (1997a); Okin (1998, 1999); Reitman (2005); Shachar (2001, 2007); Phillips and Saharso (2008); Phillips (1997, 2009).

24 Indeed, examples of the protection of religious minorities can be traced as far back as the early Middle Ages, with a number of prominent treaties that included specific religious protection also evident in the seventeenth and eighteenth centuries (Oestreich, 1999). For a useful historical overview of minority protections, and the role and influence of the League of Nations, see Duchêne (2008: 47–54).

25 It has to be said that the League of Nations did not initially encompass a formal concern for minority rights. Indeed, no provisions dealing with the protection of minorities – nor, for that matter, human rights generally – were incorporated within its original remit. However, these omissions created significant controversy and led the League of Nations subsequently to adopt and oversee the Minority Protection scheme. The scheme, however, was as much concerned with providing a mechanism for the protection of individual rights, especially the right to equality, as with the specific concerns of these national minorities. As such, the League of Nations' approach is not inconsistent with the more recent adoption of universal human rights, even though it was subsequently construed as being so (see de Varennes, 1996a: 26–7; see also below).

26 Article 2 of the Declaration states: 'Everyone is entitled to all the rights and freedoms set forth in this Declaration, without distinction of any kind, such as race [sic], color, sex, religion, political or other opinion, national or social origin, property, birth or other status'. Consequently, minorities, as such, do not enjoy rights in the Declaration. Various attempts at including a recognition of minorities in the text were strongly opposed at the draft stages, the consensus being that 'the best solution of the problems of minorities was to encourage respect for human rights' (see Thornberry, 1991b: 11–12).

27 Margalit and Raz's (1995: 81–91) discussion of encompassing groups could easily be applied to the notion of ethnicity as habitus. At one point e.g. they observe: 'familiarity with a culture determines the boundaries of the imaginable. Sharing a culture, being part of it, determines the limits of the feasible' (1995: 86).

28 The few notable exceptions, at least to date, have been in relation to the issue of Quebec – see e.g. Coulombe (1995, 1999) and, in relation to associated legal debates, Réaume (1999, 2003). Of course, one might also add Charles Taylor's (1994) seminal contribution on the 'politics of recognition' here as well, although language forms only a part of his wider discussion, and tends also to be framed primarily in relation to Quebec (see Chapter 7). Kymlicka is the only political theorist to discuss the possibility of language rights for minorities more generally, most prominently in *The Politics of the Vernacular* (2001). Even here though his engagement with related fields, such as sociolinguistics and education, is limited, as I will return to briefly in Chapter 4.

29 It is interesting to note, however, that nearly all the political theorists who contributed to the Kymlicka and Patten (2003) volume oppose minority language rights – Laitin and Reich, and Pogge e.g. dismiss such rights out of hand. Only Patten and Boran offer qualified support. I will return to Laitin and Reich's, and Pogge's, contributions in Chapter 6, since their arguments on bilingual education for Latinos in the USA are not dissimilar to Schlesinger and Barry's, discussed earlier. Those contributors to the Kymlicka and Patten volume who did support minority language rights, including myself, Rubio-Marin, Grin and Réaume, come from backgrounds in sociolinguistics or international law.

4 Language, identity, rights and representation

1 Sociolinguistics is concerned primarily with exploring societal effects on language(s) and their use. It articulates with a wide range of related disciplinary areas, including the sociology of language, applied linguistics, language ideology, language policy and linguistic anthropology, as well as subdisciplines such as research on bilingualism and second language acquisition. These other fields are research traditions in their own right, although the overlap among them is often considerable (see e.g. Gumperz and Cook-Gumperz, 2008; May, 2011c). Nonetheless, I use sociolinguistics as an overarching term in what follows for the sake of both brevity and convenience.

2 There is an extensive, longstanding, literature supporting this conclusion. For useful recent overviews see e.g. Cummins (2000); May et al. (2004a); May (2008a); García (2009); Grosjean (2010); Baker (2011).

3 And yet, many commentators do precisely that – see e.g. Glazer (1975, 1983); Eastman (1984); Rodriguez (1983, 1993). The most consistent sociolinguistic commentator to expound this position is John Edwards (see 1984, 1985, 1994, 2009, 2010) and I will return to his contributions in due course.

4 While the Sapir-Whorf hypothesis is widely known and still regularly used, recent commentators prefer the latter term, linguistic relativity, arguing that it is misleading to think that Sapir and Whorf developed this as a hypothesis (see Lee, 1996; Joseph, 2002). As such, I use linguistic relativity in what follows.

5 For a useful summary of Sapir and Whorf's development of linguistic relativity, and the subsequent tendency to misinterpret and caricature their work, see Glaser (2007: 41–5). It should be noted that the political motivations underpinning the development of their work have also been regularly overlooked. For example, Whorf's wider commitment to supporting a view of difference and diversity was largely in response to the genocide of Native American cultures and languages (Fishman, 1989d; see also Pennycook, 1994).

6 Reines and Prinz provide a fascinating overview of neo-Whorfian research, particularly over the last decade and, in so doing, outline empirical support for two forms of neo-Whorfianism. *Habitual Whorfianism*, they describe, as instilling 'habits of thought that lead us to think in certain ways by default that we would not have thought in without [particular] language learning [experiences]' (2009: 1028). This helps to explain why 'language can give us the impression that certain inferences are "natural" because we make them automatically as a result of our linguistically inculcated habits' (ibid.). *Ontological Whorfianism* suggests that 'languages influence psychological processes because they lead us to organize the world into categories that differ from those we would discover without language', thus shaping the 'categorical boundaries that constitute our subjective organization of the world' (2009: 1029). Both are clearly consonant with Fishman's account, as well as Bourdieu's notion of linguistic habitus, discussed further below.

7 The original meaning of 'Gaeltacht' was 'Irish speaking people' (Walsh, 2011) and it applies to those Irish-speaking communities that are situated mainly in rural coastal areas in the northwest, west and south of Ireland. It should be noted though that the term is now somewhat problematic since, traditionally, the Gaeltacht was viewed as a composite geographical area, whereas currently many parts of Ireland which were once part of the Gaeltacht are no longer so (see Ó Riagáin, 1997; Chapter 3). Accordingly, the plural term 'Gaeltachtaí' is increasingly used to describe present Irish-speaking communities (Ó Gadhra, 1988).

8 Article 8.1 of the Irish Constitution, passed by plebiscite in 1937, declares that: 'The Irish language as the national language is the first official language.' Ó Catháin argues, however, that a more accurate translation should be: 'As the Irish language is the national language, it is the *primary* official language' (2007: 294; my emphasis).

9 Diglossia can be defined as the pattern of language behavior within a bilingual community where one language is associated with certain (usually high-status) domains of social activity (e.g. commerce) while the other language is usually associated with low-status domains (such as family life). Ó Murchú (1988) observes that this appears to be the only instance of bilingual diglossia in Irish history.

10 The Irish Free State (1922–37) was renamed as Ireland in 1937, the name of the new state being affirmed in the Constitution at that time. In 1949, when Ireland left the Commonwealth, it became officially the Republic of Ireland.

11 As Williams (2008: 217–18) observes, the Irish government has recently weakened the rule that all secondary students should learn Irish, along with the Irish language requirement for their teachers. Meanwhile, recent restructuring of the National University has also seen a lowering of the Irish language requirement for entry.

12 Edwards has expounded this position consistently over the last thirty years. In his latest contribution (2010), he continues to construct a highly disingenuous, rhetorical argument along these lines. First, he dismisses all academic commentators who support language rights on the basis that taking such a position must necessarily involve 'activism' or 'advocacy' – thus equating all such commentary with linguistic nationalism rather than 'serious' academic inquiry. Then, in contrast, he offers his more 'reasonable', 'disinterested' – and, by implication, more 'academically rigorous' – position as the (only) alternative. If only language rights proponents could listen to the voice of academic reason (his voice, obviously), all would be well.

13 Fishman's emphasis on intergenerational transmission is important and widely accepted. However, one can also invert his argument somewhat here. Intergenerational transmission, while obviously central, also has to be supported concurrently by measures that result in minority languages re-entering, and thus being explicitly *re*valued in, the public domain. It is the latter that gives status to

minority languages and thus potentially limits language shift. I will return to this argument in the final chapter.

14 Space precludes me from discussing the Northern Ireland context further. However, for useful recent overviews of minority language developments in Northern Ireland, particularly in relation to the re-emergence of both Irish and Ulster Scots, see Nic Craith (2003); Muller (2010); Walsh (2011).

15 This includes the Irish language radio (Raidió na Gaeltachta) now being able to reach the Irish-language diaspora, via the web, and the establishment in 2001 of a high quality Irish-language e-journal, *Beo* http://www.beo.ie/ (Nic Craith, 2007).

16 The sometimes-profound cultural dislocation that accompanies language shift for the individual in this context is illustrated well by the personal accounts of Hoffman (1989) and Rodriguez (1983, 1993). Grosjean (2010) also provides examples of the psychological costs of language loss to the individual.

17 In the original formulation of this argument (1991), Fishman actually used the gendered terms 'Xmen' and 'Ymen' but changed this in his 2001 volume to 'Xians' and 'Yians'.

18 This disparity is highlighted in the Irish context by the contrasting efforts of a small bilingual elite in Dublin, who were at the heart of nationalist efforts to promote the Irish language, and the rest of the population who were far more interested in acquiring English.

19 The criticism of 'self-interested' elites, and the related dismissal of the legitimacy of the movements associated with them, is a regular trope in constructionist critiques of ethnicity, nationalism and multiculturalism, as we have seen in the previous chapters. For a critique of the 'self-interested elite' position, see Brubaker (1998: 289–92).

20 Status language planning relates to the recognition of particular languages in specific public and/or private language domains within modern nation-states (see Hornberger, 2006; May, 2006).

21 Brian Barry (2001) makes precisely this argument about Welsh vis-à-vis English in Wales, as I discuss further in Chapter 6.

22 It should be pointed out, however, that many so-called 'national' language(s) hold de facto rather than de jure status (see Ruiz, 1990). In the UK, for example, English is the only accepted language of the state (except in Wales where Welsh has recently been recognized as having equivalent status; see Chapter 7) but the role of English is not constitutionally or legislatively enshrined. A similar situation pertains in the USA, although there have been consistent attempts by pressure groups to have English made the only official language (see the discussion of the 'English Only' movement in Chapter 6). A similar de facto status for French in France was only changed by constitutional legislation in 1992.

23 The Council of Europe, established in 1949 and based in Strasbourg, is separate from the European Union (EU). Its responsibilities include European-wide legal standards, human rights, and cultural cooperation. It currently has forty-seven member states.

24 In contrast to the intent of the Charter, which focuses on territorially based regional or minority languages, France actually recognized seventy-five languages (now seventy-seven) as 'langues de France' (languages of France), including those in metropolitan France, its departments and overseas territories. This followed the recommendation of a legal response to the Poignant Report by the Director of the National Institute for the French Language, Bernard Cerquiglini (Chonaill, 2004; Judge, 2007).

5   Language, education and minority rights

1   International measures of comparative academic achievement, such as the International Association for the Evaluation of Educational Achievement (IEA), Progress in International Reading and Literacy Study (PIRLS) and, perhaps most influentially, the OECD Program for International Student Assessment (PISA), have since regularly highlighted and confirmed this general pattern of differential achievement for minority groups, both within and across nation-states.

2   As Kenneth Howe argues: 'The principle of equal educational opportunity can only be realized for cultural minorities by rendering educational opportunities worth wanting, and rendering educational opportunities worth wanting requires that minorities not be required to give up their identities in order to enjoy them' (1992: 469).

3   The term often used for this educational approach, particularly by majority language advocates, is 'immersion' education; equating it directly with second language education programs such as French immersion education programs in Canada (see Chapters 6 and 7 for further discussion). However, for reasons I will return to there, this association is entirely spurious, since immersion programs, such as those in Canada, actually have as their core aim eventual student bilingualism. In contrast, the programs highlighted here aim for the active retrenchment of student bilingualism, with the ultimate aim of monolingualism in the majority language – hence, 'submersion' or 'sink or swim' are far more accurate descriptors.

4   For example, in late 2010 over 1,000 Tibetan students rallied against the ongoing erosion of Tibetan language and culture as a result of this restrictive language policy. See http://www.bbc.co.uk/news/world-asia-pacific-11581189.

5   For analyses of Australia's official policy of multiculturalism, particularly with regard to language and education, see: Ozolins (1993); Kane (1997); Kalantzis and Cope (1999); Hill and Allan (2004); Clyne (1998, 2005). For analyses of Canada's official multiculturalism, see: Fleras and Elliot (1991); Berry (1998); Kamboureli (1998); Kymlicka (1998); Joshee and Johnson (2007).

6   For key examples of this position, which has since come to be termed 'critical multiculturalism', see Sleeter (1996); Giroux (1997); Kincheloe and Steinberg (1997); McLaren (1995, 1997); May (1999b); Sleeter and Delgado (2004); May and Sleeter (2010). Comparable, albeit distinct, arguments can also be found in antiracist education and critical race theory; see Darder and Torres (2002), and May and Sleeter (2010) for further discussion.

7   For examples of indigenous arguments along these lines, see Ignace and Ignace (1998); Perera and Pugliese (1998); Ivison et al. (2000); May (1999c, 2002); Povinelli (2002); May and Aikman (2003); see also Chapter 8. For a more general critique of multiculturalism as a form of institutional control, see the iconoclastic accounts of Australian multicultural policy by Ghassan Hage (2000, 2003).

8   This accords with now widely recognized and accepted research findings within cognitive linguistics and related bilingual research. In this research, it has been found that, *where their bilingualism is explicitly valued and promoted*, bilinguals mature earlier than monolinguals in acquiring skills for linguistic abstraction, are superior to monolinguals on divergent thinking tasks and in their analytical orientation to language, and demonstrate greater social sensitivity than monolinguals in situations requiring verbal communication (see Romaine, 1995; Corson, 2000; Cummins, 2000; May et al., 2004a; May, 2008a).

9   For useful recent overviews and analysis of maintenance bilingual education programs in these and other regions, see García et al. (2006); Skutnabb-Kangas et al. (2009); Menken and García (2010). For earlier examples, see Cenoz and Genesee (1998); May (1999c), Skutnabb-Kangas (2000); May and Aikman (2003).

10 The official language in Flanders is now standard Dutch, although a number of local Flemish dialects are also still regularly used.
11 As Mnookin and Verbeke (2009: 161) observe, a key argument for independence in this proposal is, ironically, that Flanders is now more economically prosperous than Wallonia. Wallonia has seen its coal and steel industries collapse, while Flanders's more recent industrialization, associated most prominently with shipbuilding, has seen it emerge as one of Europe's most prosperous regions.
12 The adoption of a formal Swiss Language Act in 2010 has further entrenched the importance of maintaining public multilingualism in Switzerland, with particular emphasis placed on supporting Romansh and Italian as official languages. See http://www.loc.gov/lawweb/servlet/lloc_news?disp3_l205401779_text
13 For contemporary educational examples that include a wide range of minority groups and contexts, see Skutnabb-Kangas et al. (2009); Menken and García (2010); Hornberger (2011); McCarty (2011).
14 Macías distinguishes between two broadly comparable sets of rights: the right to freedom from discrimination on the basis of language, and the right to use your language(s) in the activities of communal life (1979: 88–9).
15 As we saw in Chapter 3, this has not actually proved to be the case. Indeed, the United Nations itself has since admitted as much: The *Human Rights Fact Sheet on Minorities* (No. 18, March 1992: 1) states: 'the setting of standards which create additional rights and make special arrangements for persons belonging to minorities and for the minorities as *groups* – although a stated goal of the United Nations for more than 40 years – has made slow progress'.
16 For other examples of this position, see Thornberry (1991a, 1991b); Tollefson (1991); Pejic (1997); Skutnabb-Kangas (1998, 2000); Dunbar, (2007); May (1997b, 1999c, 2004, 2011b).
17 As of 2009, nine European nation-states have signed the Charter but not ratified it: Azerbaijan, Bosnia and Herzegovina, France (discussed in Chapter 4), Iceland, Italy, Malta, Moldova, Russia and the Former Yugoslav Republic of Macedonia.

6 Monolingualism, mobility and the pre-eminence of English

1 These developments, in turn, undermine the formerly discrete categories of first, second and foreign language learners, making these categorizations both increasingly problematic and obsolete (see Blommaert, 2010; Pennycook, 2010, for further discussion). That said, I will continue to use these categories here because they are still widely referred to as key points of reference in discussions about the number of speakers in any given language.
2 Indeed, recent trends indicate that the number of first language (L1) speakers of English is actually in decline. Some commentators have suggested as a result that over the last fifty years English has slipped from 2nd to 4th in terms of L1 speakers, behind Mandarin, Spanish and Hindi-Urdu. Arabic as the language that is currently fastest growing is also predicted to overtake English by the middle of this century with respect to L1 speakers (Graddol, 2007). The real growth and influence of English as a global language, then, lie in its ascendancy as the additional language of choice for other language speakers. In Asia, English is increasingly used as a lingua franca alongside Mandarin. In Europe, as we shall see shortly, English is increasingly the lingua franca in the European Union (EU), while English has become the 'first foreign' language in education systems across Europe.

3 Although one should note that much of the visibility for these minority languages on the web is still dependent on specific state support and/or intervention; e.g. the Basque Autonomous Government paid Microsoft a significant amount in order to have Windows and Office available in Basque (see Maurais, 2003).

4 Archibugi specifically states that he is not suggesting the actual use of Esperanto, but rather 'the idea that it is the responsibility of individuals and governments to remove language barriers that obstruct communication' (2005: 545).

5 Hispanic is the term used in the US census, and by the US government, to describe those who are Spanish speakers in the USA. Latino/Latina are more grassroots descriptors, currently favored by the various Spanish-speaking communities themselves. As such, I use Latino in my own discussion but retain Hispanic when used by other commentators. The various Latino communities, and their differing relationships with each other and the US state, will be discussed further below.

6 At the time Archibugi was writing, the official languages of the EU were: Czech, Danish, Dutch, English, Estonian, Finnish, French, German, Greek, Hungarian, Italian, Latvian, Lithuanian, Maltese, Polish, Portuguese, Slovak, Slovene, Spanish and Swedish. Irish, Bulgarian and Romanian were added in 2007.

7 De Swaan distinguishes languages on the dubious basis of their mutual unintelligibility. However, as we saw in Chapter 4, this is a highly problematic distinction, since languages are granted their (official) status as 'fully fledged' languages on the basis of political rather than linguistic criteria. Even linguistically, the continuum between languages and dialects (so called) is much more complex than this distinction allows since some languages are mutually intelligible, while some dialects are not.

8 For de Swaan, the Q value or 'communication value' of a language is measured by combining the 'prevalence' of a language (the percentage of speakers of a language within the wider constellation of languages) with its 'centrality', i.e. the percentage of its *multilingual* speakers among all multilinguals in the constellation (2001: 178).

9 For further discussion, see Phillipson, 2003; van Parijs, 2005; Ammon, 2006; Kraus, 2008; de Houwer and Wilton, 2011.

10 Diglossia presumes a stable equilibrium between/among competing languages, with clearly demarcated boundaries of language use. As I argue shortly, this presumption seldom ever holds, particularly when English is involved.

11 This is more accurately described as 'submersion' in English – see Chapter 5, n. 3.

12 While this might suggest that Pogge is not, ipso facto, opposed to ongoing bilingualism, the parentheses are a telling example of where the priorities still lie. Moreover, the underlying premises of English-only educational instruction specifically militate against the maintenance of students' bilingualism.

13 Linking bilingual education directly with child abuse is, as we shall see shortly, a key trope of the visceral politics of the 'English Only' movement in the USA. Even though Pogge attempts at one point to distance himself from this wider movement, his own position ends up being not that dissimilar. So too does his fundamental misunderstanding and misrepresentation of the educational benefits of bilingual education.

14 Similar critiques along these lines can be found in Bailey, 1991; Holborow, 1999; Rassool, 1999; Tollefson, 1995, 2000; Canagarajah, 2000.

15 This was reflected clearly in early work within sociolinguistics on the proliferation of 'world Englishes'. Up until the 1990s, for example, discussions about these developments centered largely on the perceived threat they posed to 'standard English', reflecting pre-existing language hierarchies (see Quirk, 1981, 1985; Kachru, 1982, 1986, 1990; Kachru and Nelson, 1996). More recent work in sociolinguistics would seem to ally more closely with the likes of de Swaan and Archibugi, by arguing

that multilingual speakers who speak English may be the new powerbrokers in a globalized world (see Brutt-Griffler and Evan Davies, 2006; Rubdy and Saraceni, 2006; J. Jenkins, 2006, 2007). However, this work does not account satisfactorily for the differential status still ascribed to these language varieties, which Blommaert usefully encapsulates in his description of them as context-specific, 'low-mobility' forms of English (2010: 195; see also below).

16   The impact of globalization has changed this somewhat since the 1990s, particularly with the increasing use by multinational companies of business process outsourcing (BPO) and information technology outsourcing (IPO) requiring English language expertise (Graddol, 2007). Examples here include call centers and publishing, both of which India has benefited directly from over the last decade. However, these developments also highlight the significant differentials and inequalities in pay and conditions for workers in India and other comparable contexts when compared with 'source' countries – indeed, these conditions are the principal raison d'être for the outsourcing in the first place. Meanwhile, the necessary English language expertise is still closely related to existing social class and related educational hierarchies in India, as elsewhere (Morgan and Ramanathan, 2009; Sonntag, 2009).

17   The examples where this has occurred as the result of a minority language policy remain extremely rare. The post-Soviet language policies of Latvia and Estonia, however, may be said to fall into this category. This is because the significant majority Russian-speaking population in these areas has been denied citizenship rights since independence unless they can demonstrate a conversational ability in Latvian or Estonian (see de Varennes, 1996a; Hogan-Brun et al., 2007).

18   Late-exit programs, which involve bilingual instruction for a minimum of four to six years, equate with the group maintenance bilingual education programs discussed in Chapter 5. Likewise, early-exit programs equate with transitional bilingual education programs that begin in a minority language but 'transition' to the majority language within one to two years.

19   'Official English' movement is the preferred designation adopted by its proponents in the USA. However, critics use the phrase 'English Only' movement in order to highlight the exclusionary linguistic (and political and social) motives behind the movement. These motives will be highlighted in what follows.

20   English First was formed in 1986 by Larry Pratt and, while also a mass membership organization, is smaller and more strident than US English (Schmidt, 2008).

21   In 1983, US English reported having 300 members; in 1984, 35,000 (Marshall, 1986). By 1994, its numbers had grown to some 400,000 members (J. Edwards, 1994) while, over the course of this time, the organization has also attracted to its ranks many well-known public figures.

22   See www.us-english.org for a current list of US states that have adopted English-only measures.

23   See also Crawford, 1992a, b; Schmidt, 2000; Schmid, 2001; Pavlenko, 2002; Ricento, 2005: Schildkraut, 2005; Wiley, 2005.

24   As one might expect from my discussion in Chapter 5, this assimilationist approach fostered both Native American language loss and educational 'underachievement'. Interestingly, it also stands in sharp contrast to a Cherokee educational initiative implemented prior to this policy. This self-managed policy, based on first-language principles, achieved a 90% literacy rate in Cherokee *as well as* 'a higher English literacy level than the white populations of either Texas or Arkansas' (Crawford, 1989: 25; see also Fuchs and Havighurst, 1972; Szasz, 1974; and Chapter 8).

25   There is some suggestion that Franklin's increasingly trenchant views on multilingualism were linked to his bitterness over a business failure in publishing. In the 1730s Franklin did not seem at all averse to multilingualism, teaching himself

French, German, Italian, Spanish and Latin. He also launched the first *German* language newspaper in North America, the *Philadelphische Zeitung*. It was only after this venture failed, and a 'better qualified German printer' cornered the German book market, that his writings about American 'foreign' language speakers took its sharply xenophobic turn (Shell, 1993).

26 Because New Mexico comprised predominantly 'mexicanas' (a term of self-identification among the Spanish-speaking population) and was also poor, it had to wait some sixty-four years for statehood. Statehood was only granted after fifty previously unsuccessful petitions to Congress (Hernández-Chávez, 1995).

27 However, the downside of this is that because language is not specifically mentioned in the 14th Amendment, some subsequent Supreme Court decisions have simply refused to address the issue of language discrimination at all. In *Garcia v. Spun Steak* (1993), for example, a claim of discrimination on the grounds that the employer prohibited Spanish speakers from speaking privately in Spanish to each other while at work was unsuccessful. This was because the Court declined to examine the principal point raised by the Spanish-speaking workers: i.e. if some employees have the privilege of conversing with others privately at work in their primary language, they should not be denied the same privilege (de Varennes, 1996a; del Valle, 2003).

28 A similar criticism has been leveled at those who argue for bidialectalism. The most notable example here has centered on Ebonics (African American Vernacular English) and, particularly the attempts by California's Oakland School Board in 1996–7 to formalize its recognition within its education district (Collins, 1999; Baugh, 2002).

29 The remit of the (1968) Bilingual Act was to rectify the poor educational performance of 'limited English-speaking ability' students, rather than with issues of bilingualism per se (Shannon, 1999). Nonetheless, it was a consistent target of the English Only movement because it ostensibly allowed for the development of both transitional (early exit) bilingual programs and (late exit) maintenance bilingual approaches, the latter being a particular anathema to English Only proponents. The reality, as always with the English Only movement, was somewhat different. The Act was a modest, consistently underfunded, grant in aid program that focused almost solely on transitional bilingual programs over its thirty-year history (Ricento and W. Wright, 2008). Moreover, the increasing hostility generated toward bilingual education over that period meant that each time the Act came up for reauthorization, its remit was further delimited. In short the Act's influence was far less than its opponents proclaimed. This also, perhaps, explains why it was so easily dispensed with in the end by the Bush administration.

30 A study conducted by Huddy and Sears (1990) specifically supports the argument that English Only may appeal to racist beliefs. The authors examined the attitudes of white Americans toward bilingual education and found that opposition was strongest among those who looked down on minority groups, particularly immigrants, and who opposed any federal support for them. In addition, these attitudes were most strongly represented in areas with a high Latino population (see also MacKaye, 1990).

7 The rise of regionalism

1 See e.g. Robertson (1992); Held (1995); Held et al. (1999); Kraidy (2005); Heller (2003, 2008); Hobsbawm (2008); Pieterse (2009).

2 Despite the EU's formal multilingual policy, two-thirds of EU drafts are now written in English, with this expected to increase by 2% per annum. Meanwhile,

negotiations with new member states are conducted almost entirely in English (see Phillipson, 2010: 65).

3 See Chapter 4 for discussion of these terms.

4 The Official Languages Act (OLA, 1969) declared English and French the official languages of Canada 'for all purposes of the Parliament and Government of Canada' and established the Office of the Commissioner of Official Languages. As part of this development, the OLA declared that federal services accommodate the language preferences of individuals whose first language was either English or French. This acknowledged the personality language principle for the first time in Canada. In 1988, these provisions were strengthened when federal officers were expressly granted the right to work in either official language. And in Nov. 2005, this was further strengthened by requiring all federal institutions to adopt *active* measures to ensure the equality of English and French in the provision of services, a more promotion-oriented language right (Cardinal, 2007; Colin Williams, 2008; cf. Chapter 4).

5 Interestingly, recent revisionist histories of Quebec have critiqued the regular juxtaposition of the pre- and post-Quiet Revolution eras, suggesting that the continuities between the eras are greater than many previous accounts suggest (see Cardinal and Paquet, 2005, for further discussion).

6 The 'notwithstanding clause', Section 33 of the Canadian Charter of Rights and Freedoms, allows provincial legislatures to declare a law or part of a law to apply temporarily ('notwithstanding'), countermanding sections of the Charter if need be.

7 An earlier referendum on Quebec sovereignty, conducted in 1980, saw 60% vote against. The 1995 referendum has thus far proved to be the high point of the sovereignty movement.

8 Even Kymlicka suggests, at one point, that Québécois language laws may amount to an 'over-restrictive external protection' (1995a: 205).

9 Other regions within Spain, with lesser historical claims, had first to fulfil a five-year 'restricted autonomy' period. However, once 'full autonomy' is achieved, the Constitution makes no distinction between the various autonomous regions (Guibernau, 1997).

10 In 2003 the CiU lost its absolute majority for the first time, a result that led Jordi Pujol to retire from politics. From 2003 to 2010, the CiU was the main opposition party at the Catalan autonomous level, having been replaced in the government by a left-wing tripartite coalition formed in 2003 and reformed after the 2006 Catalan regional elections, which were called due to divisions in the coalition. In 2010, however, the CiU, under its current leader Artur Mas, once again regained control of the Catalan Generalitat, albeit without an absolute majority, winning 62 out of 135 seats.

11 As Woolard (1989) observes, this led to a deliberate emphasis in political discourse on inclusive/encompassing definitions of Catalan identity – principally, via the use of 'citizens of Catalonia', rather than 'Catalans' (see also Pujolar, 2007).

12 The only exception to this was a brief rise in support for independence to near 50% in early 2010 (*The Economist*, 29 Nov. 2010). This was in response to a ruling of the Spanish Constitutional Court at that time overturning aspects of the 2006 revision of the Catalan Statute of Autonomy, which had granted further powers of devolution to Catalonia. I discuss both developments more fully below. Meanwhile, the re-establishment of the CiU at the head of Catalan regional government in 2010 has, once again, shifted the focus back to (re)gaining greater political and economic autonomy for Catalonia, rather than secession.

13 This dramatic change in the fortunes of Catalan was greatly facilitated by the linguistic closeness of Catalan and Castilian Spanish as Romance languages, thus making the learning of Catalan relatively straightforward for Spanish speakers.

14 Apart from the efforts of Welsh historians themselves, such as Gwyn Williams (1985), Morgan (1995) and John Davies (2007), Wales has been disproportionately under-represented in accounts of British history. Most have been preoccupied historically with England (Crick, 1991, 1995; Kearney, 2006). Hugh Kearney's (2006) excellent revisionist account of British history provides some semblance of balance here, by specifically including the different, and at times competing, historical trajectories of Scotland, Wales and Ireland (see also, K. Robbins, 1997; Colley, 2009).

15 Welsh emerged in the sixth century when the Brythonic branch of Celtic began to separate into distinct languages. While the first written records date back to the eighth century, it was not until the Middle Welsh period (1150–1400) that a standardized language began to develop, the result, principally, of bardic writings (V. Edwards, 1991).

16 Legislation specific to Wales included the (1881) Welsh Sunday Closing Act, the (1888) Local Government Act and the (1889) Welsh Intermediate Education Act. A range of national institutions were also created over this period, including the University of Wales (1883), the Board of Education, a national library and a national museum (all 1907), and a Department of Agriculture (1912).

17 Cymdeithas yr Iaith Gymraeg has continued to play an active advocacy role on behalf of the Welsh language up to the present day (see e.g. Williams, 2007).

18 As part of the wider constitutional changes undertaken by the British Government at that time, a Northern Ireland Assembly had also been established in the preceding year.

19 The referendum saw 63.5% vote yes, 36.5% vote no.

20 Results of the most recent (2011) British Census were not available at the time of writing.

21 In one notable case, the Criminal Records Board simply ignored repeated requests to provide bilingual registration forms in Wales, including from the WAG. Only after a public campaign and a direct appeal to the British Home Secretary did they eventually comply (Roddick, 2007).

22 These developments have occurred under a Labour Party-controlled Assembly (from 1999 to 2007) and via a formal coalition between Labour and the Welsh Nationalist Party, Plaid Cymru, since 2007. They are perhaps even more significant, therefore, because of the British Labour Party's longstanding ambivalence toward the Welsh language and Welsh nationalism over much of the twentieth century: the former, because class rather than language was the focus of most Welsh Labour Party supporters; the latter, because Plaid Cymru was, until a shift toward the political center in the 1990s, largely identified as a party of the right (May, 1999d).

23 Welsh-medium education is also increasingly available at tertiary level, albeit still in a limited capacity, while there is special provision for training teachers through the medium of Welsh at designated teachers colleges.

8 Indigenous rights

1 For discussion of comparable examples in the USA, see McCarty and Watahomigie (1999) and Okihiro (2009). For Canada, see Castellano et al. (2008).

2 Hanson gained national notoriety in 1996 when, as an Australian Liberal party nominee for Ipswich in Queensland, she repudiated government funding assistance for Aboriginal peoples as 'special pleading'. The overt racism of her remarks, and the subsequent furore that resulted, saw her deselected from the (conservative) Liberal party for the 1996 Australian election, although she still won the seat easily and sat initially as an Independent. In 1997, she founded the One Nation Party, whose influence at state level was most evident in the following year when it won 11 out of 89 seats in the Queensland Legislative Assembly. Internal differences in the party

saw its electoral influence decline rapidly, however. Hanson lost her seat in the 1998 Australian federal election and narrowly failed in her bid for an Australian Senate seat in 2003. She was also convicted of electoral fraud in that year, briefly serving time in prison. Interestingly, after some time in exile in England, she launched an attempt at a political comeback in 2011 that also narrowly failed.

3 United Nations Resolution A/61/L.67: retrieved March 2011 from http://www.iwgia.org/sw248.asp.

4 Cited in GA 10/612: retrieved March 2011 from http://www.un.org/News/Press/docs/2007/ga10612.doc.htm.

5 However, as Todal (1999) points out, it is only in Finnmark that this degree of autonomy has been achieved since, in the other areas in Norway where Sámi can be found, they live in relatively isolated settlements. Accordingly, the language varieties spoken by these groups of Sámi, notably Lule Sámi and Southern Sámi, and their cultural practices, have far less institutional support.

6 Nunavut means 'our land' in Inuktitut.

7 Pastoral leases were first granted to white farmers in 1848, allowing them access to Aboriginal lands for the purposes of (limited) grazing and cultivation. While they were not intended to deprive Aboriginal peoples of their rights to roam and hunt on the land, this is very quickly what happened. Many farmers began to treat the land as private property and began commandeering Aboriginal peoples as free labor. The ongoing genocide of Aboriginal peoples, apparent throughout the nineteenth century and well into the twentieth century, was also 'vindicated' on the basis of the 'protection' of these pastoral leases (Perera and Pugliese, 1998; Tatz, 2011).

8 Even so, the Australian Labor government, which was re-elected in 2010 under its new leader, Julia Gillard, has not changed other aspects of Howard's Aboriginal policy significantly. The Northern Territory intervention, while modified by Rudd in Labor's first term, was still in operation at time of writing.

9 See note 3.

10 Aotearoa is the most widely known and accepted Māori name for New Zealand and can be translated loosely as 'land of the long white cloud'. The name, New Zealand, in turn, is derived from the Dutch sailor, Abel Tasman, the first European to sight the country in 1642.

11 'Pākehā' is the Māori term for New Zealanders of European origin. Its literal meaning is 'stranger', although it holds no pejorative connotation in modern usage.

12 Prior to the Second World War, less than 10% of Māori had lived in cities or smaller urban centers. Fifty years later, over 80% of Māori lived in urban areas (Te Taura Whiri i te Reo Māori, 1995). Māori have thus undergone what is perhaps the most comprehensive, and certainly the most rapid, urbanization process of an indigenous people in modern times.

13 Many were still skeptical at the time about the ability of the MTS to reach anything more than a small niche audience. However, the MTS has subsequently proved its critics wrong. While still small, its innovative programming, and combination of Māori and English language programs, has seen it achieve a consistent growth in its wider audience share since its inception. In June 2010 it had its highest audience share to date – a cumulative audience of nearly 2 million people for the month (Kaa, 2010).

14 The Labour Government did retain political power in the subsequent 2005 national election, although only just, having to govern as a minority administration under New Zealand's proportional representation system. It subsequently lost power to the conservative National Party, under its new leader, John Key, in the 2008 election. Interestingly, Key specifically distanced his party from the overtly racialized politics of his National Party predecessor, Brash. This was exemplified in Key's own

coalition arrangements between 2008 and 2011, which included a formal agreement with the Māori party, a splinter group from Labour that had been established in protest at the enactment of the Foreshore and Seabed Bill. Labour had refused to work with the newly formed party in parliament in the preceding administration.

15 In April 2006, New Zealand Sign Language (NZSL) was also made an official state language.

16 Much of the initial work undertaken by Te Taura Whiri focused on corpus language issues, notably the (re)development of 'authentic' vocabulary for Māori in domains from which it had been historically excluded, such as education.

17 This includes the establishment of Wharekura (Māori language high schools), although their numbers remain small (see May and Hill, 2008).

18 These arguments are strikingly similar, both in tone and content, to the instrumentalist accounts of ethnicity discussed in Chapter 1 and the critique of indigenous identities discussed in Chapter 3.

19 The recent retrenchment of Aboriginal rights in Australia, highlighted earlier, suggests as much.

20 For example, a general language survey conducted in the early 1990s found that nine out of ten of New Zealand's then 3.8 million inhabitants were first language speakers of English – a figure that made it one of the most linguistically homogeneous countries in the world at that time (Te Taura Whiri i te Reo Māori, 1995). The marked increase in Asian migration over the last fifteen years has modified this position somewhat, with more recent projections placing the proportion of monolingual English speakers at closer to 80% (Peddie, 2003). However this is still a considerable percentage and one that is not likely to change significantly any time soon.

9 Reimagining the nation-state

1 The formal discrimination of Russian speakers in the newly independent Baltic states of Latvia and Estonia is one example. See Chapter 6, n. 17.

2 The remaining Pasifika groups did not reach the threshold of 4,500 speakers (just over 0.1% of the total New Zealand population) used by the Census in their analysis of this question.

3 A research team, led by the author, developed the LEAP resource between 2003 and 2005 (see May, 2011c, for further discussion). While aimed specifically at bilingual Pasifika students, many of the principles and practices explored in the website resource can be applied to bilingual students of any ethnicity and from any context.

4 The Samoan and Tongan communities in Aotearoa/New Zealand are best placed with respect to this criterion, given both their larger size and the considerable percentage in each community (60%) who still speak a Pasifika language. That said, there is an argument to be had that the Cook Islands Māori community, despite the much lower percentage who still speak Cook Islands Māori, along with the numerically smaller Tokelauan and Niuean communities, might also be able to claim some promotion-oriented language rights. The claim here would be via a variant of national minority rights, arising from the historical constitutional relationship of each community with New Zealand. On this basis, their respective Pasifika languages could be regarded as 'indigenous languages of the realm of New Zealand' (May, 2010).

5 In a parallel argument drawn from feminist discourse, Nira Yuval-Davis describes this process as one of 'transversal politics' in which 'perceived unity and homogeneity are replaced by dialogues that give recognition to the specific positionings of those

who participate in them, as well as to the "unfinished knowledge" ... that each such situated positioning can offer' (1997b: 204). Central to this idea of transversal politics is the interrelationship between 'rooting' and 'shifting'. Each participant in the dialogue brings with them the rooting in their own grouping and identity, but tries at the same time to shift in order to put themselves in a situation of exchange with those who have different groupings and identities.

BIBLIOGRAPHY

Acton, J. (1907). Nationality. In J. Figgis, and R. Lawrence (eds), *The History of Freedom* (pp. 270–300). London: Macmillan (original, 1862).

Adams, K., and Brink, D. (eds) (1990). *Perspectives on Official English: The Campaign for English as the Official Language of the USA*. Berlin: Mouton de Gruyter.

Adeleke, T. (2009). *The Case Against Afrocentrism*. Jackson, MS: University Press of Mississippi.

Ager, D. (1999). *Identity, Insecurity and Image: France and Language*. Clevedon, Avon: Multilingual Matters.

Ahmad, A. (1995). The politics of literary postcoloniality. *Race and Class* 36, 3, 1–20.

Aitchison, J., and Carter, H. (1994). *A Geography of the Welsh Language 1961–1991*. Cardiff: University of Wales Press.

Aitchison, J., and Carter, H. (2004). *Spreading the Word: The Welsh Language 2001*. Talybont: Y Lolfa Cyf.

AJHR (1986) *Appendices to the Journals of the House of Representatives 1858–1939*. Wellington: AHJR.

Alba, R. (1990). *Ethnic Identity: The Transformation of White America*. New Haven, CT: Yale University Press.

Albright, J., and Luke, A. (eds) (2008). *Pierre Bourdieu and Literacy Education*. New York: Routledge.

Alexander, N. (2000). Language policy and planning in South Africa: some insights. In R. Phillipson (ed.), *Rights to Language: Equity, Power and Education* (pp. 170–3). Mahwah, NJ: Lawrence Erlbaum.

Alexandre, P. (1972). *Languages and Language in Black Africa*. Evanston, IL: Northwestern University Press.

Alter, P. (1989). *Nationalism*. London: Edward Arnold.

Ammon, U. (1998). *Ist Deutsch noch internationale Wissenschaftssprache? Englisch auch für die Lehre an den deutschsprachigen Hochschulen*. Berlin: Mouton de Gruyter.

Ammon, U. (ed.) (2000). *The Dominance of English as the Language of Science: Effects on Other Languages and Language Communities*. Berlin: Mouton de Gruyter.

Ammon, U. (2006). Language conflicts in the European Union: on finding a politically acceptable and practicable solution for EU institutions that satisfies diverging interests. *International Journal of Applied Linguistics* 16, 3, 319–38.

Anaya, J. (1996). *Indigenous Peoples in International Law*. New York: Oxford University Press.

Anderson, B. (1991). *Imagined Communities: Reflections on the Origin and Spread of Nationalism* (rev. edn). London: Verso.

Anthias, F., and Yuval-Davis, N. (1992). *Racialized Boundaries: Race, Nation, Gender, Colour and Class and the Anti-Racist Struggle*. London: Routledge.

Anzaldúa, G. (1987). *Borderlands/La Frontera: The New Mestiza*. San Francisco, CA: Aunt Lute Books.

Appadurai, A. (1990). Disjuncture and difference in the global cultural economy. In M. Featherstone (ed.), *Global Culture: Nationalism, Globalization and Modernity* (pp. 295–310). London: Sage.

Archibugi, D. (2005). The language of democracy: vernacular or Esperanto? A comparison between the multiculturalist and cosmopolitan perspectives. *Political Studies* 53, 3, 537–55.

Armstrong, J. (1982). *Nations Before Nationalism*. Chapel Hill, NC: University of North California Press.

Artigal, J. (1997). The Catalan immersion program. In R. Johnson and M. Swain (eds), *Immersion Education: International Perspectives* (pp. 133–50). Cambridge: Cambridge University Press.

Bader, V. (2001). Culture and identity: contesting constructivism. *Ethnicities* 1, 1, 251–73.

Baetens Beardsmore, H. (1980). Bilingualism in Belgium. *Journal of Multilingual and Multicultural Development* 1, 145–54.

Bailey, R. (1991). *Images of English: A Cultural History of the Language*. Ann Arbor, MI: University of Michigan Press.

Baker, C. (1985). *Aspects of Bilingualism in Wales*. Clevedon, Avon: Multilingual Matters.

Baker, C. (1995). Bilingual education and assessment. In B. Morris Jones and P. Singh Ghuman (eds), *Bilingualism, Education and Identity* (pp. 130–58). Cardiff: University of Wales Press.

Baker, C. (2011). *Foundations of Bilingual Education and Bilingualism* (5th edn). Bristol: Multilingual Matters.

Baker, C., and Prys Jones, S. (eds) (1998). *Encyclopedia of Bilingualism and Bilingual Education*. Clevedon, Avon: Multilingual Matters.

Baker, K., and de Kanter, A. (1981). *Effectiveness of Bilingual Education: A Review of the Literature*. Washington, DC: US Department of Education.

Baker, K., and de Kanter, A. (eds) (1983). *Bilingual Education: A Reappraisal of Federal Policy*. Lexington, MA: Lexington Books.

Bakhtin, M. (1981). *The Dialogic Imagination: Four Essays*, tr. C. Emerson and M. Holquist, ed. M. Holquist. Austin, TX: University of Texas Press.

Balibar, E. (1991). The nation form: history and ideology. In E. Balibar and I. Wallerstein (eds), *Race, Nation, Class: Ambiguous Identities* (pp. 86–106). London: Verso.

Balthazar, L. (1990). *Bilan du nationalisme au Québec*. Montreal: l'Hexagone.

Banks, J. (ed.) (2009). *Routledge International Companion to Multicultural Education*. New York: Routledge.

Banton, M. (1983). *Racial and Ethnic Competition*. Cambridge: Cambridge University Press.

Banton, M. (1987). *Racial Theories*. Cambridge: Cambridge University Press.

Barbaud, P. (1998). French in Québec. In J. Edwards (ed.), *Language in Canada* (pp. 177–201). Cambridge: Cambridge University Press.

Barelli, M. (2010). The interplay between global and regional human rights systems in the construction of the indigenous rights regime. *Human Rights Quarterly* 32, 4, 951–79.

Barker, M. (1981). *The New Racism: Conservatives and the Ideology of the Tribe*. London: Junction.

Barkhuizen, G., and Gough, D. (1996). Language curriculum development in South Africa: what place for English? *TESOL Quarterly* 30, 453–72.

Barnard, F. (1965). *Herder's Social and Political Thought: From Enlightenment to Nationalism*. Oxford: Clarendon Press.

Baron, D. (1990). *The English-Only Question: An Official Language for America?* New Haven, CT: Yale University Press.

Barrington, J. (1992). The school curriculum, occupations and race. In G. McCulloch (ed.), *The School Curriculum in New Zealand* (pp. 57–73). Palmerston North, New Zealand: Dunmore Press.

Barrington, J., and Beaglehole, T. (1974). *Māori Schools in a Changing Society*. Wellington: New Zealand Council for Education Research.

Barry, B. (2001). *Culture and Equality: An Egalitarian Critique of Multiculturalism*. Cambridge MA: Harvard University Press.

Barry, B. (2005). *Why Social Justice Matters*. Cambridge: Polity Press.

Barsh, R. (1996). Indigenous peoples and the UN Commission on Human Rights: a case of the immovable object and the irresistible force. *Human Rights Quarterly* 18, 782–813.

Barth, F. (1969a). Introduction. *Ethnic Groups and Boundaries: The Social Organization of Culture Difference* (pp. 9–38). Boston, MA: Little, Brown & Co.

Barth, F. (1969b). *Ethnic Groups and Boundaries: The Social Organization of Culture Difference*. Boston, MA: Little, Brown & Co.

Barth, F. (1989). The analysis of culture in complex societies. *Ethnos* 54, 120–42.

Barth, F. (1994). Enduring and emerging issues in the analysis of ethnicity. In H. Vermeulen and C. Govers (eds), *The Anthropology of Ethnicity: Beyond 'Ethnic Groups and Boundaries'* (pp. 11–32). Amersterdam: Het Spinhuis.

Baugh, J. (2002). *Beyond Ebonics: Linguistic Pride and Racial Prejudice*. New York: Oxford University Press.

Bauman, R., and Briggs, C. (2003). *Voices of Modernity: Language Ideologies and the Politics of Inequality*. Cambridge: Cambridge University Press.

Bauman, Z. (1973). *Culture as Praxis*. London: Routledge & Kegan Paul.

Bauman, Z. (1998). *Globalization: The Human Consequences*. London: Sage.

Bayar, M. (2009). Reconsidering primordialism: an alternative approach to the study of ethnicity. *Ethnic and Racial Studies* 32, 9, 1639–57.

Belich, J. (1986). *The New Zealand Wars*. Auckland: Auckland University Press.

Belich, J. (1996). *Making Peoples*. Auckland: Allen Lane.

Belich, J. (2001). *Paradise Reforged*. Auckland: Allen Lane.

Bell, A., Davis, K., and Starks, D. (2000). *The Languages of the Manukau Region*. Auckland: Woolf Fisher Research Centre, University of Auckland.

Benhabib, S. (2002). *The Claims of Culture: Equality and Diversity in the Global Era*. Princeton, NJ: Princeton University Press.

Benhabib, S. (2004). *The Rights of Others: Aliens, Residents, and Citizens.* Cambridge: Cambridge University Press.

Bentahila, A., and Davies, E. (1993). Language revival: restoration or transformation? *Journal of Multilingual and Multicultural Development* 14, 355–74.

Bentley, G. (1987). Ethnicity and practice. *Comparative Studies in Society and History* 29, 24–55.

Benton, N. (1989). Education, language decline and language revitalisation: the case of Māori in New Zealand. *Language and Education* 3, 65–82.

Benton, R. (1979). *Who Speaks Māori in New Zealand.* Wellington: New Zealand Council for Educational Research.

Benton, R. (1981). *The Flight of the Amokura: Oceanic Languages and Formal Education in the South Pacific.* Wellington: New Zealand Council for Educational Research.

Benton, R. (1983). *The NZCER Māori Language Survey.* Wellington: New Zealand Council for Educational Research.

Benton, R. (1988). The Māori language in New Zealand education. *Language, Culture and Curriculum* 1, 75–83.

Benton, R. (1996). Language policy in New Zealand: defining the ineffable. In M. Herriman and B. Burnaby (eds), *Language Policies in English-Dominant Countries* (pp. 62–98). Clevedon, Avon: Multilingual Matters.

Berry, J. (1998). Official multiculturalism. In J. Edwards (ed.), *Language in Canada* (pp. 84–101). Cambridge: Cambridge University Press.

Berry, V., and McNeill, A. (2005). Raising English language standards in Hong Kong. *Language Policy* 4, 4, 371–94.

Best, G. (1982). *Honour among Men and Nations: Transformations of an Idea.* Toronto: Toronto University Press.

Best, G. (ed.) (1988). *The Permanent Revolution: The French Revolution and its Legacy.* Chicago, IL: Chicago University Press.

Bhabha, H. (1994). *The Location of Culture.* London: Routledge.

Bielefeldt, H. (2000). 'Western' versus 'Islamic' human rights conceptions? A critique of cultural essentialism in the discussion on human rights. *Political Theory* 28, 1, 90–121.

Bikales, G. (1986). Comment: the other side. *International Journal of the Sociology of Language* 60, 77–85.

Billig, M. (1995). *Banal Nationalism.* London: Sage.

Birch, A. (1989). *Nationalism and National Integration.* London: Unwin Hyman.

Bishop, R., and Glynn, T. (1999). *Culture Counts: Changing Power Relations in Education.* Palmerston North, New Zealand: Dunmore Press.

Blackledge, A. (2008). Language ecology and language ideology. In A. Creese, P. Martin and N. Hornberger (eds), Ecology of language. *Encyclopedia of Language and Education* (2nd edn, vol. 9, pp. 27–40). New York: Springer.

Blaut, J. M. (1993). *The Colonizer's Model of the World: Geographical Diffusionism and Eurocentric History.* New York: Guildford Press.

Blommaert, J. (1996). Language and nationalism: comparing Flanders and Tanzania. *Nations and Nationalism* 2, 235–56.

Blommaert, J. (1999a). The debate is open. In J. Blommaert (ed.), *Language Ideological Debates* (pp. 1–38). Berlin: Mouton de Gruyter.

Blommaert, J. (1999b). The debate is closed. In J. Blommaert (ed.), *Language Ideological Debates* (pp. 425–38). Berlin: Mouton de Gruyter.

Blommaert, J. (ed.) (1999c). *Language Ideological Debates*. Berlin: Mouton de Gruyter.

Blommaert, J. (2001).The Asmara Declaration as a sociolinguistic problem: notes in scholarship and linguistic rights. *Journal of Sociolinguistics* 5, 1, 131–142.

Blommaert, J. (2010). *The Sociolinguistics of Globalization*. New York: Cambridge University Press.

Blommaert, J., and Verschueren, J. (1998). The role of language in European nationalist ideologies. In B. Schieffelin, K. Woolard and P. Kroskrity (eds), *Language Ideologies: Practice and Theory* (pp. 189–210). New York: Oxford University Press.

Bloom, A. (1987). *The Closing of the American Mind: How Higher Education has Failed Democracy and Impoverished the Souls of Today's Students*. New York: Simon & Schuster.

Bollmann, Y. (2002). Les langues régionales et minoritaires en Europe. *Hérodote*, 2e trimestre, 105: 191–201.

Bonnett, A. (2000). *Anti-Racism*. London: Routledge.

Borges, B., and Combrisson, G. (1997). Indigenous rights in Brazil: stagnation to political impasse. Retrieved March 2011 from http://saiic.nativeweb.org/brazil.html.

Bourdieu, P. (1977). The economy of linguistic exchanges. *Social Science Information* 16, 645–68.

Bourdieu, P. (1982). *Ce que parler veut dire: L'économie des échanges linguistiques*. Paris: Arthème Fayard.

Bourdieu, P. (1984). *Distinction: A Social Critique of the Judgement of Taste*. Cambridge, MA: Harvard University Press.

Bourdieu, P. (1990a). *In Other Words: Essays towards a Reflexive Sociology*. Cambridge: Polity Press.

Bourdieu, P. (1990b). *The Logic of Practice*. Cambridge: Polity Press.

Bourdieu, P. (1991). *Language and Symbolic Power*. Cambridge: Polity Press.

Bourdieu, P., and Boltanski, L. (1975). Le fétichisme de la langue. *Actes de la Recherche en Sciences Sociales* 4, 2–23.

Bourdieu, P., and Passeron, J-C. (1990). *Reproduction in Education, Society and Culture* (2nd edn). London: Sage.

Bourdieu, P., and Wacquant, L. (1992). *An Invitation to Reflexive Sociology*. Chicago, IL: Chicago University Press.

Bourhis, R. (ed.) (1984). *Conflict and Language Planning in Québec*. Clevedon, Avon: Multilingual Matters.

Bowie, F. (1993). Wales from within: conflicting interpretations of Welsh identity. In S. Macdonald (ed.), *Inside European Identities: Ethnography in Western Europe* (pp. 167–93). Oxford: Berg Publishers.

Brah, A. (1992). Difference, diversity and differentiation. In J. Donald and A. Rattansi (eds), *'Race', Culture and Difference* (pp. 126–45). London: Sage.

Brass, P. (ed.) (1985). *Ethnic Groups and the State*. London: Croom Helm.

Brazil (1996). *Constituição da República Federativa do Brasil (CF/88)*. São Paulo: Editora Revista dos Tribunais.

Brenzinger, M. (1997). Language contact and language displacement. In F. Coulmas (ed.), *The Handbook of Sociolinguistics* (pp. 273–84). Oxford: Blackwell.

Breuilly, J. (1993). *Nationalism and the State* (2nd edn). Manchester: Manchester University Press.

Breuilly, J. (2005a). Dating the nation: how old is an old nation? In A. Ichijo and G. Uzelac (eds), *When is the Nation? Towards an Understanding of Theories of Nationalism* (pp. 15–39). New York: Routledge.

Breuilly, J. (2005b). Changes in the political uses of nations: continuity and discontinuity. In L. Scales and O. Zimmer (eds), *Power and the Nation in European History* (pp. 67–101). Cambridge: Cambridge University Press.

British Council (1995). *English in the World: The English 2000 Global Consultation.* Manchester: British Council.

Brown, D. (2000). *Contemporary Nationalism: Civic, Ethnocultural and Multicultural Politics.* New York: Routledge.

Brown, D. (2008). The ethnic majority: benign or malign? *Nations and Nationalism* 14, 4, 768–88.

Brubaker, R. (1996). *Nationalism Reframed: Nationhood and the National Question in the New Europe.* Cambridge: Cambridge University Press.

Brubaker, R. (1998). Myths and misconceptions in the study of nationalism. In J. Hall (ed.), *The State of the Nation: Ernest Gellner and the Theory of Nationalism* (pp. 272–306). Cambridge: Cambridge University Press.

Brubaker, R. (2002). Ethnicity without groups. *Archives Européennes de Sociologie* 53, 2, 163–89.

Brutt-Griffler, J. (2002). Class, ethnicity and language rights: an analysis of British colonial policy in Lesotho and Sri Lanka and some implications for language policy. *Journal of Language, Identity and Education* 1, 3, 207–34.

Brutt-Griffler, J., and Evan Davies, C. (eds) (2006). *English and Ethnicity.* Basingstoke: Palgrave Macmillan.

Buchan, B., and Heath, M. (2006). Savagery and civilization: from terra nullius to the 'tide of history'. *Ethnicities* 6, 1, 5–26.

Bucholtz, M., and Hall, K. (2004). Language and identity. In A. Duranti (ed.), *A Companion to Linguistic Anthropology* (pp. 369–94). Malden, MA: Blackwell.

Bullivant, B. (1981). *The Pluralist Dilemma in Education: Six Case Studies.* Sydney: Allen & Unwin.

Burnaby, B. (2008). Language policy and education in Canada. In S. May and N. Hornberger (eds), *Encyclopedia of Language and Education* (2nd edn), vol. 1, *Language Policy and Political Issues in Education* (pp. 331–41). New York: Springer.

Burtonwood, N. (1996). Culture, identity and the curriculum. *Educational Review* 48, 227–35.

Butt Philip, A. (1975). *The Welsh Question: Nationalism in Welsh Politics, 1945–1970.* Cardiff: University of Wales Press.

Caglar, A. (1997). Hyphenated identities and the limits of 'culture'. In T. Modood and P. Werbner (eds), *The Politics of Multiculturalism in the New Europe: Racism, Identity and Community* (pp. 169–85). London: Zed Books.

Calhoun, C. (1993a). Nationalism and ethnicity. *Annual Review of Sociology* 19, 211–39.

Calhoun, C. (1993b). Nationalism and civil society: democracy, diversity and self-determination. *International Sociology* 8, 387–411.

Calhoun, C. (1997). *Nationalism.* Buckingham, Bucks: Open University Press.

Calhoun, C. (2003). Belonging in the cosmopolitan imaginary. *Ethnicities* 3, 3, 531–53.

Calhoun, C. (2007). Social solidarity as a problem for cosmopolitan democracy. In S. Benhabib, I. Shapiro and D. Petranovic (eds), *Identities, Affiliations, and Allegiances* (pp. 285–302). Cambridge: Cambridge University Press.

Calhoun, C., LiPuma, E., and Postone, M. (eds) (1993). *Bourdieu: Critical Perspectives.* Cambridge: Polity Press.

Calvet, L.-J. (1974). *Linguistique et colonialisme: Petite traité de glottophagie.* Paris: Payot.

Canagarajah, A. S. (2000). *Resisting Linguistic Imperialism in English Teaching.* Oxford: Oxford University Press.

Canagarajah, A. S. (2007). The ecology of global English. *International Multilingual Research Journal* 1, 2, 89–100.

Caney, S. (2007). Egalitarian liberalism and universalism. In A. Laden and D. Owen (eds), *Multiculturalism and Political Theory* (pp. 151–72). Cambridge: Cambridge University Press.

Cannadine, D. (1983). The context, performance and meaning of ritual: the British monarchy and the 'invention of tradition' c. 1820–1977. In E. Hobsbawm and T. Ranger (eds), *The Invention of Tradition* (pp. 101–64). Cambridge: Cambridge University Press.

Capotorti, F. (1979). *Study on the Rights of Persons Belonging to Ethnic, Religious and Linguistic Minorities.* New York: United Nations.

Cardinal, L. (1999). Linguistic rights, minority rights and national rights: some clarifications. *Inroads* 8, 77–86.

Cardinal, L. (2005). The ideological limits of linguistic diversity in Canada. *Journal of Multilingual and Multicultural Development* 26, 6, 481–95.

Cardinal, L. (2007). New approaches for the empowerment of linguistic minorities: a study of language policy innovation in Canada since the 1980s. In C. H. Williams (ed.), *Language and Governance* (pp. 434–59). Cardiff: University of Wales Press.

Cardinal, L., and Paquet, G. (2005). Theorising small nations in the Atlantic world: Scottish lessons for Québec? *British Journal of Canadian Studies* 18, 2, 214–31.

Carens, J. (ed.) (1995). *Is Quebec Nationalism Just?* Montreal: McGill-Queens University Press.

Carens, J. (2000). *Culture, Citizenship and Community: A Contextual Exploration of Justice as Evenhandedness.* Oxford: Oxford University Press.

Carter, A., and Stokes, G. (1998). *Liberal Democracy and its Critics.* Cambridge: Polity Press.

Castellano, M., Archibald, L., and DeGagné, M. (eds) (2008). *From Truth to Reconciliation: Transforming the Legacy of Residential Schools.* Ottawa: Aboriginal Healing Foundation.

Castells, M. (1997). *The Power of Identity.* Oxford: Blackwell.

Cenoz, J., and Genesee, F. (eds) (1998). *Beyond Bilingualism: Multilingualism and Multilingual Education.* Clevedon, Avon: Multilingual Matters.

Chambers, C. (2003). Nation-building, neutrality and ethnocultural justice: Kymlicka's liberal pluralism. *Ethnicities* 3, 3, 295–319.

Chandra, K. (2006). What is ethnic identity and does it matter? *Annual Review of Political Science* 9, 397–424.

Chandra, K., and Wilkinson, S. (2008). Measuring the effects of 'ethnicity'. *Comparative Political Studies* 41, 4–5, 515–63.

Chapple, S., Jeffries, R., and Walker, R. (1997). *Māori Participation and Performance in Education: A Literature Review and Research Programme.* Wellington: Ministry of Education.

Chevannes, F., and Reeves, M. (1987). The black voluntary school movement: definition, context and prospects. In B. Troyna (ed.), *Racial Inequality in Education* (pp. 147–69). London: Tavistock.

Chomsky, N. (1972). *Language and Mind*. New York: Harcourt Brace Jovanovich.

Chomsky, N. (1979). *Language and Responsibility*. London: Harvester.

Chomsky, N. (1987). *On Power and Ideology: The Managua Lectures*. Boston, MA: South End Press.

Chonaill, B. (2004). The case of regional and minority languages in France. In F. Royall (ed.), *Contemporary French Cultures and Societies* (pp. 287–302). Berne: Peter Lang.

Chow, R. (1998). *Ethics After Idealism: Theory-Culture-Ethnicity-Reading*. Bloomington, IN: Indiana University Press.

Churchill, S. (1986). *The Education of Linguistic and Cultural Minorities in the OECD Countries*. Clevedon, Avon: Multilingual Matters.

Churchill, S. (1996). The decline of the nation-state and the education of national minorities. *International Review of Education* 42, 265–90.

CILAR (Committee on Irish Language Attitudes Research) (1975). *Report*. Dublin: Stationery Office.

Clark, D., and Williamson, R. (eds) (1996). *Self-Determination: International Perspectives*. London: Macmillan.

Claude, I. (1955). *National Minorities: An International Problem*. Cambridge, MA: Harvard University Press.

Clyne, M. (1990). *Community Languages: The Australian Experience*. Cambridge: Cambridge University Press.

Clyne, M. (1997). Multilingualism. In F. Coulmas (ed.), *The Handbook of Sociolinguistics* (pp. 301–14). Oxford: Blackwell.

Clyne, M. (1998). Managing language diversity and second language programmes in Australia. In S. Wright and H. Kelly-Holmes (eds), *Managing Language Diversity* (pp. 4–29). Clevedon, Avon: Multilingual Matters.

Clyne, M. (2005). *Australia's Language Potential*. Sydney: University of New South Wales Press.

COAG (1994). *Asian Languages and Australia's Economic Future*. (Council of Australian Governments), Brisbane: Queensland Government Printer.

Coetzee, J. M. (2007). *Diary of a Bad Year*. London: Penguin.

Cohen, A. (1974). *Two-Dimensional Man*. London: Tavistock.

Colino, C. (2009). Constitutional change without constitutional reform: Spanish federalism and the revision of Catalonia's Statute of Autonomy. *Publius: The Journal of Federalism* 39, 262–88.

Colley, L. (2009). *Britons: Forging the Nation 1707–1837* (3rd edn). New Haven, CT: Yale University Press.

Collins, J. (1999). The Ebonics controversy in context: literacies, subjectivities, and language ideologies in the United States. In J. Blommaert (ed.), *Language Ideological Debates* (pp. 201–34). Berlin: Mouton de Gruyter.

Conklin, N., and Lourie, M. (1983). *Host of Tongues: Language Communities in the United States*. New York: Free Press.

Connor, W. (1978). A nation is a nation, is a state, is an ethnic group, is a ... *Ethnic and Racial Studies* 1, 377–400.

Connor, W. (1991). From tribe to nation? *History of European Ideas* 13, 5–18.

Connor, W. (1993). Beyond reason: the nature of the ethnonational bond. *Ethnic and Racial Studies* 16, 374–89.

Conversi, D. (1997). *The Basques, the Catalans and Spain*. London: Hurst.

Conversi, D. (ed.) (2002). *Ethnonationalism in the Contemporary World: Walker Connor and the Study of Nationalism*. New York: Routledge.

Cornell, S. (1990). *The Return of the Native: American Indian Political Resurgence*. New York: Oxford University Press.

Cornell, S., and Hartmann, D. (2007). *Ethnicity and Race: Making Identities in a Changing World* (2nd edn). Newbury Park, CA: Pine Forge Press.

Corntassel, J. (2007). Partnership in action? Indigenous political mobilization and co-optation during the first UN Indigenous Peoples Decade (1995–2004). *Human Rights Quarterly* 29, 1, 137–66.

Corson, D. (1995). Norway's 'Sámi Language Act': emancipatory implications for the world's indigenous peoples. *Language in Society* 24, 493–514.

Corson, D. (2000). *Language, Diversity and Education*. Mahwah, NJ: Lawrence Erlbaum.

Costa, J. (2003). Catalan linguistic policy: liberal or illiberal? *Nations and Nationalism* 9, 413–32.

Coulmas, F. (1992). *Language and Economy*. Oxford: Blackwell.

Coulmas, F. (1998). Language rights: interests of states, language groups and the individual. *Language Sciences* 20, 63–72.

Coulombe, P. (1995). *Language Rights in French Canada*. New York: Peter Lang.

Coulombe, P. (1999). Citizenship and official bilingualism in Canada. In W. Kymlicka and W. Norman (eds), *Citizenship in Diverse Societies* (pp. 273–93). Oxford: Oxford University Press.

Council of Europe (2008). *The European Charter for Regional or Minority Languages: Legal Challenges and Opportunities*. Strasbourg: Council of Europe Publishing.

Coupland, N., and Bishop, H. (2006). Ideologies of language and community in post-devolution Wales. In J. Wilson and K. Stapleton (eds), *Devolution and Identity* (pp. 33–50). Burlington, VT: Ashgate.

Cowan, M. (1963). *Humanist without Portfolio: An Anthology of the writings of Wilhelm von Humboldt*. Detroit, MI: Wayne State University Press.

Cox, R. (1996). A perspective on globalization. In J. M. Mittelman (ed.), *Globalization: Critical Reflections* (pp. 21–30). Boulder, CO: Lynne Rienner.

Coxon, E., Anae, M., Mara, D., Wendt-Samu, T., and Finau, C. (2002). *Literature Review on Pacific Education Issues: Final Report*. Wellington: Ministry of Education.

Crawford, J. (1989). *Bilingual Education: History, Politics, Theory and Practice*. Trenton, NJ: Crane Publishing Co.

Crawford, J. (1992a). *Hold your Tongue: Bilingualism and the Politics of 'English Only'*. Reading, MA: Addison-Wesley.

Crawford, J. (ed.) (1992b). *Language Loyalties: A Source Book on the Official English Controversy*. Chicago, IL: University of Chicago Press.

Crawford, J. (1992c). What's behind Official English? In J. Crawford (ed.), *Language Loyalties: A Source Book on the Official English Controversy* (pp. 171–7). Chicago, IL: University of Chicago Press.

Crawford, J. (1994). Endangered Native American languages: what is to be done and why? *Journal of Navajo Education* 11, 3, 3–11.

Crawford, J. (2000). *At War with Diversity: US Language Policy in an Age of Anxiety*. Clevedon, Avon: Multilingual Matters.

Crawford, J. (2007). Hard sell: why is bilingual education so unpopular with the American public? In O. García and C. Baker (eds), *Bilingual Education: An Introductory Reader* (pp. 145–61). Clevedon, Avon: Multilingual Matters.

Crawford, J. (2008). *Advocating for English Learners: Selected Essays*. Clevedon, Avon: Multilingual Matters.

Crick, B. (1989). An Englishman considers his passport. In N. Evans (ed.), *National Identity in the British Isles* (pp. 23–34). Harlech: Coleg Harlech.

Crick, B. (ed.) (1991). *National Identities and the Constitution*. Oxford: Blackwell.

Crick, B. (1995). The sense of identity of the indigenous British. *New Community* 21, 167–82.

Crosby, F. (2004). *Affirmative Action is Dead; Long Live Affirmative Action*. New Haven, CT: Yale University Press.

Crowley, T. (1996). *Language in History: Theories and Texts*. London: Routledge.

Crowley, T. (2007). Language endangerment, war and peace in Ireland and Northern Ireland. In A. Duchêne and M. Heller (eds), *Discourses of Endangerment: Ideology and Interest in the Defence of Languages* (pp. 149–68). London: Continuum.

Crozier, G. (1989). Multicultural education: some unintended consequences. In S. Walker and L. Barton (eds), *Politics and the Processes of Schooling* (pp. 59–81). Milton Keynes: Open University Press.

Crystal, D. (2000). *Language Death*. Cambridge: Cambridge University Press.

Crystal, D. (2003). *English as a Global Language* (2nd edn). Cambridge: Cambridge University Press.

Crystal, D. (2010). *The Cambridge Encyclopedia of Language* (3rd edn). Cambridge: Cambridge University Press.

Cummins, J. (1986). Empowering minority students: a framework for intervention. *Harvard Educational Review* 56, 18–36.

Cummins, J. (1995). The discourse of disinformation: the debate on bilingual education and language rights in the United States. In T. Skutnabb-Kangas and R. Phillipson (eds), *Linguistic Human Rights: Overcoming Linguistic Discrimination* (pp. 159–77). Berlin: Mouton de Gruyter.

Cummins, J. (2000). *Language, Power and Pedagogy: Bilingual Children in the Crossfire*. Clevedon, Avon: Multilingual Matters.

Dalacoura, K. (2002). A critique of communitarianism with reference to post-revolutionary Iran. *Review of International Studies* 28, 1, 75–92.

Dalby, A. (2003). *Language in Danger: The Loss of Linguistic Diversity and the Threat to our Future*. New York: Columbia University Press.

Dale, R., and Ozga, J. (1993). Two hemispheres – both New Right? 1980s education reform in New Zealand and England and Wales. In B. Lingard, J. Knight and P. Porter (eds), *Schooling Reform in Hard Times* (pp. 63–87). London: Falmer Press.

Daniels, H. (1990). The roots of language protectionism. In H. Daniels (ed.), *Not Only English: Affirming America's Multilingual Heritage* (pp. 3–12). Urbana, IL: National Council of Teachers.

Daniels, R. (1991). *Coming to America: A History of Immigration and Ethnicity in American Life*. New York: Harper Perennial.

Danoff, M., Coles, G., McLaughlin, D., and Reynolds, D. (1978). *Evaluation of the Impact of ESEA Title VII Spanish/English Bilingual Education Program*. Palo Alto, CA.: American Institutes for Research.

Darder, A., and Torres, R. (2002). Shattering the 'race' lens: towards a critical theory of racism. In A. Darder, R. Torres and M. Baltodano (eds), *The Critical Pedagogy Reader* (pp. 245–61). New York: RoutledgeFalmer.

Dasgupta, P. (1993). *The Otherness of English: India's Auntie Tongue Syndrome*. London: Sage.

Daswani, C. (ed.) (2001). *Language Education in Multilingual India*. New Delhi: UNESCO.

Davidson, K. (2010). Language and identity in Switzerland: a proposal for federal status for English as a Swiss language. *English Today* 26, 1, 15–17.

Davies, Charlotte. (1989). *Welsh Nationalism in the Twentieth Century: The Ethnic Option and the Modern State*. London: Praeger.

Davies, Christie. (1997). Minority language and social division: linguistic dead-ends, linguistic time bombs and the policies of subversion. In G. Frost (ed.), *Loyalty Misplaced: Misdirected Virtue and Social Disintegration* (pp. 39–47). London: Social Affairs Unit.

Davies, J. (2007). *A History of Wales* (rev. edn). London: Penguin.

Davies, L., and Nicholl, K. (1993). *Te Māori i roto i ngā Mahi Whakaakoranga. Māori Education: A Statistical Profile of the Position of Māori across the New Zealand Education System*. Wellington: Ministry of Education.

Davis, K., Bell, A., and Starks, D. (2001). Māori and Pasifika languages in Manukau: a preliminary study. *Many Voices* 15, 8–13.

Dawkins, J. (1992). *Australia's Language: The Australian Language and Literacy Policy*. Canberra: Australian Government Publishing Service.

Deacon, R., and Sandry, A. (2007). *Devolution in the United Kingdom*. Edinburgh: Edinburgh University Press.

De Bres, J. (2008). Planning for tolerability in New Zealand, Wales and Catalonia. *Current Issues in Language Planning* 9, 4, 464–82.

de Certeau, M., Julia, D., and Revel, J. (1975). *Une politique de la langue: La Révolution Française et les patois*. Paris: Editions Gallimard.

De Houwer, A., and Wilton, A. (eds) (2011). *English in Europe Today: Sociocultural and Educational Perspectives*. Amsterdam: John Benjamins.

Del Valle, S. (2003). *Language Rights and the Law in the United States: Finding our Voices*. Clevedon, Avon: Multilingual Matters.

Dench, G. (1986). *Minorities in the Open Society: Prisoners of Ambivalence*. London: Routledge & Kegan Paul.

Denison, N. (1977). Language death or language suicide? *International Journal of the Sociology of Language* 12, 13–22.

DES (Department of Education and Science). (1985). *Education for All: Report of the Committee of Inquiry into the Education of Children from Ethnic Minority Groups* (The Swann Report). London: HMSO.

de Saussure, F. (1974). *Course in General Linguistics*, tr. W. Baskin. London: Fontana.

De Schutter, H. (2007). Language policy and political philosophy: on the emerging linguistic justice debate. *Language Problems and Language Planning* 31, 1, 1–23.

de Swaan, A. (2001). *Words of the World: The Global Language System*. Cambridge: Polity Press.

Deutsch, K. (1966). *Nationalism and Social Communication: An Inquiry into the Foundations of Nationality*. Cambridge, MA: MIT Press.

Deutsch, K. (1975). The political significance of linguistic conflicts. In J.-G. Savard and R. Vigneault (eds), *Les états multilingues: Problèmes et solutions* (pp. 7–28). Laval, Québec: Les Presses de l'Université Laval.

de Varennes, F. (1996a). *Language, Minorities and Human Rights*. The Hague: Kluwer Law International.

de Varennes, F. (1996b). Minority aspirations and the revival of indigenous peoples. *International Review of Education* 42, 309–25.

Dicker, S. (2000). Official English and bilingual education: the controversy over language pluralism in U.S. society. In J. Kelly Hall and W. Eggington (eds), *The Sociopolitics of English Language Teaching* (pp. 45–66). Clevedon, Avon: Multilingual Matters.

Dicker, S. (2003). *Languages in America* (2nd edn). Clevedon, Avon: Multilingual Matters.

DiGiacomo, S. (1999). Language ideological debates in an Olympic city: Barcelona 1992–1996. In J. Blommaert (ed.), *Language Ideological Debates* (pp. 105–42). Berlin: Mouton de Gruyter.

Di Maggio, P. (1979). Review essay on Pierre Bourdieu. *American Journal of Sociology* 84, 1460–74.

Donahue, T. (1985). 'U.S. English': its life and works. *International Journal of the Sociology of Language* 56, 99–112.

Donahue, T. (1995). American language policy and compensatory opinion. In J. Tollefson (ed.), *Power and Inequality in Language Education* (pp. 112–41). Cambridge: Cambridge University Press.

Dorian, N. (1981). *Language Death*. Philadelphia, PA: University of Pennsylvania Press.

Dorian, N. (1982). Language loss and maintenance in language contact situations. In R. Lambert and B. Freed (eds), *The Loss of Language Skills* (pp. 44–59). Rowley, MA: Newbury House.

Dorian, N. (1998). Western language ideologies and small-language prospects. In L. Grenoble and L. Whaley (eds), *Endangered Languages: Language Loss and Community Response* (pp. 3–21). Cambridge: Cambridge University Press.

D'Souza, D. (1991). *Illiberal Education: The Politics of Race and Sex on Campus*. New York: Free Press.

D'Souza, D. (1995). *The End of Racism: Principles for a Multiracial Society*. New York: Free Press.

Dua, H. (1994). *Hegemony of English*. Mysore: Yashoda Publications.

Duchêne, A. (2008). *Ideologies across Nations: The Construction of Linguistic Minorities at the United Nations*. Berlin: Mouton de Gruyter.

Dumas, G. (2007). Quebec's language policies: perceptions and realities. In C. H. Williams (ed.), *Language and Governance* (pp. 250–62). Cardiff: University of Wales Press.

Dunbar, R. (2007). Diversity in addressing diversity: Canadian and British legislative approaches to linguistic minorities and their international context. In C. H. Williams (ed.), *Language and Governance* (pp. 104–58). Cardiff: University of Wales Press.

Durie, M. (1998). *Te Mana, Te Kāwanatanga: The Politics of Māori Self-Determination*. Auckland: Oxford University Press.

Durkheim, E. (1956). *Education and Sociology*. New York: Free Press.

Dworkin, R. (1978). Liberalism. In S. Hampshire (ed.), *Public and Private Morality* (pp. 113–43). Cambridge: Cambridge University Press.

Dworkin, R. (1983). In defence of equality. *Social Philosophy and Policy*, 1, 24–40.

Dwyer, T. (1980). *Eamon de Valera*. Dublin: Gill & Macmillan.

Dyer, R. (1997). *White*. London: Routledge.

Eagleton, T. (1990). *Nationalism, Colonialism and Literature*. Minneapolis, MN: University of Minnesota Press.

Eastman, C. (1984). Language, ethnic identity and change. In J. Edwards (ed.), *Linguistic Minorities, Policies and Pluralism* (pp. 259–76). London: Academic Press.

Eastman, C. (1991). The political and sociolinguistic status of language planning in Africa. In D. Marshall (ed.), *Language Planning: Focusschrift in honour of Joshua A. Fishman* (pp. 131–51). Amsterdam: John Benjamins.

Education Counts (2008). School leavers with little or no attainment. Retrieved Feb. 2009 from http://www.educationcounts.govt.nz/indicators/education_and_learning_outcomes/qualifications/753.

Edwards, C., and Read, P. (1992). *The Lost Children: Thirteen Australians taken from their Aboriginal Families Tell of the Struggle to Find their Natural Parents*. London: Doubleday.

Edwards, J. (1984). Language, diversity and identity. In J. Edwards (ed.), *Linguistic Minorities, Policies and Pluralism* (pp. 277–310). London: Academic Press.

Edwards, J. (1985). *Language, Society and Identity*. Oxford: Basil Blackwell.

Edwards, J. (1994). *Multilingualism*. London: Routledge.

Edwards, J. (2001). The ecology of language revival. *Current Issues in Language Planning* 2, 231–41.

Edwards, J. (2009). *Language and Identity: An Introduction*. Cambridge: Cambridge University Press.

Edwards, J. (2010). *Minority Languages and Group Identity: Cases and Categories*. Amsterdam: John Benjamins.

Edwards, V. (1991). The Welsh speech community. In S. Alladina and V. Edwards (eds), *Multilingualism in the British Isles* (vol. 1, pp. 107–25). London: Longman.

Edwards, V. (2004). *Multilingualism in the English-Speaking World*. Malden, MA: Blackwell.

Eller, J. and Coughlan, R. (1993). The poverty of primordialism: the demystification of ethnic attachments. *Ethnic and Racial Studies* 16, 183–201.

Ellison, N. (1997). Towards a new social politics: citizenship and reflexivity in late modernity. *Sociology* 31, 697–717.

Eriksen, T. (1998). *Common Denominators: Ethnicity, Nation-Building and Compromise in Mauritius*. Oxford: Berg.

Eriksen, T. (2010). *Ethnicity and Nationalism: Anthropological Perspectives* (3rd edn). London: Pluto Press.

Esteve, J. (1992). Multicultural education in Spain: the autonomous communities face the challenge of European unity. *Education Review* 44, 255–72.

Evans, E. (1978). Welsh (Cymraeg). In C. James (ed.), *The Older Mother Tongues of the United Kingdom* (pp. 5–35). London: Centre for Information on Language Teaching and Research.

Evans, S. (2000). Hong Kong's new English language policy in education. *World Englishes* 19, 185–204.

Featherstone, M. (1995). *Undoing Culture: Globalization, Postmodernism and Identity*. London: Sage.

Feldman, A. (2001). Transforming peoples and subverting states: developing a pedagogical approach to the study of indigenous peoples and ethnocultural movements. *Ethnicities* 1, 2, 147–78.

Fenton, S. (1999). *Ethnicity: Racism, Class and Culture*. London: Macmillan.

Fenton, S. (2003). *Ethnicity*. Cambridge: Polity Press.

Fenton, S., and May, S. (eds) (2002). *Ethnonational Identities*. Basingstoke: Palgrave Macmillan.

Fetui, V. and Malaki-Williams, M. (1996). *Introduction of a Samoan Language Program into the School System of New Zealand*. Suva: Pacific Languages in Education, Institute of Pacific Studies.

Fichte, J. (1968). *Addresses to the German Nation.* New York: Harper & Row (original, 1807).

Figueroa, P. (1991). *Education and the Social Construction of 'Race'.* London: Routledge.

Fishman, J. (1989a). Language and ethnicity. In J. Fishman, *Language and Ethnicity in Minority Sociolinguistic Perspective* (pp. 23–65). Clevedon, Avon: Multilingual Matters (original, 1977).

Fishman, J. (1989b). Language and nationalism: two integrative essays. Part 1. The nature of nationalism. In J. Fishman, *Language and Ethnicity in Minority Sociolinguistic Perspective* (pp. 97–175). Clevedon, Avon: Multilingual Matters (original, 1972).

Fishman, J. (1989c). Language and nationalism: two integrative essays. Part 2. The impact of nationalism on language planning. In J. Fishman, *Language and Ethnicity in Minority Sociolinguistic Perspective* (pp. 269–367). Clevedon, Avon: Multilingual Matters (original, 1972).

Fishman, J. (1989d). Whorfianism of the third kind: ethnolinguistic diversity as a worldwide societal asset. In J. Fishman, *Language and Ethnicity in Minority Sociolinguistic Perspective* (pp. 564–79). Clevedon, Avon: Multilingual Matters (original, 1982).

Fishman, J. (1989e). Language, ethnicity and racism. In J. Fishman, *Language and Ethnicity in Minority Sociolinguistic Perspective* (pp. 9–22). Clevedon, Avon: Multilingual Matters (original, 1977).

Fishman, J. (1991). *Reversing Language Shift: Theoretical and Empirical Foundations of Assistance to Threatened Languages.* Clevedon, Avon: Multilingual Matters.

Fishman, J. (1992). The displaced anxieties of Anglo-Americans. In J. Crawford (ed.), *Language Loyalties: A Source Book on the Official English Controversy* (pp. 165–70). Chicago, IL: University of Chicago Press.

Fishman, J. (1995a). Good conferences in a wicked world: on some worrisome problems in the study of language maintenance and language shift. In W. Fase, K. Jaspaert and S. Kroon (eds), *The State of Minority Languages: International Perspectives on Survival and Decline* (pp. 395–403). Lisse, Netherlands: Swets & Zeitlinger.

Fishman, J. (1995b). On the limits of ethnolinguistic democracy. In T. Skutnabb-Kangas and R. Phillipson (eds), *Linguistic Human Rights: Overcoming Linguistic Discrimination* (pp. 49–61). Berlin: Mouton de Gruyter.

Fishman, J. (1997). Language and ethnicity: the view from within. In F. Coulmas (ed.), *The Handbook of Sociolinguistics* (pp. 327–43). Oxford: Blackwell.

Fishman, J. (ed.) (2001). *Can Threatened Languages be Saved? Reversing Language Shift Revisited.* Clevedon, Avon: Multilingual Matters.

Fishman, J., and García, O. (eds) (2010). *Handbook of Language and Ethnic Identity: Disciplinary and Regional Perspectives* (vol. 1, 2nd edn). New York: Oxford University Press.

Fishman, J., and Solano, F. (1989). Cross polity perspective on the importance of linguistic heterogeneity as a 'contributing factor' in civil strife. In J. Fishman, *Language and Ethnicity in Minority Sociolinguistic Perspective* (pp. 605–26). Clevedon, Avon: Multilingual Matters.

Fitjar, R. (2010). *The Rise of Regionalism: Causes of Regional Mobilization in Western Europe.* New York: Routledge.

Flaitz, J. (1988). *The Ideology of English: French Perceptions of English as a World Language.* Berlin: Mouton de Gruyter.

Fleras, A., and Elliot, J. (1991). *Multiculturalism in Canada: The Challenge of Diversity.* Toronto: Nelson.

Fleras, A., and Spoonley, A. (1999). *Recalling Aotearoa: Indigenous Politics and Ethnic Relations in New Zealand*. Auckland: Oxford University Press.

Fletcher, D. (1998). Iris Marion Young: the politics of difference, justice and democracy. In A. Carter and G. Stokes (eds), *Liberal Democracy and its Critics* (pp. 196–215). Cambridge: Polity Press.

Fought, C. (2006). *Language and Ethnicity*. Cambridge: Cambridge University Press.

Franklin, M. (2003). I define my own identity: Pacific articulations of 'race' and 'culture' on the internet. *Ethnicities* 3, 4, 465–90.

Friedman, J. (1997). Global crises, the struggle for identity and intellectual porkbarrelling: cosmopolitans versus locals, ethnics and nationals in an era of de-hegemonisation. In P. Werbner, and T. Modood (eds), *Debating Cultural Hybridity: Multicultural Identities and the Politics of Antiracism* (pp. 70–89). London: Zed Books.

Fuchs, E., and Havighurst, R. (1972). *To Live on this Earth: American Indian Education*. Garden City, NJ: Anchor Books.

Furnivall, J. (1948). *Colonial Policy and Practice: A Comparative Study of Burma and Netherlands India*. Cambridge: Cambridge University Press.

Gagnon, A. (2000). Plaidoyer pour l'interculturalisme. *Possibles* 24, 4, 11–25.

Gans, H. (1979). Symbolic ethnicity: the future of ethnic groups and cultures in America. *Ethnic and Racial Studies* 2, 1–20.

García, O. (1995). Spanish language loss as a determinant of income among Latinos in the United States: implications for language policies in schools. In J. Tollefson (ed.), *Power and Inequality in Language Education* (pp. 142–60). Cambridge: Cambridge University Press.

García, O. (2009). *Bilingual Education in the 21st Century: A Global Perspective*. Malden, MA: Blackwell.

García, O., Skutnabb-Kangas, T., and Torres-Guzmán, M. (2006). *Imagining Multilingual Schools: Languages in Education and Glocalization*. Clevedon, Avon: Multilingual Matters.

Geertz, C. (1963). The integrative revolution: primordial sentiments and civil politics in new states. In C. Geertz (ed.), *Old Societies and New States: The Quest for Modernity in Asia and Africa* (pp. 105–57). New York: Free Press.

Geertz, C. (1973). *The Interpretation of Cultures*. New York: Basic Books.

Gellner, E. (1964). *Thought and Change*. London: Weidenfeld & Nicolson.

Gellner, E. (1983). *Nations and Nationalism: New Perspectives on the Past*. Oxford: Basil Blackwell.

Gellner, E. (1987). *Culture, Identity and Politics*. Cambridge: Cambridge University Press.

Gellner, E. (1993). Nationalism. In W. Outhwaite and T. Bottomore (eds), *Blackwell Dictionary of Twentieth-Century Social Thought* (pp. 409–11). Oxford: Basil Blackwell.

Gellner, E. (1994). *Conditions of Liberty: Civil Society and its Rivals*. London: Hamish Hamilton.

Gellner, E. (1996). Reply to my critics. In J. Hall and I. Jarvie (eds), *The Social Philosophy of Ernest Gellner* (pp. 625–87). Amsterdam: Rodopi.

Gellner, E. (1997). *Nationalism*. London: Weidenfeld & Nicolson.

Gibson, M., and Ogbu, J. (eds) (1991). *Minority Status and Schooling: A Comparative Study of Immigrant and Involuntary Minorities*. New York: Garland Publishing.

Giddens, A. (1984). *The Nation State and Violence*. Berkeley, CA: University of California Press.

Gilbert, G. (1996). The Council of Europe and minority rights. *Human Rights Quarterly* 18, 1, 160–89.

Gilbert, R. (1987). The concept of social practice and modes of ideology critique in schools. *Discourse* 7, 37–54.

Giles, H., Bourhis, R., and Taylor, D. (1977). Towards a theory of language in ethnic group relations. In H. Giles (ed.), *Language, Ethnicity and Intergroup Relations* (pp. 307–48). London: Academic Press.

Gilroy, P. (1987). *There Ain't No Black in the Union Jack*. London: Hutchinson.

Gilroy, P. (1990). One nation under a groove: the cultural politics of 'race' and racism in Britain. In D. Goldberg (ed.), *Anatomy of Racism* (pp. 263–82). Minneapolis, MN: University of Minnesota Press.

Gilroy, P. (1993a). *Small Acts: Thoughts on the Politics of Black Cultures*. London: Serpent's Tail.

Gilroy, P. (1993b). *The Black Atlantic: Modernity and Double Consciousness*. London: Verso.

Gilroy, P. (2000). *Between Camps: Nations, Cultures and the Allure of Race*. London: Allen Lane/Penguin Press.

Gil-White, F. (1999). How thick is blood? The plot thickens …: If ethnic actors are primordialists, what remains of the circumstantialist/primordialist controversy? *Ethnic and Racial Studies* 22, 5, 789–820.

Ginsburgh, V., and Weber, S. (2006). La dynamique des langues en Belgique. *Regards Economiques* 42 (June).

Giroux, H. (1992). *Border Crossings*. London: Routledge.

Giroux, H. (1997). *Pedagogy and the Politics of Hope: Theory, Culture and Schooling*. Boulder, CO: Westview Press.

Glaser, K. (2007). *Minority Languages and Cultural Diversity in Europe: Gaelic and Sorbian Perspectives*. Clevedon, Avon: Multilingual Matters.

Glazer, N. (1975). *Affirmative Discrimination: Ethnic Inequality and Public Policy*. New York: Basic Books.

Glazer, N. (1983). *Ethnic Dilemmas: 1964–1982*. Cambridge, MA: Harvard University Press.

Glazer, N. (1998). *We are All Multiculturalists Now*. Cambridge, MA: Harvard University Press.

Glazer, N., and Moynihan, D. (1975). *Ethnicity: Theory and Experience*. Cambridge, MA: Harvard University Press.

Glenny, M. (1996). *The Fall of Yugoslavia: The Third Balkan War* (3rd edn). London: Penguin.

Goldberg, D. (1993). *Racist Culture: Philosophy and the Politics of Meaning*. Cambridge, MA: Blackwell.

Goldberg, D. (1994). Introduction: multicultural conditions. In D. Goldberg (ed.), *Multiculturalism: A Critical Reader* (pp. 1–41). Cambridge, MA: Blackwell.

Gordon, M. (1978). *Human Nature, Class and Ethnicity*. New York: Oxford University Press.

Gordon, M. (1981). Models of pluralism: the new American dilemma. *Annals of the American Academy of Political and Social Science* 454, 178–88.

Gorlach, M. (1986). Comment. *International Journal of the Sociology of Language* 60, 97–103.

Goulbourne, H. (1991a). *Ethnicity and Nationalism in Post-Imperial Britain*. Cambridge: Cambridge University Press.

Goulbourne, H. (1991b). Varieties of pluralism: the notion of a post-imperial Britain. *New Community* 17, 211–27.

Gould, S. (1981). *The Mismeasure of Man*. London: Penguin.

Gracia, J. (2007). *Latinos in America: Philosophy and Social Identity*. Cambridge, MA: Blackwell.

Graddol, D. (1997). *The Future of English: A Guide to Forecasting the Popularity of the English Language in the 21st Century*. London: British Council.

Graddol, D. (2007). *English Next: Why Global English may Mean the End of 'English as a Foreign Language'*. London: British Council.

Graddol, D., Leith, D., Swann, J., Rhys, M., and Gillen, J. (eds) (2006). *Changing English*. London: Routledge.

Gramsci, A. (1971). *Selections from the Prison Notebooks*, ed. Q. Hoare and G. Nowell-Smith. London: Lawrence & Wishart.

Grant, N. (1997). Democracy and cultural pluralism: towards the 21st century. In R. Watts and J. Smolicz (eds), *Cultural Democracy and Ethnic Pluralism: Multicultural and Multilingual Policies in Education* (pp. 25–50). Frankfurt: Peter Lang.

Grau, R. (1992). Le statut juridique des droits linguistiques en France. In H. Giordan (ed.), *Les minorités en Europe* (pp. 93–112). Paris: Editions Kimé.

Greenfeld, L. (1992). *Nationalism: Five Roads to Modernity*. Cambridge, MA: Harvard University Press.

Greenland, H. (1991). Māori ethnicity as ideology. In P. Spoonley, D. Pearson and C. Macpherson (eds), *Nga Take: Ethnic Relations and Racism in Aotearoa/New Zealand* (pp. 90–107). Palmerston North, New Zealand: Dunmore Press.

Grenfell, M. (ed.) (2011). *Bourdieu, Language and Linguistics*. London: Continuum.

Grenoble, L., and Whaley, L. (1996). Endangered languages: current issues and future prospects. *International Journal of the Sociology of Language* 118, 209–23.

Grenoble, L., and Whaley, L. (eds) (1998). *Endangered Languages: Language Loss and Community Response*. Cambridge: Cambridge University Press.

Griffith, W. (1950). *The Welsh*. Harmondsworth: Penguin.

Grillo, R. (1989). *Dominant Languages: Language and Hierarchy in Britain and France*. Cambridge: Cambridge University Press.

Grillo, R. (1998). *Pluralism and the Politics of Difference: State, Culture, and Ethnicity in Comparative Perspective*. Oxford: Oxford University Press.

Grin, F. (1995). Combining immigrant and autochthonous language rights: a territorial approach to multilingualism. In T. Skutnabb-Kangas and R. Phillipson (eds), *Linguistic Human Rights: Overcoming Linguistic Discrimination* (pp. 31–48). Berlin: Mouton de Gruyter.

Grin, F. (1999). *Language Policy in Multilingual Switzerland: Overview and Recent Developments*. Flensburg, Germany: European Centre for Minority Issues.

Grin, F. (2003). *Language Policy Evaluation and the European Charter for Regional or Minority Languages*. Basingstoke: Palgrave Macmillan.

Grosby, S. (2005). *Nationalism: A Very Short Introduction*. New York: Oxford University Press.

Grosjean, F. (2010). *Bilingual: Life and Reality*. Cambridge, MA: Harvard University Press.

Grugel, J., and Rees, T. (1997). *Franco's Spain*. London: Arnold.

Guibernau, M. (1996). *Nationalisms: The Nation-State and Nationalism in the Twentieth Century*. Cambridge: Polity Press.

Guibernau, M. (1997). Images of Catalonia. *Nations and Nationalism* 3, 89–111.

Guibernau, M. (1999). *Nations without States*. Cambridge: Polity Press.

Guibernau, M. (2001). Globalization and the nation-state. In M. Guibernau and J. Hutchinson (eds), *Understanding Nationalism* (pp. 242–68). Cambridge: Polity Press.

Guibernau, M. (2004). *Catalan Nationalism: Francoism, Transition and Democracy*. London: Routledge.

Gumperz, J., and Cook-Gumperz, J. (2008). Studying language, culture, and society: sociolinguistics or linguistic anthropology? *Journal of Sociolinguistics* 12, 4, 532–45.

Gunaratnam, Y. (2003). *Researching 'Race' and Ethnicity: Methods, Knowledge and Power*. London: Sage.

Gurr, T. (1993). *Minorities at Risk: A Global View of Ethnopolitical Conflicts*. Washington, DC: United States Institute of Peace Press.

Gurr, T. (2000). *People versus States: Minorities at Risk in the New Century*. Washington, DC: United States Institute of Peace.

Gutmann, A. (2003). *Identity in Democracy*. Princeton, NJ: Princeton University Press.

Habermas, J. (1994). Struggles for recognition in the democratic constitutional state. In A. Gutmann (ed.), *Multiculturalism: Examining the Politics of Recognition* (pp. 107–48). Princeton, NJ: Princeton University Press.

Hage, G. (2000). *White Nation: Fantasies of White Supremacy in a Multicultural Society*. New York: Routledge.

Hage, G. (2003). *Against Paranoid Nationalism: Searching for Hope in a Shrinking Society*. Annandale, Australia: Pluto Press.

Hakuta, K., Butler, G., and Witt, D. (2000). *How Long Does it Take Learners to Attain English Proficiency?* Santa Barbara, CA: University of California Linguistic Minority Research Institute.

Hall, J. (1993). Nationalisms: classified and explained. *Daedalus* 122, 3, 1–28.

Hall, S. (1992a). The questions of cultural identity. In S. Hall, D. Held and T. McGrew (eds), *Modernity and its Futures* (pp. 274–325). Cambridge: Polity Press.

Hall, S. (1992b). New ethnicities. In J. Donald and A. Rattansi (eds), *'Race', Culture and Difference* (pp. 252–9). London: Sage.

Halle, L. (1962). *Men and Nations*. Princeton, NJ: Princeton University Press.

Hamel, R. (ed.) (1997). Special issue: linguistic human rights in a sociolinguistic perspective. *International Journal of the Sociology of Language* 127.

Handler, R. (1988). *Nationalism and the Politics of Culture in Québec*. Madison, WI: Wisconsin University Press.

Hannerz, U. (1992). *Cultural Complexity: Studies in the Organisation of Meaning*. New York: Columbia University Press.

Hanson, A. (1989). The making of Māori: culture invention and its logic. *American Anthropologist* 91, 890–902.

Harker, R. (1984). On reproduction, habitus and education. *British Journal of Sociology of Education* 5, 117–27.

Harker, R. (1990). Bourdieu: education and reproduction. In R. Harker, C. Mahar and C. Wilkes (eds), *An Introduction to the Work of Pierre Bourdieu: The Practice of Theory* (pp. 86–108). London: Macmillan.

Harker, R., and May, S. (1993). Code and habitus: comparing the accounts of Bernstein and Bourdieu. *British Journal of Sociology of Education* 14, 169–78.

Harker, R., and McConnochie, K. (1985). *Education as Cultural Artifact: Studies in Māori and Aboriginal Education*. Palmerston North, New Zealand: Dunmore Press.

Harker, R., Mahar, C., and Wilkes, C. (eds) (1990). *An Introduction to the Work of Pierre Bourdieu: The Practice of Theory*. London: Macmillan.

Harris, J., and Murtagh, L. (1999). *Teaching and Learning Irish in Primary Schools.* Dublin: Institiúid Teangeolaíochta Éireann.

Harris, R. (1981). *The Language Myth.* London: Duckworth.

Harrison, K. (2007). *When Languages Die: The Extinction of the World's Languages and the Erosion of Human Knowledge.* Oxford: Oxford University Press.

Hastings, W. (1988). *The Right to an Education in Māori: The Case from International Law.* Wellington: Victoria University Press.

Haugen, E. (1966). Dialect, language, nation. *American Anthropologist* 68, 922–35.

Heath, S. (1977). Language and politics in the United States. In M. Saville-Troike (ed.), *Linguistics and Anthropology: Georgetown University Round Table on Language and Linguistics* (pp. 267–96). Washington, DC: Georgetown University Press.

Heath, S. (1981). English in our language heritage. In C. Ferguson and S. Heath (eds), *Language in the U.S.A.* (pp. 6–20). Cambridge: Cambridge University Press.

Hechter, M. (1975). *Internal Colonialism: The Celtic Fringe in British National Development, 1536–1966.* London: Routledge & Kegan Paul.

Hechter, M. (1986). Rational choice theory and the study of race and ethnic relations. In J. Rex and D. Mason (eds), *Theories of Race and Race Relations* (pp. 264–79). Cambridge: Cambridge University Press.

Hechter, M. (1987). *Principles of Group Solidarity.* Berkeley, CA: University of California Press.

Hechter, M. (2000). *Containing Nationalism.* Oxford: Oxford University Press.

Held, D. (1995). *Democracy and the Global Order: From the Modern State to Cosmopolitan Governance.* Cambridge: Polity Press.

Held, D., McGrew, A., Goldblatt, D., and Perraton, J. (1999). *Global Transformations: Politics, Economics and Culture.* Cambridge: Polity Press.

Heller, M. (1987). The role of language in the formation of ethnic identity. In J. Phinney and M. Rotheram (eds), *Children's Ethnic Socialisation: Pluralism and Development* (pp. 180–200). Newbury Park, CA: Sage.

Heller, M. (1999). Heated language in a cold climate. In J. Blommaert (ed.), *Language Ideological Debates* (pp. 143–70). Berlin: Mouton de Gruyter.

Heller, M. (2003). Globalization, the new economy, and the commodification of language and identity. *Journal of Sociolinguistics* 7, 4, 473–92.

Heller, M. (2008). Language and the nation-state: challenges to sociolinguistic theory and practice. *Journal of Sociolinguistics* 12, 4, 504–24.

Heller, M. (2011). *Paths to Post-Nationalism: A Critical Ethnography of Language and Identity.* Oxford: Oxford University Press.

Henderson, J. (2009). *Indigenous Diplomacy and the Rights of Peoples: Achieving UN Recognition.* Saskatoon: Purich Publishing.

Henley, J. (1999). Chirac defends pure French tongue against regional Tower of Babel. *Observer* (27 June), 25.

Henrard, K. (2000). *Devising an Adequate System of Minority Protection.* The Hague: Kluwer Law.

Henze, R., and Davis, K. (1999). Special issue. Authenticity and identity: lessons from indigenous language education. *Anthropology and Education Quarterly* 30, 1.

Herder, J. (1969). *On Social and Political Culture,* ed. F. Barnard. Cambridge: Cambridge University Press.

Hernández-Chávez, E. (1995). Language policy in the United States: a history of cultural genocide. In T. Skutnabb-Kangas and R. Phillipson (eds), *Linguistic Human Rights: Overcoming Linguistic Discrimination* (pp. 141–58). Berlin: Mouton de Gruyter.

Herriman, M. (1996). Language policy in Australia. In M. Herriman and B. Burnaby (eds), *Language Policies in English-Dominant Countries* (pp. 35–61). Clevedon, Avon: Multilingual Matters.

Heugh, K. (1997). Disabling and enabling: implications of language policy in South Africa. In R. Watts and J. Smolicz (eds), *Cultural Democracy and Ethnic Pluralism: Multicultural and Multilingual Policies in Education* (pp. 243–70). Frankfurt: Peter Lang.

Heugh, K. (2000). Giving good weight to multilingualism in South Africa. In R. Phillipson (ed.), *Rights to Language: Equity, Power and Education* (pp. 234–8). Mahwah NJ: Lawrence Erlbaum.

Heugh, K. (2002). The case against bilingual and multicultural education in South Africa: laying bare the myths. *Perspectives in Education* 20, 1, 171–96.

Heugh, K. (2008). Language policy in Southern Africa. In S. May and N. Hornberger (eds), *Encyclopedia of Language and Education* (2nd edn), vol. 1, Language Policy and Political Issues in Education (pp. 355–67). New York: Springer.

Heugh, K., Siegrühn, A., and Plüddermann, P. (eds) (1995). *Multilingual Education for South Africa*. Johannesburg: Heinemann.

Higham, J. (1963). *Strangers in the Land: Patterns of American Nativism, 1860–1925*. New York: Atheneum.

Hill, B., and Allan, R. (2004). Multicultural education in Australia: historical development and current status. In J. Banks and C. Banks (eds.) (2004). *Handbook of Research on Multicultural Education* (2nd edn, pp.979–96). San Francisco, CA: Jossey Bass.

Hill, C. (2004). English demand Welsh-medium school places. *Wales Online*. Retrieved March 2011 from http://www.walesonline.co.uk/news/wales-news/content_objectid=14027289_method=full_siteid=50082_headline=-English-demand-Welsh-medium-school-places-name_page.html.

Hill, J. (1978). Language death, language contact, and language evolution. In W. McCormack and S. Wurm (eds), *Approaches to Language: Anthropological Issues* (pp. 45–78). The Hague: Mouton.

Hindley R. (1990). *The Death of the Irish Language: A Qualified Obituary*. London: Routledge.

Hinsley, F. (1986). *Sovereignty*. Cambridge: Cambridge University Press.

Hintjens, H. (2001). When identity becomes a knife: reflecting on the genocide in Rwanda. *Ethnicities* 1, 1, 25–55.

Hintjens, H. (2008). Post-genocide identity politics in Rwanda. *Ethnicities* 8, 1, 5–41.

Hinton, L., and Hale, K. (eds) (2001). *The Green Book of Language Revitalization in Practice*. San Diego, CA: Academic Press.

Hirsch, E. (1987). *Cultural Literacy: What Every American Needs to Know*. Boston, MA: Houghton Mifflin.

Hobhouse, L. (1928). *Social Evolution and Political Theory*. New York: Columbia University Press.

Hobsbawm, E. (1990). *Nations and Nationalism Since 1780*. Cambridge: Cambridge University Press.

Hobsbawm, E. (1992). Ethnicity and nationalism in Europe today. *Anthropology Today* 8, 3–8.

Hobsbawm, E. (1995). *Age of Extremes: The Short Twentieth Century, 1914–1991*. London: Abacus.

Hobsbawm, E. (2008). *Globalisation, Democracy and Terrorism*. London: Abacus.

Hobsbawm, E., and Ranger, T. (eds) (1983). *The Invention of Tradition*. Cambridge: Cambridge University Press.

Hoffman, E. (1989). *Lost in Translation: A Life in a New Language*. New York: E. P. Dutton.

Hoffmann, C. (1999). Language autonomy and national identity in Catalonia. In D. Smith and S. Wright (eds), *Whose Europe? The Turn Towards Democracy* (pp. 48–78). Oxford: Blackwell/Sociological Review.

Hoffmann, C. (2000). Balancing language planning and language rights: Catalonia's uneasy juggling act. *Journal of Multilingual and Multicultural Development* 21, 5: 425–41.

Hogan-Brun, G., Ozolins, U., Ramonien, M., and Rannut, M. (2007). Language politics and practices in the Baltic states. *Current Issues in Language Planning* 8, 4, 469–631.

Holborow, M. (1999). *The Politics of English: A Marxist View of Language*. London: Sage.

Honneth, A. (1995). *The Struggle for Recognition*. Cambridge: Polity Press.

Hornberger, N. (1997). Literacy, language maintenance, and linguistic human rights: three telling cases. *International Journal of the Sociology of Language* 127, 87–103.

Hornberger, N. (1998). Language policy, language education, language rights: indigenous, immigrant, and international perspectives. *Language in Society* 27, 439–58.

Hornberger, N. (2006). Frameworks and models in language policy and planning. In T. Ricento (ed.), *An Introduction to Language Policy* (pp. 24–41). New York: Blackwell.

Hornberger, N. (ed.) (2011). *Can Schools Save Indigenous Languages? Policy and Practice on Four Continents*. Basingstoke: Palgrave Macmillan.

Hornberger, N., and King, K. (1999). Authenticity and unification in Quechua language planning. In S. May (ed.), *Indigenous Community-Based Education* (pp. 160–80). Clevedon, Avon: Multilingual Matters.

Horowitz, D. (2000). *Ethnic Groups in Conflict* (2nd edn). Berkeley, CA: University of California Press.

Horowitz, D. (2002). The primordialists. In D. Conversi (ed.), *Ethnonationalism in the Contemporary World: Walker Connor and the Study of Nationalism* (pp. 72–82). New York: Routledge.

Howe, K. (1992). Liberal democracy, equal opportunity, and the challenge of multiculturalism. *American Educational Research Journal* 29, 455–70.

Howe, S. (1998). *Afrocentrism: Mythical Pasts and Imagined Homes*. London: Verso.

Hroch, M. (1985). *Social Preconditions of National Revival in Europe*. Cambridge: Cambridge University Press.

Hroch, M. (1993). From national movement to the fully-formed nation: the nation-building process in Europe. *New Left Review* 198, 3–20.

Hroch, M. (1998). Real and constructed: the nature of the nation. In J. Hall (ed.), *The State of the Nation: Ernest Gellner and the Theory of Nationalism* (pp. 91–106). Cambridge: Cambridge University Press.

Huddy, L., and Sears, J. (1990). Qualified public support for bilingual education: some policy implications. *Annals of the American Academy of Political and Social Science* 505 (March), 119–34.

Hughes, R. (1993). *Culture of Complaint: The Fraying of America*. New York: Oxford University Press.

Humboldt, W. von (1988). *On Language: The Diversity of Human Language Structure and its Influence on the Mental Development of Mankind*, tr. P. Heath. Cambridge: Cambridge University Press (original, 1836).

Hunkin-Tuiletufuga, G. (2001). Pasefika languages and Pasefika identities: contemporary and future challenges. In C. Macpherson, P. Spoonley and M. Anae (eds), *Tangata O Te Moana Nui: The Evolving Identities of Pacific Peoples in Aotearoa/New Zealand* (pp. 196–211). Palmerston North, New Zealand: Dunmore Press.

Hunn, J. (1961). *Report on the Department of Māori Affairs.* Wellington: Government Printer.

Hunt, G., Maloney, M., and Evans, K. (2010). 'How Asian am I'? Asian American youth cultures, drug use, and ethnic identity construction. *Youth and Society.* Published 17 March at: http://yas.sagepub.com/content/early/2010/03/17/0044118X10364044.

Huntingdon, S. (2005). *Who Are We? America's Great Debate.* New York: Free Press.

Huss, L. (1999). *Reversing Language Shift in the Far North: Linguistic Revitalization in Northern Scandinavia and Finland.* Uppsala: Acta Universitatis Upsaliensis.

Hutchinson, J. (1987). *The Dynamics of Cultural Nationalism: The Gaelic Revival and the Creation of the Irish Nation State.* London: Allen & Unwin.

Hutchinson, J. (1994). *Modern Nationalism.* London: Fontana.

Hutchinson, J. (2000). Ethnicity and modern nations. *Ethnic and Racial Studies* 23, 4, 651–69.

Hutchinson, J. (2005). *Nations as Zones of Conflict.* London: Sage.

Hutchinson, J. (2008). In defence of transhistorical ethno-symbolism: a reply to my critics. *Nations and Nationalism* 14, 1, 18–28.

Hutnyk, J. (2005). Hybridity. *Ethnic and Racial Studies* 28, 1, 79–102.

Ignace, M., and Ignace, R. (1998). 'The old wolf in sheep's clothing': Canadian Aboriginal peoples and multiculturalism. In D. Haselbach (ed.), *Multiculturalism in a World of Leaking Boundaries* (pp. 101–32). New Brunswick, NJ: Transaction Publishers.

Imhoff, G. (1990). The position of U.S. English on bilingual education. *Annals of the American Academy of Political and Social Science* 505 (March), 48–61.

Irwin, K. (1989). Multicultural education: the New Zealand response. *New Zealand Journal of Educational Studies* 24, 3–18.

Irwin, K. (1990). The politics of Kōhanga Reo. In S. Middleton, J. Codd and A. Jones (eds), *New Zealand Education Policy Today: Critical Perspectives* (pp. 110–20). Wellington: Allen & Unwin.

Isaacs, H. (1975). *Idols of the Tribe: Group Identity and Political Change.* New York: Harper & Row.

Isajiw, W. (1980). Definitions of ethnicity. In J. Goldstein and R. Bienvenue (eds), *Ethnicity and Ethnic Relations in Canada* (pp. 5–17). Toronto: Butterworth.

Ives, P. (2010). Cosmopolitanism and global English: language politics in globalisation debates. *Political Studies* 58, 3, 516–35.

Ivison, D., Patton, D., and Sanders, W. (eds) (2000). *Political Theory and the Rights of Indigenous Peoples.* Cambridge: Cambridge University Press.

Jakšić, B. (ed.) (1995). *Interkulturalnost/Interculturality.* Beograd: Savo Bjelajac.

James, P. (2006). *Globalism, Nationalism, Tribalism: Bringing Theory Back In.* London: Sage.

Janulf, P. (1998). *Kommer finskan i Sverige att fortleva?* Stockholm, Sweden: Almqvist & Wiksell.

Jenkins, J. (2006). Points of view and blind spots: ELF and SLA. *International Journal of Applied Linguistics* 16, 2, 137–62.

Jenkins, J. (2007). *English as a Lingua Franca: Attitude and Identity.* Oxford: Oxford University Press.

Jenkins, P. (1992). *A History of Modern Wales, 1536–1990.* London: Longman.

Jenkins, R. (1986). Social anthropological models of inter-ethnic relations. In J. Rex and D. Mason (eds), *Theories of Race and Race Relations* (pp. 170–86). Cambridge: Cambridge University Press.

Jenkins, R. (1991). Violence, language and politics: nationalism in Northern Ireland and Wales. *North Atlantic Studies* 3, 31–40.

Jenkins, R. (1994). Rethinking ethnicity: identity, categorization and power. *Ethnic and Racial Studies* 17, 197–223.

Jenkins, R. (1995). Nations and nationalisms: towards more open models. *Nations and Nationalism* 1, 369–90.

Jenkins, R. (1996). 'Us' and 'them': ethnicity, racism and ideology. In R. Barot (ed.), *The Racism Problematic: Contemporary Sociological Debates on Race and Ethnicity* (pp. 69–88). Lampeter, Wales: Edward Mellen Press.

Jenkins, R. (2003). *Pierre Bourdieu* (rev. edn). London: Routledge.

Jenkins, R. (2007). *Rethinking Ethnicity: Arguments and Explorations* (2nd edn). London: Sage.

Jespersen, O. (1968). *Growth and Structure of the English Language.* Toronto: Collier-Macmillan (original, 1938).

Jiménez, T. (2004). Negotiating ethnic boundaries: multiethnic Mexican Americans and ethnic identity in the United States. *Ethnicities* 4, 1, 75–97.

Johnson, D. (1993). The making of the French nation. In M. Teich and R. Porter (eds), *The National Question in Europe in Historical Context* (pp. 35–62). Cambridge: Cambridge University Press.

Jones, B., and Keating, M. (eds) (1995). *The European Union and the Regions.* Oxford: Clarendon Press.

Jones, G. (1997). *The Education of a Nation.* Cardiff: University of Wales Press.

Joppke, C. (2004). The retreat of multiculturalism in the liberal state: theory and policy. *British Journal of Sociology* 55, 2, 237–57.

Joppke, C. (2010). *Citizenship and Immigration.* Cambridge: Polity Press.

Joppke, C., and Lukes, S. (eds) (1999). *Multicultural Questions.* Oxford: Oxford University Press

Joseph, J. (1996). English in Hong Kong: emergence and decline. *Current Issues in Language and Society* 3, 166–79.

Joseph, J. (2002). *From Whitney to Chomsky: Essays in the History of American Linguistics.* Amsterdam: John Benjamins.

Joseph, J. (2004). *Language and Identity: National, Ethnic, Religious.* Basingstoke: Palgrave Macmillan.

Joshee, R., and Johnson, L. (eds) (2007). *Multicultural Education Policies in Canada and the United States.* Vancouver: University of British Columbia Press.

Joy, R. (1992). *Canada's Official Languages: The Progress of Bilingualism.* Toronto: University of Toronto Press.

Judge, A. (2007). *Linguistic Policies and the Survival of Regional Languages in France and Britain.* Basingstoke: Palgrave Macmillan.

Juteau, D. (1996). Theorising ethnicity and ethnic communalisms at the margins: from Québec to the world system. *Nations and Nationalism* 2, 45–66.

Kaa, J. (2010). In the ring with Māori television. *Indigenous Business Magazine*, Koha. Retrieved March 2011 from http://www.koha.biz/2010/06/in-the-ring-with-maori-television.

Kā'ai, T. (1990). Te hiringa taketake: mai i te Kōhanga Reo ki te kura. Māori pedagogy: te Kōhanga Reo and the transition to school. Unpublished MPhil thesis, University of Auckland.

Kachru, B. (ed.) (1982). *The Other Tongue: English Across Cultures*. Urbana, IL: University of Illinois Press.

Kachru, B. (1986). *The Alchemy of English: The Spread, Functions and Models of Non-Native Englishes*. Oxford: Pergamon Press.

Kachru, B. (1990). World Englishes and applied linguistics. *World Englishes* 9, 3–20.

Kachru, B. (2004). *Asian Englishes: Beyond the Canon*. Hong Kong: Hong Kong University Press.

Kachru, B., and Nelson, C. (1996). World Englishes. In S. McKay and N. Hornberger (eds), *Sociolinguistics and Language Teaching* (pp. 71–102). Cambridge: Cambridge University Press.

Kalantzis, M., and Cope, B. (1999). Multicultural education: transforming the mainstream. In S. May (ed.), *Critical Multiculturalism: Rethinking Multicultural and Antiracist Education* (pp. 245–76). London: RoutledgeFalmer.

Kamboureli, S. (1998). The technology of ethnicity: Canadian multiculturalism and the language of the law. In D. Bennett (ed.), *Multicultural States: Rethinking Difference and Identity* (pp. 208–22). London: Routledge.

Kane, J. (1997). From ethnic exclusion to ethnic diversity: the Australian path to multiculturalism. In I. Shapiro and W. Kymlicka (eds), *Ethnicity and Group Rights* (pp. 540–71). New York: New York University Press.

Kaufmann, E. (ed.) (2004). *Rethinking Ethnicity: Majority Groups and Dominant Minorities*. London: Routledge.

Kaufmann, E., and Haklai, O. (2008). Dominant ethnicity: from minority to majority. *Nations and Nationalism* 14, 4, 743–67.

Kawharu, I. (ed.) (1989). *Waitangi: Māori and Pākehā Perspectives of the Treaty of Waitangi*. Auckland: Oxford University Press.

Kay, G. (1993). Ethnicity, the cosmos and economic development, with special reference to Central Africa. Mimeo.

Kearney, H. (2006). *The British Isles: A History of Four Nations* (2nd edn). Cambridge: Cambridge University Press.

Keating, M. (1996). *Nations Against the State: The New Politics of Nationalism in Québec, Catalonia and Scotland*. London: Macmillan Press.

Keating, M. (1997). Stateless nation-building: Québec, Catalonia and Scotland in the changing state system. *Nations and Nationalism* 3, 689–717.

Keating, M. (2009). Social citizenship, solidarity and welfare in regionalized and plurinational states. *Citizenship Studies* 13, 501–13.

Kedourie, E. (1960). *Nationalism*. London: Hutchinson.

Kellas, J. (1998). *The Politics of Nationalism and Identity* (2nd edn). London: Macmillan.

Kellough, J. (2006). *Understanding Affirmative Action: Politics, Discrimination, and the Search for Justice*. Washington, DC: Georgetown University Press.

Khleif, B. (1979). Insiders, outsiders and renegades: towards a classification of ethnolinguistic labels. In H. Giles and B. Saint-Jacques (eds), *Language and Ethnic Relations* (pp. 159–72). Oxford: Pergamon Press.

Khubchandani, L. (2008). Language policy and education in the Indian subcontinent. In S. May and N. Hornberger (eds), *Encyclopedia of Language and Education* (2nd edn), vol. 1, *Language Policy and Political Issues in Education* (pp. 369–81). New York: Springer.

Kincheloe, J., and Steinberg, S. (1997). *Changing Multiculturalism*. Buckingham: Open University Press.

King, M. (2003). *The Penguin History of New Zealand*. Auckland: Penguin.

Kingsbury, B. (1989). The Treaty of Waitangi: some international law aspects. In I. Kawharu (ed.), *Waitangi: Māori and Pākehā Perspectives of the Treaty of Waitangi* (pp. 121–57). Auckland: Oxford University Press.

Kirisci, K., and Winrow, G. (1997). *The Kurdish Question and Turkey: An Example of a Trans-State Ethnic Conflict*. London: Frank Cass.

Kivisto, P. (2002). *Multiculturalism in a Global Society*. Cambridge, MA: Blackwell.

Kloss, H. (1971). The language rights of immigrant groups. *International Migration Review* 5, 250–68.

Kloss, H. (1977). *The American Bilingual Tradition*. Rowley, MA: Newbury House.

Kohn, H. (1961). *The Idea of Nationalism: A Study in its Origins and Background*. New York: Macmillan.

Kohn, M. (1995). *The Race Gallery: The Return of Racial Science*. London: Jonathan Cape.

Kraidy, M. (2002). Hybridity in cultural globalization. *Communication Theory*, 12, 3, 316–39.

Kraidy, M. (2005). *Hybridity, or the Cultural Logic of Globalization*. Philadelphia, PA: Temple University Press.

Krashen, S. (1996). *Under Attack: The Case Against Bilingual Education*. Culver City, CA: Language Education Associates.

Krashen, S. (1999). *Condemned without Trial: Bogus Arguments Against Bilingual Education*. Portsmouth, NH: Heinemann.

Kraus, P. (2008). *A Union of Diversity: Language, Identity and Polity-Building in Europe*. Cambridge: Cambridge University Press.

Krauss, M. (1992). The world's languages in crisis. *Language* 68, 4–10.

Krumova, K. (2010). Catalonia protests 'one nation' in Spain. *The Epoch Times* (11 July). Retrieved July 2010 from http://www.theepochtimes.com/n2/content/view/38989.

Kumar, K. (2003). *The Making of English National Identity*. Cambridge: Cambridge University Press.

Kuppe, R. (2009). The three dimensions of the rights of indigenous peoples. *International Community Law Review* 11, 1, 103–118.

Kymlicka, W. (1989). *Liberalism, Community and Culture*. Oxford: Clarendon Press.

Kymlicka, W. (1995a). *Multicultural Citizenship: A Liberal Theory of Minority Rights*. Oxford: Clarendon Press.

Kymlicka, W. (1995b). Introduction. In W. Kymlicka (ed.), *The Rights of Minority Cultures* (pp. 1–27). Oxford: Oxford University Press.

Kymlicka, W. (1998). *Finding our Way: Rethinking Ethnocultural Relations in Canada*. Toronto: Oxford University Press.

Kymlicka, W. (1999a). Response to Okin. In J. Cohen, M. Howard and M. Nussbaum (eds), *Is Multiculturalism Bad for Women?* (pp. 31–4). Princeton, NJ: Princeton University Press.

Kymlicka, W. (1999b). Comments on Shachar and Spinner-Halev: an update from the multiculturalism wars. In C. Joppke and S. Lukes (eds), *Multicultural Questions* (pp. 112–29). Oxford: Oxford University Press.

Kymlicka, W. (1999c). Theorizing indigenous rights. *University of Toronto Law Journal* 49, 281–93.

Kymlicka, W. (2001). *Politics in the Vernacular: Nationalism, Multiculturalism, Citizenship.* Oxford: Oxford University Press.

Kymlicka, W. (2007). *Multicultural Odysseys: Navigating the New International Politics of Diversity.* Oxford: Oxford University Press.

Kymlicka, W., and Opalski, M. (eds) (2001). *Can Liberalism be Exported? Western Political Theory and Ethnic Relations in Eastern Europe.* Oxford: Oxford University Press.

Kymlicka, W., and Patten, A. (eds) (2003). *Language Rights and Political Theory.* Oxford: Oxford University Press.

Ladefoged, P. (1992). Another view of endangered languages. *Language* 68, 809–811.

Laitin, D. (1998). Nationalism and language: a post-Soviet perspective. In J. Hall (ed.), *The State of the Nation: Ernest Gellner and the Theory of Nationalism* (pp. 135–57). Cambridge: Cambridge University Press.

Laitin, D., and Reich, R. (2003). A liberal democratic approach to language justice. In W. Kymlicka and A. Patten (eds) *Language Rights and Political Theory* (pp. 80–104). Oxford: Oxford University Press.

Lamy, M-N. (1996). Franglais. In D. Graddol, D. Leith and J. Swann (eds), *English History, Diversity and Change* (pp. 32–6). London: Routledge.

Language Plan Task Group (LANGTAG) (1996). *Towards a Language Plan for South Africa.* Pretoria: Ministry of Arts, Culture, Science and Technology.

Larner, W., and Spoonley, P. (1995). Post-colonial politics in Aotearoa/New Zealand. In D. Stasiulus and N. Yuval-Davis (eds), *Unsettling Settler Societies* (pp. 39–64). London: Sage.

Larrivée, P. (ed.) (2003). *Linguistic Conflict and Language Laws: Understanding the Québec Question.* Basingstoke: Palgrave Macmillan.

Leap, W. (1981). American Indian languages. In C. Ferguson and S. Heath (eds), *Language in the U.S.A.* (pp. 116–44). Cambridge: Cambridge University Press.

Lee, P. (1996). *The Whorf Theory Complex: A Critical Reconstruction.* Amsterdam: John Benjamins.

Légaré, A. (2002). Nunavut: the construction of a regional collective identity in the Canadian Arctic. *Wicazo Sa Review* 17, 2, 65–89.

Légaré, A. (2008). Canada's experiment with Aboriginal self-determination in Nunavut: from vision to illusion. *International Journal on Minority and Group Rights* 15, 2–3, 335–67.

Leibowitz, A. (1969). English literacy: legal sanction and discrimination. *Notre Dame Lawyer* 45, 7–66.

Leith, D., and Graddol, D. (1996). Modernity and English as a national language. In D. Graddol, D. Leith and J. Swann (eds), *English History, Diversity and Change* (pp. 136–79). London: Routledge.

Levine, H. (1999). Reconstructing ethnicity. *Journal of the Royal Anthropological Institute* 5, 165–80.

Lévi Strauss, C. (1994). Anthropology, race, and politics: a conversation with Didier Eribon. In R. Borofsky (ed.), *Assessing Cultural Anthropology* (pp. 420–9). New York: McGraw Hill.

Levy, J. (2001). *The Multiculturalism of Fear*. New York: Oxford University Press.

Levy, J. (2007). Contextualism, constitutionalism, and *modus vivendi* approaches. In A. Laden and D. Owen (eds), *Multiculturalism and Political Theory* (pp. 173–97). Cambridge: Cambridge University Press.

Lewis, M. (ed.) (2009). *Ethnologue: Languages of the World* (16th edn). Dallas, TX: SIL International.

Likhachev, V. (2009). Parliamentary diplomacy. *International Affairs* 3, 153–65.

Lind, M. (1995). *The Next American Nation*. New York: Free Press.

Little, D. (1994). *Sri Lanka: The Invention of Enmity*. Washington, DC: United States Institute of Peace Press.

Lisée, J-F. (2007). How Quebec became a North American region state. In C. H. Williams (ed.), *Language and Governance* (pp. 460–502). Cardiff: University of Wales Press.

Lo Bianco, J. (1987). *National Policy on Languages*. Canberra: Australian Government Publishing Service.

Lo Bianco, J. (2004). *A Site for Debate, Negotiation and Contest of National Identity: Language Policy in Australia*. Strasbourg: Council of Europe.

Lo Bianco, J. (2008). Language policy and education in Australia. In S. May and N. Hornberger (eds), *Encyclopedia of Language and Education* (2nd edn), vol. 1, *Language Policy and Political Issues in Education* (pp. 343–53). New York: Springer.

Lo Bianco, J., and Rhydwen, M. (2001). Is the extinction of Australia's indigenous languages inevitable? In J. Fishman (ed.), *Can Threatened Languages be Saved? Reversing Language Shift Revisited* (pp. 391–423). Clevedon, Avon: Multilingual Matters.

Lodge, R. (1993). *French: From Dialect to Standard*. London: Routledge.

Loobuyck, P. (2005). Liberal multiculturalism: A defence of liberal multicultural measures without minority rights. *Ethnicities* 5, 1, 108–23.

Louarn, T. (1998). Poignant Report on the regional languages and culture of France delivered to Jospin. *Contact Bulletin* 15, 1, 4–5 (Nov.).

Lukes, S. (1996). Humiliation and the politics of identity. *Social Research* 64, 36–51.

Lyotard, J. (1984). *The Postmodern Condition: A Report on Knowledge,* tr. G. Bennington and B. Massumi. Manchester: Manchester University Press.

McCarty, T. (2002). *A Place to be Navajo: Rough Rock and the Struggle for Self-Determination in Indigenous Schooling*. Mahwah, NJ: Lawrence Erlbaum.

McCarty, T. (ed.) (2011). *Ethnography and Language Policy*. New York: Routledge.

McCarty, T., and Watahomigie, L. (1999). Indigenous community-based education in the USA. In S. May (ed.), *Indigenous Community-Based Education* (pp. 79–94). Clevedon, Avon: Multilingual Matters.

McCarty, T., and Zepeda, O. (eds) (1995). Special Issue. Indigenous language education and literacy. *Bilingual Research Journal* 19, 1.

McCrone, D. (1992). *Understanding Scotland: The Sociology of a Stateless Nation*. London: Routledge.

McCrone, D. (1998). *The Sociology of Nationalism: Tomorrow's Ancestors*. London: Routledge.

McCrum, R. (2011). *Globish: How the English Language Became the World's Language*. London: Penguin.

McCrum, R., MacNeil, R., and Cran, W. (2011). *The Story of English*. London: Faber & Faber.

Mac Donnacha, S., Chualáin, F., Shéaghdha, A., and Mhainín, T. (2005). *Staid Reatha na Scoileanna Gaeltachta/A Study of Gaeltacht Schools*. Dublin: An Chomhairle um Oideachas Gaeltachta & Gaelscolaíochta.

Macedo, D. (1994). *Literacies of Power: What Americans are Not Allowed to Know*. Boulder, CO: Westview Press.

Macedo, D., Dendrinos, B., and Gounari, P. (2003). *The Hegemony of English*. Boulder, CO: Paradigm Publishers.

McGoldrick, D. (2005). Multiculturalism and its discontents. *Human Rights Law Review* 5, 1, 27–56.

Macías, R. (1979). Language choice and human rights in the United States. In J. Alatis and G. Tucker (eds), *Language in Public Life: Georgetown University Round Table on Language and Linguistics* (pp. 86–101). Washington, DC: Georgetown University Press.

McKay, S., and Wong, S. (1988). *Language Diversity: Problem or Resource?* Boston, MA: Heinle & Heinle.

MacKaye, S. (1990). California Proposition 63: language attitudes reflected in the public debate. *Annals of the American Academy of Political and Social Science* 505 (March), 135–46.

MacLachlan, C. (1988). *Spain's Empire in the New World: The Role of Ideas in Institutional and Social Change*. Berkeley, CA: University of California Press.

McLaren, P. (1995). *Critical Pedagogy and Predatory Culture*. New York: Routledge.

McLaren, P. (1997). *Revolutionary Multiculturalism: Pedagogies of Dissent for the New Millennium*. Boulder, CO: Westview Press.

McLaren, P., and Torres, R. (1999). Racism and multicultural education: rethinking 'race' and 'whiteness' in late capitalism. In S. May (ed.), *Critical Multiculturalism: Rethinking Multicultural and Antiracist Education* (pp. 42–76). London and New York: RoutledgeFalmer.

McLoughlin, D. (1993). The Māori Burden. *North and South* (Nov.), 60–71.

MacMillan, C. M. (2003). Federal language policy in Canada and the Quebec challenge. In P. Larrivée (ed.), *Linguistic Conflict and Language Laws: Understanding the Québec Question* (pp. 87–117). Basingstoke: Palgrave Macmillan.

Macpherson, C. (1996). Pacific Islands identity and community. In. P. Spoonley, C. Macpherson, and D. Pearson (eds), *Nga Patai: Racism and Ethnic Relations in Aotearoa/New Zealand* (pp. 124–43). Palmerston North, New Zealand: Dunmore Press.

Macpherson, C. (2004). From Pacific Islanders to Pacific people and beyond. In P. Spoonley, C. Macpherson and D. Pearson (eds), *Tangata Tangata: The Changing Contours of New Zealand* (pp. 135–56). Southbank, Australia: Thompson.

Macpherson, C., Spoonley, P., and Anae, M. (2001). *Tangata o te Moana Nui: The Evolving Identities of Pacific Peoples in Aotearoa/New Zealand*. Palmerston North, New Zealand: Dunmore Press.

McQuillan, J., and Tse, L. (1996). Does research matter? An analysis of media opinion on bilingual education 1984–1994. *Bilingual Research Journal* 20, 1–27.

McRoberts, K. (1999). *Québec: Social Change and Political Crisis* (3rd edn.). Toronto: Oxford University Press.

Maffi, L. (ed.) (2000). *Language, Knowledge and the Environment: The Interdependence of Biological and Cultural Diversity*. Washington, DC: Smithsonian Institute Press.

Maffi, L. (2001). *On Biocultural Diversity: Linking Language, Knowledge, and the Environment.* Washington, DC: Smithsonian Institution Press.

Magga, O. (1996). Sámi past and present and the Sámi picture of the world. In E. Helander (ed.), *Awakened Voice: The Return of Sámi Knowledge* (pp. 74–80). Kautokeino, Norway: Nordic Sámi Institute.

Magnet, J. (1995). *Official Language of Canada: Perspectives from Law, Policy and the Future.* Cowansville, Québec: Editions Yvon Blais.

Makoni, S., and Pennycook, A. (2007). Disinventing and reconstituting languages. In S. Makoni and A. Pennycook (eds), *Disinventing and Reconstituting Languages* (pp. 1–41). Clevedon, Avon: Multilingual Matters.

Mallea, J. (1989). *Schooling in Plural Canada.* Clevedon, Avon: Multilingual Matters.

Mann, R. (2007). Negotiating the politics of language: language learning and civic identity in Wales. *Ethnicities* 7, 2, 208–24.

Margalit, A., and Raz, J. (1995). National self-determination. In W. Kymlicka (ed.), *The Rights of Minority Cultures* (pp. 79–92). Oxford: Oxford University Press.

Mar-Molinero, C. (2000). *The Politics of Language in the Spanish-Speaking World.* London: Routledge.

Marshall, D. (1986). The question of an official language: language rights and the English Language Amendment. *International Journal of the Sociology of Language* 60, 7–75.

Marshall, D., and Gonzalez, R. (1990). Una lingua, una patria? Is monolingualism beneficial or harmful to a nation's unity? In K. Adams and D. Brink (eds), *Perspectives on Official English: The Campaign for English as the Official Language of the USA* (pp. 29–51). Berlin: Mouton de Gruyter.

Marshall, N., Caygill, R., and May, S. (2008). *PISA 2006 Reading Literacy.* Wellington: Ministry of Education.

Marx, K., and Engels, F. (1976a). *Marx and Engels Collected Works.* London: Lawrence & Wishart.

Marx, K., and Engels, F. (1976b). *Basic Writings on Politics and Philosophy,* ed. L. Feuer. Glasgow: Collins.

Mason, A. (2007). Multiculturalism and the critique of essentialism. In A. Laden and D. Owen (eds), *Multiculturalism and Political Theory* (pp. 221–43). Cambridge: Cambridge University Press.

Maurais, J. (ed.) (1996). *Québec's Aboriginal Languages: History, Planning, Development.* Clevedon, Avon: Multilingual Matters.

Maurais, J. (1997). Regional majority languages, language planning, and linguistic rights. *International Journal of the Sociology of Language* 127, 135–60.

Maurais, J. (2003). Towards a new global linguistic order? In J. Maurais and M. Morris (eds), *Languages in a Globalising World* (pp. 13–36). Cambridge: Cambridge University Press.

Maxwell, A. (1998). Ethnicity and education: biculturalism in New Zealand. In D. Bennett (ed.), *Multicultural States: Rethinking Difference and Identity* (pp. 195–207). London: Routledge.

May, S. (1994). *Making Multicultural Education Work.* Clevedon, Avon: Multilingual Matters.

May, S. (1995). Deconstructing traditional discourses of schooling: an example of school reform. *Language and Education* 9, 1–29.

May, S. (1997a). Critical ethnography. In N. Hornberger and D. Corson (eds), *Research Methods and Education: The Encyclopedia of Language and Education* (vol. 8, pp. 197–206). Dordrecht: Kluwer.

May, S. (1997b). Indigenous language rights and education. In J. Lynch, C. Modgil and S. Modgil (eds) *Education and Development: Tradition and Innovation* (vol. 1, pp. 149–71). London: Cassell.

May, S. (1998). Just how safe is Australia's multilingual language policy? In S. Wright and H. Kelly-Holmes (eds), *Managing Language Diversity* (pp. 54–7). Clevedon, Avon: Multilingual Matters.

May, S. (1999a). Critical multiculturalism and cultural difference: avoiding essentialism. In S. May (ed.), *Critical Multiculturalism: Rethinking Multicultural and Antiracist Education* (pp. 11–41). London and New York: RoutledgeFalmer.

May, S. (ed.) (1999b). *Critical Multiculturalism: Rethinking Multicultural and Antiracist Education*. London and New York: RoutledgeFalmer.

May, S. (ed.) (1999c). *Indigenous Community-Based Education*. Clevedon, Avon: Multilingual Matters.

May, S. (1999d). Extending ethnolinguistic democracy in Europe: the case of Wales. In D. Smith and S. Wright (eds), *Whose Europe? The Turn Towards Democracy* (pp. 142–67). Oxford: Blackwell/Sociological Review.

May, S. (2000). Accommodating and resisting minority language policy: the case of Wales. *International Journal of Bilingual Education and Bilingualism* 3, 2, 101–28.

May, S. (2001). Multiculturalism. In D. Goldberg and J. Solomos (eds), *The Blackwell Companion to Racial and Ethnic Studies*. Cambridge MA: Blackwell.

May, S. (2002). Indigenous rights and the politics of self-determination: the case of Aotearoa/New Zealand. In S. Fenton and S. May (eds), *Ethnonational Identities* (pp. 84–108). Basingstoke: Palgrave Macmillan.

May, S. (2003a). Rearticulating the case for minority language rights. *Current Issues in Language Planning*, 4, 2, 95–125.

May, S. (2003b). Misconceiving minority language rights: implications for liberal political theory. In W. Kymlicka and A. Patten (eds) *Language Rights and Political Theory* (pp. 123–52). Oxford: Oxford University Press.

May S. (2004). Medium of instruction policy in New Zealand. In J. Tollefson and A. Tsui (eds) *Medium of Instruction Policies: Which Agenda? Whose Agenda?* (pp. 21–41). Mahwah, NJ: Lawrence Erlbaum Associates.

May, S. (2005a). Language rights: moving the debate forward. *Journal of Sociolinguistics* 9, 3, 319–47.

May, S. (2005b). Language planning and minority language rights. In E. Hinkel (ed.), *Handbook of Research in Second Language Teaching and Learning* (pp. 1055–74). Mahwah, NJ: Lawrence Erlbaum Associates.

May, S. (2006). Language policy and minority rights. In T. Ricento (ed.), *An Introduction to Language Policy* (pp. 255–72). New York: Blackwell.

May, S. (2008a). Bilingual/immersion education: what the research tells us. In J. Cummins and N. Hornberger (eds), *Encyclopedia of Language and Education* (2nd edn), vol. 5, *Bilingual Education* (pp. 19–34). New York: Springer.

May, S. (2008b). Language education, pluralism and citizenship. In S. May and N. Hornberger (eds), *Encyclopedia of Language and Education* (2nd edn), vol. 1, Language Policy and Political Issues in Education (pp. 15–29). New York: Springer.

May, S. (2009). Critical multiculturalism and education. In J. Banks (ed.) *Routledge International Companion to Multicultural Education* (pp. 33–48). New York: Routledge.

May, S. (2010). Aotearoa/New Zealand. In J. Fishman and O. García (eds), *Handbook of Language and Ethnicity* (pp. 501–17). New York: Oxford University Press.

May, S. (2011a). Bourdieu and language policy. In M. Grenfell (ed.) *Bourdieu, Language and Linguistics* (pp. 147–69) London: Continuum.

May, S. (2011b). Language rights: the 'Cinderella' human right. *Journal of Human Rights* 10, 3, 265–89.

May, S. (2011c). The disciplinary constraints of SLA and TESOL: additive bilingualism and second language acquisition, teaching and learning. *Linguistics and Education.* 22, 3, 233–47.

May, S., and Aikman, S. (eds) (2003). Special issue. Indigenous education: addressing current issues and developments. *Comparative Education,* 39, 2.

May, S., and Hill, R. (2008). Māori-medium education: current issues and challenges. In N. Hornberger (ed.), *Can Schools Save Indigenous Languages?* (pp. 66–98). London: Palgrave Macmillan.

May, S., and Sleeter, C. (2010). Introduction. Critical multiculturalism: theory and praxis. In S. May and C. Sleeter (eds), *Critical Multiculturalism: Theory and Praxis* (pp. 1–16). New York: Routledge.

May, S., Hill, R., and Tiakiwai, S. (2004a). *Bilingual/Immersion Education: Indicators of Good Practice.* Wellington: Ministry of Education: http://www.educationcounts.govt.nz/publications/pasifika_education/5079.

May, S., Modood, T., and Squires, J. (eds) (2004b). *Ethnicity, Nationalism and Minority Rights.* Cambridge: Cambridge University Press.

Mayo, P. (1979). *The Roots of Identity: Three National Movements in Contemporary European Politics.* London: Allen Lane.

Mazrui, A. (1975). *The Political Sociology of the English Language: An African Perspective.* The Hague: Mouton.

Melucci, A. (1989). *Nomads in the Present.* London: Hutchinson Radius.

Menken, K., and García, O. (eds). (2010). *Negotiating Language Policies in Schools: Educators as Policymakers.* New York: Routledge.

Metge, J. (1990). *Te Kōhao o te Ngira: Culture and Learning.* Wellington: Learning Media, Ministry of Education.

Mey, J. (1985). *Whose Language? A Study in Linguistic Pragmatics.* Amsterdam: John Benjamins.

Michaels, W. (2006). *The Trouble with Diversity: How We Learned to Love Identity and Ignore Inequality.* New York: Metropolitan Books.

Michelet, J. (1946). *The People,* tr. C. Cooks. London: Longman (original, 1846).

Mignolo, W. (1995). *The Darker Side of the Renaissance: Literacy, Territoriality, and Colonization.* Ann Arbor, MI: University of Michigan Press.

Mignolo, W. (2000). *Coloniality, Subaltern Knowledges, and Border Thinking.* Princeton, NJ: Princeton University Press.

Miles, R. (1993). *Racism After 'Race Relations'.* London: Routledge.

Miles, R. (1996). Racism and nationalism in the United Kingdom: a view from the periphery. In R. Barot (ed.), *The Racism Problematic: Contemporary Sociological Debates on Race and Ethnicity* (pp. 231–55). Lampeter, Wales: Edward Mellen Press.

Miles, R., and Brown, M. (2003). *Racism* (2nd edn). London: Routledge.

Miles, R., and Spoonley, P. (1985). The political economy of labour migration: an alternative to the sociology of 'race' and 'ethnic relations' in New Zealand. *Australian and New Zealand Journal of Sociology* 21, 3–26.

Mill, J. (1972). *Considerations on Representative Government*, ed. H. Acton. London: J. M. Dent (original, 1861).

Miller, D. (1995). Reflections on British national identity. *New Community* 21, 153–66.

Miller, D. (2002). Doctrinaire liberalism versus multicultural democracy. *Ethnicities* 2, 2, 261–5.

Miller, H., and Miller, K. (1996). Language policy and identity: the case of Catalonia. *International Studies in Sociology of Education* 6, 113–28.

Milward, A. (1992). *The European Rescue of the Nation-State*. London: Routledge.

Minority Rights Group (1997). *World Directory of Minorities* (2nd edn). London: Longman.

Mnookin, R., and Verbeke, A. (2009). Persistent non-violent conflict with no reconciliation: the Flemish and Walloons in Belgium. *Law and Contemporary Problems* 72, 2, 151–86.

Modood, T. (1992). *Not Easy Being British: Colour, Culture and Citizenship*. Stoke-on-Trent: Runnymede Trust and Trentham Books.

Modood, T. (1997). Culture and identity. In T. Modood, R. Berthoud, J. Lakey, J. Nazroo, P. Smith, S. Virdee and S. Beishon, *Ethnic Minorities in Britain: Diversity and Disadvantage* (pp. 290–338). London: Policy Studies Institute.

Modood, T. (1998a). Anti-essentialism, multiculturalism and the 'recognition' of religious groups. *Journal of Political Philosophy* 6, 378–99.

Modood, T. (1998b). Multiculturalism, secularism and the state. *Critical Review of International Social and Political Philosophy* 1, 79–97.

Modood, T. (2007). *Multiculturalism: A Civic Idea*. Cambridge, UK: Polity Press.

Modood, T., and May, S. (2001). Multiculturalism and education in Britain: an internally contested debate. *International Journal of Educational Research*. 35, 3, 305–17.

Moerman, M. (1965). Who are the Lue: ethnic identification in a complex civilization. *American Anthropologist* 67, 1215–29.

Moerman, M. (1974). Accomplishing ethnicity. In R. Turner (ed.), *Ethnomethodology* (pp. 54–68). New York: Penguin Education.

Mohan, R. (1995). Multiculturalism in the nineties: pitfalls and possibilities. In C. Newfield and R. Strickland (eds), *After Political Correctness: The Humanities and Society in the 1990s* (pp. 372–88). Boulder, CO: Westview Press.

Moïse, C. (2007). Protecting French: the view from France. In A. Duchêne and M. Heller (eds), *Discourses of Endangerment: Ideology and Interest in the Defence of Languages* (pp. 216–41). London: Continuum.

Moodley, K. (1999). Antiracist education through political literacy: the case of Canada. In S. May (ed.), *Critical Multiculturalism: Rethinking Multicultural and Antiracist Education* (pp. 138–52). London and New York: RoutledgeFalmer.

Moore, M. (1991). Liberalism and the ideal of the good life. *Review of Politics* 53, 687–8.

Morgan, B., and Ramanathan, V. (2009). Outsourcing, globalizing economics, and shifting language policies: issues in managing Indian call centers. *Language Policy* 8, 1, 69–80.

Morgan, K. (1981). *Rebirth of a Nation: Wales 1880–1980*. Oxford: Clarendon Press.

Morgan, K. (1995). Welsh nationalism: the historical background. In K. Morgan, *Modern Wales: Politics, Places and People* (pp. 197–213). Cardiff: University of Wales Press.

Moss, S. (1994). Lost for words. *Guardian Weekend* (30 July), 26–30.

Mouffe, C. (1993). *The Return of the Political*. London: Verso.

Mufwene, S. (2001). *The Ecology of Language Evolution*. Cambridge: Cambridge University Press.

Mufwene, S. (2004). Language birth and death. *Annual Review of Anthropology* 33, 201–22.

Mühlhäusler, P. (1996). *Linguistic Ecology: Language Change and Linguistic Imperialism in the Pacific Region*. London: Routledge.

Mühlhäusler, P. (2000). Language planning and Language ecology. *Current Issues in Language Planning* 1, 3, 306–67.

Mulgan, R. (1989). *Māori, Pākehā and Democracy*. Auckland: Oxford University Press.

Muller, J. (2010). *Language and Conflict in Northern Ireland and Canada: A Silent War*. Basingstoke: Palgrave Macmillan.

Nagel, J. (1994). Constructing ethnicity: creating and recreating ethnic identity and culture. *Social Problems* 41, 152–76.

Nairn, T. (1981). *The Break-up of Britain: Crisis and Neo-Nationalism* (rev. edn). London: Verso.

Nakamura, L. (2002). *Cybertypes: Race, Ethnicity, and Identity on the Internet*. New York: Routledge.

Nash, M. (1989). *The Cauldron of Ethnicity in the Modern World*. Chicago, IL: Chicago University Press.

Nash, R. (1990). Bourdieu on education and social and cultural reproduction. *British Journal of Sociology of Education* 11, 431–47.

Nathan, D. (n.d.). *Aboriginal Languages of Australia*: http://www.dnathan.com/VL/austLang.htm.

Ndebele, N. (1987). The English language and social change in South Africa. *English Academy Review* 4, 1–16.

Nelde, P. (1997). Language conflict. In F. Coulmas (ed.), *The Handbook of Sociolinguistics* (pp. 285–300). London: Blackwell.

Nelde, P., Strubell, M., and Williams, G. (1996). *Euromosaic: The Production and Reproduction of the Minority Language Groups in the European Union*. Luxembourg: Office for Official Publications of the European Communities.

Nettle, D., and Romaine, S. (2000). *Vanishing Voices: The Extinction of the World's Languages*. Oxford: Oxford University Press.

New Zealand Department of Education (1984a). *Taha Māori: Suggestions for Getting Started*. Wellington: Department of Education.

New Zealand Department of Education (1984b). *A Review of the Core Curriculum for Schools*. Wellington: Department of Education.

New Zealand Ministerial Advisory Committee (1986). *Pūao-Te-Atatu* (The Report of the Ministerial Advisory Committee on a Māori Perspective for the Department of Social Welfare). Wellington: Government Printer.

New Zealand Ministry of Education (1993). *The New Zealand Curriculum Framework*. Wellington: Learning Media, Ministry of Education.

New Zealand Ministry of Education (1998). *Nga Haeata Mātauranga: Annual Report on Māori Education 1997/98 and Direction for 1999*. Wellington: Ministry of Education.

New Zealand Ministry of Education (2001). *More than Words*. Wellington: Ministry of Education.

New Zealand Ministry of Education (2007). *Nga Haeata Matauranga: Annual Report on Māori Education 2006/2007*. Wellington: Ministry of Education.

New Zealand Ministry of Pacific Island Affairs (2002). *Social and Economic Report.* Wellington: Ministry of Pacific Island Affairs.

Ngũgĩ, wa Thiong'o (1993). *Moving the Centre: The Struggle for Cultural Freedoms.* London: James Currey.

Nic Craith, M. (2003). *Culture and Identity Politics in Northern Ireland.* Basingstoke: Palgrave Macmillan.

Nic Craith, M. (2006) *Europe and the Politics of Language: Citizens, Migrants, and Outsiders.* London: Palgrave-Macmillan.

Nic Craith, M. (2007). Rethinking language policies: challenges and opportunities. In C. H. Williams (ed.), *Language and Governance* (pp. 159–84). Cardiff: University of Wales Press.

Nielsson, G. (1985). States and 'nation-groups': a global taxonomy. In E. Tiryakian and R. Rugowski (eds), *New Nationalisms of the Developed West: Towards Explanations* (pp. 27–56). Boston, MA: Allen & Unwin.

Nieto, S., and Bode, P. (2007). *Affirming Diversity: The Sociopolitical Context of Multicultural Education* (5th edn). New York: Allyn & Bacon.

Nimni, E. (1995). Marx, Engels, and the national question. In W. Kymlicka (ed.), *The Rights of Minority Cultures* (pp. 57–75). Oxford: Oxford University Press.

NOP (1995). *Public Attitudes to the Welsh Language.* London: NOP Social and Political.

Norman, W. (1999). Theorizing nationalism (normatively): the first steps. In R. Beiner (ed.), *Theorizing Nationalism* (pp. 51–66). Albany, NY: SUNY Press.

Norton, B. (2000). *Identity and Language Learning: Gender, Ethnicity and Educational Change.* London: Longman.

Nunberg, G. (1989). Linguists and the official language movement. *Language* 65, 579–87.

Nunberg, G. (1992). Afterword: the official language movement: reimagining America. In J. Crawford (ed.), *Language Loyalties: A Source Book on the Official English Controversy* (pp. 479–94). Chicago, IL: University of Chicago Press.

Nussbaum, M. (1997). *Cultivating Humanity.* Cambridge, MA: Harvard University Press.

Nussbaum, M. (2001). *Upheavals in Thought.* Cambridge: Cambridge University Press.

Oakes, L. (2004). French: a language for everyone in Québec? *Nations and Nationalism* 10, 4, 539–58.

Oakes, L., and Warren, J. (2007). *Language, Citizenship and Identity in Quebec.* Basingstoke: Palgrave Macmillan.

Ó Catháin, L. (2007). Language, law and governance: an Irish perspective. In C. H. Williams (ed.), *Language and Governance* (pp. 293–313). Cardiff: University of Wales Press.

O'Cinnéide, M., Keane, M., and Cawley, M. (1985). Industrialisation and linguistic change among Gaelic-speaking communities in the West of Ireland. *Language Problems and Language Planning* 9, 3–16.

Ó Ciosáin, S. (1988). Language planning and Irish. *Language, Culture and Curriculum* 1, 263–79.

Oestreich, J. (1999). Liberal theory and minority group rights. *Human Rights Quarterly* 21, 1, 108–32.

Office for National Statistics (2003). Census 2001: Wales and its people. Retrieved April 2011 from http://www.statistics.gov.uk/census2001/profiles/commentaries/wales.asp.

Ó Gadhra, N. (1988). Irish government policy and political development of the Gaeltacht. *Language, Culture and Curriculum* 1, 251–61.

Ogbu, J. (1987). Variability in minority school performance: a problem in search of an explanation. *Anthropology and Education Quarterly* 18, 312–34.

Ogunwole, S. (2006). *We the People: American Indians and Alaska Natives in the United States. Census 2000 Special Report*. Washington, DC: US Census Bureau.

Okihiro, G. (2009). *Island World: A History of Hawai'i and the United States*. Berkeley, CA: University of California Press.

Okin, S. (1998). Feminism and multiculturalism: some tensions. *Ethics* 108, 661–84.

Okin, S. (1999). Is multiculturalism bad for women? In J. Cohen, M. Howard and M. Nussbaum (eds), *Is Multiculturalism Bad for Women?* (pp. 9–24). Princeton, NJ: Princeton University Press.

O'Leary, B. (1998). Ernest Gellner's diagnoses of nationalism: a critical overview, or, what is living and what is dead in Ernest Gellner's philosophy of nationalism. In J. Hall (ed.), *The State of the Nation: Ernest Gellner and the Theory of Nationalism* (pp. 40–90). Cambridge: Cambridge University Press.

Omi, M., and Winant, H. (1986). *Racial Formation in the United States: From the 1960s to the 1980s*. New York: Routledge & Kegan Paul.

Ó Murchú, M. (1988). Diglossia and interlanguage contact in Ireland. *Language, Culture and Curriculum* 1, 243–9.

Oommen, T. (1994). State, nation, and ethnie: the processual linkages. In P. Ratcliffe (ed.), *'Race', Ethnicity and Nation: International Perspectives on Social Conflict* (pp. 26–46). London: UCL Press.

Orange, C. (1987). *The Treaty of Waitangi*. Wellington: Allen & Unwin.

Ó Riagáin, P. (1988a). Bilingualism in Ireland 1793–1983: an overview of national sociolinguistic surveys. *International Journal of the Sociology of Language* 70, 29–51.

Ó Riagáin, P. (1988b). Introduction. *International Journal of the Sociology of Language* 70, 5–9.

Ó Riagáin, P. (1996). Reviving the Irish language 1893–1993: the first hundred years. In M. Nic Craith (ed.), *Watching one's Tongue: Issues in Language Planning* (pp. 33–56). Liverpool: Liverpool University Press.

Ó Riagáin, P. (1997). *Language Policy and Social Reproduction: Ireland 1893–1993*. Oxford: Clarendon Press.

Ó Riagáin, P. (2008). Irish-language policy 1922–2007: balancing maintenance and revival. In C. Pháidín and S. Ó Cearnaigh (eds), *A New View of the Irish Language* (pp. 55–65). Dublin: Cois Life.

Osava, M. (2006). Indigenous people fight for their rights. Retrieved March 2011 from http://ipsnews.net/news.asp?idnews=32029.

Osmond, J. (1988). *The Divided Kingdom*. London: Constable.

O'Sullivan, D. (2007). *Beyond Biculturalism: The Politics of an Indigenous Minority*. Wellington: Huia Publishers.

Ozolins, U. (1993). *The Politics of Language in Australia*. Cambridge: Cambridge University Press.

Packer, J. (1999). Problems in defining minorities. In D. Fottrell and B. Bowring (eds), *Minority and Group Rights in the New Millennium* (pp. 223–73). The Hague: Kluwer Law International.

Padilla, A. (1991). English only vs. bilingual education: ensuring a language-competent society. *Journal of Education* 173, 38–51.

Padilla, F. (1985). *Latino Ethnic Consciousness: The Case of Mexican Americans and Puerto Ricans in Chicago*. Notre Dame, IN: Notre Dame Press.

Paine, R. (2000). Aboriginality, authenticity and the settler world. In A. Cohen (ed.), *Signifying Identities: Anthropological Perspectives on Boundaries and Contested Values* (pp. 77–116). London: Routledge.

Parekh. B. (1995). The concept of national identity. *New Community* 21, 255–68.

Parekh, B. (2000). *Rethinking Multiculturalism: Cultural Diversity and Political Theory*. London: Macmillan.

París, M. (2007). Language policy as social policy: the role of languages in an open society. Retrieved Dec. 2009 from http://www20.gencat.cat/docs/Llengcat/Documents/Publicacions/Publicacions%20en%20linea/Arxius/conf_spl2007_ang.pdf.

Patrick, D. (2004). The politics of language rights in the Eastern Canadian Arctic. In J. Freeland and D. Patrick (eds), *Language Rights and Language Survival* (pp. 171–90). Manchester: St Jerome Press.

Patrick, D. (2007). Indigenous language endangerment and the unfinished business of nation-states. In A. Duchêne and M. Heller (eds), *Discourses of Endangerment: Ideology and Interest in the Defence of Languages* (pp. 35–55). London: Continuum.

Pattanayak, D. (1969). *Aspects of Applied Linguistics*. London: Asia Publishing House.

Pattanayak, D. (1985). Diversity in communication and languages; predicament of a multilingual nation state: India, a case study. In N. Wolfson and J. Manes (eds), *Language of Inequality* (pp. 399–407). Berlin: Mouton de Gruyter.

Pattanayak, D. (ed.) (1990). *Multilingualism in India*. Clevedon, Avon: Multilingual Matters.

Patton, P. (1995). Post-structuralism and the Mabo debate: difference, society and justice. In M. Wilson and A. Yeatman (eds), *Justice and Identity: Antipodean Practices* (pp. 153–71). Wellington: Bridget Williams Books.

Paulston, C. (1993). Language regenesis: a conceptual overview of language revival, revitalisation and reversal. *Journal of Multilingual and Multicultural Development* 14, 275–86.

Pavlenko, A. (2002). 'We have room for but one language here'. Language and national identity in the US at the turn of the twentieth century. *Multilingua* 21, 163–96.

Pearson, D. (1990). *A Dream Deferred: The Origins of Ethnic Conflict in New Zealand*. Wellington: Allen & Unwin.

Pearson, D. (2000a). The ties that unwind: civic and ethnic imaginings in New Zealand. *Nations and Nationalism* 6, 91–110.

Pearson, D. (2000b). *The Politics of Ethnicity in Settler Societies: States of Unease*. New York: Palgrave.

Peddie, R. (2003). Languages in New Zealand: population, politics and policy. In R. Barnard and T. Glynn (eds), *Bilingual Children's Language and Literacy Development* (pp. 8–35). Clevedon, Avon: Multilingual Matters.

Pejic, J. (1997). Minority rights in international law. *Human Rights Quarterly* 19, 3, 666–85.

Pennycook, A. (1994). *The Cultural Politics of English as an International Language*. London: Longman.

Pennycook, A. (1995). English in the world/the world in English. In J. Tollefson (ed.), *Power and Inequality in Language Education* (pp. 34–58). Cambridge: Cambridge University Press.

Pennycook, A. (1998a). The right to language: towards a situated ethics of language possibilities. *Language Sciences* 20, 73–87.

Pennycook, A. (1998b). *English and the Discourses of Colonialism*. London: Routledge.

Pennycook, A. (2004). Language policy and the ecological turn. *Language Policy* 3, 3, 213–39.

Pennycook, A. (2007). *Global Englishes and Transcultural Flows*. New York: Routledge.

Pennycook, A. (2010). *Language as a Local Practice*. New York: Routledge.

Perera, S., and Pugliese, J. (1998). Wogface, anglo-drag, contested aboriginalities: making and unmaking identities in Australia. *Social Identities* 4, 39–72.

Pericay, G. (2010). The Spanish Constitutional Court shortens the Catalan Statute of Autonomy. *Catalan News Agency* (28 June). Retrieved July 2010 from http://www.catalannewsagency.com/news/politics/the-spanish-constitutional-court-shortens-the-current-catalan-statute-of-autonom.

Pew Hispanic Center (2011). Demographic profile of Hispanics in California, 2008. Retrieved Feb. 2011 at http://pewhispanic.org/states/?stateid=CA.

Peyre, H. (1933). *La royauté et les langues provinciales*. Paris: Les Presses Modernes.

Phillips, A. (1995). Democracy and difference: some problems for feminist theory. In W. Kymlicka (ed.), *The Rights of Minority Cultures* (pp. 288–99). Oxford: Oxford University Press.

Phillips, A. (1997). Why worry about multiculturalism? *Dissent* 44, 57–63.

Phillips, A. (2009). *Multiculturalism Without Culture*. Princeton, NJ: Princeton University Press.

Phillips, A., and Saharso, S. (eds) (2008). The rights of women and the crisis of multiculturalism. Special Issue. *Ethnicities* 8, 3.

Phillipson, R. (1992). *Linguistic Imperialism*. Oxford: Oxford University Press.

Phillipson, R. (1998). Globalizing English: are linguistic human rights an alternative to linguistic imperialism? *Language Sciences* 20, 101–12.

Phillipson, R. (ed.) (2000). *Rights to Language: Equity, Power and Education*. Mahwah, NJ: Lawrence Erlbaum.

Phillipson, R. (2003). *English-Only Europe? Challenging Language Policy*. London: Routledge.

Phillipson, R. (2010). *Linguistic Imperialism Continued*. New York: Routledge.

Phillipson, R., and Skutnabb-Kangas, T. (1994). English, panacea or pandemic? *Sociolinguistica* 8, 73–87.

Pieterse, J. (2007). *Ethnicities and Global Multiculture: Pants for an Octopus*. Lanham, MD: Rowman & Littlefield.

Pieterse, J. (2009). *Globalization and Culture: Global Mélange* (2nd edn). Lanham, MD: Rowman & Littlefield.

Pinker, S. (1995). *The Language Instinct*. London: Penguin.

Pogge, T. (2003). Accommodation rights for Hispanics in the US. In W. Kymlicka and A. Patten (eds) *Language Rights and Political Theory* (pp. 105–22). Oxford: Oxford University Press.

Porter, J. (1965). *The Vertical Mosaic*. Toronto: Toronto University Press.

Porter, J. (1972). Dilemmas and contradictions of a multi-ethnic society. *Transactions of the Royal Society of Canada* 10, 193–205.

Porter, J. (1975). Ethnic pluralism in Canadian perspective. In N. Glazer and D. Moynihan (eds), *Ethnicity: Theory and Experience* (pp. 267–304). Cambridge, MA: Harvard University Press.

Porter, R. (1990). *Forked Tongue: The Politics of Bilingual Education*. New York: Basic Books.

Portes, A., and Hao, L. (1998). E pluribis unum: bilingualism and loss of language in the second generation. *Sociology of Education* 71, 269–94.

Povinelli, E. (2002). *The Cunning of Recognition: Indigenous Alterities and the Making of Australian Multiculturalism*. Durham, NC: Duke University Press.

Preece, J. (1998). *National Minorities and the European Nation-States System*. Oxford: Clarendon Press.

Pujolar, J. (2007). The future of Catalan: language endangerment and nationalist discourses in Catalonia. In A. Duchêne and M. Heller (eds), *Discourses of Endangerment: Ideology and Interest in the Defence of Languages* (pp. 121–48). London: Continuum.

Quiniou-Tempereau, R. (1988). *The Breton Language in Primary Education in Brittany, France*. Leeuwarden, Netherlands: Fryske Akodemy.

Quirk, R. (1981). International communication and the concept of nuclear English. In L. Smith (ed.), *English for Cross-Cultural Communication* (pp. 151–65). London: Macmillan.

Quirk, R. (1985). The English language in a global context. In R. Quirk and H. Widdowson (eds), *English in the World* (pp. 1–6). Cambridge: Cambridge University Press.

Raj, D. (2003). *Where Are You From? Middle-Class Migrants in the Modern World*. Berkeley, CA: University of California Press.

Ramírez, J., Yuen, S., and Ramey D. (1991). *Final Report: Longitudinal Study of Structured English Immersion Strategy, Early-Exit and Late-Exit Transitional Bilingual Education Programs for Language-Minority Children*. San Mateo, CA: Aguirre International.

Rassool, N. (1999). *Literacy for Sustainable Development in the Age of Information*. Clevedon, Avon: Multilingual Matters.

Rata, E. (2000). *A Political Economy of Neotribal Capitalism*. Lanham, MA: Lexington Books.

Rata, E. (2005). Rethinking biculturalism. *Anthropological Theory* 5, 3, 267–84.

Rata, E., and Openshaw, R. (eds) (2006). *Public Policy and Ethnicity: The Politics of Ethnic Boundary-Making*. Basingstoke: Palgrave Macmillan.

Ravitch, D. (1992). Diversity in education. *Dialogue* 95, 39–47.

Ravitch, D. (2001). *Left Back: A Century of Battles over School Reform*. New York: Simon and Schuster.

Rawkins, P. (1987). The politics of benign neglect: education, public policy, and the mediation of linguistic conflict in Wales. *International Journal of the Sociology of Language* 66, 27–48.

Rawls, J. (1971). *A Theory of Justice*. Oxford: Oxford University Press.

Rawls, J. (1985). Justice as fairness: political not metaphysical. *Philosophy and Public Affairs* 14, 223–51.

Réaume, D. (1999). Official language rights: intrinsic value and the protection of difference. In W. Kymlicka and W. Norman (eds), *Citizenship in Diverse Societies* (pp. 245–72). Oxford: Oxford University Press.

Réaume, D. (2003). Beyond personality: the territorial and personal principles of language policy reconsidered. In W. Kymlicka and A. Patten (eds), *Language Rights and Political Theory* (pp. 271–95). Oxford: Oxford University Press.

Reay, D. (1995a). 'They employ cleaners to do that': habitus in the primary classroom. *British Journal of Sociology of Education* 16, 353–71.

Reay, D. (1995b). Using habitus to look at 'race' and class in primary school classrooms. In M. Griffiths and B. Troyna (eds), *Antiracism, Culture and Social Justice in Education* (pp. 115–32). Stoke-on-Trent: Trentham Books.

Reines, M., and Prinz, J. (2009). Reviving Whorf: the return of linguistic relativity. *Philosophy Compass* 4, 6, 1022–32.

Reitman, O. (2005). Multiculturalism and feminism: incompatibility, compatibility, or synonymity? *Ethnicities*, 5, 2, 216–47.

Renan, E. (1990). What is a nation? In H. Bhabha (ed.), *Nation and Narration* (pp. 8–22). London: Routledge (original, 1882).

Rex, J. (1973). *Race, Colonialism and the City.* Oxford: Oxford University Press.

Rex, J. (1991). *Ethnic Identity and Ethnic Mobilisation in Britain.* Coventry: Centre for Research in Ethnic Relations, University of Warwick.

Rex, J., and Mason, D. (eds) (1986). *Theories of Race and Race Relations.* Cambridge: Cambridge University Press.

Ricento, T. (1996). Language policy in the United States. In M. Herriman and B. Burnaby (eds), *Language Policies in English-Dominant Countries* (pp. 122–58). Clevedon, Avon: Multilingual Matters.

Ricento, T. (2005). Problems with the 'language-as-resource' discourse in the promotion of heritage languages in the U.S.A., *Journal of Sociolinguistics* 19, 3, 348–68.

Ricento, T., and Wright, W. (2008). Language policy and education in the United States. In S. May and N. Hornberger (eds.), *Encyclopedia of Language and Education,* 2nd ed., Vol. 1, Language Policy and Political Issues in Education (pp. 285–300). New York: Springer.

Robbins, D. (1991). *The Work of Pierre Bourdieu: Recognizing Society.* Milton Keynes: Open University Press.

Robbins, D. (2000). *Bourdieu and Culture.* London: Sage.

Robbins, J. (2007). The Howard government and indigenous rights: an imposed national unity? *Australian Journal of Political Science* 42, 2, 315–28.

Robbins, J. (2010). A nation within? Indigenous peoples, representation and sovereignty in Australia. *Ethnicities* 10, 2, 257–74.

Robbins, K. (1997). *Great Britain: Identities, Institutions and the Idea of Britishness.* London: Longman.

Robertson, R. (1992). *Globalization: Social Theory and Global Culture.* London: Sage.

Robertson, R. (1995). Globalization: time-space and homogeneity-heterogeneity. In M. Featherstone, S. Lash and R. Robertson (eds), *Global Modernities* (pp. 25–44). London: Sage.

Roddick, W. (2007). One nation – two voices? The Welsh language in the governance of Wales. In C. H. Williams (ed.), *Language and Governance* (pp. 263–92). Cardiff: University of Wales Press.

Rodriguez. R. (1983). *Hunger of Memory.* New York: Bantam.

Rodriguez, R. (1993). *Days of Obligation: An Argument with my Mexican Father.* London: Penguin.

Roediger, D. (1999). *The Wages of Whiteness: Race and the Making of the American Working Class* (rev edn). London: Verso.

Rogel, C. (2004). *The Breakup of Yugoslavia and its Aftermath* (2nd edn). Westport, CT: Greenwood Press.

Rokkan, S., and Urwin, D. (1983). *Economy, Territory, Identity.* London: Sage.

Romaine, S. (1995). *Bilingualism* (2nd edn). Oxford: Blackwell.

Romaine, S. (2000). *Language in Society: An Introduction to Sociolinguistics* (2nd edn). Oxford: Oxford University Press.

Roosens, E. (1989). *Creating Ethnicity: The Process of Ethnogenesis.* London: Sage.

Rorty, R. (1991). *Objectivity, Relativism, and Truth: Philosophical Papers I.* Cambridge: Cambridge University Press.

Rosaldo, R. (1989). *Culture and Truth.* London: Routledge.

Rossell, C., and Baker, K. (1996). The effectiveness of bilingual education. *Research in the Teaching of English* 30, 7–74.

Rothschild, J. (1981). *Ethnopolitics: A Conceptual Framework*. New York: Columbia University Press.

Royal Commission on Social Policy (1988). *April Report*, vols. 1–4. Wellington: Government Printer.

Rubdy, R., and Saraceni, M. (eds) (2006). *English in the World: Global Rules, Global Roles*. London: Continuum.

Ruiz, R. (1984). Orientations in language planning. *NABE Journal* 8, 2, 15–34.

Ruiz, R. (1990). Official languages and language planning. In K. Adams and D. Brink (eds), *Perspectives on Official English: The Campaign for English as the Official Language of the USA* (pp. 11–24). Berlin: Mouton de Gruyter.

Rynard, P. (2000). 'Welcome in, but check your rights at the door': the James Bay and Nisga'a Agreements in Canada. *Canadian Journal of Political Science/Revue Canadienne de Science Politique* 33, 2, 211–43.

Safran, W. (2004). Introduction: the political aspects of language. *Nationalism and Ethnic Politics* 10, 1, 1–14.

Safran, W. (2010). Political science and politics. In J. Fishman and O. García (eds), *Handbook of Language and Ethnic Identity: Disciplinary and Regional Perspectives* (2nd edn, vol. 1, pp. 49–69). New York: Oxford University Press.

Said, E. (1994). *Culture and Imperialism*. London: Vintage.

Salée, D. (1995). Identities in conflict: the Aboriginal question and the politics of recognition in Québec. *Ethnic and Racial Studies* 18, 277–314.

Sandall, R. (2001). *The Culture Cult: Designer Tribalism and Other Essays*. Boulder, CO: Westview Press.

Sandel, M. (1982). *Liberalism and the Limits of Justice*. Cambridge: Cambridge University Press.

San Juan, E. (2006). Ethnic identity and popular sovereignty: notes on the Moro struggle in the Philippines. *Ethnicities* 6, 3, 391–422.

San Miguel, G., and Valencia, R. (1998). From the Treaty of Guadalupe Hidalgo to Hopwood: the educational plight and struggle of Mexican Americans in the Southwest. *Harvard Educational Review* 68, 353–412.

Sapir, E. (1929). The status of linguistics as a science. *Language* 5, 4, 207–14.

Schermerhorn, R. (1970). *Comparative Ethnic Relations*. New York: Random House.

Schiffman, H. (1996). *Linguistic Culture and Language Policy*. London: Routledge.

Schildkraut, D. (2005). *Press One for English: Language Policy, Public Opinion, and American Identity*. Princeton, NJ: Princeton University Press.

Schlesinger, A. (1991). The disuniting of America: what we all stand to lose if multicultural education takes the wrong approach. *American Educator* 15, 14–33.

Schlesinger, A. (1992). *The Disuniting of America: Reflections on a Multicultural Society*. New York: W. W. Norton & Co.

Schmid, C. (2001). *The Politics of Language: Conflict, Identity, and Cultural Pluralism in Comparative Perspective*. New York: Oxford University Press.

Schmidt, R. Sr. (2000). *Language Policy and Identity Politics in the United States*. Philadelphia, PA: Temple University Press.

Schmidt, R. Sr. (2002). Racialisation and language policy: the case of the USA. *Multilingua* 21, 2–3, 141–62.

Schmidt, R. Sr. (2008). Defending English in an English-dominant world: the ideology of the 'Offical English' movement in the United States. In A. Duchêne and M. Heller (eds), *Discourses of Endangerment: Ideology and Interest in the Defence of Languages* (pp. 197–215). London: Continuum.

Schmidtke, O. (2002). Naïve universalism. *Ethnicities* 2, 2, 274–83.

Schmied, J. (1991). *English in Africa: An Introduction*. London: Longman.

Scott, C. (1996). Indigenous self-determination and decolonization of the international imagination: a plea. *Human Rights Quarterly* 18, 814–20.

Scourfield, J., and Davies, A. (2005). Children's accounts of Wales as racialized and inclusive. *Ethnicities* 5, 1, 83–107.

Secada, W., and Lightfoot, T. (1993). Symbols and the political context of bilingual education in the United States. In M. Arias and U. Casanova (eds), *Bilingual Education: Politics, Practice, and Research* (pp. 36–64). Chicago, IL: National Society for the Study of Education/University of Chicago Press.

Semb, A. (2005). Sami self-determination in the making? *Nations and Nationalism* 11, 4, 531–49.

Semprini, A. (1997). *Le Multiculturalisme*. Paris: Que sais je? PUF.

Seton-Watson, H. (1977). *Nations and States*. London: Methuen.

Shachar, A. (2001). *Multicultural Jurisdictions: Culture Differences and Women's Rights*. Cambridge: Cambridge University Press.

Shachar, A. (2007). Feminism and multiculturalism: mapping the terrain. In A. Laden and D. Owen (eds), *Multiculturalism and Political Theory* (pp. 115–47). Cambridge: Cambridge University Press.

Shannon, S. (1999). The debate on bilingual education in the U.S: language ideology as reflected in the practice of bilingual teachers. In J. Blommaert (ed.), *Language Ideological Debates* (pp. 171–99). Berlin: Mouton de Gruyter.

Sharp, A. (1990). *Justice and the Māori: Māori Claims in New Zealand Political Argument in the 1980s*. Auckland: Oxford University Press.

Sharples, P. (1988). *Kura Kaupapa Māori: Recommendations for Policy*. Auckland: Te Kura o Hoani Waititi Marae.

Shell, M. (1993). Babel in America: the politics of language diversity in the United States. *Critical Inquiry* 20, 103–27.

Shields, C., Bishop, R., and Mazawi, A. (2005). *Pathologizing Practices: The Impact of Deficit Thinking on Education*. New York: Peter Lang.

Shils, E. (1957). Primordial, personal, sacred and civil ties. *British Journal of Sociology* 8, 130–45.

Shils, E. (1980). *Tradition*. Glencoe, IL: Free Press.

Shin, H. (2003). *Language Use and English-Speaking Ability: 2000. Census 2000 Brief*. Washington, DC: US Census Bureau.

Silverstein, M. (1996). Monoglot 'standard' in America: standardization and metaphors of linguistic hegemony. In D. Brenneis and R. Macaulay (eds), *The Matrix of Language: Contemporary Linguistic Anthropology* (pp. 284–306). Boulder, CO: Westview Press.

Silverstein, M. (1998). The uses and utility of ideology: a commentary. In B. Schieffelin, K. Woolard and P. Kroskrity (eds), *Language Ideologies: Practice and Theory* (pp. 123–45). New York: Oxford University Press.

Silverstein, M. (2000). Whorfianism and the linguistic imagination of nationality. In P. Kroskrity (ed.), *Regimes of Language: Ideologies, Politics and Identities* (pp. 85–138). Santa Fe, NM: School of American Research Press.

Simon, J. (1989). Aspirations and ideology: biculturalism and multiculturalism in New Zealand education. *Sites* 18, 23–34.

Simon, J., and Smith, L. (eds) (2001). *A Civilising Mission? Perceptions and Representations of the New Zealand Native Schools System.* Auckland: Auckland University Press.

Sinclair, K. (ed.) (1993). *The Oxford Illustrated History of New Zealand.* Oxford: Oxford University Press.

Skutnabb-Kangas, T. (1988). Multilingualism and the education of minority children. In T. Skutnabb-Kangas and J. Cummins (eds), *Minority Education: From Shame to Struggle* (pp. 9–44). Clevedon, Avon: Multilingual Matters.

Skutnabb-Kangas, T. (1998). Human rights and language wrongs – a future for diversity? *Language Sciences* 20, 5–27.

Skutnabb-Kangas, T. (2000). *Linguistic Genocide in Education – or Worldwide Diversity and Human Rights?* Mahwah, NJ: Lawrence Erlbaum.

Skutnabb-Kangas, T. (2008). Human rights and language policy in education. In S. May and N. Hornberger (eds), *Encyclopedia of Language and Education* (2nd edn), vol. 1, Language Policy and Political Issues in Education, (pp. 107–119). New York: Springer.

Skutnabb-Kangas, T., and Bucak, S. (1995). Killing a mother tongue – how the Kurds are deprived of linguistic human rights. In T. Skutnabb-Kangas and R. Phillipson (eds), *Linguistic Human Rights: Overcoming Linguistic Discrimination* (pp. 347–70). Berlin: Mouton de Gruyter.

Skutnabb-Kangas, T., and Fernandes, D. (2008). Kurds in Turkey and in (Iraqi) Kurdistan: a comparison of Kurdish educational language policy in two situations of occupation. *Genocide Studies and Prevention* 3, 1, 4–73.

Skutnabb-Kangas, T., and Phillipson, R. (1995). Linguistic human rights, past and present. In T. Skutnabb-Kangas and R. Phillipson (eds), *Linguistic Human Rights: Overcoming Linguistic Discrimination* (pp. 71–110). Berlin: Mouton de Gruyter.

Skutnabb-Kangas, T., Phillipson, R., Mohanty, A., and Panda, M. (eds) (2009). *Social Justice through Multilingual Education.* Bristol: Multilingual Matters.

Sleeter, C. (1996). *Multicultural Education as Social Activism.* Albany, NY: SUNY Press.

Sleeter, C., and Delgado, Bernal D. (2004). Critical pedagogy, critical race theory, and antiracist education: their implications for multicultural education. In J. Banks and C. McGee Banks (eds), *Handbook of Research on Multicultural Education* (2nd edn, pp. 240–60). San Francisco: Jossey Bass.

Smaje, C. (1997). Not just a social construct: theorising race and ethnicity. *Sociology* 31, 307–27.

Small, S. (1994). *Racialised Barriers: The Black Experience in the United States and England in the 1980s.* London: Routledge.

Smith, Andrea (2009). *Indigenous Peoples and Boarding Schools: A Comparative Study.* New York: Secretariat of the United Nations Permanent Forum on Indigenous Issues.

Smith, Anthony (1981). *The Ethnic Revival.* Cambridge: Cambridge University Press.

Smith, Anthony (1983). *Theories of Nationalism* (2nd edn). London: Harper & Row.

Smith, Anthony (1986). *The Ethnic Origin of Nations.* Oxford: Basil Blackwell.

Smith, Anthony (1991). *National Identity.* London: Penguin.

Smith, Anthony (1994). The problem of national identity: ancient, medieval and modern? *Ethnic and Racial Studies* 17, 375–99.

Smith, Anthony (1995a). *Nations and Nationalism in a Global Era.* London: Polity Press.

Smith, Anthony (1995b). Gastronomy or geology? The role of nationalism in the construction of nations. *Nations and Nationalism* 1, 3–23.

Smith, Anthony (1998). *Nationalism and Modernism.* London: Routledge.

Smith, Anthony (2001). State and nation. In A. Leoussi (ed.), *Encyclopaedia of Nationalism* (pp. 286–8). New Brunswick, NJ: Transaction Publishers.

Smith, Anthony (2004a). Ethnic cores and dominant ethnies. In E. Kaufmann (ed.), *Rethinking Ethnicity: Majority Groups and Dominant Minorities* (pp. 17–30). London: Routledge.

Smith, Anthony (2004b). *The Antiquity of Nations.* Cambridge: Polity Press.

Smith, Anthony (2008). *The Cultural Foundations of Nations: Hierarchy, Covenant, and Republic.* Cambridge, MA: Blackwell.

Smith, Anthony (2009). *Ethno-Symbolism and Nationalism.* London: Routledge.

Smith, Anthony (2010). *Nationalism* (2nd edn). Cambridge: Polity Press.

Smith, D., and Wright, S. (eds) (1999). *Whose Europe? The Turn towards Democracy.* Oxford: Blackwell.

Smith, G. (1989). Kura Kaupapa Māori: innovation and policy development in Māori education. *Access* 8, 26–43.

Smith, G. (1990a). The politics of reforming Māori Education: the transforming potential of Kura Kaupapa Māori. In H. Lauder and C. Wylie (eds), *Towards Successful Schooling* (pp. 73–87). London: Falmer Press.

Smith, G. (1990b). Taha Māori: Pākehā capture. In J. Codd, R. Harker and R. Nash (eds), *Political Issues in New Zealand Education* (2nd edn, pp. 183–97). Palmerston North, New Zealand: Dunmore Press.

Smith, G. (1997). Kaupapa Māori as transformative practice. Unpublished PhD thesis, University of Auckland.

Smith, L. (1989). Te reo Māori: Māori language and the struggle to survive. *Access* 8, 3–9.

Smith, L. (1992). Kura kaupapa and the implications for curriculum. In G. McCulloch (ed.), *The School Curriculum in New Zealand: History, Theory, Policy and Practice* (pp. 219–31). Palmerston North, New Zealand: Dunmore Press.

Smith, L. (1999). *Decolonizing Methodologies: Research and Indigenous Peoples.* London: Zed Books.

Smith, M. (1965). *The Plural Society of the British West Indies.* London: Sangster's.

Smolicz, J. (1979). *Culture and Education in a Plural Society.* Canberra: Curriculum Development Centre.

Smolicz, J. (1993). The monolingual myopia and minority rights: Australia's language policies from an international perspective. *Muslim Education Quarterly* 10, 44–61.

Smolicz, J. (1995). Australia's language policies and minority rights. In T. Skutnabb-Kangas and R. Phillipson (eds), *Linguistic Human Rights: Overcoming Linguistic Discrimination* (pp. 235–52). Berlin: Mouton de Gruyter.

Smolicz, J., and Secombe, M. (1988). Community languages, core values and cultural maintenance: the Australian experience with special reference to Greek, Latvian and Polish groups. In M. Clyne (ed.), *Australia, Meeting Place of Languages* (pp. 11–38). Canberra: Australian National University, Pacific Linguistics.

Sollors, W. (ed.) (1989). *The Invention of Ethnicity.* Oxford: Oxford University Press.

Sollors, W. (ed.) (1998). *Multilingual America: Transnationalism, Ethnicity and the Languages of American Literature.* New York: New York University Press.

Song, M. (2001). Comparing minorities' ethnic options: do Asian Americans possess 'more' ethnic options than African Americans? *Ethnicities* 1, 1, 57–82.

Song, M. (2003). *Choosing Ethnic Identity.* Cambridge: Polity Press.

Sonntag, S. (2009). Linguistic globalization and the call center industry: imperialism, hegemony or cosmopolitanism? *Language Policy* 8, 1, 5–25.

Spinner, J. (1994). *The Boundaries of Citizenship: Race, Ethnicity and Nationality in the Liberal State*. Baltimore, MD: Johns Hopkins Press.

Spinner-Halev, J. (1999). Cultural pluralism and partial citizenship. In C. Joppke and S. Lukes (eds), *Multicultural Questions* (pp. 65–86). Oxford: Oxford University Press.

Spolsky, B. (2004). *Language Policy*. Cambridge: Cambridge University Press.

Spoonley, P. (1993). *Racism and Ethnicity* (rev. edn). Auckland: Oxford University Press.

Spoonley, P. (1996). Mahi Awatea? The racialisation of work in Aotearoa/New Zealand. In P. Spoonley, C. Macpherson and D. Pearson (eds), *Nga Pātai: Racism and Ethnic Relations in Aotearoa/New Zealand* (pp. 55–78). Palmerston North, New Zealand: Dunmore Press.

Spoonley, P., McPherson, C., and Pearson, D. (eds) (2004). *Tangata, Tangata. The Changing Ethnic Contours of Aotearoa/New Zealand*. Southbank, Victoria: Thomson/Dunmore Press.

Squires, J. (2002). Hybridity and multiculturalism. *Ethnicities* 2, 2, 265–73.

Stack, J. (1986). Ethnic mobilization in world politics: the primordial perspective. In J. Stack (ed.), *The Primordial Challenge: Ethnicity in the Contemporary World* (pp. 1–11). Westport, CT: Greenwood Press.

Stannard, D. (1989). *Before the Horror*. Honolulu: University of Hawai'i Press.

Statistics New Zealand (2007). Pacific Profiles 2006. Retrieved Jan. 2009 from http://www.stats.govt.nz/analytical-reports/pacific-profiles-2006/default.htm.

Statistics New Zealand (2009). Quickstats about New Zealand. Retrieved March 2011 from http://www.statisticsnz.govt.nz/Census/2006CensusHomePage/QuickStats/AboutAPlace/SnapShot.aspx?id=9999999&tab=Agesex&type=region&p=y&printall=true.

Statistics New Zealand (2010). Demographic trends 2010: deaths and life expectancy. Retrieved March 2011 from http://www.stats.govt.nz/browse_for_stats/population/estimates_and_projections/demographic-trends-2010/chapter4.aspx.

Stavenhagen, R., and Charters, C. (eds) (2009). *Making the Declaration Work: The Declaration on the Rights of Indigenous Peoples*. Copenhagen: IWGIA.

Steinberg, S. (1981). *The Ethnic Myth: Race, Ethnicity and Class in America*. New York: Atheneum.

Stepan, A. (1998). Modern multinational democracies: transcending a Gellnerian oxymoron. In J. Hall (ed.), *The State of the Nation: Ernest Gellner and the Theory of Nationalism* (pp. 219–39). Cambridge: Cambridge University Press.

Stone, M. (1981). *The Education of the Black Child in Britain: The Myth of Multiracial Education*. London: Collins Fontana.

Strubell, M. (1998). Language, democracy and devolution in Catalonia. *Current Issues in Language and Society* 5, 146–80.

Swartz. D. (1997). *Culture and Power: The Sociology of Pierre Bourdieu*. Chicago: University of Chicago Press.

Szasz, M. (1974). *Education and the American Indian: The Road to Self Determination, 1928–1973*. Albuquerque, NM: University of New Mexico Press.

Tabouret-Keller, A. (1997). Language and identity. In F. Coulmas (ed.), *The Handbook of Sociolinguistics* (pp. 315–26). Oxford: Blackwell.

Tamir, Y. (1993). *Liberal Nationalism*. Princeton, NJ: Princeton University Press.

Tarrow, N. (1992). Language, interculturalism and human rights: three European cases. *Prospects* 22, 489–509.

Tarver, H. (1994). Language and politics in the 1980s. The story of U.S. English. In F. Pincus and H. Ehrlich (eds.), *Race and Ethnic Conflict: Contending Views on Prejudice, Discrimination and Ethnoviolence* (pp. 206–218). Boulder, CO: Westview Press.

Tatz, C. (2011). The destruction of Aboriginal society in Australia. In S. Totten and R. Hitchcock (eds), *Genocide of Indigenous Peoples* (pp. 87–116). New Brunswick, NJ: Transaction Publishers.

Taylor, C. (1994). The politics of recognition. In A. Gutmann (ed.), *Multiculturalism: Examining the Politics of Recognition* (pp. 25–73). Princeton, NJ: Princeton University Press.

Taylor, C. (1998). Nationalism and modernity. In J. Hall (ed.), *The State of the Nation: Ernest Gellner and the Theory of Nationalism* (pp. 191–218). Cambridge: Cambridge University Press.

Te Paepae Motuhake (2011). *Te Reo Mauriora: te arotakenga o te rāngai reo Māori me te rautaki reo Māori.* Retrieved April 2011 from http://themaorilanguage.wordpress.com/2011/04/13/review-of-the-maori-language-sector-released-13-april-2011.

Te Puni Kōkiri (1994). *Mana Tangata: Draft Declaration on the Rights of Indigenous Peoples, 1993: Background and Discussion on Key Issues.* Wellington: Te Puni Kōkiri (Ministry of Māori Development).

Te Puni Kōkiri (2001). *National Māori Language Survey: Summary Report.* Wellington: Te Puni Kōkiri

Te Taura Whiri i te Reo Māori, (1995). *He Taonga te Reo.* Wellington: Te Taura Whiri i te Reo Māori (Māori Language Commission).

Thomas, R. (1992). *Cymru or Wales?* Llandysul: Gomer Press.

Thomas, W., and Collier, V. (2002). *A National Study of School Effectiveness for Language Minority Students' Long-Term Academic Achievement.* Santa Cruz, CA: Center for Research on Education, Diversity and Excellence (CREDE): http://crede.berkeley.edu/research/llaa/1.1_final.html.

Thompson, J. (1991). Editor's introduction. In P. Bourdieu, *Language and Symbolic Power* (pp. 1–31). Cambridge: Polity Press.

Thornberry, P. (1991a). *International Law and the Rights of Minorities.* Oxford: Clarendon Press.

Thornberry, P. (1991b). *Minorities and Human Rights Law.* London: Minority Rights Group.

Thornberry, P. (1997). Minority rights. In Academy of European Law (ed.), *Collected Courses of the Academy of European Law* (vol. 6, book 2, pp. 307–90). The Hague: Kluwer Law International.

Thornberry, P. (2002). Minority and indigenous rights at 'the end of history', *Ethnicities*, 2, 4, 515–37.

Thornton, R. (1988). Culture: a contemporary definition. In E. Boonzaier and J. Sharp (eds), *South African Keywords: The Uses and Abuses of Political Concepts* (pp. 17–28). Cape Town: David Philip.

Tickoo, M. (1993). When is language worth teaching? Native languages and English in India. *Language, Culture and Curriculum* 6, 225–39.

Tilly, C. (ed.) (1975). *The Formation of National States in Western Europe.* Princeton, NJ: Princeton University Press.

Tilly, C. (1984). *Big Structures, Large Processes, Huge Comparisons.* New York: Russell Sage.

Tishkov, V. (1997). *Ethnicity, Nationalism and Conflict In and After the Soviet Union: The Mind Aflame*. Oslo: International Peace Research Institute.

Tishkov, V. (2000). Forget the 'nation': post-nationalist understanding of nationalism. *Ethnic and Racial Studies* 23, 4, 625–50.

Todal, J. (1999). Minorities within a minority: language and the school in the Sámi areas of Norway. In S. May (ed.), *Indigenous Community-Based Education* (pp. 124–36). Clevedon, Avon: Multilingual Matters.

Todal, J. (2003). The Sámi school system in Norway and international cooperation. *Comparative Education* 39, 2, 185–92.

Tollefson, J. (1991). *Planning Language, Planning Inequality: Language Policy in the Community*. London: Longman.

Tollefson, J. (ed.) (1995). *Power and Inequality in Language Education*. Cambridge: Cambridge University Press.

Tollefson, J. (2000). Policy and ideology in the spread of English. In J. Kelly Hall and W. Eggington (eds), *The Sociopolitics of English Language Teaching* (pp. 7–21). Clevedon, Avon: Multilingual Matters.

Tomasi, J. (1995). Kymlicka, liberalism and respect for cultural minorities, *Ethics* 105, 580–603.

Torres, J. (1984). Problems of linguistic normalization in the Països Catalans: from the Congress of Catalan Culture to the present day. *International Journal of the Sociology of Language* 47: 59–63.

Tovey, H., Hannan, D., and Abramson, H. (1989). *Why Irish? Irish Identity and the Irish Language*. Dublin: Bord na Gaeilge.

Toynbee, A. (1953). *A Study of History* (vols 7–9). London: Oxford University Press.

Trenz, H. (2007). Reconciling diversity and unity: language minorities and European integration. *Ethnicities* 7, 157–85.

Trevor-Roper, H. (1983). The invention of tradition: the highland tradition of Scotland. In E. Hobsbawm and T. Ranger (eds), *The Invention of Tradition* (pp. 15–42). Cambridge: Cambridge University Press.

Troebst, S. (1998). *The Council of Europe's Framework Convention for the Protection of National Minorities Revisited*. Flensburg, Germany: European Centre for Minority Issues.

Trommer, S., and Chari, R. (2006). The Council of Europe: interest groups and ideological missions? *West European Politics* 29, 665–86.

Truchot, C. (1990). *L'anglais dans le monde contemporaine*. Paris: Robert.

Tully, J. (1995). *Strange Multiplicity: Constitutionalism in an Age of Diversity*. Cambridge: Cambridge University Press.

Twine, F. (2010). White like who? The value of whiteness in British interracial families. *Ethnicities* 10, 3, 292–312.

UNESCO (1953). *The Use of Vernacular Languages in Education*. Paris: UNESCO.

United Nations (2009). *State of the World's Indigenous Peoples*. New York: Dept of Economic and Social Affairs, United Nations.

US Census Bureau (2010). Hispanic Americans by the numbers. Retrieved Feb. 2010 from at http://www.infoplease.com/spot/hhmcensus1.html.

Ussher, A. (1949). *The Face and Mind of Ireland*. London: Gollancz.

Vaish, V. (2008). *Biliteracy and Globalization: English Language Education in India*. Clevedon, Avon: Multilingual Matters.

Valadez, J. (2007). The continuing significance of ethnocultural identity. In S. Benhabib, I. Shapiro, and D. Petranovic (eds), *Identities, Affiliations, and Allegiances* (pp. 303–24). Cambridge: Cambridge University Press.

Valencia, R. (ed.) (1997). *The Evolution of Deficit Thinking: Educational Thought and Practice.* New York: Falmer Press.

Valencia, R. (2010). *Dismantling Contemporary Deficit Thinking: Educational Thought and Practice.* New York: Routledge.

van den Berghe, P. (1979). *The Ethnic Phenomenon.* New York: Elsevier Press.

van den Berghe, P. (1995). Does race matter? *Nations and Nationalism* 1, 357–68.

van Dijk, T. (1993). *Elite Discourse and Racism.* London: Sage.

Van Dyke, V. (1977). The individual, the state, and ethnic communities in political theory. *World Politics* 29, 343–69.

van Parijs, P. (2005). Europe's linguistic challenge. *European Journal of Sociology* 45, 1, 113–45.

Veltman, C. (1983). *Language Shift in the United States.* Berlin: Mouton de Gruyter.

Veltman, C. (1988). Modelling the language shift process of Hispanic immigrants. *International Migration Review* 22, 545–62.

Venne, M. (ed.) (2000). *Penser la Nation Québécoise.* Montreal: Le Devoir/Québec Amérique.

Verma, G. (ed.) (1989). *Education for All: A Landmark in Pluralism.* Lewes: Falmer Press.

Vološinov, V. (1973). *Marxism and the Philosophy of Language.* Cambridge, MA: Harvard University Press (original, 1929).

Waitangi Tribunal (1986). *Findings of the Waitangi Tribunal Relating to Te Reo Māori and a Claim Lodged by Huirangi Waikerepuru and Nga Kaiwhakapumau i te Reo Incorporated Society (Wellington Board of Māori Language).* Wellington: Government Printer.

Waitangi Tribunal (2010). *Te Reo Māori.* Wellington: Waitangi Tribunal.

Waldron, J. (1993). *Liberal Rights.* Cambridge: Cambridge University Press.

Waldron, J. (1995). Minority cultures and the cosmopolitan alternative. In W. Kymlicka (ed.), *The Rights of Minority Cultures* (pp. 93–119). Oxford: Oxford University Press.

Waldron, J. (2000). Cultural identity and civic responsibility. In W. Kymlicka and W. Norman (eds), *Citizenship in Diverse Societies* (pp. 155–74). Oxford: Oxford University Press.

Waldron, J. (2002). Redressing historic injustice. *University of Toronto Law Journal,* 52, 135–60.

Walker, R. (2004). *Ka Whawhai Tonu Mātou: Struggle without End* (rev edn). Auckland: Penguin.

Wallerstein, I. (1979). *The Capitalist World Economy.* Cambridge: Cambridge University Press.

Wallerstein, I. (1983). *Historical Capitalism.* London: New Left Books.

Wallerstein, I. (1991). The construction of peoplehood: racism, nationalism, ethnicity. In E. Balibar and I. Wallerstein (eds), *Race, Nation, Class: Ambiguous Identities* (pp. 71–85). London: Verso.

Wallerstein, I. (2001). *Unthinking Social Science: The Limits of Nineteenth Century Paradigms.* Philadelphia, PA: Temple University Press.

Wallman, S. (1986). Ethnicity and the boundary process in context. In J. Rex and D. Mason (eds), *Theories of Race and Race Relations* (pp. 226–35). Cambridge: Cambridge University Press.

Walsh, J. (2002). Language, culture and development: the Gaeltacht commissions 1926 and 2002. In J. Kirk and D. Ó Baoill (eds), *Language Planning and Education: Linguistic*

Issues in Northern Ireland, the Republic of Ireland, and Scotland (pp. 300–18). Belfast: Cló Ollscoil na Ríana.

Walsh, J. (2006). Language and socio-economic development: towards a theoretical framework. *Language Problems and Language Planning* 30, 2, 127–48.

Walsh, J. (2011). *Contests and Contexts: The Irish Language and Ireland's Socio-Economic Development.* Oxford: Peter Lang.

Walzer, M. (1982). Pluralism in political perspective. In M. Walzer (ed.), *The Politics of Ethnicity* (pp. 1–28). Cambridge, MA: Harvard University Press.

Walzer, M. (1992). *What it Means to be an American.* New York: Marsilio.

Walzer, M. (1994). Comment. In A. Gutmann (ed.), *Multiculturalism: Examining the Politics of Recognition* (pp. 99–103). Princeton, NJ: Princeton University Press.

Ward, A. (1974). *A Show of Justice: Racial 'Amalgamation' in Nineteenth Century New Zealand.* Auckland: Auckland University Press.

Waters, M. (1990). *Ethnic Options: Choosing Identities in America.* Berkeley, CA: University of California Press.

Watts, R. (1997). Language policies and education in Switzerland. In R. Watts and J. Smolicz (eds), *Cultural Democracy and Ethnic Pluralism: Multicultural and Multilingual Policies in Education* (pp. 271–302). Frankfurt: Peter Lang.

Webber, J. (2000). Beyond regret: Mabo's implications for Australian constitutionalism. In D. Ivison, D. Patton and W. Sanders (eds), *Political Theory and the Rights of Indigenous Peoples* (pp. 60–88). Cambridge: Cambridge University Press.

Webber, J., and Strubell, M. (1991). *The Catalan Language: Progress towards Normalisation.* London: Anglo-Catalan Society.

Weber, E. (1976). *Peasants into Frenchmen: The Modernization of Rural France 1870–1914.* Stanford, CA: Stanford University Press.

Weber, M. (1968). *Economy and Society,* ed. G. Roth and C. Wittich. Berkeley CA: University of California Press.

Wee, L. (2010). *Language without Rights.* Oxford: Oxford University Press.

Weinstein, B. (1983). *The Civic Tongue: Political Consequences of Language Choices.* New York: Longman.

Werbner, P. (1997a). Introduction: the dialectics of cultural hybridity. In P. Werbner and T. Modood (eds), *Debating Cultural Hybridity: Multicultural Identities and the Politics of Antiracism* (pp. 1–26). London: Zed Books.

Werbner, P. (1997b). Essentialising essentialism, essentialising silence: ambivalence and multiplicity in the constructions of racism and ethnicity. In P. Werbner and T. Modood (eds), *Debating Cultural Hybridity: Multicultural Identities and the Politics of Antiracism* (pp. 226–54). London: Zed Books.

Whorf, B. (1956). Science and linguistics. In J. Carrol (ed.), *Language, Thought and Reality: Selected Writings of Benjamin Lee Whorf* (pp. 207–19). Cambridge, MA: MIT Press.

Wicker, H-R. (1997). From complex culture to cultural complexity. In P. Werbner, and T. Modood (eds), *Debating Cultural Hybridity: Multicultural Identities and the Politics of Antiracism* (pp. 29–45). London: Zed Books.

Wiley, T. (2005). *Literacy and Language Diversity in the United States* (2nd edn). Washington, DC: Center for Applied Linguistics and Delta Systems.

Wiley, T., and Wright, W. (2004). Against the undertow: the politics of language instruction in the United States. *Educational Policy* 18, 1, 142–68.

Wilkinson, I. (1998). Dealing with diversity: achievement gaps in reading literacy among New Zealand students. *Reading Research Quarterly* 33, 144–67.

Williams, Charlotte (1995). 'Race' and racism: some reflections on the Welsh context. *Contemporary Wales* 8, 113–32.

Williams, Charlotte, and De Lima, P. (2006). Devolution, multicultural citizenship and race equality: from laissez faire to nationally responsive policies. *Critical Social Policy* 26, 3, 498–522.

Williams, Colin (1990). The anglicisation of Wales. In N. Coupland (ed.), *English in Wales: Diversity, Conflict and Change* (pp. 19–47). Clevedon, Avon: Multilingual Matters.

Williams, Colin (1994). *Called Unto Liberty: On Language and Nationalism*. Clevedon, Avon: Multilingual Matters.

Williams, Colin (1996). Ethnic identity and language issues in development. In D. Dwyer and D. Drakakis-Smith (eds), *Ethnicity and Development: Geographical Perspectives* (pp. 45–85). London: John Wiley & Sons.

Williams, Colin (2007). Articulating the horizons of Welsh. In C. H. Williams (ed.), *Language and Governance* (pp. 387–433). Cardiff: University of Wales Press.

Williams, Colin (2008). *Linguistic Minorities in Democratic Context*. Basingstoke: Palgrave Macmillan.

Williams, Colin, and Raybould, W. (1991). *Welsh Language Planning: Opportunities and Constraints*. Cardiff: PDAG.

Williams, E. (1989). The dynamic of Welsh identity. In N. Evans (ed.), *National Identity in the British Isles* (pp. 46–59). Harlech: Coleg Harlech.

Williams, Glyn (1987). Bilingualism, class dialect, and social reproduction. *International Journal of the Sociology of Language* 66, 85–98.

Williams, Glyn (1994). Discourses on 'nation' and 'race'. *Contemporary Wales* 6, 87–103.

Williams, Glyn (2005). *Sustaining Language Diversity in Europe: Evidence from the Euromosaic Project*. Basingstoke: Palgrave Macmillan.

Williams, Gwyn (1982). *The Welsh in their History*. London: Croom Helm.

Williams, Gwyn (1985). *When was Wales?* London: Penguin.

Williams, J. (1969). *Politics of the New Zealand Māori: Protest and Cooperation*. Auckland: Auckland University Press.

Williams, R. (1976). *Keywords*. London: Flamingo.

Williamson, D. (2010). Welsh-medium education gains government strategy. *Wales Online* (20 April). Retrieved March 2011 from http://www.walesonline.co.uk/news/wales-news/2010/04/20/welsh-medium-education-gains-government-strategy-91466-26283004.

Willig, A. (1985). A meta-analysis of selected studies on the effectiveness of bilingual education. *Review of Educational Research* 55, 269–317.

Willig, A. (1987). Examining bilingual education research through meta-analysis and narrative review: a response to Baker. *Review of Educational Research* 57, 363–76.

Wilmer, F. (2002). *Construction of Man, the State, and War: Identity, Conflict, and Violence in the former Yugoslavia*. London: Routledge.

Wilson, M., and Yeatman, A. (eds) (1995). *Justice and Identity: Antipodean Practices*. Wellington: Bridget Williams Books.

Wimmer, A. (2004). Dominant ethnicity and nationhood. In E. Kaufmann (ed.), *Rethinking Ethnicity: Majority Groups and Dominant Minorities* (pp. 40–58). London: Routledge.

Wimmer, A. (2008). The making and unmaking of ethnic boundaries: a multilevel process theory. *American Journal of Sociology* 113, 4, 970–1022.

Wimmer, A., and Schiller, N. (2002). Methodological nationalism and the study of migration. *Archives Européennes de Sociologie* 53, 2, 217–40.

Wolfrum, R. (1993). The emergence of 'new minorities' as a result of migration. In C. Brölmann, R. Lefeber and M. Zieck (eds), *Peoples and Minorities in International Law* (pp. 153–66). Dordrecht: Martinus Nijhoff Publishers.

Woolard, K. (1989). *Double Talk: Bilingualism and the Politics of Ethnicity in Catalonia*. Stanford, CA: Stanford University Press.

Woolard, K. (1998). Introduction: language ideology as a field of inquiry. In B. Schieffelin, K. Woolard and P. Kroskrity (eds), *Language Ideologies: Practice and Theory* (pp. 3–47). New York: Oxford University Press.

Worsley, P. (1984). *The Three Worlds: Culture and World Development*. London: Weidenfeld & Nicolson.

Wright, A. (2004). The politics of multiculturalism. *Studies in Philosophy and Education* 23, 4, 299–311.

Wright, S. (2000). *Community and Communication: The Role of Language in Nation State Building and European Integration*. Clevedon, Avon: Multilingual Matters.

Wright, S. (2004). *Language Policy and Language Planning: From Nationalism to Globalisation*. Basingstoke: Palgrave Macmillan.

Wright, W. (2005). The political spectacle of Arizona's Proposition 203. *Educational Policy* 19, 5, 662–700.

Xanthaki, A. (2007). *Indigenous Rights and United Nations Standards*. Cambridge: Cambridge University Press.

Yates, A. (1998). Language, democracy and devolution in Catalonia: a response to Miquel Strubell. *Current Issues in Language and Society* 5, 204–9.

Young, I. (1989). Polity and group difference: a critique of the ideal of universal citizenship. *Ethics* 99, 250–74.

Young, I. (1990). *Justice and the Politics of Difference*. Princeton, NJ: Princeton University Press.

Young, I. (1993). Together in difference: transforming the logic of group political conflict. In J. Squires (ed.), *Principled Positions: Postmodernism and the Rediscovery of Value* (pp. 121–50). London: Lawrence & Wishart.

Young, I. (2000). *Inclusion and Democracy*. Oxford: Oxford University Press.

Young, I. (2004). Two concepts of self-determination. In S. May, T. Modood and J. Squires (eds), *Ethnicity, Nationalism and Minority Rights* (pp. 176–98). Cambridge: Cambridge University Press.

Young, I. (2005). Self-determination as non-domination: ideals applied to Palestine/ Israel. *Ethnicities* 5, 2, 139–59.

Young, I. (2007). Structural injustice and the politics of difference. In A. Laden and D. Owen (eds), *Multiculturalism and Political Theory* (pp. 60–88). Cambridge: Cambridge University Press.

Yuval-Davis, N. (1997a). *Gender and the Nation*. London: Sage.

Yuval-Davis, N. (1997b). Ethnicity, gender relations and multiculturalism. In P. Werbner and T. Modood (eds), *Debating Cultural Hybridity: Multicultural Identities and the Politics of Antiracism* (pp. 193–208). London: Zed Books.

Zentella, A. (1997). The hispanophobia of the Official English movement in the US. *International Journal of the Sociology of Language* 127, 71–86.

INDEX

An environmentally friendly book printed and bound in England by www.printondemand-worldwide.com

PEFC Certified

This product is
from sustainably
managed forests
and controlled
sources

www.pefc.org

MIX
Paper from
responsible sources

www.fsc.org   FSC® C004959

This book is made entirely of chain-of-custody materials; FSC materials for the cover and PEFC materials for the text pages

#0056 - 191112 - C0 - 229/152/24 [26] - CB